Lecture Notes in Artificial Intelligence   8857

Subseries of Lecture Notes in Computer Science

LNAI Series Editors

Randy Goebel
   University of Alberta, Edmonton, Canada
Yuzuru Tanaka
   Hokkaido University, Sapporo, Japan
Wolfgang Wahlster
   DFKI and Saarland University, Saarbrücken, Germany

LNAI Founding Series Editor

Joerg Siekmann
   DFKI and Saarland University, Saarbrücken, Germany

T0212820

Alexander Gelbukh
Félix Castro Espinoza
Sofía N. Galicia-Haro (Eds.)

Nature-Inspired Computation and Machine Learning

13th Mexican International Conference
on Artificial Intelligence, MICAI 2014
Tuxtla Gutiérrez, Mexico, November 16-22, 2014
Proceedings, Part II

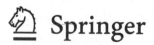
Springer

Volume Editors

Alexander Gelbukh
Centro de Investigación en Computación
Instituto Politécnico Nacional
Mexico City, Mexico
E-mail: gelbukh@gelbukh.com

Félix Castro Espinoza
Universidad Autónoma del Estado de Hidalgo
Área Académica de Computación y Electrónica
Hidalgo, Mexico
E-mail: fcastroe@gmail.com

Sofía N. Galicia-Haro
Universidad Autónoma Nacional de México
Facultad de Ciencias
Mexico City, Mexico
E-mail: sngh@fciencias.unam.mx

ISSN 0302-9743   e-ISSN 1611-3349
ISBN 978-3-319-13649-3   e-ISBN 978-3-319-13650-9
DOI 10.1007/978-3-319-13650-9
Springer Cham Heidelberg New York Dordrecht London

Library of Congress Control Number: 2014955199

LNCS Sublibrary: SL 7 – Artificial Intelligence

Typesetting: Camera-ready by author, data conversion by Scientific Publishing Services, Chennai, India

Printed on acid-free paper

Springer is part of Springer Science+Business Media (www.springer.com)

Preface

The Mexican International Conference on Artificial Intelligence (MICAI) is a yearly international conference series organized by the Mexican Society of Artificial Intelligence (SMIA) since 2000. MICAI is a major international artificial intelligence forum and the main event in the academic life of the country's growing artificial intelligence community.

MICAI conferences publish high-quality papers in all areas of artificial intelligence and its applications. The proceedings of the previous MICAI events have been published by Springer in its *Lecture Notes in Artificial Intelligence* series, vols. 1793, 2313, 2972, 3789, 4293, 4827, 5317, 5845, 6437, 6438, 7094, 7095, 7629, 7630, 8265, and 8266. Since its foundation in 2000, the conference has been growing in popularity and improving in quality.

According to two main areas of artificial intelligence—modeling human mental abilities on the one hand and optimization and classification on the other hand—the proceedings of MICAI 2014 have been published in two volumes. The first volume, *Human-Inspired Computing and Its Applications*, contains 44 papers structured into seven sections:

- Natural Language Processing
- Natural Language Processing Applications
- Opinion Mining, Sentiment Analysis, and Social Network Applications
- Computer Vision
- Image Processing
- Logic, Reasoning, and Multi-agent Systems
- Intelligent Tutoring Systems

The second volume, *Nature-Inspired Computation and Machine Learning*, contains 44 papers structured into eight sections:

- Genetic and Evolutionary Algorithms
- Neural Networks
- Machine Learning
- Machine Learning Applications to Audio and Text
- Data Mining
- Fuzzy Logic
- Robotics, Planning, and Scheduling
- Biomedical Applications

This two-volume set will be of interest to researchers in all areas of artificial intelligence, students specializing in related topics, and to the general public interested in recent developments in artificial intelligence.

The conference received for evaluation 350 submissions by 823 authors from a record high number of 46 countries: Algeria, Argentina, Australia, Austria,

Brazil, Bulgaria, Canada, Chile, China, Colombia, Cuba, Czech Republic, Ecuador, Egypt, France, Germany, India, Iran, Ireland, Israel, Italy, Jordan, Kazakhstan, Lithuania, Malaysia, Mexico, Morocco, Nepal, Norway, Pakistan, Panama, Paraguay, Peru, Poland, Portugal, Russia, Singapore, Slovakia, South Africa, Spain, Sweden, Turkey, UK, Ukraine, USA, and Virgin Islands (USA); the distribution of papers by tracks is shown in Table 1. Of these submissions, 87 papers were selected for publication in these two volumes after a peer-reviewing process carried out by the international Program Committee. The acceptance rate was 24.8%.

In addition to regular papers, the second volume contains an invited paper by Oscar Castillo, Patricia Mclin, and Fevrier Valdez: "Nature-Inspired Optimization of Type-2 Fuzzy Systems."

The international Program Committee consisted of 201 experts from 34 countries: Australia, Austria, Azerbaijan, Belgium, Brazil, Canada, China, Colombia, Czech Republic, Denmark, Finland, France, Germany, Greece, India, Israel, Italy, Japan, Mexico, The Netherlands, New Zealand, Norway, Poland, Portugal, Russia, Singapore, Slovenia, Spain, Sweden, Switzerland, Tunisia, Turkey, UK, and USA.

Table 1. Distribution of papers by tracks

Track	Submissions	Accepted	Rate
Natural Language Processing	59	19	32%
Machine Learning and Pattern Recognition	42	12	29%
Logic, Knowledge-Based Systems, Multi-Agent Systems and Distributed AI	40	8	20%
Computer Vision and Image Processing	38	13	34%
Evolutionary and Nature-Inspired Metaheuristic Algorithms	33	6	18%
Data Mining	29	7	24%
Neural Networks and Hybrid Intelligent Systems	28	7	25%
Robotics, Planning and Scheduling	24	5	21%
Fuzzy Systems and Probabilistic Models in Decision Making	23	4	17%
Bioinformatics and Medical Applications	18	3	17%
Intelligent Tutoring Systems	16	3	19%

MICAI 2014 was honored by the presence of such renowned experts as Hojjat Adeli of The Ohio State University, USA, Oscar Castillo of Instituto Tecnológico de Tijuana, Mexico, Bonnie E. John of IBM T.J. Watson Research Center, USA, Bing Liu of the University of Illinois, USA, John Sowa of VivoMind Research, USA, and Vladimir Vapnik of the NEC Laboratories, USA, who gave excellent keynote lectures. The technical program of the conference also featured tutorials presented by Roman Bartak of Charles University, Czech Republic; Oscar Castillo of Tijuana Institute of Technology, Mexico; Héctor G. Ceballos of Clark & Parsia LLC, USA, and Héctor Pérez Urbina of Tecnológico de Monterrey, Mexico; Sanjoy Das of Kansas State University, USA; Alexander Gelbukh of

Instituto Politécnico Nacional, Mexico; Bonnie E. John of IBM T. J. Watson Research Center, USA; Bing Liu of University of Illinois, USA; Raúl Monroy of Tecnológico de Monterrey, Mexico; John Sowa of VivoMind Research, USA; and Luis Martín Torres Treviño of Universidad Autónoma de Nuevo León, Mexico, among others. Three workshops were held jointly with the conference: the 7th International Workshop on Hybrid Intelligent Systems, HIS 2014; the 7th International Workshop on Intelligent Learning Environments, WILE 2014, and the First International Workshop on Recognizing Textual Entailment and Question Answering, RTE-QA 2014.

The authors of the following papers received the Best Paper Award on the basis of the paper's overall quality, significance, and originality of the reported results:

1st place: "The Best Neural Network Architecture," by Angel Kuri-Morales (Mexico)

2nd place: "Multisensor-Based Obstacles Detection in Challenging Scenes," by Yong Fang, Cindy Cappelle, and Yassine Ruichek (France)

"Intelligent Control of Induction Motor-Based Comparative Study: Analysis of Two Topologies," by Moulay Rachid Douiri, El Batoul Mabrouki, Ouissam Belghazi, Mohamed Ferfra, and Mohamed Cherkaoui (Morocco)

3rd place: "A Fast Scheduling Algorithm for Detection and Localization of Hidden Objects Based on Data Gathering in Wireless Sensor Networks," by Eugene Levner, Boris Kriheli, Amir Elalouf, and Dmitry Tsadikovich (Israel)

The authors of the following papers selected among all papers of which the first author was a full-time student, excluding the papers listed above, received the Best Student Paper Award:

1st place: "Solving Binary Cutting Stock with Matheuristics," by Ivan Adrian Lopez Sanchez, Jaime Mora Vargas, Cipriano A. Santos, and Miguel Gonzalez Mendoza (Mexico)

"Novel Unsupervised Features for Czech Multi-label Document Classification," by Tomáš Brychcín and Pavel Král (Czech Republic)

We want to thank everyone involved in the organization of this conference. In the first place, these are the authors of the papers published in this book: It is their research work that gives value to the book and to the work of the organizers. We thank the track chairs for their hard work, the Program Committee members, and additional reviewers for their great effort spent on reviewing the submissions.

We are grateful to the Dean of the Instituto Tecnológico de Tuxtla Gutiérrez (ITTG), M.E.H. José Luis Méndez Navarro, the Dean of the Universidad Autónoma de Chiapas (UNACH), Professor Jaime Valls Esponda, and M.C. Francisco de Jesús Suárez Ruiz, Head of IT Department, for their instrumental support of MICAI and for providing the infrastructure for the keynote talks, tutorials, and workshops, and to all professors of the Engineering School of Computational Systems for their warm hospitality and hard work, as well as for their active participation in the organization of this conference. We greatly appreciate the generous sponsorship provided by the Government of Chiapas via the Conventions and Visitors Office (OCV).

We are deeply grateful to the conference staff and to all members of the Local Committee headed by Imelda Valles López. We gratefully acknowledge support received from the project WIQ-EI (Web Information Quality Evaluation Initiative, European project 269180). The entire submission, reviewing, and selection process, as well as preparation of the proceedings, was supported for free by the EasyChair system (www.easychair.org). Finally, yet importantly, we are very grateful to the staff at Springer for their patience and help in the preparation of this volume.

October 2014

Alexander Gelbukh
Félix Castro Espinoza
Sofía N. Galicia-Haro

Conference Organization

MICAI 2014 was organized by the Mexican Society of Artificial Intelligence (SMIA, Sociedad Mexicana de Inteligencia Artificial) in collaboration with the Instituto Tecnológico de Tuxtla Gutiérrez (ITTG), the Universidad Autónoma de Chiapas (UNACH), the Centro de Investigación en Computación del Instituto Politécnico Nacional (CIC-IPN), the Universidad Autónoma del Estado de Hidalgo (UAEH), and the Universidad Nacional Autónoma de México (UNAM).

The MICAI series website is www.MICAI.org. The website of the Mexican Society of Artificial Intelligence, SMIA, is www.SMIA.org.mx. Contact options and additional information can be found on these websites.

Conference Committee

General Chairs

Alexander Gelbukh	Instituto Politécnico Nacional, Mexico
Grigori Sidorov	Instituto Politécnico Nacional, Mexico

Program Chairs

Alexander Gelbukh	Instituto Politécnico Nacional, Mexico
Félix Castro Espinoza	Universidad Autónoma del Estado de Hidalgo, Mexico
Sofía N. Galicia Haro	Universidad Autónoma Nacional de México, Mexico

Workshop Chairs

Obdulia Pichardo Lagunas	Instituto Politécnico Nacional, Mexico
Noé Alejandro Castro Sánchez	Centro Nacional de Investigación y Desarrollo Tecnológico, Mexico

Tutorials Chair

Félix Castro Espinoza	Universidad Autónoma del Estado de Hidalgo, Mexico

Doctoral Consortium Chairs

Miguel Gonzalez Mendoza	Tecnológico de Monterrey CEM, Mexico
Antonio Marín Hernandez	Universidad Veracruzana, Mexico

Keynote Talks Chair

Sabino Miranda Jiménez	INFOTEC, Mexico

Publication Chair

Miguel Gonzalez Mendoza   Tecnológico de Monterrey CEM, Mexico

Financial Chair

Ildar Batyrshin   Instituto Politécnico Nacional, Mexico

Grant Chairs

Grigori Sidorov   Instituto Politécnico Nacional, Mexico
Miguel Gonzalez Mendoza   Tecnológico de Monterrey CEM, Mexico

Organizing Committee Chair

Imelda Valles López   Instituto Tecnológico de Tuxtla Gutiérrez,
                                 Mexico

Track Chairs

Natural Language Processing

Grigori Sidorov   Instituto Politécnico Nacional, Mexico

Machine Learning and Pattern Recognition

Alexander Gelbukh   Instituto Politécnico Nacional, Mexico

Data Mining

Miguel Gonzalez-Mendoza   Tecnológico de Monterrey CEM, Mexico
Félix Castro Espinoza   Universidad Autónoma del Estado de Hidalgo,
                                 Mexico

Intelligent Tutoring Systems

Alexander Gelbukh   Instituto Politécnico Nacional, Mexico

Evolutionary and Nature-Inspired Metaheuristic Algorithms

Oliver Schütze   CINVESTAV, Mexico
Jaime Mora Vargas   Tecnológico de Monterrey CEM, Mexico

Computer Vision and Image Processing

Oscar Herrera Alcántara   Universidad Autónoma Metropolitana
                                 Azcapotzalco, Mexico

Robotics, Planning and Scheduling

Fernando Martin
  Montes-Gonzalez   Universidad Veracruzana, Mexico

Neural Networks and Hybrid Intelligent Systems

Sergio Ledesma-Orozco   Universidad de Guanajuato, Mexico

Logic, Knowledge-Based Systems, Multi-Agent Systems and Distributed AI

Mauricio Osorio   Universidad de las Américas, Mexico
Jose Raymundo   Universidad Autónoma del Estado de México,
  Marcial Romero   Mexico

Fuzzy Systems and Probabilistic Models in Decision Making

Ildar Batyrshin   Instituto Politécnico Nacional, Mexico

Bioinformatics and Medical Applications

Jesus A. Gonzalez   Instituto Nacional de Astrofísica, Óptica y
                                  Electrónica, Mexico
Felipe Orihuela-Espina   Instituto Nacional de Astrofísica, Óptica y
                                  Electrónica, Mexico

Program Committee

Juan C. Acosta-Guadarrama   Universidad Autónoma del Estado de México,
                                  Mexico
Teresa Alarcón   Universidad de Guadalajara, Mexico
Fernando Aldana   Universidad Veracruzana, Mexico
Guillem Alenya   IRI (CSIC-UPC), Spain
Adel Alimi   University of Sfax, Tunisia
Jesus Angulo   Ecole des Mines de Paris, France
Marianna Apidianaki   LIMSI-CNRS, France
Alfredo Arias-Montaño   Instituto Politécnico Nacional, Mexico
Jose Arrazola   Universidad Autónoma de Puebla, Mexico
Gustavo Arroyo   Instituto de Investigaciones Eléctricas, Mexico
Victor Ayala-Ramirez   Universidad de Guanajuato, Mexico
Alexandra Balahur   European Commission Joint Research Centre,
                                Italy
Sivaji Bandyopadhyay   Jadavpur University, India
Maria Lucia Barrón-Estrada Instituto Tecnológico de Culiacán, Mexico
Ildar Batyrshin   Instituto Politécnico Nacional, Mexico
Anastasios Bezerianos   University of Patras, Greece

Anilu Franco-Arcega   Instituto Nacional de Astrofísica, Óptica y
                           Electrónica, Mexico
Claude Frasson   University of Montreal, Canada
Alfredo Gabaldon   Carnegie Mellon University, USA
Sofia N. Galicia-Haro   Universidad Nacional Autónoma de México,
                           Mexico
Ana Gabriela   Universidad Nacional Autónoma de México,
  Gallardo-Hernández   Mexico
Carlos Garcia-Capulin   Instituto Tecnológico Superior de Irapuato,
                           Mexico
Ma. de Guadalupe
  Garcia-Hernandez   Universidad de Guanajuato, Mexico
Arturo Garcia-Perez   Universidad de Guanajuato, Mexico
Alexander Gelbukh   Instituto Politécnico Nacional, Mexico
Onofrio Gigliotta   University of Naples Federico II, Italy
Roxana Girju   University of Illinois at Urbana-Champaign,
                           USA
Eduardo Gomez-Ramirez   Universidad La Salle, Mexico
Arturo Gonzalez   Universidad de Guanajuato, Mexico
Miguel Gonzalez-Mendoza   Tecnológico de Monterrey CEM, Mexico
Felix F. Gonzalez-Navarro Universidad Autónoma de Baja California,
                           Mexico
Efren Gorrostieta   Universidad Autónoma de Querétaro, Mexico
Carlos Arturo Gracios-Marin CERN, Switzerland
Joaquin Gutierrez   Centro de Investigaciones Biológicas del
                           Noroeste S.C., Mexico
Yasunari Harada   Waseda University, Japan
Mark Hasegawa-Johnson   University of Illinois at Urbana-Champaign,
                           USA
Rogelio Hasimoto   Centro de Investigación en Matemáticas,
                           Mexico
Antonio Hernandez   Instituto Politécnico Nacional, Mexico
Oscar Herrera   Universidad Autónoma Metropolitana
                           Azcapotzalco, Mexico
Dieter Hutter   DFKI GmbH, Germany
Pablo H. Ibarguengoytia   Instituto de Investigaciones Eléctricas, Mexico
Rodolfo Ibarra   Tecnológico de Monterrey, Mexico
Oscar G. Ibarra-Manzano   Universidad de Guanajuato, Mexico
Diana Inkpen   University of Ottawa, Canada
Héctor Jiménez Salazar   Universidad Autónoma Metropolitana, Mexico
Laetitia Jourdan   Inria/LIFL/CNRS, France
Pinar Karagoz   Middle East Technical University, Turkey
Olga Kolesnikova   Instituto Politécnico Nacional, Mexico
Valia Kordoni   Humboldt University Berlin, Germany

Konstantinos Koutroumbas	National Observatory of Athens, Greece
Vladik Kreinovich	University of Texas at El Paso, USA
Angel Kuri-Morales	Instituto Tecnológico Autónomo de México, Mexico
Mathieu Lafourcade	Le Laboratoire d'Informatique, de Robotique et de Microélectronique de Montpellier (UM2/CNRS), France
Ricardo Landa	CINVESTAV Tamaulipas, Mexico
Dario Landa-Silva	University of Nottingham, UK
Bruno Lara	Universidad Autónoma del Estado de Morelos, Mexico
Yulia Ledeneva	Universidad Autónoma del Estado de México, Mexico
Sergio Ledesma	Universidad de Guanajuato, Mexico
Yoel Ledo Mezquita	Universidad de las Américas, Mexico
Eugene Levner	Ashkelon Academic College, Israel
Aristidis Likas	University of Ioannina, Greece
Rocio Lizarraga-Morales	Universidad de Guanajuato, Mexico
Aurelio Lopez	Instituto Nacional de Astrofísica, Óptica y Electrónica, Mexico
Virgilio Lopez-Morales	Universidad Autónoma del Estado de Hidalgo, Mexico
Omar López-Ortega	Universidad Autónoma del Estado de Hidalgo, Mexico
Tanja Magoc	University of Texas at El Paso, USA
Stephane Marchand-Maillet	University of Geneva, Switzerland
J. Raymundo Marcial-Romero	Universidad Autónoma del Estado de México, Mexico
Ricardo Martinez	Instituto Tecnológico de Tijuana, Mexico
Luis Martí	Pontifícia Universidade Católica do Rio de Janeiro, Brazil
Lourdes Martínez	Tecnológico de Monterrey CEM, Mexico
Francisco Martínez-Álvarez	Universidad Pablo de Olavide, Spain
María Auxilio Medina Nieto	Universidad Politécnica de Puebla, Mexico
R. Carolina Medina-Ramirez	Universidad Autónoma Metropolitana Iztapalapa, Mexico
Patricia Melin	Instituto Tecnológico de Tijuana, Mexico
Ivan Vladimir Meza Ruiz	Universidad Nacional Autónoma de México, Mexico
Efrén Mezura-Montes	Universidad Veracruzana, Mexico
Mikhail Mikhailov	University of Tampere, Finland
Sabino Miranda	INFOTEC, Mexico
Dieter Mitsche	Universitat Politècnica de Catalunya, Spain

Dunja Mladenic	Jozef Stefan Institute, Slovenia
Raul Monroy	Tecnologico de Monterrey CEM, Mexico
Manuel Montes-y-Gómez	Instituto Nacional de Astrofísica, Óptica y Electrónica, Mexico
Carlos Montoro	Universidad de Guanajuato, Mexico
Jaime Mora-Vargas	Tecnológico de Monterrey CEM, Mexico
Guillermo Morales-Luna	CINVESTAV, Mexico
Masaki Murata	Tottori University, Japan
Victor Muñiz	Centro de Investigación en Matemáticas, Mexico
Michele Nappi	Dipartimento di Matematica e Informatica, Italy
Jesús Emeterio Navarro-Barrientos	Society for the Promotion of Applied Computer Science (GFaI e.V.), Germany
Juan Carlos Nieves	Umeå University, Sweden
Roger Nkambou	Université du Québec à Montréal, Canada
Juan Arturo Nolazco Flores	Tecnológico de Monterrey CM, Mexico
Leszek Nowak	Jagiellonian University, Poland
C. Alberto Ochoa-Zezatti	Universidad Autónoma de Ciudad Juárez, Mexico
Ivan Olmos	Benemérita Universidad Autónoma de Puebla, Mexico
Sonia Ordoñez	Universidad Distrital Francisco Jose de Caldas, Colombia
Felipe Orihuela-Espina	Instituto Nacional de Astrofísica, Óptica y Electrónica, Mexico
Eber Enrique Orozco Guillén	Universidad Politécnica de Sinaloa, Mexico
Magdalena Ortiz	Vienna University of Technology, Austria
Mauricio Osorio	Universidad de Las Américas, Mexico
Ekaterina Ovchinnikova	Information Sciences Institute, University of Southern California, USA
Partha Pakray	Norwegian University of Science and Technology, Norway
Ivandre Paraboni	University of Sao Paulo, Brazil
Mario Pavone	University of Catania, Italy
Ted Pedersen	University of Minnesota Duluth, USA
Obdulia Pichardo	Instituto Politécnico Nacional, Mexico
David Pinto	Benemérita Universidad Autónoma de Puebla, Mexico
Volodymyr Ponomaryov	Instituto Politécnico Nacional, Mexico
Héctor Pérez-Urbina	Clark & Parsia, LLC, USA
Marta R. Costa-Jussà	Institute For Infocomm Research, Singapore
Risto Fermin Rangel Kuoppa	Universidad Autónoma Metropolitana Azcapotzalco, Mexico

Ivan Razo	Université libre de Bruxelles, Belgium
Alberto Reyes	Instituto de Investigaciones Eléctricas, Mexico
Orion Reyes	University of Alberta Edmonton AB, Canada
Bernardete Ribeiro	University of Coimbra, Portugal
Alessandro Ricci	University of Bologna, Italy
Erik Rodner	Friedrich Schiller University of Jena, Germany
Arles Rodriguez	Universidad Nacional de Colombia, Colombia
Eduardo Rodriguez-Tello	CINVESTAV Tamaulipas, Mexico
Alejandro Rosales	Instituto Nacional de Astrofísica, Óptica y Electrónica, Mexico
Paolo Rosso	Technical University of Valencia, Spain
Horacio Rostro Gonzalez	Universidad de Guanajuato, Mexico
Salvador Ruiz Correa	Centro de Investigación en Matemáticas, Mexico
Jose Ruiz-Pinales	Universidad de Guanajuato, Mexico
Klempous Ryszard	Wroclaw University of Technology, Poland
Chaman Sabharwal	Missouri University of Science and Technology, USA
Abraham Sánchez López	Benemérita Universidad Autónoma de Puebla, Mexico
Luciano Sanchez	Universidad de Oviedo, Spain
Guillermo Sanchez-Diaz	Universidad Autónoma de San Luis Potosí, Mexico
Jose Santos	University of A Coruña, Spain
Oliver Schuetze	CINVESTAV, Mexico
Friedhelm Schwenker	Ulm University, Germany
Shahnaz Shahbazova	Azerbaijan Technical University, Azerbaijan
Bernadette Sharp	Staffordshire University, UK
Oleksiy Shulika	Universidad de Guanajuato, Mexico
Patrick Siarry	Université de Paris 12, France
Grigori Sidorov	Instituto Politécnico Nacional, Mexico
Bogdan Smolka	Silesian University of Technology, Poland
Jorge Solis	Waseda University, Japan
Thamar Solorio	University of Alabama at Birmingham, USA
Juan Humberto Sossa Azuela	Instituto Politécnico Nacional, Mexico
Efstathios Stamatatos	University of the Aegean, Greece
Josef Steinberger	University of West Bohemia, Czech Republic
Vera Lúcia Strube de Lima	Pontifícia Universidade Católica do Rio Grande do Sul, Brazil
Luis Enrique Sucar	Instituto Nacional de Astrofísica, Óptica y Electrónica, Mexico
Shiliang Sun	East China Normal University, China
Johan Suykens	Katholieke Universiteit Leuven, Belgium
Antonio-José Sánchez-Salmerón	Universitat Politècnica de València, Spain

Anastasios Tefas	Aristotle University of Thessaloniki, Greece
Gregorio Toscano Pulido	CINVESTAV Tamaulipas, Mexico
Kostas Triantafyllopoulos	University of Sheffield, UK
Leonardo Trujillo	Instituto Tecnológico de Tijuana, Mexico
Alexander Tulupyev	St. Petersburg Institute for Informatics and Automation of Russian Academy of Sciences, Russia
Fevrier Valdez	Instituto Tecnológico de Tijuana, Mexico
Edgar Vallejo	Tecnológico de Monterrey CEM, Mexico
Manuel Vilares Ferro	University of Vigo, Spain
Aline Villavicencio	Universidade Federal do Rio Grande do Sul, Brazil
Francisco Viveros Jiménez	Instituto Politécnico Nacional, Mexico
Panagiotis Vlamos	Ionian University, Greece
Piotr W. Fuglewicz	TiP Sp. z o. o., Poland
Fanhai Yang	University of Massachusetts Lowell, USA
Nicolas Younan	Mississippi State University, USA
Carlos Mario Zapata Jaramillo	Universidad Nacional de Colombia, Colombia
Ramon Zatarain	Instituto Tecnológico de Culiacán, Mexico
Claudia Zepeda Cortes	Benemérita Universidad Autónoma de Puebla, Mexico
Reyer Zwiggelaar	Aberystwyth University, UK

Additional Reviewers

Roberto Alonso	Homero Miranda
Ricardo Alvarez Salas	Soujanya Poria
Igor Bolshakov	Pedro Reta
Michael Emmerich	Daniel Rivera
Victor Ferman	Carlos Rodriguez-Donate
Esteban Guerrero	Salvador Ruiz-Correa
Goffredo Haus	Chrysostomos Stylios
Misael Lopez Ramirez	Yasushi Tsubota
José Lozano	Dan-El Vila-Rosado
Ana Martinez	

Organizing Committee

Local Chair

Imelda Valles López	Instituto Tecnológico de Tuxtla Gutiérrez, Mexico

Logistics Chairs

Delina Culebro Farrera — Instituto Tecnológico de Tuxtla Gutiérrez, Mexico

Adolfo Solís — Universidad Autónoma de Chiapas, Mexico

Marketing Chair

Aida Cossio Martínez — Instituto Tecnológico de Tuxtla Gutiérrez, Mexico

Registration Chair

Héctor Guerra Crespo — Instituto Tecnológico de Tuxtla Gutiérrez, Mexico

Workshop Chair

Octavio Guzmán Sánchez — Instituto Tecnológico de Tuxtla Gutiérrez, Mexico

International Relations Chair

María Candelaria Gutiérrez Gómez — Instituto Tecnológico de Tuxtla Gutiérrez, Mexico

Finance Chair

Jacinta Luna Villalobos — Instituto Tecnológico de Tuxtla Gutiérrez, Mexico

Student Chair

Sebastián Moreno Vázquez — Instituto Tecnológico de Tuxtla Gutiérrez, Mexico

Table of Contents – Part II

Genetic and Evolutionary Algorithms

Performance Classification of Genetic Algorithms on Continuous
Optimization Problems 1
  Noel E. Rodriguez-Maya, Mario Graff, and Juan J. Flores

A Multi-objective Genetic Algorithm for the Software Project
Scheduling Problem 13
  Abel García-Nájera and María del Carmen Gómez-Fuentes

An Effective Method for MOGAs Initialization to Solve the
Multi-Objective Next Release Problem. 25
  Thiago Gomes Nepomuceno Da Silva, Leonardo Sampaio Rocha,
  and José Everardo Bessa Maia

Extension of the Method of Musical Composition for the Treatment of
Multi-objective Optimization Problems 38
  José Roberto Méndez Rosiles, Antonin Ponsich,
  Eric Alfredo Rincón García,
  and Roman Anselmo Mora Gutiérrez

k-Nearest-Neighbor by Differential Evolution for Time Series
Forecasting. 50
  Erick De la Vega, Juan J. Flores, and Mario Graff

A Binary Differential Evolution with Adaptive Parameters Applied to
the Multiple Knapsack Problem. 61
  Leanderson André and Rafael Stubs Parpinelli

Neural Networks

Best Paper Award, First Place

The Best Neural Network Architecture 72
  Angel Fernando Kuri-Morales

On the Connection Weight Space Structure of a Two-Neuron Discrete
Neural Network: Bifurcations of the Fixed Point at the Origin 85
  Jorge Cervantes-Ojeda and María del Carmen Gómez-Fuentes

Stability of Modular Recurrent Trainable Neural Networks 95
  Sergio Miguel Hernández Manzano and Ieroham Baruch

Best Paper Award, Second Place

Intelligent Control of Induction Motor Based Comparative Study:
Analysis of Two Topologies 105
  *Moulay Rachid Douiri, El Batoul Mabrouki, Ouissam Belghazi,
  Mohamed Ferfra, and Mohamed Cherkaoui*

Auto-Adaptive Neuro-Fuzzy Parameter Regulator for Motor Drive 116
  *Moulay Rachid Douiri, Mohamed Ferfra, Ouissam Belghazi,
  and Mohamed Cherkaoui*

Machine Learning

Voting Algorithms Model with a Support Sets System by Class 128
  *Dalia Rodríguez-Salas, Manuel S. Lazo-Cortés, Ramón A. Mollineda,
  J. Arturo Olvera-López, Jorge de la Calleja,
  and Antonio Benitez*

A Meta Classifier by Clustering of Classifiers 140
  *Mohammad Iman Jamnejad, Sajad Parvin, Ali Heidarzadegan,
  and Mohsen Moshki*

Multiple Kernel Support Vector Machine Problem Is NP-Complete 152
  *Luis Carlos Padierna, Juan Martín Carpio,
  María del Rosario Baltazar, Héctor José Puga,
  and Héctor Joaquín Fraire*

Feature Analysis for the Classification of Volcanic Seismic Events Using
Support Vector Machines 160
  *Millaray Curilem, Fernando Huenupan, Cesar San Martin,
  Gustavo Fuentealba, Carlos Cardona, Luis Franco, Gonzalo Acuña,
  and Max Chacón*

A Hierarchical Reinforcement Learning Based Artificial Intelligence for
Non-Player Characters in Video Games 172
  Hiram Ponce and Ricardo Padilla

Wind Power Forecasting Using Dynamic Bayesian Models 184
  *Pablo H. Ibargüengoytia, Alberto Reyes, Inés Romero-Leon,
  David Pech, Uriel A. García, Luis Enrique Sucar,
  and Eduardo F. Morales*

Predictive Models Applied to Heavy Duty Equipment Management..... 198
  *Gonzalo Acuña, Millaray Curilem, Beatriz Araya,
  Francisco Cubillos, Rodrigo Miranda, and Fernanda Garrido*

Customer Churn Prediction in Telecommunication Industry: With and
without Counter-Example.. 206
  Adnan Amin, Changez Khan, Imtiaz Ali, and Sajid Anwar

Machine Learning Applications to Audio and Text

Audio-to-Audio Alignment for Performances Tracking 219
   Alain Manzo-Martínez and Jose Antonia Camarena-Ibarrola

Statistical Features Based Noise Type Identification 231
   Sohail Masood, Ismael Soto, Ayyaz Hussain, and M. Arfan Jaffar

Using Values of the Human Cochlea in the Macro and Micro Mechanical
Model for Automatic Speech Recognition 242
   José Luis Oropeza Rodríguez and Sergio Suárez Guerra

Identification of Vowel Sounds of the Choapan Variant of Zapotec
Language 252
   Gabriela Oliva-Juarez, Fabiola Martinez-Licona,
   Alma Martinez-Licona, and John Goddard-Close

An Open-Domain Cause-Effect Relation Detection
from Paired Nominals 263
   Partha Pakray and Alexander Gelbukh

An Alignment Comparator for Entity Resolution with Multi-valued
Attributes 272
   Pablo N. Mazzucchi-Augel and Héctor G. Ceballos

Data Mining

Data Mining for Discovering Patterns in Migration 285
   Anilu Franco-Arcega, Kristell D. Franco-Sánchez,
   Felix A. Castro-Espinoza, and Luis H. García-Islas

Horizontal Partitioning of Multimedia Databases Using Hierarchical
Agglomerative Clustering 296
   Lisbeth Rodríguez-Mazahua, Giner Alor-Hernández,
   Ma. Antonieta Abud-Figueroa, and S. Gustavo Peláez-Camarena

Classification with Graph-Based Markov Chain 310
   Ping He and Xiaohua Xu

Best Student Paper Award

Solving Binary Cutting Stock with Matheuristics.................... 319
   Ivan Adrian Lopez Sanchez, Jaime Mora Vargas,
   Cipriano A. Santos, and Miguel Gonzalez Mendoza

Fuzzy Logic

Invited Paper

Nature-Inspired Optimization of Type-2 Fuzzy Systems 331
   Oscar Castillo, Patricia Melin, and Fevrier Valdez

Hierarchical Genetic Algorithms for Fuzzy Inference
System Optimization Applied to Response Integration
for Pattern Recognition 345
   Daniela Sánchez, Patricia Melin, and Oscar Castillo

Low-Cost Fuzzy-Based Obstacle Avoidance Method for Autonomous
Agents 357
   *Luis Carlos Gonzalez-Sua, Ivan Gonzalez, Leonardo Garrido,
   and Rogelio Soto*

Fuzzy Controller for a Pneumatic Positioning Nonlinear System 370
   *Omar Rodríguez-Zalapa, Antonio Hernández-Zavala,
   and Jorge Adalberto Huerta-Ruelas*

Yager–Rybalov Triple Π Operator as a Means of Reducing the
Number of Generated Clusters in Unsupervised Anuran Vocalization
Recognition 382
   *Carol Bedoya, Julio Waissman-Villanova,
   and Claudia Victoria Isaza-Narvaez*

Robotics, Planning, and Scheduling

AI-Based Design of a Parallel Robot Used as a Laser Tracker System:
Intelligent vs. Nonlinear Classical Controllers 392
   *Ricardo Zavala-Yoé, Ricardo A. Ramírez-Mendoza,
   and Daniel Chaparro-Altamirano*

Simple Direct Propositional Encoding of Cooperative Path Finding
Simplified Yet More 410
   Pavel Surynek

Pendulum Position Based Fuzzy Regulator of the Furuta Pendulum –
A Stable Closed-Loop System Design Approach 426
   *Nohe Ramon Cazarez-Castro, Luis T. Aguilar,
   Selene L. Cardenas-Maciel, and Carlos A. Goribar-Jimenez*

Best Paper Award, Third Place

A Fast Scheduling Algorithm for Detection and Localization of Hidden
Objects Based on Data Gathering in Wireless Sensor Networks 436
   Eugene Levner, Boris Kriheli, Amir Elalouf, and Dmitry Tsadikovich

A Constraint-Based Planner for Mars Express Orbiter   451
    Martin Kolombo and Roman Barták

Biomedical Applications

Glucose Oxidase Biosensor Modeling by Machine Learning Methods   464
    *Livier Rentería-Gutiérrez, Félix F. González-Navarro,
    Margarita Stilianova-Stoytcheva, Lluís A. Belanche-Muñoz,
    Brenda L. Flores-Ríos, and Jorge Eduardo Ibarra-Esquer*

On the Breast Mass Diagnosis Using Bayesian Networks   474
    Verónica Rodríguez-López and Raúl Cruz-Barbosa

Predicting the Occurrence of Sepsis by *In Silico* Simulation   486
    *Flávio Oliveira de Sousa, Alcione Oliveira de Paiva,
    Luiz Alberto Santana, Fábio Ribeiro Cerqueira,
    Rodrigo Siqueira-Batista, and Andréia Patrícia Gomes*

Data Mining and Machine Learning on the Basis from Reflexive
Eye Movements Can Predict Symptom Development in Individual
Parkinson's Patients   499
    *Andrzej W. Przybyszewski, Mark Kon, Stanislaw Szlufik,
    Justyna Dutkiewicz, Piotr Habela, and Dariusz M. Koziorowski*

Agents That Help to Avoid Hyperthermia in Young Children Left in a
Baby Seat Inside an Enclosed Car   510
    *Juan Pablo Soto, Julio Waissman, Pedro Flores-Pérez,
    and Gilberto Muñoz-Sandoval*

Author Index   519

Table of Contents – Part I

Natural Language Processing

Finding the Most Frequent Sense of a Word by the Length of Its
Definition 1
   Hiram Calvo and Alexander Gelbukh

Complete Syntactic N-grams as Style Markers for Authorship
Attribution 9
   Juan-Pablo Posadas-Duran, Grigori Sidorov, and Ildar Batyrshin

Extracting Frame-Like Structures from Google Books NGram
Dataset 18
   Vladimir Ivanov

Modeling Natural Language Metaphors with an Answer Set
Programming Framework 28
   Juan Carlos Acosta-Guadarrama, Rogelio Dávila-Pérez,
   Mauricio Osorio, and Victor Hugo Zaldivar

Whole-Part Relations Rule-Based Automatic Identification: Issues from
Fine-Grained Error Analysis 37
   Ilia Markov, Nuno Mamede, and Jorge Baptista

Statistical Recognition of References in Czech Court Decisions 51
   Vincent Kríž, Barbora Hladká, Jan Dědek, and Martin Nečaský

LSA Based Approach to Domain Detection 62
   Diego Uribe

Natural Language Processing Applications

Best Student Paper Award

Novel Unsupervised Features for Czech Multi-label Document
Classification 70
   Tomáš Brychcín and Pavel Král

Feature Selection Based on Sampling and C4.5 Algorithm to Improve
the Quality of Text Classification Using Naïve Bayes 80
   Viviana Molano, Carlos Cobos, Martha Mendoza,
   Enrique Herrera-Viedma, and Milos Manic

Detailed Description of the Development of a MOOC in the Topic
of Statistical Machine Translation   92
    Marta Ruiz Costa-jussà, Lluís Formiga, Jordi Petit,
    and José A.R. Fonollosa

NEBEL: Never-Ending Bilingual Equivalent Learner   99
    Thiago Lima Vieira and Helena de Medeiros Caseli

RI for IR: Capturing Term Contexts Using Random Indexing
for Comprehensive Information Retrieval   104
    Rajendra Prasath, Sudeshna Sarkar, and Philip O'Reilly

Data Extraction Using NLP Techniques and Its Transformation to
Linked Data   113
    Vincent Kríž, Barbora Hladká, Martin Nečaský, and Tomáš Knap

A New Memetic Algorithm for Multi-document Summarization Based
on CHC Algorithm and Greedy Search   125
    Martha Mendoza, Carlos Cobos, Elizabeth León, Manuel Lozano,
    Francisco Rodríguez, and Enrique Herrera-Viedma

How Predictive Is Tense for Language Profiency? A Cautionary Tale ...   139
    Alexandra Panagiotopoulos and Sabine Bergler

Evaluating Term-Expansion for Unsupervised Image Annotation   151
    Luis Pellegrin, Hugo Jair Escalante, and Manuel Montes-y-Gómez

Opinion Mining, Sentiment Analysis, and Social Network Applications

Gender Differences in Deceivers Writing Style   163
    Verónica Pérez-Rosas and Rada Mihalcea

Extraction of Semantic Relations from Opinion Reviews in Spanish.....   175
    Sofía N. Galicia-Haro and Alexander Gelbukh

Evaluating Polarity for Verbal Phraseological Units   191
    Belém Priego Sánchez, David Pinto, and Salah Mejri

Restaurant Information Extraction (Including Opinion Mining
Elements) for the Recommendation System   201
    Ekaterina Pronoza, Elena Yagunova, Svetlana Volskaya,
    and Andrey Lyashin

Aggressive Text Detection for Cyberbullying   221
    Laura P. Del Bosque and Sara Elena Garza

A Sentiment Analysis Model: To Process Subjective Social Corpus
through the Adaptation of an Affective Semantic Lexicon   233
  Guadalupe Gutiérrez, Lourdes Margain, Carlos de Luna,
  Alejandro Padilla, Julio Ponce, Juana Canul, and Alberto Ochoa

Towards Automatic Detection of User Influence in Twitter by Means
of Stylistic and Behavioral Features   245
  Gabriela Ramírez-de-la-Rosa, Esaú Villatoro-Tello,
  Héctor Jiménez-Salazar, and Christian Sánchez-Sánchez

Computer Vision

Best Paper Award, Second Place

Multisensor Based Obstacles Detection in Challenging Scenes   257
  Yong Fang, Cindy Cappelle, and Yassine Ruichek

GP-MPU Method for Implicit Surface Reconstruction   269
  Manuel Guillermo López, Boris Mederos, and Oscar S. Dalmau

Monocular Visual Odometry Based Navigation for a Differential Mobile
Robot with Android OS   281
  Carla Villanueva-Escudero, Juan Villegas-Cortez,
  Arturo Zúñiga-López, and Carlos Avilés-Cruz

Comparison and Analysis of Models to Predict the Motion of Segmented
Regions by Optical Flow   293
  Angel Juan Sanchez Garcia, Maria de Lourdes Velasco Vazquez,
  Homero Vladimir Rios Figueroa, Antonio Marin Hernandez,
  and Gerardo Contreras Vega

Image Based Place Recognition and Lidar Validation for Vehicle
Localization   304
  Yongliang Qiao, Cindy Cappelle, and Yassine Ruichek

Image Processing

Frequency Filter Bank for Enhancing Carbon Nanotube Images   316
  José de Jesús Guerrero Casas, Oscar S. Dalmau, Teresa E. Alarcón,
  and Adalberto Zamudio

A Supervised Segmentation Algorithm for Crop Classification Based on
Histograms Using Satellite Images................................   327
  Francisco E. Oliva, Oscar S. Dalmau, and Teresa E. Alarcón

An Effective Visual Descriptor Based on Color and Shape Features for
Image Retrieval   336
    Atoany Fierro-Radilla, Karina Perez-Daniel,
    Mariko Nakano-Miyatakea, Hector Perez-Meana,
    and Jenny Benois-Pineau

Compressive Sensing Architecture for Gray Scale Images   349
    Gustavo Gonzalez-Garcia, Alfonso Fernandez-Vazquez,
    and Rodolfo Romero-Herrera

A Novel Approach for Face Authentication Using Speeded Up Robust
Features Algorithm   356
    Cyntia Mendoza-Martinez, Jesus Carlos Pedraza-Ortega,
    and Juan Manuel Ramos-Arreguin

On-Line Dense Point Cloud Generation from Monocular Images with
Scale Estimation   368
    Ander Larranaga-Cepeda, Jose Gabriel Ramirez-Torres,
    and Carlos Alberto Motta-Avila

An Improved Colorimetric Invariants and RGB-Depth-Based Codebook
Model for Background Subtraction Using Kinect   380
    Julian Murgia, Cyril Meurie, and Yassine Ruichek

Novel Binarization Method for Enhancing Ancient and Historical
Manuscript Images   393
    Saad M. Ismail and Siti Norul Huda Sheikh Abdullah

Logic, Reasoning, and Multi-agent Systems

Preferences for Argumentation Semantics   407
    Mauricio Osorio, Claudia Zepeda, and José Luis Carballido

Computing Preferred Semantics: Comparing Two ASP Approaches vs
an Approach Based on 0-1 Integer Programming   419
    Mauricio Osorio, Juan Díaz, and Alejandro Santoyo

Experimenting with SAT Solvers in Vampire   431
    Armin Biere, Ioan Dragan, Laura Kovács, and Andrei Voronkov

Onto Design Graphics (ODG): A Graphical Notation to Standardize
Ontology Design   443
    Rafaela Blanca Silva-López, Mónica Silva-López,
    Iris Iddaly Méndez-Gurrola, and Maricela Bravo

A Logic for Context-Aware Non-monotonic Reasoning Agents   453
    Abdur Rakib and Hafiz Mahfooz Ul Haque

MAS-td: An Approach to Termination Detection of Multi-agent
Systems 472
    Ammar Lahlouhi

Intelligent Tutoring Systems

Intelligent Tutoring System with Affective Learning for Mathematics ... 483
    Ramón Zataraín Cabada, María Lucía Barrón Estrada,
    Francisco González Hernández, and Raúl Oramas Bustillos

Emotion Recognition in Intelligent Tutoring System for Android-Based
Mobile Devices 494
    Ramón Zataraín Cabada, María Lucía Barrón Estrada,
    Giner Alor-Hernández, and Carlos Alberto Reyes-García

Author Index 505

Performance Classification of Genetic Algorithms on Continuous Optimization Problems

Noel E. Rodriguez-Maya, Mario Graff, and Juan J. Flores

Universidad Michoacana de San Nicolas de Hidalgo,
Av. Francisco J. Mugica S/N Ciudad Universitaria, Morelia, Michoacan, Mexico
{nrodriguez,mgraffg}@dep.fie.umich.mx,
juanf@umich.mx

Abstract. Modelling the behaviour of algorithms is the realm of Evolutionary Algorithm theory. From a practitioner's point of view, theory must provide some guidelines regarding which algorithm/parameters to use in order to solve a particular problem. Unfortunately, most theoretical models of evolutionary algorithms are difficult to apply to realistic situations. Recently, there have been works that addressed this problem by proposing models of performance of different Genetic Programming Systems. In this work, we complement previous approaches by proposing a scheme capable of classifying the hardness of optimization problems based on different difficulty measures such as Negative Slope Coefficient, Fitness Distance Correlation, Neutrality, Ruggedness, Basins of Attraction, and Epistasis. The results indicate that this procedure is able to accurately classify the performance of the GA over a set of benchmark problems.

Keywords: Algorithm Performance Classification, Genetic Algorithms, Optimization Problems.

1 Introduction

Evolutionary Algorithms (EAs) are popular forms of search and optimisation [10,5]. Their invention dates back many decades (e.g., see [3]). Consequently, one might expect that, by now, there would be a rich set of theoretically-sound guidelines to decide which EAs and its parameters to use in order to solve a particular problem. The problem is that sound theoretical models of EAs and precise mathematical results are hard to obtain. A key reason for this is that each component of a EA requires a different theoretical model.

Perhaps, the first works that can give some sort of guidelines to a practitioner are the works related to the problem of understanding what makes a problem easy or hard for EAs. The notion of *fitness landscape*, originally proposed in [39], underlies many recent approaches to problem difficulty. It is clear, for example, that a smooth landscape with a single optimum will be relatively easy to search for many algorithms, while a very rugged landscape, with many local optima, may be more problematic [11,15]. Nonetheless, a graphical visualisation of the

A. Gelbukh et al. (Eds.): MICAI 2014, Part II, LNAI 8857, pp. 1–12, 2014.

fitness landscape (FL) is rarely possible given the size and dimensions of a typical search space.

Given the inability to depict a traditional fitness landscape and the subjective that would be to draw conclusions from observation of fitness landscapes, there have been proposed descriptors, i.e. *hardness measures*, that try to capture the characteristics of the fitness landscape. Perhaps, one of the first hardness measures is the Fitness Distance Correlation (FDC) proposed in [13]. The FDC has been successfully applied to measure the hardness of different problems solved by GA. The drawback is that the FDC requires to know beforehand the problem's optimum solution. This is unrealistic in any practical application. A measure that tries to overcome the FDC limitation is the *negative slope coefficient* NSC proposed by Vanneschi *et al.* [34]. NSC is based on the concept of fitness cloud which is a scatter plot of parent/offspring fitness pairs. Different characteristics of the fitness landscape have been related to the hardness of the problem. In this category one can find *neutrality* [17], which is related to the flatness of the landscape. On the opposite site it is found *ruggedness* [18], which is related to the number of local optima. Related to the smoothness of a landscape is *Basins of Attraction* [22,19], which describes the areas that lead the search to a local optimum. Another measure relating the phenotype with the genotype is *Epistasis* [4,26].

Although, the aforementioned hardness measures have shown success in estimating the difficulty of different problems, there are a number of open questions that can be addressed. Firstly, these measures have been tested on different classes of problems, so a direct comparison between them has not been made. Secondly, these measures mostly have only been tested to discern between easy and hard problems. And thirdly, to the best of our knowledge, these have not been used together to estimate the difficulty of a particular problem solved by a GA.

In this contribution, we start filling these research gaps by first comparing the capacity of the aforementioned difficulty measures to estimate the hardness of continuous optimization problems solved by a GA. Secondly, we compare these indicators using a finer granularity of hardness, that is, these indicators are tested on whether these are capable of categorizing the problem hardness into three categories: easy, medium, and hard problems. Thirdly, these hardness measures are combined in a machine learning algorithm in order to classify the problem hardness in the three classes mentioned above. The results show that the hardness measures are capable of correctly estimating the hardness of an unseen problem approximately 70% to 80% of the time, and using a combination of all the features the correct classification reaches to 96%.

This paper are organized as follow: Section 2 reviews the related work. Section 3 defines the difficulty indicators used in this work. Section 4 describes the proposed procedure to classify the performance of Genetic Algorithms. Section 5 presents the experimental design, and the results. A discussion and the conclusions of the present work are presented in Section 6.

2   Related Work

Our work is related to estimate the performance of an EA when solving a particular problem. In the field of Genetic Programming (GP) there has been a number of models that are able to estimate the performance of GP on different classes of problems. Graff and Poli proposed a model of performance [20]; the idea is that the performance of a GP system on problem can be estimated using a set of points from the search space. Later on, Graff et. al proposed a different model of performance [7], based on the the discrete derivative of a function, and, consequently, it has only been tested on symbolic regression problems. These two models have been successfully applied to different symbolic regression problems, Boolean induction problems, and time series forecasters [6], among other classes of problems. Continuing with estimating the performance of GP Trujillo et. al [30,31,29] proposed different approaches to estimate the performance of GP on classification problems.

Moving away from the evolutionary computation literature, this work is also related to the *algorithm selection problem* [27] and *algorithm portfolios* [28]. The algorithm selection problem is the problem of deciding which algorithm to use to solve a particular problem from a set of available algorithms. An algorithm portfolio is a particular way of solving the algorithm selection problem based on choosing a collection of algorithms that are run in parallel or in sequence to solve a particular problem. The connection between these problems and our current work is that in order to solve the algorithm selection problem or to create an algorithm portfolio, a model of performance is created to select the algorithm.

The methodology proposed here complements the related work by the following facts. First, the models of performance developed for GP uses the fact that GP is used in the context of supervised learning and consequently one has a function or a set of cases that needs to be learned by GP. The hardness measures used in these works rely on this assumption. Secondly, the works used to solve the algorithm selection problem in general use hardness measures that are specific to the problem being solved, for example, Xu et. al [40] used descriptors related to SAT problems. Instead, our approach uses hardness measures that can be applied to any optimization algorithm, consequently, these measures are not specific to a particular problem neither these features rely on problems of supervised learning.

3   Difficulty Indicators

Let us start describing in more detail the different hardness measures used in this contribution.

Fitness Distance Correlation (FDC). Deceptive problems in Evolutionary Computation Algorithms (ECA) usually mislead the search to some local optima rather to the global optima [2]. The more deceptive the problem is, the harder to solve [2]. A way to measure the level of deceptiveness is to get the Fitness Distance Correlation (Jones and Forrest [13]). The FDC measures the extent to which the fitness function values are correlated with distance to a global optimum. FDC takes a sample of individuals and computes the level of correlation between the set of fitnesses and distances to the optimum [35]. The most important flaw presented by FDC it the fact that it is not predictive; the global optima must be known beforehand; this is unrealistic in real optimisation problems [32]. Implementation details can be found in [13].

Negative Slope Coefficient (NSC). The Negative Slope Coefficient is a tool that based on the concept of evolvability, gives a measure of problem difficulty in ECA [36,21]. The term evolvability is the capacity of genetic operators to improve its fitness quality [34]; the most common form of study of evolvability is to plot the fitness values of neighbours against the fitness values of individuals, where the neighbours are obtained by applying one step of a genetic operator; the set of neighbors is called fitness cloud [24]. The main advantage of this method is that it is predictive and it is not necessary to know a prior an optimal solution [21]. The main disadvantages of NSC is how to tune the bins in the fitness cloud and that there is no technique to normalize the NSC values into a given range [33,24]. Implementation details can be found in [36,34].

Neutrality. The lack of improvement in fitness is not due to the population being trapped in local optima. In many real-world problems it is possible (or even common) to have a large amount of neutrality, so the dynamics of evolution must be seen in terms of navigating among neutral networks that eventually lead to higher-fit neutral networks [17]. FL which include neutrality have been conceptualized as containing neutral networks [14,23]. A neutral network is sometimes defined as a set of points in the search space with identical fitness [23]. Implementation details can be found in [37].

Ruggedness. Ruggedness is a metric related to the number of local optima on a FL [18]. A rugged landscape corresponds to a search space with an irregular topography consisting of numerous peaks (local optima) [16]. In general, search algorithms struggle to optimise very rugged landscapes, because the algorithms can get trapped in local optima [19,38]. Implementation details can be found in [18].

Basins of Attraction. Basins of Attraction and Smoothness are related concepts; basins of attraction are areas that lead to a local optimum [22,19]. A smooth landscape is one where neighbouring points have nearly the same fitness value. Smoothness also relates to the size of the basins of attraction. A landscape is smooth if the number of optima is small and the optima have large basins of attraction [19]. The number of local optima in a landscape clearly has some bearing on the difficulty of finding the global optimum. However, it is not the only indicator, the size of the basins of attraction of the various optima is also an important influence [25]. Implemenation details can be foun in [22].

Epistasis. In genetics, the term Epistasis refers to the masking (phenotype) effects of a set of genes by another set of genes. This concept was introduced by Davidor [4] as a tool for the evaluation of interdependences between genes. Epistasis can be thought of as expressing a degree of non-linearity in the fitness function, and roughly speaking, the more epistatic the problem is, the harder it may be for a genetic algorithm to find its optimum [1]. Analysis of Variance (ANOVA) is usually employed to evaluate the characteristic of model with real coded parameters [1]. Implementation details can be found in [1].

4   Performance Classification for Genetic Algorithms

This section explains the main contribution of the paper, which is the classification of the performance of Genetic Algorithms in the optimization of two dimensions problems. To classify the hardness of a problem, we consider as problem features a set of features that characterizes its fitness landscape.

This section formally defines the problem and provides algorithms that allows us to perform the classification task we have in mind.

4.1   Problem Definition

The problem addressed by this contribution is to learn a function Performance Classification PC which establishes a map from the set of problems F to the set of difficulty indicators DI. The mapping is defined in Equation 1.

$$PC : F \to DI \tag{1}$$

4.2   Measure of Relative Performance

It turns out that the set of measures of problem difficulty are not sufficient to determine the hardness of a problem by themselves. To complement the information in the training set and being able to predict the difficulty of a new problem, we execute GA on each problem and measure its performance. The ability of GA to solve a problem depends mainly on two parameters: precision and population size. GA is executed on each problem for different values of those parameters and measure its performance on each case. The performance of GA on each setting of those parameters is then discretized and converted into a label of difficulty. Now the problem is to determine a function that maps the complete set of problem features to a label that indicates the difficulty of the problem. All these notions will be formally defined in the rest of this section.

Definition 1. *Function MoD computes the measures of difficulty defined in Section 3 for a problem, specified by its objective function.*

$$MoD : F \to \mathbb{R}^6 \tag{2}$$

GA may or may not be successful in determining the optimum of a given problem. Since both the domain and range of the set of problems addressed in this work are real-valued, it is very unlikely that any metaheuristic used for this optimization process to get the exact optimum. Given that, we need to relax the optimization problem and obtain a quasi-optimal value, to a given precision. The success of GA to determine a quasi-optimal solution of a problem up to a precision value, depends on the population size (given a constant number of generations for all problems). Population-based metaheuristics, particularly GA, are stochastic in nature, so we need to run the same experiment a number of times, to determine the statistical success rate of GA on every function. Let us call the success rate of GA on solving function f at precision c, $\mathcal{P}_\epsilon(f)$. This success rate is relative to the values of those parameters, therefore it will be called relative performance; this relative performance indicator will be computed for all the functions analyzed in this work for given sets of precision values PV and population sizes PS. The relative performance is only a preliminary step towards the computation of an indicator of Relative Difficulty, to measure how hard it is for GA to solve that problem at the indicated precision level and population size. Let us call the set of indicators of Relative Difficulty RD.

Definition 2. *Given a problem f, function RD determines its Relative Difficulty level at given precision level and population size.*

$$RD : F \times PV \times PS \to DI \qquad (3)$$

In this contribution, we are considering a coarse granularity for the Relative Difficulty indicator; i.e., easy, medium, difficult. This indicator can be determined as indicated by Equation 4.

$$RD = \begin{cases} \text{difficult,} & \text{if } 0 \le \mathcal{P}_\epsilon(f) \le \frac{1}{3} \\ \text{medium,} & \text{if } \frac{1}{3} < \mathcal{P}_\epsilon(f) \le \frac{2}{3} \\ \text{easy,} & \text{if } \frac{2}{3} < \mathcal{P}_\epsilon(f) \le 1.0 \end{cases} \qquad (4)$$

Once the relative performance has been computed for the set of functions included in the training set, function RD can be determined using any machine learning classification method (see [9]). Section 5 provides details of performance of several classification methods used to implement RD.

5   Results

In order to test our approach, we decided to measure the performance of a generation GA with tournament selection on a set of 110 continuous optimization two dimensional problems $\mathcal{F}$ (see [12]). Their short names are: $\mathcal{F} = \{$ *Ackley, Beale, Bohachevsky, Booth, Branin, Dixonprice, Goldsteinprice, Griewank, Hump, Michalewicz, Rastrigin, Rosenbrock, Schwefel, Shubert, Sphere, Trid, Zakharov,*

Dropwave, Eggholder, Holder, Levy13, Styblinskitang, Randompeaks, Sumofdif-ferentpower, Levy, Dejong, Langermann, Himmelblau, Sumsquares, Schaffer2, Easom, Matyas, Crossintray, Bukin, Schaffer4, Equalpeaks, Ackley2, Ackley3, Ackley4, Adjiman, Alpine1, Alpine2, Bartels, Biggexp2, Bird, Bohachevsky2, Bohachevsky3, Braninrcos, Braninrcos2, Brent, Brown, Bukin2, Bukin4, Three-humpcamel, Sixhumpcamel, Chenbird, Chenv, Chichinadze, Chungreynolds, Cosinemixture, Csendes, Cube, Damavandi, Deckkersaarts, Elattarvidyasagar-dutta, Eggcrate, Exponential, Exp2, Freudensteinroth, Giunta, Hansen, Hosaki, Jennrichsampson, Keane, Leon, Mccormick, Mishra3, Mishra4, Mishra5, Mishra6, Mishra8, Penholder, Pathological, Periodic, Powellsum, Price1, Price2, Price3, Price4, Qing, Quadratic, Quartic, Quintic, Rosenbrockmodified, Rotat-edellipse, Rotatedellipse2, Rump, Salomon, Sargan, Schaffer3, Schumersteiglitz, Schwefel24, Schwefel222, Schwefel236, Strechedvsinewave, Testtubeholder, Tre-canni, Trefethen, Trigonometric, Trigonometric2}.

Table 1 shows the parameters used in the experiments. We used 10 different values of population size (PS) and also 10 different values of precision (PV). For each combination of parameters $(PV \times PS)$, we perform 100 independent runs to estimate the success rate for each problem, then, the hardness of problems is computed using Equation (4).

Table 1. GA Parameters

Parameter	Value
Population Size	$\{50, 100, \ldots, 500\}$
Precision	$\{1 \times 10^{-1}, 1 \times 10^{-2}, \ldots, 1 \times 10^{-10}\}$
Number of Generations	1000
Crossover rate	70%
Mutation rate	30%
Selection	Tournament of size 10

Once the hardness of the problems is estimated, we computed the difficulty indicators for each of the 110 problems using Equation (2). This gives us 110 different difficulty indicators, and 11,000 labels, let us remember that each problem was run with different values of population size and precision. In order to create 11,000 difficulty indicators, we included in each of the vectors returned by Equation (2) the values of population size and precision, i.e., each vector is cloned 100 times for each combination of PS and PV.

As can be seen this procedure gives us a data set of 11,000 different vectors with 8 dimensions and 11,000 different classes. Consequently, this information can be treated by any machine learning algorithm that performs classification. In this contribution we decided to test four different classification algorithms: Naïve Bayes, Multilayer Perceptron, Decision Trees, and Random Forests. All these algorithms were used with the default parameters used in WEKA [8].

In order to measure the accuracy of the different algorithms, we shuffle the data, and, then, performed a 10-fold crossvalidation. Table 2 shows the accuracy of the different classification algorithms used with different difficulty indicators. The first seven rows of the table present the accuracy when the learning algorithm only uses the difficulty indicator indicated in the first column and the different values of PS and PV. It can be observed from the table that FDC had the best accuracy with 84%, this is followed by Epistasis (81%) and Ruggedness (80%) all of those results produced using decision trees.

Table 2. Accuracy results using different classification methods

	Naive Bayes	Multilayer Perceptron	Decision Tree	Random Forest
FDC	70%	73%	84%	78%
NSC	65%	68%	78%	78%
Neutrality	68%	69%	75%	68%
Ruggedness	71%	72%	80%	75%
Basins of Attraction	69%	71%	78%	71%
Epistasis	69%	71%	81%	77%
All the features	66%	80%	95%	96%
All except FDC	66%	79%	95%	96%

The last two rows of Table 2 presents the accuracy when all the difficulty indicators are used, and with all these indicators except FDC. It is observed that Random Forest obtained the best accuracy (96%) with either all the features or all except FDC. Random forest is closely followed by decision trees. Comparing the performance of the different configurations, it is evident that the use of all the features with and without FDC improves the accuracy. It is very interesting that although the FDC obtained the best accuracy over all difficulty indicators, this feature can be removed and the accuracy is not affected when all the features are combined. This is an important characteristic given that one needs to know the optimum in order to apply FDC, and, clearly, this is unrealistic in any practical application.

In order to complement our analysis, Table 3 shows the confusion matrix and detail of accuracy of random forest with all the features except the FDC on a 10-fold cross validation. The table shows that the classifier is performing accurate predictions where the *easy* and *difficult* problems have the best classification rates.

Table 3. Random Forest, confusion matrix using cross validation with 10 folds

	Predicted					
	difficult	*medium*	*easy*	*Precision*	*Recall*	*Roc Area*
difficult	2920	90	30	0.95	0.96	0.99
medium	110	391	121	0.68	0.63	0.92
easy	36	95	7207	0.98	0.98	0.99
				0.96	0.96	0.99	*Mean*

6 Conclusions and Future Work

This work presented a procedure to classify the performance of Genetic Algorithms when solving problems with two dimensions on continuous domains. The performance was classified in three different classes: easy, medium, and difficult. The results showed that a Random Forest with a set of difficult indicators obtained an accuracy of 96% of correct classification on a 10-fold cross validation.

The main contributions of this work are: (1) the use of different types of problems in two dimensions on the continuous domain, this gives us a set of problems with distinct characteristics and complexity, (2) the use of GA real-coded implementation to assess performance experiments, and (3) the use of a model based on Random Forests to label the performance of GA problems. The input data set uses a mixture of characteristics or metrics of difficulty (MoD) and GA parameters (precision and population size). The output data set or ideal values where obtained by measuring the success rate of GAs and then codified into three classes: easy, medium, and difficult.

The main improvements of this work might be: (1) the use of problems in higher dimensions; real applications are in higher dimensions, (2) the use of another type of sampling of the search space, given that some metrics of difficulty only give us descriptive information about the FL, which is not enough for ECA, (3) use a larger data set to train the model, this might give us more general features about problems.

As future work we will work on real-valued n-dimensional problems, given that real applications are in the n-dimensional spaces. Another work is to select (add or remove) features from the model, taking in consideration the most relevant characteristics of the pairs metaheuristic-problem. Finally, another topic of our interest is the integration of more optimization algorithms based on ECA.

References

1. Chan, K.Y., Aydin, M.E., Fogarty, T.C.: An epistasis measure based on the analysis of variance for the real-coded representation in genetic algorithms. In: IEEE Congress on Evolutionary Computation, pp. 297–304. IEEE (2003)
2. Chen, Y., Hu, J., Hirasawa, K., Yu, S.: Solving deceptive problems using a genetic algorithm with reserve selection. In: IEEE Congress on Evolutionary Computation, CEC 2008, IEEE World Congress on Computational Intelligence, pp. 884–889 (2008)
3. Fogel, D.B. (ed.): Evolutionary Computation. The Fossil Record. Selected Readings on the History of Evolutionary Computation. IEEE Press (1998)
4. Fonlupt, C., Robilliard, D., Preux, P.: A bit-wise epistasis measure for binary search spaces. In: Eiben, A.E., Bäck, T., Schoenauer, M., Schwefel, H.-P. (eds.) PPSN 1998. LNCS, vol. 1498, pp. 47–56. Springer, Heidelberg (1998)
5. Goldberg, D.E.: Genetic Algorithms in Search, Optimization and Machine Learning. Addison-Wesley (1989)

6. Graff, M., Escalante, H.J., Cerda-Jacobo, J., Avalos Gonzalez, A.: Models of performance of time series forecasters. Neurocomputing 122, 375–385 (2013) 00001
7. Graff, M., Poli, R., Flores, J.J.: Models of performance of evolutionary program induction algorithms based on indicators of problem difficulty. In: Evolutionary Computation (November 2012)
8. Hall, M., Frank, E., Holmes, G., Pfahringer, B., Reutemann, P., Witten, I.H.: The weka data mining software: An update. SIGKDD Explor. Newsl. 11(1), 10–18 (2009)
9. Han, J., Kamber, M.: Data Mining: Concepts and Techniques. Elsevier (2012)
10. Holland, J.H.: Adaptation in Natural and Artificial Systems. University of Michigan Press, Ann Arbor (1975)
11. Horn, J., Goldberg, D.E.: Genetic algorithm difficulty and the modality of the fitness landscapes. In: Whitley, L.D., Vose, M.D. (eds.) Foundations of Genetic Algorithms Workshop, vol. 3, pp. 243–269. Morgan Kaufmann (1995)
12. Jamil, M., Yang, X.-S.: A literature survey of benchmark functions for global optimisation problems. International Journal of Mathematical Modelling and Numerical Optimisation 4(2), 150–194 (2013)
13. Jones, T., Forrest, S.: Fitness distance correlation as a measure of problem difficulty for genetic algorithms. In: Proceedings of the 6th International Conference on Genetic Algorithms, pp. 184–192. Morgan Kaufmann Publishers Inc., San Francisco (1995)
14. Katada, Y., Ohkura, K., Ueda, K.: Measuring neutrality of fitness landscapes based on the nei's standard genetic distance. In: Proceedings of 2003 Asia Pacific Symposium on Intelligent and Evolutionary Systems: Technology and Applications, pp. 107–114 (2003)
15. Kauffman, S.A., Johnsen, S.: Coevolution to the edge of chaos: Coupled fitness landscapes, poised states, and coevolutionary avalanches. Journal of Theoretical Biology 149(4), 467–505 (1991)
16. Lobo, J., Miller, J.H., Fontana, W.: Neutrality in Technological Landscapes. Technical report, working paper, Santa Fe Institute, Santa Fe (2004)
17. López, E.G., Poli, R., Kattan, A., O'Neill, M., Brabazon, A.: Neutrality in evolutionary algorithms.. what do we know? Evolving Systems 2(3), 145–163 (2011)
18. Malan, K., Engelbrecht, A.P.: Quantifying ruggedness of continuous landscapes using entropy. In: IEEE Congress on Evolutionary Computation, pp. 1440–1447. IEEE (2009)
19. Malan, K.M., Engelbrecht, A.P.: A survey of techniques for characterising fitness landscapes and some possible ways forward. Information Sciences 241, 148–163 (2013)
20. Graff, M., Poli, R.: Practical performance models of algorithms in evolutionary program induction and other domains. Artificial Intelligence 174(15), 1254–1276 (2010)
21. Picek, S., Golub, M.: The new negative slope coefficient measure. In: Proceedings of the 10th WSEAS International Conference on Evolutionary Computing, EC 2009, pp. 96–101. World Scientific and Engineering Academy and Society (WSEAS), Stevens Point (2009)
22. Pitzer, E., Affenzeller, M., Beham, A.: A closer look down the basins of attraction. In: 2010 UK Workshop on Computational Intelligence (UKCI), pp. 1–6 (September 2010)

23. Poli, R., López, E.G.: The effects of constant and bit-wise neutrality on problem hardness, fitness distance correlation and phenotypic mutation rates. IEEE Trans. Evolutionary Computation 16(2), 279–300 (2012)
24. Poli, R., Vanneschi, L.: Fitness-proportional negative slope coefficient as a hardness measure for genetic algorithms. In: Proceedings of the 9th Annual Conference on Genetic and Evolutionary Computation, GECCO 2007, pp. 1335–1342. ACM, New York (2007)
25. Reeves, C.: Fitness landscapes and evolutionary algorithms. In: Fonlupt, C., Hao, J.-K., Lutton, E., Schoenauer, M., Ronald, E. (eds.) AE 1999. LNCS, vol. 1829, pp. 3–20. Springer, Heidelberg (2000)
26. Reeves, C.R., Wright, C.C.: Epistasis in genetic algorithms: An experimental design perspective. In: Proc. of the 6th International Conference on Genetic Algorithms, pp. 217–224. Morgan Kaufmann (1995)
27. Rice, J.R.: The algorithm selection problem. Advances in Computers 15, 65–118 (1976)
28. Smith-Miles, K.A.: Cross-disciplinary perspectives on meta-learning for algorithm selection. ACM Comput. Surv. 41(1), 1–25 (2008)
29. Trujillo, L., Martínez, Y., Galván-López, E., Legrand, P.: Predicting problem difficulty for genetic programming applied to data classification. In: Proceedings of the 13th Annual Conference on Genetic and Evolutionary Computation, GECCO 2011, pp. 1355–1362. ACM, New York (2011)
30. Trujillo, L., Martínez, Y., López, E.G., Legrand, P.: A comparative study of an evolvability indicator and a predictor of expected performance for genetic programming. In: Soule, T., Moore, J.H. (eds.) GECCO (Companion), pp. 1489–1490. ACM (2012)
31. Trujillo, L., Martínez, Y., Melin, P.: Estimating Classifier Performance with Genetic Programming. In: Silva, S., Foster, J.A., Nicolau, M., Machado, P., Giacobini, M. (eds.) EuroGP 2011. LNCS, vol. 6621, pp. 274–285. Springer, Heidelberg (2011)
32. Vanneschi, L.: Genetic programming theory and practice V. In: Riolo, R.L., Soule, T., Worzel, B. (eds.) Genetic Programming Theory and Practice V, May 17–19, pp. 107–125. Springer, Ann Arbor (2007)
33. Vanneschi, L.: Investigating problem hardness of real life applications. In: Riolo, R., Soule, T., Worzel, B. (eds.) Genetic Programming Theory and Practice V. Genetic and Evolutionary Computation Series, pp. 107–124. Springer US (2008)
34. Vanneschi, L., Clergue, M., Collard, P., Tomassini, M., Vérel, S.: Fitness clouds and problem hardness in genetic programming. In: Deb, K., Tari, Z. (eds.) GECCO 2004. LNCS, vol. 3103, pp. 690–701. Springer, Heidelberg (2004)
35. Vanneschi, L., Tomassini, M.: A study on fitness distance correlation and problem difficulty for genetic programming. In: Luke, S., Ryan, C., O'Reilly, U.-M. (eds.) Graduate Student Workshop, New York, July 8, pp. 307–310. AAAI Press (2002)
36. Vanneschi, L., Tomassini, M., Collard, P., Vérel, S.: Negative Slope Coefficient: A Measure to Characterize Genetic Programming Fitness Landscapes. In: Collet, P., Tomassini, M., Ebner, M., Gustafson, S., Ekárt, A. (eds.) EuroGP 2006. LNCS, vol. 3905, pp. 178–189. Springer, Heidelberg (2006)
37. Verel, S.: Fitness landscapes and graphs: multimodularity, ruggedness and neutrality. In: Proceedings of the Fifth International Conference on Genetic and Evolutionary Computation Conference Companion, Amsterdam, Pays-Bas, pp. 1013–1034. ACM (2013)
38. Weise, T.: Global Optimization Algorithms – Theory and Application. it-weise.de (self-published): Germany (2009)

39. Wright, S.J.: The roles of mutation, inbreeding, crossbreeding and selection in evolution. In: Jones, F. (ed.) Proceedings of the Sixth International Congress on Genetics, vol. 1, pp. 356–366 (1932)
40. Xu, L., Hutter, F., Hoos, H.H., Leyton-Brown, K.: SATzilla: portfolio-based algorithm selection for SAT. Journal of Artificial Intelligence Research 32, 565–606 (2008)

A Multi-objective Genetic Algorithm
for the Software Project Scheduling Problem

Abel García-Nájera and María del Carmen Gómez-Fuentes

Departamento de Matemáticas Aplicadas y Sistemas,
Universidad Autónoma Metropolitana, Cuajimalpa
Av. Vasco de Quiroga 4871, Col. Santa Fe Cuajimalpa, 05300, México, D.F., México
{agarcian,mgomez}@correo.cua.uam.mx

Abstract. The software project scheduling problem considers the assignment of employees to project tasks with the aim of minimizing the project cost and delivering the project on time. Recent research takes into account that each employee is proficient in some development tasks only, which requiere specific skills. However, this cannot be totally applied in the Mexican context due to software companies do not categorize their employees by software skills, but by their skill level instead. In this study we propose a model that is closer to how software companies operate in Mexico. Moreover, we propose a multi-objective genetic algorithm for solving benchmark instances of this model. Results show that our proposed genetic algorithm performs similarly to two recent approaches and that it finds better multi-objective solutions when they are compared to those found by a well-known multi-objective optimizer.

Keywords: Search-based software engineering, software project scheduling problem, genetic algorithm, multi-objective optimization.

1 Introduction

Managing a software project involves planning and monitoring the project by using the required resources, in the shortest possible time and with a minimum number of failures. The main objectives to be achieved are: meeting the requirements, and finishing the project on time and within budget [14]. The process of managing a project consists of four phases: initiation, planning, execution and closing. Moreover, the control phase allows to make adjustments in planning throughout the entire process.

Project planning consists of refining the project scope, defining tasks and activities to achieve the goals, establishing a sequence of activities to further develop a schedule, cost estimation and budget. One of the key problems in software project planning is the scheduling, which involves resource allocation and scheduling activities on time, optimizing the cost and/or duration of the project. The scheduling is a complex constrained optimization problem, because for the optimization of resources, time and cost, it is necessary to consider a combination of variables, rules and restrictions that cause the problem to be NP-hard [2].

A. Gelbukh et al. (Eds.): MICAI 2014, Part II, LNAI 8857, pp. 13–24, 2014.

Search-based software engineering (SBSE) is an emerging area focused on solving software engineering problems by using search-based optimization algorithms. SBSE has been applied to a number of problems which arise during the software life cycle [10]. However, as Harman states [9], in order to affirm that it is valid to use search algorithms to solve such problems, it is necessary to continue doing experiments to establish baseline data and more evidence. Hence, this work demonstrates the usefulness of a metaheuristic algorithm in software project management, particularly, in project planning. We propose a multi-objective genetic algorithm which assigns the available developers to project tasks, taking into account the time each developer dedicates to a task, and the salary and the level of experience of each employee. Furthermore, we present a model that better reflects the operation of some Mexican software development companies, with the aim of bridging the gap between SBSE research and real software projects.

This study is structured as follows. Section 2 introduces the software project scheduling problem and our model of the problem. In Section 3 we describe what optimization problems are and how we can compare the performance of multi-objective optimizers. Our proposed multi-objective genetic algorithm for solving the problem under study is explained in Section 4. Section 5 summarizes the experimental setup, our results and their analysis. Finally, Section 6 presents our conclusions and motivates some ideas for future work.

2　The Software Project Scheduling Problem

The software project scheduling problem (SPSP) can be stated as follows. A software project can be divided into n tasks $t_1, \ldots, t_n$, where each task t_i has an associated effort estimation t_i^e and a set of skills t_i^l required to carry it out. These tasks have to be performed according to a precedence constraint, which indicate what tasks must be completed before starting another task. With the aim of executing all tasks, i.e. conclude the project, there is a staff available which comprises m employees $e_1, \ldots, e_m$. Employee e_i has a salary e_i^s and is proficient in a set of skills e_i^l. The problem consists in finding a suitable assignment of employees to tasks, such that the project can be delivered in the shortest possible time and with the minimum cost. In principle, each employee can execute any task which requires any of the skills the employee is competent in. Moreover, each employee can be assigned to two or more simultaneous tasks, distributing the workday among the assigned tasks. An assignment of employees to tasks is feasible if: (i) each task t_i has at least one employee assigned, (ii) the set of skills t_i^l required to carry out task t_i is included in the union of the sets of skills of the employees assigned to task t_i, and (iii) all employees do not work overtime.

Some studies on project scheduling by means of search-based optimization is review next. With the purpose of minimizing the length and cost of the project and maximizing product quality, Chang et al. [2] solved the SPSP by using genetic algorithms (GAs) already coded in an existing library. Chang et al. [2] based their study on the assumption that the time for completing the project is inversely proportional to the number of people involved, however, this assumption is not entirely realistic [14]. They found results which demonstrate the feasibility of solving scheduling problems using GAs. In the resource-constrained project scheduling problem resources are not limited to staff, i.e. they also take into account other factors. For example, Alba and Chicano [1] solved the SPSP considering time, staff skills, budget, and project complexity. They designed a GA for minimizing a composite objective function that involves project cost and duration, and a penalization which takes into account the number of unattended tasks, the number of missing skills and the overtime. They tested their approach on five benchmark sets which differ in the number of tasks, number of employees, number of skills, and task precedence. Recently, Xiao et al. [17] tackled SPSP in the same manner as Alba and Chicano [1] and designed an ant colony optimization-based approach for solving a number of benchmark instances.

There are other studies which consider the SPSP a bi-objective problem. For example, Chicano et al. [4] considered five well-known multi-objective optimizers to find solutions which minimize project cost and project duration simultaneously. This is an improvement on the work of Alba and Chicano [1] since cost and duration are objectives that are in conflict, and combining them in a single objective function is not most appropriate method to tackle the problem. Luna et al. [12,13] continued the research of Chicano et al. [4] by studying the scalability performance of several multi-objective optimizers.

A different formulation of the SPSP is that of Chicano et al. [3]. Here, additionally to the skills each employee is proficient in, productivity is considered, i.e. the higher the productivity of an employee, the less time is spent by that employee to finish a task. Furthermore, task delay is taken into consideration in order to avoid infeasible solutions, which are those with overtime.

Although staff skills and productivity make the problem more realistic, the skills quantification based on the ability of employees to perform different types of activities (design, databases, programming, etc.) could not be feasible in practice, since it is difficult to imagine, for example, a person with advanced databases skills but with basic programming skills, and vice versa. We expect that people who are competent in one aspect of software development also have considerable skills in the other areas, i.e. if one person masters the high-level design, most likely she also has good skills in programming. For example, developers at Google understand client, web, browser, and mobile technologies, and can program effectively in multiple languages and on a variety of platforms [16].

We propose a formulation of the problem of assigning tasks to employees, inspired in how some software development companies work in Mexico, our country, which implies a different way to classify the kind of tasks and the developers skills. With this model we intend to bring closer to practice the theoretical work that has been done on software project scheduling in SBSE.

2.1 Proposed Problem Formulation

Software life cycle standard tasks are: requirements analysis and specification, design, coding and testing. We assume that documentation is part of each task.

Usually, novice staff starts in the testing phase, since it is the simplest task (beginner level). When the employee acquires some experience, he is assigned to coding tasks (junior level). The experienced staff performs the design (senior level), and it is an expert person who normally take over the requirements analysis and specification (expert level), since an error in the requirements specification is much more expensive than errors in the later stages [15].

In order to assist the project manager with ranking of the staff skills, we propose four levels: a person with expert level (EL) can perform any task and she has the highest salary. An employee with senior level (SL) can design, implement and test, and his or her salary is the second highest. Staff with junior level (JL) is able to do good coding and testing and their salary is lower than that of SL. Finally, employees with beginner level (BL) are only able to do testing and their salary is the lowest.

Considering the staff classification described above, we define the SPSP as follows. Given a list of n tasks $t_1, \ldots, t_n$, representing the coding and testing of the designed modules and the corresponding modules integration testing, we denote the effort estimation of task i as t_i^e. The required skill level to perform task t_i is denoted as $t_i^l \in \{$BL, JL, SL, EL $\}$. These tasks have to be performed according to a precedence constraint, which indicate what tasks must be completed before starting a new task. This precedence constraint can be seen as an acyclic directed graph $G\{V, A\}$, where the vertex set V is the set of all tasks t_i, i.e. $\{t_1, \ldots, t_n\}$ and the elements $(t_i, t_j) \in A$ establishes which task t_i must be completed, with no other intervening tasks, before starting task t_j. With the aim of completing all tasks, there is a staff available which comprises m employees $e_1, \ldots, e_m$. Employee i has a salary e_i^s and a skill level $e_i^l \in \{$BL, JL, SL, EL $\}$.

A solution to the SPSP can be seen as a table with m rows, where row i corresponds to employee e_i, and n columns, where column j corresponds to task t_j. Cell (i, j) represents the time d_{ij}, based on the workday, employee e_i dedicates to task t_j. Once this table is filled, since we know the employee dedication to each task, we can calculate the duration t_j^d of task t_j as

$$t_j^d = t_j^e \Big/ \sum_{i=1}^m d_{ij} \, . \tag{1}$$

At this point we know the length of each task, hence, given that we have the precedence restriction, we can calculate the times t_j^b and t_j^f when each task t_j begins and finishes, respectively. Consequently, we can obtain the project duration P_d which will be the maximum finishing time of any task, that is

$$P_d = \max \{t_j^f \mid j = 1, \ldots, n\} \, . \tag{2}$$

We can also calculate the project cost P_c as the sum of the salary paid to each employee for their dedication to each task of the project, which is

$$P_c = \sum_{i=1}^m \sum_{j=1}^n d_{ij} \, t_j^d \, e_i^s \, . \tag{3}$$

Furthermore, for each employee e_i we define $e_i^w(\tau)$ as the working function

$$e_i^w(\tau) = \sum_{\{j \mid t_j^b \le \tau \le t_j^f\}} d_{ij} \, . \tag{4}$$

If $e_i^w(\tau)$ exceeds the workday at time τ, then the scheduling incurs in overwork. The overwork e_i^o of employee e_i is

$$e_i^o = \int_0^{P_d} \text{ramp } (e_i^w(\tau) - \text{workday})d\tau . \tag{5}$$

Finally, the total overwork of the project P_o is the sum of the overwork done by each employee, which is

$$P_o = \sum_{i=1}^m e_i^o \tag{6}$$

In this study, we aim at minimizing P_d, P_c and P_o simultaneously, subject to (i) there cannot be any task left unattended and (ii) each task must be assigned to at least one employee who has the required skill level.

3   Multi-Objective Optimization Problems

Without loss of generality, any multi-objective optimization problem can be defined as the minimization problem

$$\text{minimize } \mathbf{f}(\mathbf{x}) = (f_1(\mathbf{x}), \ldots, f_k(\mathbf{x})) \tag{7}$$

subject to the constraints

$$g_i(\mathbf{x}) \leq 0, \qquad \forall\, i = 1, \ldots, p , \tag{8}$$
$$h_j(\mathbf{x}) = 0, \qquad \forall\, j = 1, \ldots, q , \tag{9}$$

where $\mathbf{x} \in \mathcal{X}$ is a solution to the problem, $\mathcal{X}$ is the solution space, and $f_i : \mathcal{X} \to \mathbb{R}$, for $i = 1, \ldots, k$, are k objective functions. The constraint functions $g_i, h_j : \mathcal{X} \to \mathbb{R}$ in (8) and (9) restrict $\mathbf{x}$ to a feasible region $\mathcal{X}' \subseteq \mathcal{X}$.

We say that a solution $\mathbf{x} \in \mathcal{X}$ *dominates* solution $\mathbf{y}$, written as $\mathbf{x} \prec \mathbf{y}$, if and only if $f_i(\mathbf{x}) \leq f_i(\mathbf{y}), \forall\, i \in \{1, \ldots, k\}$ and $\exists\, j \in \{1, \ldots, k\} : f_j(\mathbf{x}) < f_j(\mathbf{y})$. Consequently, we say that a solution $\mathbf{x} \in \mathcal{S} \subseteq \mathcal{X}$ is *non-dominated* with respect to $\mathcal{S}$ if there is no solution $\mathbf{y} \in \mathcal{S}$ such that $\mathbf{y} \prec \mathbf{x}$. A solution $\mathbf{x} \in \mathcal{X}$ is said to be *Pareto optimal* if it is non-dominated with respect to $\mathcal{X}$, and the *Pareto optimal set* is defined as $\mathcal{P}_s = \{\mathbf{x} \in \mathcal{X} \mid \mathbf{x} \text{ is Pareto optimal}\}$. Finally, the *Pareto front* is defined as $\mathcal{P}_f = \{\mathbf{f}(\mathbf{x}) \in \mathbb{R}^k \mid \mathbf{x} \in \mathcal{P}_s\}$. The aim of the optimization process is to find the best representation of the Pareto front for the given problem instance, called the *Pareto approximation*.

To measure the performance of mulit-objective optimizers, we have to use proper multi-objective performance indicators. One of such indicators is the *hypervolume* metric $\mathcal{H}(\mathcal{A}, \mathbf{z})$ [18], which measures the size of the objective space defined by the approximation set $\mathcal{A}$ of solutions and a suitable reference point $\mathbf{z}$. The idea is that a greater hypervolume indicates that the approximation set offers a closer representation of the true Pareto front. For a two-dimensional objective space $\mathbf{f}(\mathbf{x}) = (f_1(\mathbf{x}), f_2(\mathbf{x}))$, each solution $\mathbf{x}_i \in \mathcal{A}$ delimits a rectangle defined by its coordinates $(f_1(\mathbf{x}_i), f_2(\mathbf{x}_i))$ and the reference point $\mathbf{z} = (z_1, z_2)$, and the size of the union of all such rectangles delimited by the solutions is the hypervolume $\mathcal{H}(\mathcal{A}, \mathbf{z})$. This idea can be extended to any number k of dimensions to give the general hypervolume metric:

$$\mathcal{H}(\mathcal{A}, \mathbf{z}) = \lambda \left(\bigcup_{\mathbf{x}_i \in \mathcal{A}} \left\{ [f_1(\mathbf{x}_i), z_1] \times \cdots \times [f_k(\mathbf{x}_i), z_k] \right\} \right) , \qquad (10)$$

where $\lambda(\cdot)$ is the standard Lebesgue measure [6]. When using this metric to compare the performance of two or more algorithms, the one providing solutions with the largest delimited hypervolume is regarded to be the best.

In this study we focus on two topics. The first is related to the ability of our algorithm to find feasible solutions, that are those solutions with no overtime. The second is related to compare the performance of our proposed GA with that of a well-known multi-objective optimizer.

4   Multi-Objective GA for Solving the SPSP

As with all GAs, the basic idea is to maintain a population (set) of individuals (solutions), and evolve them (recombine and mutate) by survival of the fittest (natural selection). The following defines all stages of our proposal.

Our multi-objective (MO) GA uses an integer solution encoding which length is $m \times n$: the first n integers corresponds to the dedication time d_{1j} of employee e_1 to each task t_j, the next n integers corresponds to the dedication time d_{2j} of employee e_2 to each task t_j, etc. The dedication time d_{ij} is measured in hours according to the workday, that is, $t_{ij} \in \{0, 1, \ldots, wd\}$, where wd is the maximum number of hours an employee can work per day.

The initial population is filled with feasible randomly generated solutions. Each solution is built by randomly selecting d_{ij} from the interval $[0, wd]$, where $i = 1, \ldots, m$, and $j = 1, \ldots, n$.

In this study, we consider the three objective functions project cost, project duration and project overtime to be minimized, and all individuals in the population are evaluated with respect to them. Since we are interested in the evaluation of all three functions, an appropriate fitness assignment is the non-dominance sorting criterion [8], whereby the population is divided into non-dominated fronts, and the depth of each front determines the fitness of the individuals in it. That is, individuals that are not dominated belong to the first front, and from the rest of the population, those non-dominated solutions belong to the second front, and so on. Individuals belonging to the first front are the fittest, followed by those in the second front, etc. We use the specific algorithm of Deb et al. [5], which is used in their NSGA-II algorithm.

In a previous study, it was demonstrated that measuring solution similarity in the solution space and using this information to boost solution diversity leads to a wider exploration of the search space, and, consequently, to an improved performance of the multi-objective optimizer [7]. Following this idea, we measure the similarity $\mathcal{S}_{\mathcal{P}\mathcal{Q}}$ of solution $\mathcal{P}$ with solution $\mathcal{Q}$ as the normalized difference between each dedication time of employee e_i to task t_j, that is

$$\mathcal{S}_{\mathcal{P}\mathcal{Q}} = 1.0 - \tfrac{1}{n \times m \times wd} \sum_{i=1}^{m} \sum_{j=1}^{n} |d_{ij}^{\mathcal{P}} - d_{ij}^{\mathcal{Q}}| , \qquad (11)$$

where $d_{ij}^{\mathcal{P}}$ and $d_{ij}^{\mathcal{Q}}$ are the dedication times of employee e_i to task t_j in solutions $\mathcal{P}$ and $\mathcal{Q}$, respectively. Hence, if solutions $\mathcal{P}$ and $\mathcal{Q}$ consider exactly the same dedication times d_{ij}, $\mathcal{S}_{\mathcal{PQ}} = 1$. On the contrary, if dedication times $d_{ij}^{\mathcal{P}}$ and $d_{ij}^{\mathcal{Q}}$ are on the opposite extremes, $\mathcal{S}_{\mathcal{PQ}} = 0$. Afterward, we compute the average similarity $\mathcal{S}_{\mathcal{P}}$ of solution $\mathcal{P}$ with all other solutions in the population P as

$$\mathcal{S}_{\mathcal{P}} = \tfrac{1}{|P|-1} \sum_{\mathcal{Q} \in P \backslash \mathcal{P}} \mathcal{S}_{\mathcal{PQ}} . \tag{12}$$

A standard binary tournament selection method is applied for choosing two parents for crossover. This tournament method randomly selects two individuals from the population, and the fittest will be chosen as one of the parents. This procedure is repeated for selecting the second parent, however, the less similar on average is chosen.

The evolution continues with the crossover of the two selected parents. We implemented two different crossover operators, which we will call *flat* crossover (F) and *simple* crossover (S) [11]. Flat crossover generates an offspring in the following manner. A random number between the dedication times d_{ij} of each parent is chosen and it is assigned as the dedication time d_{ij} in the offspring. On the other hand, simple crossover works as follows. From the first parent, a random number of employees are selected, and their dedication times to each task are copied into the offspring. The dedication times for the remaining employees are copied from the second parent.

Once the offspring has been built, it is subjected to mutation with a probability of 10%, and randomly selects and employee e_i and a task t_j, which dedication time d_{ij} is to be changed. Here we implemented two different mutation operators [11], which we will call *gradient* mutation (G) and *random* mutation (R). Gradient mutation randomly adds or subtracts one hour from the dedication time d_{ij}, while random mutation assigns a random number taken from the interval $[0, wd]$ as the dedication time d_{ij}.

After the offspring has been created, it could represent an infeasible solution, thus a repair operator is applied. This operator validates, first, that all tasks have at least one employee assigned and, second, that the employees assigned to each task have the aggregated skills needed to perform the task. For the first situation, the repair operator sums all dedication times $d_{ij}, i = 1, \ldots, m$, for each task t_j. If the sum is zero, it is an infeasible solution, and an employee e_i with at least one of the skills required t_j^s to perform task t_j is randomly selected and a dedication time t_{ij} is randomly assigned. In the second situation, for each task t_j, the union of the sets of skills e_i^s is computed, $i = 1, \ldots, m$. If the union does not contain all the skills required t_j^s by task t_j, it is an infeasible solution, and an employee e_i with at least one of the skills required t_j^s to perform task t_j is randomly selected and a dedication time t_{ij} is randomly assigned. This procedure is repeated until all the required skills are contained in the union.

The final stage of each evolutionary cycle is the selection of individuals to form the next generation. Here, the offspring and parent populations are combined and individual fitness determined as described above. Those solutions having the highest fitness, i.e. falling in the outermost fronts, are taken to survive and form the next generation. The process of parent selection, crossover, mutation, repair and survivor selection is repeated for a prefixed number of generations.

5 Experimental Setup and Results

The experimental study is two-fold. On the one hand, we are going to compare our results with those obtained by two recent proposals. On the other hand, we are interested in the performance of our algorithm when it is applied to the problem formulated in Section 2.1.

5.1 Performance on the Original Problem Formulation

Alba and Chicano [1] and Xiao et al. [17] evaluated the performance of their approaches by measuring the hit rate, which is the ratio of the number of runs where the algorithm found at least one feasible solution to the total number of runs. Hence, we are going to compare our results using the same methodology.

We used 36 benchmark instances generated by Alba and Chicano [1], which are divided into two groups. Instances in group g are labeled as in-mgs, where n is the number of tasks, m is the number of employees, and s is the total number of skills required to complete the project. Here, employees have 2 or 3 skills. Instances in group p are labeled as in-mps, where s here is 5, if employees have 4 or 5 skills, and 7 if employees have 6 or 7 skills. In these cases, the total number of skills is 10.

Table 1 shows the hit rate from Alba and Chicano [1] (study key AC) and from Xiao et al. [17] (study key K) compared to the results from our MO GA when it is set with different crossover and mutation operators. The algorithm of Xiao et al. [17] obtained a hit rate that is comparable with that of our MO GA for the instances they tested on their approach, however they did not use all the instances with 20 and 30 tasks, hence we cannot compare completely with their results. The approach of Alba and Chicano [1] obtained a lower hit rate than our GA for the instances with 10 tasks, however, their approach obtains a slightly higher hit rate for the instances with 20 tasks. Moreover, we can observe that no approach is able to obtain feasible solutions for the instances with 30 tasks. We can also see that, when our MO GA is set to use the random mutation, it obtains the highest hit rate: for instances in group g, combined with the simple crossover, and for instances in group p, combined with the flat crossover. Overall, we can conclude that the performance of our MO GA is comparable to that of previous approaches.

5.2 Performance on the Proposed Problem Formulation

We used the instance generator of Alba and Chicano [1] to generate 45 benchmark problems with $n = 10, 20, 30$ tasks, and $m = 5, 10, 15$ employees. We labeled these instances as in-m-j, with $j = 1, \ldots, 5$. In these instances, each task requires a minimum skill level and each employee has a certain skill level.

Table 1. Hit rate from previous studies compared to the hit rate from our MO GA

Instance	Study		MO GA				Instance	Study		MO GA			
	AC	X	FG	SG	FR	SR		AC	X	FG	SG	FR	SR
i10-5g5	98	100	100	100	100	100	i10-5p5	94	100	100	100	100	100
i10-5g10	61	100	100	100	100	100	i10-5p7	84	100	83	37	83	30
i10-10g5	99	95	100	100	100	100	i10-10p5	97	100	100	100	100	100
i10-10g10	85	100	100	100	100	100	i10-10p7	100	100	100	100	100	100
i10-15g5	100	96	100	100	100	100	i10-15p5	97	100	77	83	83	90
i10-15g10	85	93	97	97	90	83	i10-15p7	97	89	100	100	100	100
i20-5g5	6	-	0	0	0	0	i20-5p5	0	-	0	0	0	0
i20-5g10	8	-	0	0	0	100	i20-5p7	0	-	0	0	0	0
i20-10g5	9	25	0	0	0	0	i20-10p5	6	67	0	0	0	0
i20-10g10	1	64	0	0	0	0	i20-10p7	76	65	53	47	67	30
i20-15g5	12	-	90	90	83	67	i20-15p5	43	-	100	100	100	100
i20-15g10	6	-	0	0	0	0	i20-15p7	0	-	0	0	0	0
i30-5g5	0	-	0	0	0	0	i30-5p5	0	-	0	0	0	0
i30-5g10	0	-	0	0	0	0	i30-5p7	0	-	0	0	0	0
i30-10g5	0	-	0	0	0	0	i30-10p5	0	-	0	0	0	0
i30-10g10	0	-	0	0	0	0	i30-10p7	0	-	0	0	0	0
i30-15g5	0	-	0	0	3	0	i30-15p5	0	-	0	0	0	0
i30-15g10	0	-	0	0	0	0	i30-15p7	0	-	0	0	0	0
Average	32	-	38	38	38	42	Average	39	-	40	37	42	36

Tasks can be executed by an employee with the required skill level or higher. We assume that an employee can perform several tasks each day and that the minimum amount of time an employee can dedicate to a task is one hour. Thus, an employee can be assigned to wd different tasks. We believe that this situation is not efficient, since the employee can be distracted from one task to another. Therefore, additionally to consider the original scheme, we restrict the number of tasks an employee can perform per day to $4, 2$, and 1. Results for the hit rate is shown in Table 2. For these experiments, we set our MO GA to use simple crossover and random mutation.

We can see that, when the employees are allowed to perform 2, 4 and 8 tasks per day, our GA is able to obtain feasible solutions for all but one instance. On the other hand, if we restrict employees to perform only one task per day, solutions found by our GA to the majority of the instances are infeasible. With these results we can conclude that our MO GA do find feasible solutions to the instances of the proposed model that is closer to real software projects.

We now analyze our MO GA multi-objective performance, specifically, we are going to compare the hypervolume delimited by the non-dominated solutions found by our MO GA to that covered by the non-dominated solutions found by the popular and successful NSGA-II [5]. We decided to use NSGA-II due to the high similarity of the algorithms, which difference resides in how parent selection and survival are accomplished: while NSGA-II selects both parents

Table 2. Hit rate from our MO GA to instances of the proposed model

Instance	No. of tasks				Instance	No. of tasks				Instance	No. of tasks			
	1	2	4	8		1	2	4	8		1	2	4	8
i10-5-1	0	100	100	100	i20-5-1	0	100	100	100	i30-5-1	0	100	100	100
i10-5-2	3	100	100	100	i20-5-2	0	100	100	100	i30-5-2	0	100	100	100
i10-5-3	20	100	100	100	i20-5-3	0	100	100	100	i30-5-3	0	100	100	100
i10-5-4	0	100	100	100	i20-5-4	0	100	100	100	i30-5-4	0	100	100	100
i10-5-5	0	100	100	100	i20-5-5	0	100	100	100	i30-5-5	0	100	100	100
i10-10-1	7	100	100	100	i20-10-1	0	100	100	100	i30-10-1	0	100	100	100
i10-10-2	0	100	100	100	i20-10-2	0	100	100	100	i30-10-2	0	100	100	100
i10-10-3	100	100	100	100	i20-10-3	0	100	100	100	i30-10-3	0	100	100	100
i10-10-4	0	100	100	100	i20-10-4	0	100	100	100	i30-10-4	0	0	0	0
i10-10-5	10	100	100	100	i20-10-5	0	100	100	100	i30-10-5	0	100	100	100
i10-15-1	87	100	100	100	i20-15-1	0	100	100	100	i30-15-1	0	100	100	100
i10-15-2	0	100	100	100	i20-15-2	0	100	100	100	i30-15-2	0	100	100	100
i10-15-3	0	100	100	100	i20-15-3	0	100	100	100	i30-15-3	0	100	100	100
i10-15-4	0	100	100	100	i20-15-4	0	100	100	100	i30-15-4	0	100	100	100
i10-15-5	0	100	100	100	i20-15-5	0	100	100	100	i30-15-5	0	100	100	100
Average	15	100	100	100	Average	0	100	100	100	Average	0	93	93	93

according to fitness, our MO GA selects one of the parents according to the similarity measure. On the other hand, NSGA-II measures solution similarity in the objective space during the survival process, while our MO GA measures similarity in the solution space.

In order to compute the hypervolume metric, we need to define a suitable reference point **z**. For every problem instance, we extracted the maximal values for the three objective functions from the Pareto approximations found by both algorithms, our MO GA and NSGA-II, and these maximal values played the role of **z** for each instance. Then, for each instance and repetition, the hypervolume metric was computed for the Pareto approximation found by both, our MO GA and NSGA-II. Finally, for each instance, a *t-test* was calculated in order to know if the hypervolumes are significantly different. Table 3 shows the number of instances in each category for which solutions from our MO GA delimited a significantly larger hypervolume than that covered by those from NSGA-II.

We can see that, when employees are restricted to perform 2, 4, and 8 tasks, our MO GA found Pareto approximations which delimit a significantly larger hypervolume than that covered by the Pareto approximations found by NSGA-II for all instances and, when the employee can perform only one task, solutions from our MO GA still delimit a significantly larger hypervolume for some instances. Remarkably, solutions from NSGA-II did not cover a significantly larger hypervolume than that delimited by solutions from our MO GA for any instance. We can conclude, then, that the performance of our proposed MO GA is suitable for finding good solutions in both perspectives, feasible solutions with no overtime and multi-objective solutions that are closer to the true Pareto front.

Table 3. Number of instances (out of five) for which solutions from our MO GA delimited a significantly larger hypervolume

Instance	No. of tasks				Instance	No. of tasks				Instance	No. of tasks			
	1	2	4	8		1	2	4	8		1	2	4	8
i10-5	2	5	5	5	i20-5	1	5	5	5	i30-5	0	5	5	5
i10-10	0	5	5	5	i20-10	3	5	5	5	i30-10	0	5	5	5
i10-15	3	5	5	5	i20-15	1	5	5	5	i30-15	0	5	5	5
Total	5	15	15	15	Total	5	15	15	15	Total	0	15	15	15

6 Conclusions

We have proposed a model for the software project scheduling problem that better represents the operation of some Mexican software development firms. This model considers the employees skill level (beginner, junior, senior, expert) in order to assign employees to project tasks. The objectives of this problem are the minimization of the project cost and the minimization of the project duration. To this end, we have proposed a multi-objective genetic algorithm that, additionally to minimizing both objetives, it also considers the overtime as an objective to be minimized. Only solutions with no overtime are feasible solutions.

Our proposed approach uses standard crossover and mutation operators, however, it differs from traditional genetic algorithms in the mating selection process: while the first parent is chosen according to fitness, the second is selected according to the average similarity of the individuals to the rest of the population. Our approach was tested in three ways. Firstly, it was set to solve previously proposed instances of the original problem formulation and results showed that our algorithm is comparable to two recent approaches in the sense that they find a similar quantity of feasible solutions. Secondly, it was set to solve instances from our proposed model and it was able to find feasible solutions to all but one instance. Finally, the multi-objective solutions to the vast majority of the problem instances of the proposed problem formulation are significantly better than those found by the popular and successful NSGA-II.

There is still work to do in this respect. For example, software development companies regularly train their employees with the purpose to increase their skill level. Thus, we believe that it is important to consider this training as a further objective to be optimize, since training means additional cost. We are also interested in studying the dynamic problem, that is, for example, when an employee quit the job in the middle of a project.

Acknowledgements. This project is supported by the Mexican Dirección de Superación Académica under grant 47510356.

References

1. Alba, E., Chicano, J.F.: Software project management with GAs. Inform. Sciences 177(11), 2380–2401 (2007)
2. Chang, C.K., Christensen, M.J., Zhang, T.: Genetic algorithms for project management. Ann. Softw. Eng. 11(1), 107–139 (2001)
3. Chicano, F., Cervantes, A., Luna, F., Recio, G.: A novel multiobjective formulation of the robust software project scheduling problem. In: Di Chio, C., et al. (eds.) EvoApplications 2012. LNCS, vol. 7248, pp. 497–507. Springer, Heidelberg (2012)
4. Chicano, F., Luna, F., Nebro, A.J., Alba, E.: Using multi-objective metaheuristics to solve the software project scheduling problem. In: Genetic and Evolutionary Computation Conference 2011, pp. 1915–1922. ACM (2011)
5. Deb, K., Pratap, A., Agarwal, S., Meyarivan, T.: A fast and elitist multiobjective genetic algorithm: NSGA-II. IEEE T. Evolut. Comput. 6(2), 182–197 (2002)
6. Franks, J.: A (Terse) Introduction to Lebesgue Integration. AMS (2009)
7. Garcia-Najera, A., Bullinaria, J.A.: An improved multi-objective evolutionary algorithm for the vehicle routing problem with time windows. Comput. Oper. Res. 38(1), 287–300 (2011)
8. Goldberg, D.E.: Genetic algorithms in search, optimization and machine learning. Addison-Wesley (1989)
9. Harman, M.: The current state and future of search based software engineering. In: 2007 Future of Software Engineering, pp. 342–357. IEEE Computer Society (2007)
10. Harman, M., Mansouri, S.A., Zhang, Y.: Search-based software engineering: Trends, techniques and applications. ACM Comput. Surv. 45(1), 11 (2012)
11. Herrera, F., Lozano, M., Verdegay, J.L.: Tackling real-coded genetic algorithms: Operators and tools for behavioural analysis. Artif. Intell. Rev. 12(4), 265–319 (1998)
12. Luna, F., Gonzalez-Alvarez, D.L., Chicano, F., Vega-Rodriguez, M.: On the scalability of multi-objective metaheuristics for the software scheduling problem. In: 11th International Conference on Intelligent Systems Design and Applications, pp. 1110–1115. IEEE Press (2011)
13. Luna, F., González-Álvarez, D.L., Chicano, F., Vega-Rodríguez, M.A.: The software project scheduling problem: A scalability analysis of multi-objective metaheuristics. Appl. Soft Comput. 15, 136–148 (2014)
14. McConnell, S.: Software project survival guide. Microsoft Press (1997)
15. Pfleeger, S.L., Atlee, J.M.: Software engineering: Theory and practice. Prentice-Hall (2006)
16. Whittaker, J., Arbon, J., Carollo, J.: How Google Tests Software. Addison-Wesley (2012)
17. Xiao, J., Ao, X.T., Tang, Y.: Solving software project scheduling problems with ant colony optimization. Comput. Oper. Res. 40(1), 33–46 (2013)
18. Zitzler, E., Thiele, L.: Multiobjective optimization using evolutionary algorithms - A comparative case study. In: Eiben, A.E., Bäck, T., Schoenauer, M., Schwefel, H.-P. (eds.) PPSN 1998. LNCS, vol. 1498, pp. 292–304. Springer, Heidelberg (1998)

An Effective Method for MOGAs Initialization to Solve the Multi-Objective Next Release Problem

Thiago Gomes Nepomuceno Da Silva, Leonardo Sampaio Rocha,
and José Everardo Bessa Maia

Universidade Estadual do Ceará
Av. Dr. Silas Munguba, 1700, Fortaleza, Brazil
{thi.nepo,leonardo.sampaio,bessa.maia}@gmail.com

Abstract. In this work we evaluate the usefulness of a Path Relinking based method for generating the initial population of Multi-Objective Genetic Algorithms and evaluate its performance on the Multi-Objective Next Release Problem.The performance of the method was evaluated for the algorithms MoCell and NSGA-II, and the experimental results have shown that it is consistently superior to the random initialization method and the extreme solutions method, considering the convergence speed and the quality of the Pareto front, that was measured using the Spread and Hypervolume indexes.

Keywords: Search Based Software Engineering, Next Release Problem, MOGA Initialization.

1 Introduction

A problem that is faced by companies developing complex software systems is the one of deciding what are the software requirements that are going to be implemented in their next release. There are many things that need to be considered in order to make this choice including the cost of implementing the requirements, costumers satisfaction and dependency between requirements.

Bagnall et al. [3] was the first to give a model this problem, the (mono-objective) Next-Release Problem (NRP). In his model, there is a set of binary variables $X = \{x_1, x_2, \ldots, x_m\}$ and $Y = \{y_1, y_2, \ldots, y_n\}$ representing the set of requirements and the set of costumers. For every requirement x_i there is an associated cost c_i, and for every costumer y_i there is a *weight of importance to the company* w_i. For a costumer y_i there is an associated subset $R_i \subseteq R$, the requirements requested by costumer y_i. The model ensures that if $y_i = 1$, for every $x_k \in R_i$ we have $x_k = 1$. In other words, if a costumer is chosen, all its requirements must be satisfied. They use a dependency graph for the dependency between requirements, with vertex set R and with an edge (x_i, x_j) for every x_i that is a prerequisite to x_j. Finally, one important constraint of the model is that there is a fixed, pre-determined budget, $B \in \mathbb{Z}^+$, to be respected by the

A. Gelbukh et al. (Eds.): MICAI 2014, Part II, LNAI 8857, pp. 25–37, 2014.
© Springer International Publishing Switzerland 2014

company. This is translated by the constraint $\sum_{i=1}^{n} c_i x_i \leq B$. The objective of the problem is to maximize costumers satisfaction $\sum_{i=1}^{m} w_i y_i$.

If we eliminate the dependency constraints and consider only instances in which no requirement is requested by more than one company, it can be show that the problem corresponds to the classic, well-known knapsack problem, one of the first problems to be shown NP-complete [9]. As a consequence, unless P = NP, there is no polynomial time algorithm for solving NRP.

In the Multi-Objective Next Release Problem (MONRP) [15], the budget is no longer a constraint, and a set of requirements is to be found that maximizes costumer satisfaction and minimizes the total cost. The multi-objective formulation of NRP, as proposed by Zhang [15], is given by:

$$\left\langle \text{maximize} \sum_{i=1}^{n} score_i \cdot r_i, \text{minimize} \sum_{i=1}^{n} cost_i \cdot r_i \right\rangle$$

In this formulation, $R = \{r_1, r_2, \ldots, r_n\}$ are the binary variables corresponding to the requirements, with the *importance value* and *cost* of a requirement represented by $score_i$ and $cost_i$, respectively. Zhang's model is different from Bagnall's model in the way that costumers choices of requirements are taken in consideration. When modelling the problem, one needs to ensure that $score_i$ takes into account that costumers may value requirement i differently, and also that costumers have different *degrees of importance* to the company. This can be done by as follows. Assume $C = \{c_1, c_2, \ldots, c_m\}$ is the set of costumers, and that $W = \{w_1, w_2, \ldots, w_m\}$ is the degree of importance of these costumers to the company. Then costumer c_j assigns requirement r_i a value $value(r_i, c_j)$, which is positive whenever requirement r_j was chosen by costumer c_j. Therefore the importance given to requirement r_i is:

$$score_i = \sum_{j=1}^{m} w_j \cdot value(r_i, c_j)$$

In this multi-objective formulation, there is no longer an optimal solution, but a set of solutions known as the *Pareto optimal set*. When this set of solutions is plotted in the objective space, it is called *Pareto Front*. Having the Pareto Front can be very helpful to the software engineer, since it can give a clear idea of the trade-offs between the score and cost of requirements. Multi-Objective Genetic algorithms (MOGA's) like NSGA-II [5, 8, 15], MOCell [8], Pareto GA [15] and SPEA2 [5] have been used to solve the MONRP.

The effects of the initial population in the quality of the final solution has been vastly studied [11, 14], even in the context of multi-objective approaches [13]. All studies are consistent to demonstrate the significant impact the initial sampling process plays in the general performance of the genetic algorithm, related both to the convergence of the algorithm as well as to the quality of the final solution, pointing out to the importance of employing intelligent sampling techniques to select individuals to be added to this population.

The main contribution of this paper is a method to generate the inital population for MOGA's for the MONRP. The method can be seen as an adaptation of the Path Relinking method [4], that constructs new solutions by recombining the features of other good solutions. In this work, Path Relinking is only applied to generate the initial population, based on some *extreme* solutions for the MONRP. A detaied presentation of the method is given in Section 2. In Section 3 we study the performance of MoCell and NSGA-II with distinct initialization methods, including the proposed one, and compare their performance. The conclusion of this work is presented in Section 4.

2   The Proposed Method

The MONRP described in the previous section is a Constrained Multi-Objective Optimization Problem.The population-based paradigm of genetic algorithms makes them extremely suitable for determining a representative subset of the Pareto optimal solution set of a multi-objective optimization problem [10].

On the other hand, many constraint-handling techniques have been adopted over the years to multi-objective genetic algorithms [12, 6]. Two of the most used are the repair algorithms and various types of penalty functions (static, dynamic, adaptive or death). In this work, penalty functions are used in the NSGA-II and MoCell algorithms, while a repair algorithm is used over the infeasible solutions to make them feasible, when generating the initial population.

Multi-Objetice Genetic Algorithms (MOGAs) are iterative optimization techniques [10]. It has been observed that the convergence of population-based algorithms is heavily dependent on the initial population. Furthermore, using a random sampling for the initial population often results in infeasible solutions.

Many methods were proposed to improve the convergence and quality of the solutions of the genetic algorithm. One of the most efficient is called *Path Relinking* (PR) [4]. Path Relinking shares with genetic algorithms (GAs) the idea of constructing new solutions by recombining the features of other good solutions (parents).

The initialization method we propose initially feeds the initial population with extreme mono-objective solutions, and then randomly generate solutions in the path linking the first solutions. Before including these solutions on the population, a repair algorithm is used to make sure that only feasible solutions are included. The method is only applied to generate the initial population, what makes it different to the Path Relinking heuristic that is applyed periodically throughout the evolutionary process. In addition to the solutions obtained by path linking between point solutions, the initial population is also composed of random feasible solutions obtained by the repair algorithm.

The penalty strategy for infeasible solutions used in the NSGA-II and MoCell algorithms ensure that, starting with a initial population of feasible solutions, the generations in the following iterations of the genetic algorithm are feasible even when mutations or crossover generate infeasible offspring.

The complete pseudo-code of the proposed initial population generation algorithm is presented in Algorithm 3. Some relevant points in the pseudocode are discussed below.

Algorithm 1. fixSolution

---

input : A integer M that represent the quantity of requirements, a *solution* to be fixed and a graph of dependences G (Where G[u][v] says that requisite u depends of requisite v).
output: A feasible *solution*.

while *solution is not feasible* **do**
  for $i \leftarrow 1$ **to** M **do**
    if *solution*[i] $== 1$: /* The requirement i was implemented */
      for $j \leftarrow 1$ **to** M **do**
        if $G[i][j] == 1$ *and solution*[j] $== 0$:   /* requirement i depends of requirement j and requirement j was not implemented */
          choose $x \in \{0, 1\}$ *at random*;
          if $x == 0$: /* Implement the requirement j or not implement the requirement i */
            | *solution*[j] $= 1$;
          else:
            | *solution*[i] $= 0$;
      end for
  end for
end while

A Linking Path (LP) is a set of feasible solutions that lie close to the line that binds two Pareto optimal (PO) solutions in the objective space.

N stands for the total number of solutions in initial population, N_{lp} stands for the number of solutions in the LP between the extreme solutions, and N_r stands for the number of feasible random solutions in the initial population. Thus, $N = 2 + N_{lp} + N_r$.

First, a path between the solutions $extreme_0$ (solution where all the requirements are not implemented) and $extreme_1$ (solution where all requirements are implemented) is created according to Algorithm 2. Then, these solutions are added to the population that will be used as initial population of the MOGA. Approximately N_{lp} solutions are created in this process.

The second loop completes the initial population with feasible solutions that are chosen at random. The $fixSolution()$ method described in Algorithm 1 is used to transform the generated solutions that are infeasible into feasible ones.

In Figure 1 the initial populations of NSGA-II and MoCell are presented. It shows the distribution in the objective space of the Pareto front of the initial populations for Random initialzation and PathRelinking intialization methods. In (1a) random solutions are generated and are made feasible by a repair algorithm. The only difference between the Extreme Solutions initialization method

---

Algorithm 2. createPath

---

input : A integer M that represent the quantity of requirements, a integer E that represent the quantity of solutions that are expected to be created, a *initial* solution and a *guiding* solution.

output: A new population.

Solution newSolution = new Solution(initial) ; /* solution became a copy of initial */

$D = distance(initial, guiding)$;   /* distance(a,b) returns how many variables solution a differ of the solution b */

step = ceil(D/(E+1));

for $k \leftarrow 1$ **to** D**do**

   starting = random() % M;

   for $i \leftarrow 1$ **to** M**do**

      index = (i + starting) % M;

      if *newSolution[index]* $\neq$ *guiding[index] and change value of newSolution[index] to guiding[index] don't break a constraint*:

         newSolution[index] = guiding[index];

         break;

   end for

   if $k \% step == 0$:

      population.add(newSolution);

end for

Algorithm 3. Create Initial Population

---

input : A integer N that represent the quantity of solutions in initial population.

output: A initial *population* that will be used in Genetic Algorithm.

$N_c = 0$;   /* The quantity of solutions created */

$PR_{set} = createPath(extreme_0, extreme_1)$; /* $extreme_0$ is the solution that don't have any requirements implemented and $extreme_1$ have all requirements implemented */

for $j \leftarrow 1$ **to** $PR_{set}.size()$**do**

   population.add(PR_{set}.get(j));

   $N_c++;$

end for

while $N_c < N$**do**   /* Random Feasible Solutions */

   individual = new Solution(problem);

   problem.fixSolution(individual) ;   /* Make the solution feasible */

   population.add(individual);

   $N_c++;$

end while

---

and the Random method is that the first adds extreme mono-objective solutions in the front. Therefore, the figures are very similar (And it was not included in this paper due to space restriction). Finally, in (1b) we see the initial population generated by the proposed method.

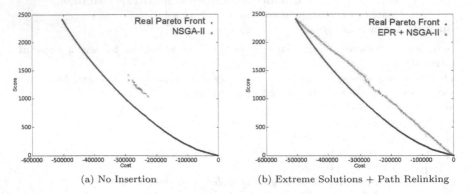

(a) No Insertion   (b) Extreme Solutions + Path Relinking

Fig. 1. Feasible Initial Populations

3   Experiments and Discussion

3.1   Details of the Instances and Genetic Algorithms

The experiments were made using 24 instances of the NRP. We considered the following choices of values for the number of requirements, costumers and edges in the dependency graphs of the instances:

Number of requirements: {200, 300, 500, 800};
Number of costumers: {10, 20};
Percentual of edges in the dependency graph: {20%, 30%, 40%} (The number
    of dependencies is indicated as a percentage of the number of requirements).

There are 24 possible settings of these parameters, and for each one, an instance was generated at random. We use the nomenclature rX_cY_dZ to describe the instance that is generated with a set of X requirements, Y clients and Z% of edges in the dependency graph.

In [8] they consider that a typical instance of the NRP has a number of costumers ranging from 15 to 100 and requirements from 40 to 140. This is in agreement to the instances that are considered in other experimental works on the NRP. In this work we have focused on instances that are more complex and therefore harder to solve than in these previous works. As we will show later, the quality of the solutions obtained by the genetic algorithms with the proposed initialization method is superior to the ones using the common initialization methods. The instances used to this work can be found in [1]. The tests were run in a computer with the following specification: Windows 7 Ultimate Edition, Processor AMD FX-8120, RAM 8Gb (1600MHz), Hard Drive Vertex 3 Max IOPs 120GB.

Every solution of the NRP consists of a set of requirements that are to be chosen to the next release of a software. We encode the solutions (chromosome) using an integer vector ranging in $\{0, 1\}$ and of length equal to the number of requirements from the instance. We used binary tournament for the selection scheme. For the crossover operator we used single point crossover. The probability of the crossover operator was set to 0.9. Random mutation was used as the mutation operator. The probability of the mutation operator was set to $\frac{1}{n}$, where n is the number of requirements. The initial population was always set to 1024 solutions, this being also the maximum population size. The algorithms have been implemented using jMetal [7], an object-oriented Java-based framework for multi-objective optimization with metaheuristics.

3.2   Quality Indicators

In order to evaluate convergence and diversity of our algorithm, we use the following quality indicators:

Spread [2]: We desire Pareto fronts with a smaller Spread. The zero value corresponds to a perfect spread of the solutions in the Pareto front.

Hypervolume (HV) [16]: Used to measure both diversity and convergence of the solutions. A Pareto front has a higher HV than another one either because solutions from the second front are dominated by solutions in the first front, or because the ones from the first front are better distributed. Therefore we desire Pareto fronts with larger values of HV.

To calculate the spread and hypervolume of a Pareto front, we need the real Pareto front. In our experiments we used an approximated one. The approximation was obtained by taking 50 equaly distant points in the interval [0, SUM-COST] (SUMCOST is simply the sum of the costs from all requirements, a trivial upper bound to the maximum cost of a valid solution) and then, for each point value, solve the mono-objective NRP problem using the point value as the limit value to cost constraint (We use a Linear Programming solver to do it). We have now 50 optimal solutions in Pareto front, for each of the 50 different cost values, we have the maximum score possible. After, Path Relinking is used to generated interpolated solutions based on the ones that were generated first and then is used the MoCell with 5000000 evaluations. The same process was used with NSGA-II. Then, the two populations was put together and we got the Pareto front of this new population.

3.3   Results

For our tests we considered MoCell and NSGA-II with the following initialization procedures:

Random Solutions (RS): The initial population is generated at random.

Valid Solutions (VS): The initial population is generated at random and a repair procedure is applied to ensure only valid solutions are kept.

Extreme Solutions (EXT): In this method, we inserted the two extreme solutions in the initial population, one with all requirements implemented and another with no requirement implemented.

Extreme Solutions with Path Relinking (EPR): This is the method proposed in this article, that behaves similarly to EXT, with the difference that now Path Relinking is used to generate new interpolated solutions.

In Table 1, we have calculated the mean and standart deviation to HV and Spread. The tables were made by running each instance 10 times and with 300000 evaluations. The first columns of Table 1 show that the hypervolume of the solutions obtained by NSGA-II with the EPR initialization method is already higher when considering the experiments with smaller instances. For the more complex instances the difference becomes even more evident, with the HV of the EPR algorithms being almost twice the one of the solutions using RS or VS. A similar conclusion can be taken looking at last columns of the Table 2 where the EPR initialization method outperforms the RS, VS and EXT methods.

We should highlight that in some instances the Pareto front of the initial population is only the two extreme solutions and the MoCell with EXT method have problems with that, because MoCell always make a crossover beteween a individual that is not in the Pareto front with a individual that can or not be in Pareto front. But when we use Path Reliking that is not a problem, since the Pareto front is a well distributed front and MoCell can work properly. From this we conclude that, although the proposed initialization procedure with extreme solutions and Path Relinking increases the computational work, the impact in the total time is low, since the initial population is only generated once.

Table 1. Hypervolume and Spread - NSGA-II (mean, (standard deviation))

Instance	Hypervolume				Spread			
	NSGA-II (RS)	NSGA-II (VS)	EXT + NSGA-II	EPR + NSGA-II	NSGA-II (RS)	NSGA-II (VS)	EXT + NSGA-II	EPR + NSGA-II
r200_c10_d20	0.5961 (0.0050)	0.5988 (0.0094)	**0.6372** (0.0014)	0.6349 (0.0022)	0.5358 (0.0230)	0.5216 (0.0278)	**0.4068** (0.0192)	0.4290 (0.0230)
r200_c10_d40	0.5549 (0.0068)	0.5593 (0.0053)	**0.6057** (**0.0034**)	0.6027 (0.0026)	0.5798 (0.0264)	0.5766 (0.0193)	**0.4315** (0.0318)	0.4448 (0.0228)
r200_c20_d20	0.5820 (0.0061)	0.5888 (0.0026)	**0.6271** (**0.0007**)	0.6239 (0.0013)	0.5454 (0.0211)	0.5306 (0.0199)	**0.3821** (**0.0099**)	0.4045 (0.0149)
r200_c20_d40	0.5633 (0.0099)	0.5685 (0.0072)	**0.6141** (**0.0019**)	0.6134 (0.0018)	0.5953 (0.0284)	0.5850 (0.0213)	0.4129 (0.0211)	**0.4128** (**0.0163**)
r500_c10_d20	0.4936 (0.0068)	0.4881 (0.0101)	0.5613 (0.0131)	**0.5914** (**0.0021**)	0.7924 (0.0152)	0.7988 (0.0108)	0.6360 (0.0707)	**0.5108** (**0.0189**)
r500_c10_d40	0.4737 (0.0075)	0.4530 (0.0079)	0.4821 (0.0166)	**0.5792** (**0.0025**)	0.8208 (0.0122)	0.8295 (0.0140)	1.0562 (0.0916)	**0.4987** (**0.0091**)
r500_c20_d20	0.5026 (0.0035)	0.4935 (0.0069)	0.5765 (0.0122)	**0.5970** (**0.0038**)	0.7890 (0.0099)	0.8052 (0.0164)	0.5691 (0.0716)	**0.5055** (**0.0194**)
r500_c20_d40	0.4639 (0.0046)	0.4488 (0.0094)	0.4913 (0.0135)	**0.5750** (**0.0020**)	0.8240 (0.0053)	0.8346 (0.0173)	0.9826 (0.0803)	**0.4979** (**0.0195**)
r800_c10_d20	0.4375 (0.0052)	0.4216 (0.0111)	0.5044 (0.0176)	**0.5707** (**0.0028**)	0.8691 (0.0104)	0.8775 (0.0129)	0.9069 (0.1025)	**0.4587** (**0.0238**)
r800_c10_d40	0.3935 (0.0093)	0.3769 (0.0053)	0.4015 (0.0082)	**0.5465** (**0.0018**)	0.8965 (0.0073)	0.8905 (0.0076)	1.3624 (0.0372)	**0.4731** (**0.0168**)
r800_c20_d20	0.4400 (0.0046)	0.4199 (0.0117)	0.4804 (0.0120)	**0.5734** (**0.0029**)	0.8661 (0.0055)	0.8781 (0.0093)	1.0316 (0.0743)	**0.4664** (**0.0225**)
r800_c20_d40	0.3841 (0.0237)	0.3783 (0.0042)	0.4065 (0.0056)	**0.5441** (**0.0029**)	0.9004 (0.0178)	0.8870 (0.0090)	1.3593 (0.0374)	**0.4593** (**0.0292**)

To give a clear idea of the behaviour of the algorithms, in all the Figures we are considering instance r800_c20_d40, which is the largest one that was used in the experiments.

Table 2. Hypervolume and Spread - MoCell(mean, (standard deviation))

Instance	Hypervolume				Spread			
	MoCell (RS)	MoCell (VS)	EXT + MoCell	EPR + MoCell	MoCell (RS)	MoCell (VS)	EXT + MoCell	EPR + MoCell
r200_c10_d20	0.6043 (0.0054)	0,6083 (0,0067)	0.1194 (0.00003)	0.6326 (0.0015)	0.5186 (0.0171)	0,5109 (0,0194)	0.8620 (0.0022)	0.4407 (0.0187)
r200_c10_d40	0.5601 (0.0096)	0,5761 (0,0042)	0.1135 (0.00007)	0.6031 (0.0026)	0.5541 (0.0262)	0,5310 (0,0234)	0.8675 (0.0038)	0.4127 (0.0223)
r200_c20_d20	0.5843 (0.0056)	0,5949 (0,0053)	0.2142 (0.00017)	0.6222 (0.0008)	0.5476 (0.0198)	0,5324 (0,0129)	0.8427 (0.0036)	0.3984 (0.0055)
r200_c20_d40	0.5740 (0.0060)	0,5807 (0,0105)	0.2270 (0.00074)	0.6114 (0.0018)	0.5584 (0.0174)	0,5407 (0,0238)	0.8472 (0.0043)	0.4072 (0.0199)
r500_c10_d20	0.4985 (0.0055)	0,5045 (0,0072)	0.1717 (0.00080)	0.5662 (0.0034)	0.7837 (0.0092)	0,7815 (0,0106)	0.7856 (0.0080)	0.5260 (0.0237)
r500_c10_d40	0.4849 (0.0079)	0,4764 (0,0054)	0.2342 (0.00128)	0.5552 (0.0036)	0.8022 (0.0157)	0,8102 (0,0158)	0.8396 (0.0319)	0.4989 (0.0232)
r500_c20_d20	0.5084 (0.0042)	0,5133 (0,0055)	0.4992 (0.00203)	0.5731 (0.0038)	0.7829 (0.0094)	0,7764 (0,0109)	0.6636 (0.0303)	0.5225 (0.0294)
r500_c20_d40	0.4788 (0.0067)	0,4678 (0,0080)	0.4075 (0.00261)	0.5494 (0.0052)	0.8013 (0.0102)	0,8187 (0,0219)	0.8400 (0.0439)	0.5085 (0.0255)
r800_c10_d20	0.4473 (0.0273)	0,4454 (0,0078)	0.1248 (0.00203)	0.5306 (0.0045)	0.8622 (0.0185)	0,8601 (0,0089)	0.8452 (0.0328)	0.5839 (0.0232)
r800_c10_d40	0.4293 (0.0078)	0,3936 (0,0061)	0.2572 (0.00271)	0.5137 (0.0022)	0.8717 (0.0085)	0,8883 (0,0146)	1.1296 (0.0201)	0.5275 (0.0162)
r800_c20_d20	0.4586 (0.0047)	0,4415 (0,0063)	0.4393 (0.00938)	0.5322 (0.0038)	0.8561 (0.0083)	0,8617 (0,0113)	0.8330 (0.0833)	0.5806 (0.0180)
r800_c20_d40	0.4142 (0.0286)	0,4037 (0,0084)	0.4420 (0.00592)	0.5108 (0.0039)	0.8782 (0.0176)	0,8741 (0,0089)	1.1635 (0.0334)	0.5523 (0.0110)

In Figure 1 we can see the difference between initial populations. Where the path relinking was not used, most of the solutions are generated at random and stay in the center of the search space. In contrast, the use of extreme solutions combined with path relinking provided a initial population that represented the search space in a much better way.

The Figure 2a presents the evolution of the spread of the fronts obtained by NSGA-II with the initialization procedures. A higher number of function evaluations was considered. We used 1000000 function evaluations, in order to study the behaviour of the algorithms for a large number of function evaluations. The Spread of the algorithms with the EPR initialization method is remarkably smaller than the other ones already in the early generations. The same can be said about the HV indicator, as can be seen in Figure 2b.

The Figure 2c presents the evolution of the spread of the fronts obtained by MoCell with the initialization procedures. Again, we used 1000000 function evaluations and chose the largest instance. The Spread of the algorithms with the EPR initialization method is remarkably smaller than the other ones already in the early generations. The same can be said about the HV indicator, as can be seen in Figure 2d.

Statistical evaluation of the results used the two-sample t-test with a significance level equal to 2%. The null hypothesis for both algorithms is that the Spread or Hypervolume distributions are independent random samples from normal distributions with equal means and equal but unknown variances. The alternative hypothesis is that the means are not equal. Tables 3 and 4 presents the results for each metric to both algorithms, NSGA-II and MoCell. Each table entry shows three values: the mean, the standard deviation and the p-value (To values below 1e-10 we used the zero value.) obtained with the t-test. For all tests the reference sample is that one achieved by algorithm with random initialization i.e., the t-test of each column always matches with the random initialization

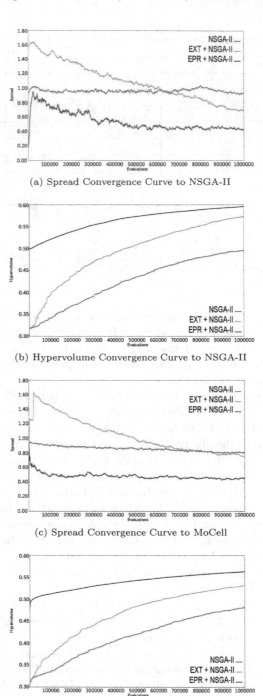

(a) Spread Convergence Curve to NSGA-II

(b) Hypervolume Convergence Curve to NSGA-II

(c) Spread Convergence Curve to MoCell

(d) Hypervolume Convergence Curve to MoCell

Fig. 2. Convergence Curves

Table 3. Hypervolume Statistics(mean, standard deviation, p-value)

	NSGA-II	EPR + NSGA-II [402]	EPR + NSGA-II [1024]	MoCell	EPR + MoCell [402]	EPR + MoCell [1024]
Mutation: 1/N Crossover: 0.2	0.5327 0.032	0.587 0.06 ✗(1.42e-5)	0.592 0.13 ✗(9.19e-3)	0.535 0.023	0.5287 0.04 ✓(0.197)	0.5389 0.024 ✓(0.190)
Mutation: 1/N Crossover: 0.5	0.5163 0.019	0.5969 0.11 ✗(1.92e-4)	0.5934 0.15 ✗(4.33e-3)	0.5296 0.036	0.5433 0.034 ✗(1.76e-2)	0.551 0.027 ✗(7.86e-5)
Mutation: 1/N Crossover: 0.8	0.4884 0.042	0.5973 0.24 ✗(9.47e-3)	0.5875 0.35 6.58e-2	0.5034 0.002	0.5523 0.052 ✗(8.34e-6)	0.5537 0.035 ✗(5.55e-9)
Mutation: 3/N Crossover: 0.2	0.5556 0.028	0.5929 0.03 ✗(8.86e-8)	0.6013 0.07 ✗(6.24e-4)	0.5363 0.02	0.5448 0.021 ✗(1.73e-2)	0.5462 0.017 ✗(1.70e-3)
Mutation: 3/N Crossover: 0.5	0.5362 0.0027	0.5983 0.07 ✗(1.87e-5)	0.5989 0.14 ✗(1.02e-2)	0.534 0.032	0.556 0.022 ✗(3.36e-6)	0.5557 0.014 ✗(1.17e-9)
Mutation: 3/N Crossover: 0.8	0.501 0.0054	0.5977 0.019 ✗(0)	0.5902 0.022 ✗(0)	0.5102 0.0034	0.5624 0.027 ✗(0)	0.5594 0.029 ✗(1.697e-10)
Mutation: 5/N Crossover: 0.2	0.5472 0.004	0.5929 0.005 ✗(0)	0.5981 0.006 ✗(0)	0.5163 0.0019	0.545 0.015 ✗(0)	0.5437 0.01 ✗(0)
Mutation: 5/N Crossover: 0.5	0.5285 0.0027	0.5958 0.001 ✗(0)	0.5943 0.005 ✗(0)	0.5148 0.0035	0.5553 0.017 ✗(0)	0.5518 0.015 ✗(0)
Mutation: 5/N Crossover: 0.8	0.4984 0.0038	0.5956 0.011 ✗(0)	0.5856 0.016 ✗(0)	0.5021 0.0023	0.5606 0.023 ✗(0)	0.5573 0.019 ✗(0)

Table 4. Spread Statistics(mean, standard deviation, p-value)

	NSGA-II	EPR + NSGA-II [402]	EPR + NSGA-II [1024]	MoCell	EPR + MoCell [402]	EPR + MoCell [1024]
Mutation: 1/N Crossover: 0.2	0.7489 0.0823	0.4169 0.736 ✗(9.80e-3)	0.3959 0.38 ✗(9.92e-6)	0.6135 0.0102	0.2633 0.136 ✗(0)	0.4962 0.21 ✗(2.36e-3)
Mutation: 1/N Crossover: 0.5	0.7935 0.0761	0.3866 0.711 ✗(1.95e-3)	0.3885 0.906 ✗(1.03e-2)	0.6579 0.0128	0.2456 0.17 ✗(0)	0.4977 0.21 ✗(1.23e-4)
Mutation: 1/N Crossover: 0.8	0.8735 0.0892	0.3725 0.492 ✗(2.55e-6)	0.4026 0.671 ✗(3.05e-4)	0.7446 0.0124	0.2226 0.104 ✗(0)	0.5204 0.249 ✗(1.53e-5)
Mutation: 3/N Crossover: 0.2	0.6451 0.0481	0.3777 0.294 ✗(1.33e-5)	0.3427 0.472 ✗(7.44e-4)	0.6116 0.0128	0.1889 0.127 ✗(0)	0.4673 0.19 ✗(1.29e-4)
Mutation: 3/N Crossover: 0.5	0.74 0.0618	0.3502 0.21 ✗(0)	0.3571 0.462 ✗(4.55e-5)	0.6595 0.0137	0.2001 0.129 ✗(0)	0.4869 0.202 ✗(3.08e-5)
Mutation: 3/N Crossover: 0.8	0.8536 0.0876	0.3293 0.187 ✗(0)	0.377 0.367 ✗(3.96e-8)	0.7435 0.0116	0.2107 0.135 ✗(0)	0.5123 0.162 ✗(6.38e-9)
Mutation: 5/N Crossover: 0.2	0.6821 0.0431	0.3306 0.15 ✗(0)	0.3193 0.231 ✗(8.93e-10)	0.6618 0.0118	0.1867 0.16 ✗(0)	0.4739 0.161 ✗(2.73e-7)
Mutation: 5/N Crossover: 0.5	0.7791 0.0766	0.3133 0.095 ✗(0)	0.3288 0.206 ✗(0)	0.7059 0.0115	0.1897 0.162 ✗(0)	0.4982 0.135 ✗(1.37e-9)
Mutation: 5/N Crossover: 0.8	0.8219 0.0581	0.2858 0.085 ✗(0)	0.4026 0.262 ✗(5.99e-10)	0.7573 0.01	0.2072 0.097 ✗(0)	0.5153 0.151 ✗(5.81e-10)

algorithm result. In order to facilitate the tables comprehension, each table cell indicates, using a symbol, if the hypothesis has been rejected (✗) or not (✓).

The Table 3 shows the statistics analise to Hypervolume metric where the null hypothesis is not rejected in only one case. In all other cases ERP is superior when applied to MoCell and NSGA-II, in both the configurations of population 1024 or 402 chromosomes. Also note in Table 4 for the Spread results in which the null hypothesis is rejected in all cases tested.

In this experiment 30 different initial populations randomly chosen with the configuration r800_c20_d40 were used.

4   Conclusions

In this paper we face the problem of solving the Multi-Objective Next Release Problem via evolutionary algorithms. Three objectives are to be sought by MO-GAs: achieve good convergence, maintain the diversity of the population and reducing the computational effort. The achievement of these goals is strongly dependent on the initial population, with our experiments showing that for large instances of the problem, evolutionary algorithms such as NSGA-II and MoCell with random initialization do not give good results even with long processing times, as shown in Figure 2 and 3.

We propose to use Extreme solutions and Path Relinking (EPR) to obtain a set of interpolated solutions in the initial population. This work showed that the proposed method has a big impact on the three above-mentioned goals, where we used hypervolume and spread as measures for diversity and convergence.

In any future attempts to solve MONRP with this formulation, the possibility of inserting extreme solutions should be taken into account. In case one needs to solve complex instances, with a big quantity of requirements and dependencies, using the EPR method should be a good choice, since it presents the best Spread and Hypervolume in all tested instances, with little impact on the total running time of the algorithms.

References

1. Multi-objective next release problem instances, `https://mega.co.nz/#!OoJXCbZI!R5cCl4r4KGGTI2f-yXjacBiSQphdeAv6SrOgvv6a-1Q` (updated: March 25, 2014)
2. Azarm, S., Wu, J.: Metrics for Quality Assessment of a Multiobjective Design Optimization Solution Set. Journal of Mechanical Design 123(1), 18–25 (2001)
3. Bagnall, A., Rayward-Smith, V., Whittley, I.: The next release problem. Information and Software Technology 43(14), 883–890 (2001)
4. Basseur, M., Seynhaeve, F., Talbi, E.-G.: Path relinking in pareto multi-objective genetic algorithms. In: Coello Coello, C.A., Aguirre, A.H., Zitzler, E. (eds.) EMO 2005. LNCS, vol. 3410, pp. 120–134. Springer, Heidelberg (2005)
5. Cai, X., Wei, O., Huang, Z.: Evolutionary approaches for multi-objective next release problem. Computing and Informatics 31(4), 847 (2012)
6. Coello Coello, C.A.: Theoretical and numerical constraint-handling techniques used with evolutionary algorithms: a survey of the state of the art. Computer Methods in Applied Mechanics and Engineering 191(11-12), 1245–1287 (2002)
7. Durillo, J.J., Nebro, A.J.: jmetal: A java framework for multi-objective optimization. Advances in Engineering Software 42(10), 760–771 (2011)
8. Durillo, J.J., Zhang, Y., Alba, E., Nebro, A.J.: A study of the multi-objective next release problem. In: Proceedings of the 2009 1st International Symposium on Search Based Software Engineering, SSBSE 2009, pp. 49–58. IEEE Computer Society, Washington, DC (2009)
9. Karp, R.M.: Reducibility among combinatorial problems. In: Miller, R.E., Thatcher, J.W., Bohlinger, J.D. (eds.) Complexity of Computer Computations. The IBM Research Symposia Series, pp. 85–103. Springer US (1972)

10. Konak, A., Coit, D.W., Smith, A.E.: Multi-objective optimization using genetic algorithms: A tutorial. Reliability Engineering & System Safety 91(9), 992–1007 (2006)
11. Maaranen, H., Miettinen, K., Penttinen, A.: On initial populations of a genetic algorithm for continuous optimization problems. Journal of Global Optimization 37(3), 405–436 (2007)
12. Michalewicz, Z.: A survey of constraint handling techniques in evolutionary computation methods. In: Proceedings of the 4th Annual Conference on Evolutionary Programming, pp. 135–155 (1995)
13. Poles, S., Fu, Y., Rigoni, E.: The effect of initial population sampling on the convergence of multi-objective genetic algorithms. In: Barichard, V., Ehrgott, M., Gandibleux, X., T'Kindt, V. (eds.) Multiobjective Programming and Goal Programming. Lecture Notes in Economics and Mathematical Systems, vol. 618, pp. 123–133. Springer, Heidelberg (2009)
14. Rahnamayan, S., Tizhoosh, H.R., Salama, M.M.: A novel population initialization method for accelerating evolutionary algorithms. Computers and Mathematics with Applications 53(10), 1605 (2007)
15. Zhang, Y., Harman, M., Mansouri, S.: The multi-objective next release problem. In: Proceedings of the 9th Annual Conference on Genetic and Evolutionary Computation, pp. 1129–1137. ACM (2007)
16. Zitzler, E.: Evolutionary Algorithms for Multiobjective Optimization: Methods and Applications. PhD thesis, Swiss Federal Institute of Technology (ETH) (November 1999)

Extension of the Method of Musical Composition for the Treatment of Multi-objective Optimization Problems

José Roberto Méndez Rosiles, Antonin Ponsich, Eric Alfredo Rincón García, and Roman Anselmo Mora Gutiérrez

Universidad Autónoma Metropolitana - Azcapotzalco
Dpto. de Sistemas, C.P. 02200, México DF

Abstract. This work proposes a new technique for the treatment of Multi-objective Optimization Problems (MOPs), based on the extension of a socio-cultural algorithm, the Method of Musical Composition (MMC). The MMC uses a society of agents, called composers, who have their own creative ability, maintain a memory of their previous artwork and are also able to exchange information.

According to this analogy, a decomposition approach implemented through a Tchebycheff function is adapted, assigning each composer to the solution of a particular scalar sub-problem. Agents with similar parameterization of the original MOP may share their solutions. Furthermore, the generation of new tunes was modified, using the Differential Evolution mutation operator. Computational experiments performed on the ZDT and DTLZ test suite highlight the promising performances obtained by the resulting MO-MMC algorithm, when compared with the NSGA-II, MOEA/D and two swarm intelligence based techniques.

1 Introduction

The treatment of Multi-objective Optimization Problems (MOPs) has become, in the two last decades, a main research area, particulary in Evolutionary Computation. A MOP accounts for the simultaneous optimization (without lack of generality, we will assume minimization in the remainder of this paper) of m objectives: $\min \{f_1(x), \ldots, f_m(x)\}$. The aim is therefore to determine an approximation of the set $\mathcal{P}^*$ of Pareto (or non-dominated) solutions, which represent a trade-off between the m objectives: $\mathcal{P}^* = \{x \in \mathcal{F} \mid \nexists x' \in \mathcal{F} : x' \prec x\}$, where $\mathcal{F}$ is the set of feasible solutions of the tackled problem and $x' \prec x$ (x' dominates x) means that $\forall i \in \{1, \ldots, m\}, f_i(x') \leq f_i(x)$ and $\exists j \in \{1, \ldots, m\} : f_j(x') < f_j(x)$. The representation of $\mathcal{P}^*$ in the objective space is commonly denoted as the Pareto front $\mathcal{PF}^*$. In practice, not all the Pareto-optimal set is usually desirable. The aim is rather to obtain a limited number of solutions, as close as possible and well (uniformly) distributed along the Pareto front $\mathcal{PF}^*$.

Redefining optimality in those terms has involved the design of adapted optimization methods. Furthermore, the need to obtain, in a single run, a set of

A. Gelbukh et al. (Eds.): MICAI 2014, Part II, LNAI 8857, pp. 38–49, 2014.

non-dominated solutions, led to the use of population-based techniques, particularly Evolutionary Algorithms (EAs). The integration of non-dominance and elitism concepts, as well as the design of refined techniques for diversity preservation, allowed significant advances, illustrated by the development of state-of-the art techniques whose results are still currently reported in many applications (see for instance the SPEA2 [1]) and NSGA-II [2] algorithms).

More recently, the weakness of dominance-based methods for solving many-objectives problems has attracted the interest of researchers on alternative techniques. First, the decomposition approach, introduced in the MOEA/D [3], consists in dividing a MOP into a set of scalar subproblems, each one being associated with a specific parameterization of the original MOP. On the other hand, the design of different measures assessing the algorithmic performances led to the idea of optimizing these metrics instead of directly minimizing the problem objectives (see for instance the SMS-EMOA [4]). Finally, the extension of other metaheuristics has also constituted a promising research line, like for example the Particle Swarm Optimization (MOPSO, [5]).

Following these guidelines, the present work proposes the extension of a novel socio-cultural algorithm for the solution of MOPs, namely the Method of Musical Composition (MMC, [6]). Regarding the remainder of this paper, Section 2 proposes a short outline on multi-objective socially-motivated algorithms. In section 3, the Method of Musical Composition is briefly described, while the proposed modifications for dealing with MOPs are provided in section 4. Computational experiments and numerical results are discussed in section 5 and some conclusions are drawn in section 6.

2   Multi-objective Socially-Motivated Algorithms

As above-mentioned, a great amount of research effort was carried out for the extension of different kinds of metaheuristics to the treatment of MOPs. Because of their conceptual similarity with the MMC (defined as a socio-cultutural optimization algorithm), the so-called "socially-motivated" techniques are of particular interest in the framework of this study: Particle Swarm Optimization (PSO), Ant Colony Optimization (ACO) and Cultural Algorithms (CAs).

Many multi-objective PSO implementations have been proposed since 1999 (see [7] for a complete overview on this topic). Among these techniques, which are mainly based on the Pareto dominance strategy, the most quoted one is MOPSO, introduced in [5]. MOPSO maintains an external archive of non-dominated solutions used to guide the particles' flight, and includes a mutation operator to promote exploration.

Also, some works based on the decomposition approach introduced in [3] were proposed more recently. For instance, dMOPSO [8] builds a set of *global best* particles according to the decomposition approach and uses it to update particles' position. Furthermore, a memory reinitialization is carried out to provide diversity to the swarm. [9] and [10] are other illustrations applying decomposition and combining it with either a crowding distance or the creation of sub-swarms in order to promote diversity. Note that the two former works use a Penalty Boundary Intersection decomposition scheme for decomposition, while the latter one is based on Tchebycheff approach. However, in [11], the authors propose a min-max strategy for decomposition and a *local best* solution updating performed for each sub-region associated to each sub-problem. This approach seems to clearly outperform the dominance-based MOPSO [5] for several 2 and 3-objective continuous test functions.

Regarding multi-objective implementations of ACO, only a few approaches use the Pareto dominance concept while a great majority rely on the metaheuristic specific features (using, for instance, several ant colonies, or different pheromone or heuristic matrices). Besides, due to the nature of the metaheuristic, a great majority of studies deal with combinatorial optimization problems. However, two recent works are based on a decomposition approach, such as [12] and [13] that showed good performances on several instances of the multi-objective knapsack and TSP problems.

Finally, very few multi-objective implementations of Cultural Algorithms are reported in the specialized literature. The most relevant one is based on Evolutionary Programming, uses Pareto ranking and enforces elitism through an external archive storing the non-dominated solutions [14]. Evaluated on some test functions, this technique is successfully compared with NSGA-II [2]. Apart from this proposal, other works [15,16] exclusively present qualitative studies of the CAs' internal features. None of them propose any consistent results on classical benchmarks. In this sense, the extension of MMC, as a socio-cultural algorithm, is part of the contribution of the present work.

3   Description of the MMC

The MMC [6] is an algorithm based on a multiagent model that mimics a creativity system, such as musical composition. The MMC considers a social network, composed of N_c agents, called composers, and a set E of edges, that represent relationships between composers. Note that this society is dynamic: at the end of each iteration, the social network is updated in such a way that some edges may be probabilistically created or removed from the associated graph.

According to the MMC model, each composer has his/her own artwork, i.e. a set of N_s "tunes" (solutions) that he/she previously created. Moreover, any agent is able to learn tunes from other agents he/she shares a link with, within the previously defined social network. All these tunes are stored in a matrix denoted as the acquired knowledge. Both personal and acquired knowledge may be used by each agent to create new tunes, by performing a crossover/mutation-like technique. However, composers also have creative abilities, allowing them to invent new tunes (complete solutions) or tune fragments (partial solutions) in a completely random way.

Summarizing for a n-dimension search space, the social network is first randomly initialized and a set of N_c artworks is created. Each composer stores his/her personal knowledge in the corresponding *score matrix*, $P_{i,\star,\star}$ ($i = 1, \ldots, N_c$). Then, a complete cycle of the MMC algorithm is as follows:

1. Each composer i receives information from all the composers j he/she is connected with.
2. Composer i accepts or rejects a tune randomly selected from composer j's artwork, in order to build his/her acquired knowledge matrix $ISC_{i,\star,\star}$: the selected tune $P_{j,sel,\star}$ is accepted if composer j's worst tune $P_{j,worst,\star}$ is better than composer i's worst tune $P_{i,worst,\star}$.
3. Each composer i builds his/her background knowledge matrix by concatenating personal and acquired knowledges: $KM_{i,\star,\star} = P_{i,\star,\star} \cup ISC_{i,\star,\star}$.
4. Each composer i probabilistically decides whether generating a new tune on the basis of the background knowledge matrix, or in a random way (composer's inspiration).
5. If the tune is created from the background knowledge, crossover is applied to three tunes selected from composer i's matrix $KM_{i,\star,\star}$. A normal perturbation is subsequently added to the resulting child.
6. Composer i accepts the new tune if it is better than $P_{i,worst,\star}$.
7. The social network is updated: every edge in E (respectively in $\overline{E}$) is probabilistically removed from (resp. added to) the social network.

This operation cycle is repeated until the stopping criterion is met, e.g. when a maximum number of iterations have been computed. The MMC has been evaluated on various test function benchmarks, including unrestricted [6] and restricted [17] problems. The promising results reached by this novel optimization technique make it a very effective socially motivated algorithm.

In the general framework of population-based search techniques, the MMC can be related to Evolutionary Algorithms and Particle Swarm Optimization. However, the fact that each agent represents a set of solutions (which can be seen as an extended memory) and the dynamically updated topology of the artificial society constitute its main differences with the above-mentioned algorithms.

4 A Multi-objective MMC

The MO-MMC algorithm proposed in this paper is based on the decomposition approach, which appears as one of the best performing. This strategy involved the design of new selection mechanisms and acceptance functions. Furthermore, since MMC can be considered as a cultural algorithm, it has been necessary to deal with multiple interactions between agents to update their knowledge about the problem (as a population) and also to use information collected from the population (as individuals).

4.1 Decomposition Approach

In this first implementation of the MO-MMC, the Tchebycheff approach was selected for the decomposition of the global MOP into several parameterized scalar subproblems, which are in the form:

$$\text{minimize } g^{te}(x|\lambda, z^*) = \max_{1 \leq j \leq m} \{\lambda_j | f_j(x) - z_j^*|\} \tag{1}$$

where $z^* = (z_1^*, \ldots, z_m^*)^T = \min\{f_j(x)|x \in \Omega\}$ is the ideal vector, $\lambda = (\lambda_1, \ldots, \lambda_m)^T$ is a weight vector and Ω is the variable decision space. For every Pareto optimal point x^*, there exists a weight vector λ such that x^* is an optimal solution. In the proposed algorithm, every composer has a weight vector λ assigned, meaning that every composer solves a specific scalar problem and searches a sub-region of the Pareto front. A consequence of this operating mode is that solutions from different composers cannot be easily compared, since their fitness $g^{te}(x|\lambda, z^*)$ is computed according to different weights. Note that previous MOCAs usually rely on Pareto dominance schemes to evaluate solutions, so that the MO-MMC represents the first decomposition-based Multi-Objective Cultural Algorithm.

4.2 Initialization

The initialization phase of the algorithm consists of building the social network and creating a personal artwork for each composer. In this first implementation, it has been considered (as in the MOEA/D [3]) that collaboration between composers having very different weight vectors might not be useful since they are respectively optimizing very different scalar sub-problems. Since each composer's weight vector is constant, the society is static and not dynamically updated as in the original MMC. Therefore, N_c weight vectors are generated uniformly over the search direction space and assigned to the N_c composers. A link between two composers is then created only if their weight vectors are significantly close. This configuration does not change during a run.

Besides, every composer's artwork, consisting of N_s tunes, is initialized, meaning that $N_c \times N_s$ solutions should be generated. However, only one solution is randomly created for each composer and N_s copies of this solution are assigned to him/her. Preliminary experiments proved that this allows a slight reduction of the number of objective evaluations, without deteriorating the technique's performance. These solutions are subsequently evaluated for each objective, allowing the computation of a first estimation of the ideal vector: $\forall j \in \{1, \ldots, m\}$, $z_j^* = \min\{f_j(x)|x = P_{i,k,\star}, i = 1, \ldots, N_c, k = 1, \ldots, N_s\}$. The tunes can then be evaluated according to the composer's weight vectors in $g^{te}(x|\lambda, z^*)$.

4.3 Main Cycle

The main cycle consists of four steps performed by each composer.

  (i) Updating the Acquired Knowledge Matrix
Each composer randomly selects exactly one tune from each of his/her neighbors and includes it to his/her acquired knowledge matrix $ISC_{i,\star,\star}$, whatever its associated value of the Tchebycheff function.

  (ii) Creating a New Tune
As in the original MMC, each composer can generate new tunes according to

either his/her personal knowledge, the knowledge acquired from other agents or his/her own inspiration (a flash of genius). Thus, with probability cfg, each variable of the new solution is randomly set within its bound. Otherwise, it is built from solutions drawn from the composer's background knowledge (including both personal and acquired knowledges, see section 3). In this second case, the variable value is not computed, as in the initial MMC, through a three parent-crossover, but rather through the classical Differential Evolution mutation operator:

$$y_k = x_k^a + F \cdot (x_k^b - x_k^c) \tag{2}$$

where y_k is the kth variable of the mutant solution and x_k^a, x_k^b, x_k^c are drawn from $KM_{i,\star,k}$, e.g. the kth variable of three solutions of composer i's background knowledge. In any case, x^a is selected from composer i's personal artwork through a tournament technique. This tournament involves a random number of solutions from $P_{i,\star,\star}$ and the winner is the solution with the best value of the Tchebycheff fitness function. Regarding x^b and x^c, with probability ifg, these latter are randomly chosen from $P_{i,\star,\star}$; otherwise, they are randomly chosen from $ISC_{i,\star,\star}$, e.g. composer i's acquired knowledge. If the resulting variable value lies outside its bounds, it is randomly reset inside them.

(iii) Sharing the New Tune

The tune just created by composer i is subsequently proposed to his/her neighbors (composers having a similar weight vector). In order to avoid convergence to a single point, the new tune can be accepted by only one composer, in addition to the one who created it. The new solution should logically be assigned to the composer whose search is focused on the corresponding sub-region of the Pareto front, i.e. the composer that most benefits him/herself from this tune. This means that composer i and his/her neighbors first re-calculate the Tchebycheff fitness function according to their own weight vector and normalized objective values. The composer with the lowest resulting $g^{te}(x|\lambda, z^*)$ value can accept the new tune. If he/she rejects it, the tune is then proposed to the composer with the second lowest $g^{te}(x|\lambda, z^*)$ value, who may accept it, and so on. If no composer accepts the new tune, this one is thrown away.

(iv) Accepting the New Tune

Every time a recently created tune is proposed to a composer, this latter can accept o reject it. The acceptance criterion is performed with respect to his/her personal artwork. If the Tchebycheff fitness function of the new tune is lower than that of the composer's worst tune, $P_{i,worst,\star}$, then the new tune replaces $P_{i,worst,\star}$ in the composer's artwork. Otherwise, the tune is either proposed to another neighboring composer or thrown away.

The above-described instructions are repeated until a user-defined number of iterations is reached. When concluding, the final number of solutions in the society is still $N_c \times N_s$. This number must be reduced to N_c in order to produce only one solution for each search direction (weight vector). Therefore, the fast Pareto sorting procedure from the NSGA-II technique [2] is applied. If the resulting number of non-dominated solutions is still higher than N_c, it is further reduced through a clustering procedure similar to that introduced in [1].

Note that, in contrast with a great majority of state-of-the-art techniques, no diversity preservation technique is included in the MO-MMC since it appears that the weight-based decomposition approach provides by itself means for diversifying the search. In the same way, no external archive maintenance nor Pareto sorting procedure are carried out during the search process, but at the end of the execution, which just involves a marginal increase in the run time. However, as previously mentioned, the proposed MO-MMC represents a first version, which might be improved including the above mentioned features if necessary.

4.4   Algorithm

Summarizing, the MO-MMC algorithm can be stated as follows:

Step 1. Initialization.
 1.1 Create a set of N_c uniformly distributed weight vectors, $\{\lambda^1, \ldots, \lambda^N\}$.
 1.2 Create an artificial society of N_c composers and assign a weight vector λ^i to each composer i.
 1.3 Create the social network as undirected links between each composer and the $N_c \times c_{fla}$ composers with closest weight vectors.
 1.4 For each composer i, randomly initialize one tune within the bounds of each variable of the considered n-dimensional MOP. Store N_s copies of this tune in $P_{i,\star,\star}$. Compute objective functions of the created tunes.
 1.5 Initialize $z^* = (z_1^*, \ldots, z_m^*)^T$ and the iteration counter $t = 0$.

Step 2. Main cycle. While $t < t_{max}$, do for each composer i:
 2.1 Update the acquired knowledge matrix $ISC_{i,\star,\star}$ by randomly selecting one tune of each of composer i's neighbors.
 2.2 Select tune x^a from $P_{i,\star,\star}$ through a random size tournament using the Tchebycheff function as a criterion.
 2.3 If $rnd < ifg$, randomly select x^b and x^c in $P_{i,\star,\star}$; otherwise, randomly select x^b and x^c in $ISC_{i,\star,\star}$.
 2.4 For each variable $k = 1, \ldots, n$, if $rnd < cfg$ create randomly a new variable y_k; otherwise, compute y_k from equation 2.
 2.5 Compute objective functions of the new tune and possibly update z^*.
 2.6 Composer i accepts the new tune if it is better that the worst one of his/her artwork, $P_{i,worst,\star}$, in terms of the Tchebycheff function.
 2.7 For each composer i' neighbor of i, compute $g^{te}(y|\lambda^{i'}, z^*)$.
 2.8 Propose the new tune to composer i' in increasing order of $g^{te}(y|\lambda^{i'}, z^*)$:
  - if $g^{te}(y|\lambda^{i'}, z^*) < g^{te}(P_{i',worst,\star}|\lambda^{i'}, z^*)$ then y replaces $P_{i',worst,\star}$.
  - otherwise, either propose y to another neighbor or throw it away.
 2.9 Increment the iteration counter $t \leftarrow t + 1$.

Step 3. Conclusion.
 3.1 Apply the fast Pareto sorting procedure to the $N_c \times N_s$ final solutions to obtain the approximated Pareto set $\mathcal{P}$.
 3.2 If the number of non-dominated solutions is higher than N_c, apply clustering to $\mathcal{P}$. Output $\mathcal{P}$.

In the previous description, rnd is a uniform random number generated in [0,1].

5   Computational Experiments

In order to assess the performance of the proposed MO-MMC, it is evaluated on several test-suites commonly used in the specialized literature: five of the two-objective ZDT test functions from [18] (ZDT5 is not considered since it is a binary problem) and the three-objective DTLZ2 function from [19]. 30 decision variables were used for ZDT1, ZDT2 and ZDT3, while ZDT4, ZDT6 and DTLZ2 were tested using 10 decision variables. The MO-MMC performance level is subsequently compared with other techniques whose results are available in the specialized literature. Two state-of-the-art MOEAs, namely NSGA-II [2] and MOEA/D [3] were considered, as well as two multi-objective PSO implementations, MOPSO [5] and MOPSO-PD [11]. Note that these techniques include different paradigms (EA and PSO), as well as different approaches for dealing with MOPs (dominance and decomposition).

In order to compare the above-mentioned algorithms, the Inverted Generational Distance ($\mathcal{IGD}$) is used in this study. The advantage of this metric is that it does not only account for convergence to the real Pareto front $\mathcal{PF}^*$ but also for the even distribution of the approximated front $\mathcal{PF}_{ap}$ when a uniform sample of $\mathcal{PF}^*$ is known.

5.1   Experimental Settings

For each test function, 30 independent runs were performed with each algorithm. The parameters used in MO-MMC are summarized in Table 1. In addition to these parameters, the maximum iteration number was set in order to provide a fair number of objective evaluations, regarding the algorithms MO-MMC is compared with. Thus, 250 (resp. 500) iterations were used when comparing with the EAs for two-objective (resp. three-objective) test functions, while 200 iterations were used when comparing with the MOPSOs.

Regarding the EAs, they use a population size of 100 (resp. 300) solutions for two-objective test instances (resp. three-objective test instances). They report a 100 (resp. 300) for points approximate Pareto front after 250 generations, therefore using 25,000 (resp. 75,000) objective evaluations [3]. Both EAs use SBX crossover and polynomial mutation. The $\mathcal{IGD}$ metric is computed with 500 points in $\mathcal{PF}^*$ for 2-objective functions and 990 points for 3-objective functions.

With respect to the two PSO-based algorithms, the results in [11] were reported for swarm sizes of 100 particles. The global archive contains 100 solutions, obtained after 20,000 objective evaluations. However in this case, the authors do not indicate the number of points in $\mathcal{PF}^*$ used to compute the $\mathcal{IGD}$ metric, so the results reported here for the MO-MMC are for 100 points (which looked like the most difficult conditions).

5.2   Results and Discussion

Figure 1 shows the final Pareto fronts obtained by the MO-MMC algorithm for the tackled test functions. These plots show the final set of non-dominated

Table 1. Parameters for MO-MMC

	Parameter	Value
N	Number of composers and weight vectors	100 (2-obj.) or 150 (3-obj.)
N_s	Tunes in artwork	3
ifg	Factor for creating tunes based on own artwork	0.35
cfg	Factor for creating random tunes (genius)	0.01
c_{fla}	Proportion of neighbors in artificial society	0.1
F	Parameter for DE mutation operator	0.5

solutions found for a random run out of the 30 performed for each problem. In addition, the results obtained for the $\mathcal{IGD}$ metric, compared with those of the above-mentioned challenging algorithms, are presented in tables 2 and 3. In both tables, the reported data are the mean value and, in parentheses, the standard deviation, computed over the 30 runs.

From table 2, MO-MMC clearly outperforms the NSGA-II and the MOEA/D for all test functions but ZDT3, for which the NSGA-II obtains the best results. However on this problem, the MO-MMC still provides a better $\mathcal{IGD}$ value than MOEA/D. Regarding standard deviation, the very low values of MO-MMC confirm the robustness of the proposed algorithm.

Table 2. MO-MMC $\mathcal{IGD}$ values compared with EAs

Instance	NSGA-II	MOEA/D	MO-MMC
ZDT1	0.0050 (0.0002)	0.0055 (0.0039)	**0.0040** (0.0000)
ZDT2	0.0049 (0.0002)	0.0079 (0.0109)	**0.0038** (0.0000)
ZDT3	**0.0065** (0.0054)	0.0143 (0.0091)	0.0103 (0.0001)
ZDT4	0.0182 (0.0237)	0.0076 (0.0023)	**0.0041** (0.0001)
ZDT6	0.0169 (0.0028)	0.0042 (0.0003)	**0.0032** (0.0000)
DTLZ2	0.0417 (0.0013)	0.0389 (0.0001)	**0.0373** (0.0011)

Concerning the comparison with the two PSO-based techniques, MOPSO is clearly outperformed for all test problems. MOPSO-PD obtains the best results for ZDT3 and ZDT4 functions, although with a very marginal difference with MO-MMC. This latter outperforms MOPSO-PD for all the remaining instances, in some cases with a significant difference (particularly for ZDT2 and ZDT6). So, the conclusions of the computational experiments are clearly in favor of the MO-MMC algorithm. The $\mathcal{IGD}$ metric confirms the quality of the proposed approach, as well as the graphs of the obtained Pareto fronts showed in figure 1. In all cases,

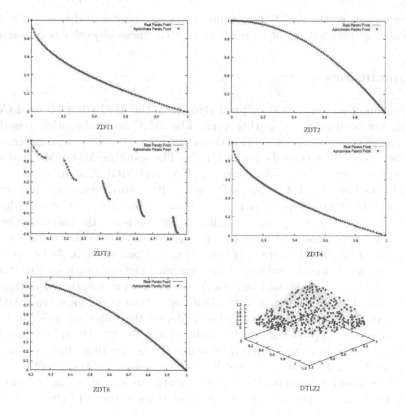

Fig. 1. Pareto fronts obtained by the MO-MMC

Table 3. MO-MMC $\mathcal{IGD}$ values compared with MOPSOs

Instance	MOPSO-PD	MOPSO	MO-MMC
ZDT1	0.0053 –	0.1248 –	**0.0039** (0.0001)
ZDT2	0.2782 –	0.5530 –	**0.0041** (0.0000)
ZDT3	**0.0099** –	0.5524 –	0.0100 (0.0001)
ZDT4	**0.0040** –	0.0775 –	0.0045 (0.0004)
ZDT6	0.0459 –	0.0534 –	**0.0031** (0.0001)
DTLZ2	0.0717 –	0.4079 –	**0.0569** (0.0040)

the convergence to the real Pareto front seems excellent and dispersion is also satisfactory, although it might be improved for the three-objective test function.

6 Conclusions

An extension of a recent socio-cultural algorithm, the Method of Musical Composition, has been proposed in this work. The MMC is an algorithm based on both creativity and social interaction concepts, whose main internal procedures had to be modified for the solution of MOPs. The resulting MO-MMC was able to outperform several state-of-the-art MOEAs and MOPSOs, in most of the test problems considered, for the IGD metric. It is worth recalling that, given a uniformly distributed sample of the real Pareto front, this metric provides an assessment for both convergence and uniform distribution of the points in the approximated Pareto front, justifying that it was the only one required for the MO competition of the 2009 Congress on Evolutionary Computation. As perspective of future works, however, additional performance metrics (such as the Pareto compliant hypervolume) should be considered. Besides, as mentioned in this paper, the present MO-MMC is the first adaptation of the MMC for solving MOPs, and the technique might be improved considering the following guidelines: *(i)* the decomposition approach might be changed to a Penalty Boundary Intersection strategy, *(ii)* some technique promoting the search diversification should be integrated in order to improve results for three-objective test functions, and *(iii)* more exhaustive computational experimentation should be carried out, for instance with small populations to study regularities in the approximated front.

References

1. Zitzler, E., Laumanns, M., Thiele, L.: SPEA2: Improving the Strength Pareto Evolutionary Algorithm. In: Giannakoglou, K., Tsahalis, D., Periaux, J., Papailou, P., Fogarty, T. (eds.) EUROGEN 2001. Evolutionary Methods for Design, Optimization and Control with Applications to Industrial Problems, Athens, Greece, pp. 95–100 (2002)
2. Deb, K., Pratap, A., Agarwal, S., Meyarivan, T.: A fast elitist multi-objective genetic algorithm: NSGA-II. IEEE Transactions on Evolutionary Computation 6, 182–197 (2002)
3. Zhang, Q., Li, H.: MOEA/D: A multiobjective evolutionary algorithm based on decomposition. IEEE Transactions on Evolutionary Computation 11, 712–731 (2007)
4. Emmerich, M., Beume, N., Naujoks, B.: An EMO algorithm using the hypervolume measure as selection criterion. In: Coello Coello, C.A., Hernández Aguirre, A., Zitzler, E. (eds.) EMO 2005. LNCS, vol. 3410, pp. 62–76. Springer, Heidelberg (2005)
5. Coello Coello, C.A., Pulido, G.T., Lechuga, M.S.: Handling multiple objectives with particle swarm optimization. IEEE Transactions on Evolutionary Computation 8, 256–279 (2004)
6. Mora Gutiérrez, R., Ramírez-Rodríguez, J., García, E.R.: An optimization algorithm inspired by musical composition. Artificial Intelligence Review (2012)

7. Coello Coello, C.A., Lamont, G., Veldhuizen, D.V.: Evolutionary Algorithms for Solving Multi-Objective Problems, 2nd edn. Springer, New York (2007) ISBN 978-0-387-33254-3
8. Zapotecas Martínez, S., Coello Coello, C.A.: A multi-objective particle swarm optimizer based on decomposition. In: Proceedings of the 13th Annual Conference on Genetic and Evolutionary Computation (GECCO 2011), pp. 69–76. ACM (2011)
9. Al Moubayed, N., Petrovski, A., McCall, J.: D^2MOPSO: Multi-objective particle swarm optimizer based on decomposition and dominance. In: Hao, J.-K., Middendorf, M. (eds.) EvoCOP 2012. LNCS, vol. 7245, pp. 75–86. Springer, Heidelberg (2012)
10. Liu, Y., Niu, B.: A multi-objective particle swarm optimization based on decomposition. In: Huang, D.-S., Gupta, P., Wang, L., Gromiha, M. (eds.) ICIC 2013. CCIS, vol. 375, pp. 200–205. Springer, Heidelberg (2013)
11. Zhao, Y., Liu, H.L.: Multi-objective particle swarm optimization algorithm based on population decomposition. In: Yin, H., et al. (eds.) IDEAL 2013. LNCS, vol. 8206, pp. 463–470. Springer, Heidelberg (2013)
12. Cheng, J., Zhang, G., Li, Z., Li, Y.: Multi-objective ant colony optimization based on decomposition for bi-objective traveling salesman problems. Soft Computing 16, 597–614 (2012)
13. Ke, L., Zhang, Q., Battiti, R.: MOEA/D-ACO: A multiobjective evolutionary algorithm using decomposition and ant colony. IEEE Transactions on Cybernetics 43, 1845–1859 (2013)
14. Coello Coello, C.A., Becerra, R.L.: Evolutionary multiobjective optimization using a cultural algorithm. In: Proceedings of the 2003 IEEE Swarm Intelligence Symposium, Indianapolis, USA, pp. 6–13. IEEE service center (2003)
15. Best, C., Che, X., Reynolds, R.G., Liu, D.: Multi objective cultural algorithm. In: Proceedings of the 2010 IEEE Congress on Evolutionary Computation (CEC 2010), Barcelona, Spain, pp. 1–9. IEEE service center (2010)
16. Reynolds, R.G., Liu, D.: Multi-objective cultural algorithm. In: Proceedings of the 2011 IEEE Congress on Evolutionary Computation (CEC 2011), New Orleans, USA, pp. 1233–1241. IEEE service center (2011)
17. Mora Gutiérrez, R., Ramírez-Rodríguez, J., García, E.R., Ponsich, A., Herrera, O.: Adaptation of the musical composition method for solving constrained optimization problems. Soft Computing (in press, 2014)
18. Zitzler, E., Deb, K., Thiele, L.: Comparison of multiobjective evolutionary algorithms: Empirical results. Evolutionary Computation 8, 173–195 (2000)
19. Deb, K., Thiele, L., Laumanns, M., Zitzler, E.: Scalable test problems for evolutionary multiobjective optimization. In: Abraham, A., Jain, L., Goldberg, R. (eds.) Evolutionary Multiobjective Optimization. Theoretical Advances and Applications, pp. 15–145. Springer, USA (2005)

k-Nearest-Neighbor by Differential Evolution for Time Series Forecasting

Erick De La Vega, Juan J. Flores,
and Mario Graff

Universidad Michoacana de San Nicolás de Hidalgo
División de Estudios de Posgrado, Facultad de Ingeniería Eléctrica
Santiago Tapia 403 Centro, Morelia, Michoacán, México, CP 58000
edelavega@dep.fie.umich.mx, juanf@umich.mx, mgraffg@gmail.com

Abstract. A framework for time series forecasting that integrates k-Nearest-Neighbors (kNN) and Differential Evolution (DE) is proposed. The methodology called NNDEF (Nearest Neighbor - Differential Evolution Forecasting) is based on knowledge shared from nearest neighbors with previous similar behaviour, which are then taken into account to forecast. NNDEF relies on the assumption that observations in the past similar to the present ones are also likely to have similar outcomes. The main advantages of NNDEF are the ability to predict complex nonlinear behavior and handling large amounts of data. Experiments have shown that DE can optimize the parameters of kNN and improve the accuracy of the predictions.

Keywords: Time Series Forecasting, Prediction, k-Nearest-Neighbor, Differential Evolution.

1 Introduction

A time series is defined as a set of quantitative observations arranged in chronological order [9], where we generally assume that time is a discrete variable. Examples of time series are commonly found in the fields of engineering, science, sociology, and economics, among others [3]; time series are analysed to understand the past and to predict the future [5]. This forecast must be as accurate as possible, since it can be linked to activities involving marketing decisions, product sales, stock market indices, and electricity load demand, among others.

In many occasions, it is fairly simple and straightforward to forecast the next value of the time series. But the further we delve into the future, the more uncertain we are and the bigger forecast errors we get.

Some statistical models such as autoregressive models [20] can be used for time series modelling and forecasting. These traditional forecasting techniques are based on linear models, however many of the time series encountered in practice exhibit characteristics not shown by linear processes. If the time series is confirmed to be nonlinear, very rich dynamic possibilities can emerge, including sensibility to initial conditions, known as chaotic behaviour [13].

A. Gelbukh et al. (Eds.): MICAI 2014, Part II, LNAI 8857, pp. 50–60, 2014.
© Springer International Publishing Switzerland 2014

In the past, several methods have been proposed to predict chaotic time series. One of the first methods proposed was the modeling of the system using Nonlinear Models (NLM) [8], but the main problems of this approach are proper model selection and data-dependency.

Another approach to solve the time series forecasting problem is Artificial Neural Networks (ANNs) [15]. The ANNs are trained to learn the relationships between the input variables and historical patterns, however the main disadvantage of ANNs is the required learning procedure.

More recently, classification techniques based on the nearest neighbours have been successfully applied in different areas from the traditional pattern recognition. The k-Nearest-Neighbors (kNN) [4] is an algorithm that can be employed in time series forecasting due to its simplicity and intuitiveness. kNN searches for similar instances recovering them from large dimensional feature spaces and incomplete data [8]. The kNN algorithm assumes that subsequences of the time series that emerged in the past are likely to have a resemblance to the future subsequences and can be used for generating kNN-based forecasts.

One significant drawback of the kNN forecasting method is the sensitivity to changes in the input parameters, (i.e the number of nearest neighbors and the embedding dimension). If the input parameters are not selected appropriately, it could decrease the accuracy of the forecasts.

One way to select the best posible input parameters for the kNN method is using an algorithm of the Evolutionary Computation (EC) family [16]. EC is a computational technology made up of a collection of randomized global search paradigms for finding the optimal solutions to a given problem. In particular, Differential Evolution (DE) is a population-based search strategy that has recently proven to be a valuable method for optimizing real valued multi-modal objective functions [19,22]. It is a parallel direct search method having good convergence properties and simplicity in implementation.

In this work, we propose a combination of two techniques: kNN, applied to time series forecasting and DE for parameter optimization. The rest of the work is organized as follows: a brief introduction to the kNN forecasting methods is described in Section 2. The proposed technique is discussed in Section 3. Section 4 contains the explanation of the datasets used in this work and discusses the results obtained using the proposed approach. Finally, Section 5 presents the conclusions of the proposed methods and experiments.

2   k-Nearest-Neighbors Forecast

The kNN approximation method is a very simple, but powerful one. It has been used in many different applications and particularly in classification tasks [21]. For this purpose, kNN uses the average of the forecast of the k objects, without taking into account assumptions on the distribution of predicting variables during the learning process.

The key idea behind the kNN is that similar training samples most likely will have similar output values. One has to look for a certain number of nearest neighbors, according to some distance. The distance usually used to determine the similarity metric between the objects is the Euclidean distance. However, the method also permits the use of other distance measures like Chebyshev, Manhattan, and Mahalanobis [1]. Once we find the neighbors, we compute an estimation of the output simply by using the average of the outputs of the neighbors in the neighborhood.

In contrast to statistical methods that try to identify a model from the available data, the kNN method uses the training set as the model [14]. The main advantage of kNN is the effectiveness in situations where the training dataset is large and contains deterministic structures.

2.1   One-Step-Ahead Forecasting

Let $\mathbb{S} = \{s_1, s_2, \ldots, s_t \ldots, s_N\}$ be a time series, where s_t is the recorded value of variable s at time t. The forecasting problem targets the estimation of Δn consecutive future values, i.e. $\{s_{N+1}, s_{N+2}, \ldots s_{N+\Delta n}\}$, using any of the currently available observations from $\mathbb{S}$ [7].

If we choose a delay time τ and an embedding dimension m, it is possible to construct delay vectors of the form $\mathbf{S}_t = [s_{t-(m-1)\tau}, s_{t-(m-2)\tau}, \ldots, s_{t-\tau}, s_t]$, where $m > 0$ and $t > 0$. The time series is then organized in a training set by running a sliding window $\mathbf{S}_N$ of size m along each delay vector. To retrieve the k nearest neighbors of $\mathbf{S}_N$ we choose the parameter ϵ and calculate the distance to every delay vector $\mathbf{S}_t$, where $t = (m-1)\tau + 1, (m-1)\tau + 2, \ldots, N - 1$.

For all the k vectors $\mathbf{S}_t$ that satisfy Equation (1) we look up the individual values $s_{t+\Delta n}$.

$$|\mathbf{S}_N - \mathbf{S}_t| \leq \epsilon \tag{1}$$

The forecast is then the average of all these individual values, expressed by Equation (2),

$$\hat{s}_{N+\Delta n} = \frac{1}{k} \sum_{j=1}^{k} s_{t+\Delta n} \tag{2}$$

where $\hat{s}_{N+\Delta n}$ is the forecasted value at time N.

In the case where we do not find any neighbors, we just pick the closest vector to $\mathbf{S}_N$. In order to forecast a sequence of future values we use real data as input, that is, $FS(s_t) = \hat{s}_{t+\Delta n}$, where FS is the one-step-ahead forecasting function.

Note that when $\Delta n = 1$, Equation (2) produces only one forecast, however in many occasions, it is neccesary to forecast more than one value at the time. For this purpose, two strategies have been used in the past, the iterative or recursive scheme and the simultaneous or direct scheme [21].

2.2   Iterative Forecasting

In the iterative forecasting strategy, a single point is predicted at a time and it is afterwards appended to $\mathbb{S}$ for subsequent forecasts. Iterative forecasting can be computed by Equation (3).

$$FS(\dot{s}_t) = s_{t+k\Delta n} \quad k \in [1, \ldots, m]$$
$$\text{where} \quad \dot{s}_t \begin{cases} s_t \text{ if } t \leq N \\ \hat{s}_t \text{ otherwise} \end{cases} \tag{3}$$

This process is repeated until the number of forecasts is reached. In this way, we are applying a one-step-ahead forecast many times, iteratively. This scheme presents a caveat: if the errors are non-zero and the forecasts are used as inputs repeatedly, a cumulative prediction error is included in the forecasts. Iterative predictions are more accurate for short horizons, but since the prediction error accumulates, this method is not recommended for long horizons.

2.3 Simultaneous Forecasting

Compared to the iterative strategy, it is possible to forecast Δn from the same input data as can be seen from Equation (4).

$$\hat{s}_{N+r\Delta n} = \frac{1}{k} \sum_{j=1}^{k} s_{t+r\Delta n} \quad r \in [1, \ldots, m] \tag{4}$$

The simultaneous strategy always uses the real measured data as inputs. No forecasts are introduced to $\mathbb{S}$, also, there is no cumulative error introduced through the inputs, because only original data values are used in the forecast of future values. Each time step only the normal prediction error is present and there is no cumulative prediction errors.

2.4 Forecast Model Accuracy

A measure of forecast accuracy must always be evaluated as part of a model validation effort. To evaluate the forecast performance we measure the mean absolute percentage error (MAPE) between the real and the forecasted value. The usage of MAPE is to measure the derivation between the predicted and actual values, the smaller values of MAPE, the closer the predicted and real values are. See [6] for more details.

3   Optimizing kNN with DE

As mentioned before, in order to generate an accurate output, it is necessary to optimize the value of the parameters of kNN (m, τ, and ϵ). For this purpose, we use DE to minimize the prediction error on the training set.

DE was developed by Storn and Price [19,22] around 1995 as an efficient and robust meta-heuristic to optimize functions of arbitrary complexity. Like most algorithms in EC, DE is a population-based optimizer. Most of these methods produce new individuals, by different heuristic techniques, as perturbations of old ones. In this work, we focus on the classical version of DE, which applies the simple arithmetic operations: mutation, crossover, and selection to evolve the population.

The kNN parameters $[m, \tau] \in \mathbb{Z}^+$, while $\epsilon \in \mathbb{R}^+$. When using DE as an optimizer, there are two considerations about these parameters: parameter types and boundary constraints.

The optimization task of the kNN parameters is a mixed-variable problem, because it contains both continuous and discrete parameters. DE handles this kind of problems by representing all parameters internally as real values and quantizing the discrete parameters values to the nearest allowed point [12]. For m and τ we use the quantizing function round i.e. $\lfloor \rceil$ to transform their continuous values to discrete values [18]. When working with discrete parameters, the objective function is evaluated once DE's continuous parameters values are quantized to (but not overwritten by) their nearest allowed discrete values. Equation (5) shows how the evaluation function of a kNN-DE vector is proposed,

$$f(x^{(g,i)}) = \text{kNN}(\lfloor m \rceil, \lfloor \tau \rceil, \epsilon) \tag{5}$$

where $x^{(g,i)}$ is the i-th individual of generation g.

In particular, we are trying to find $x^{(g,i)} = [x_1, x_2, \ldots, x_D]^T$, where $x^{(g,i)} \in \mathbb{R}^D$, to minimize the outcome of Equation (5) subject to $x_j^L \leq x_j^{(g,i)} \leq x_j^U$, where L is the set that contains the lower bounds of the parameters and U is the set that contains the upper bounds of the parameters. However, to satisfy the boundary constraints of the kNN parameters we have to take a look at DE's mutation scheme. In DE, each population vector is crossed with a randomly generated mutant vector. The mutation process is computed using Equation (6),

$$v^{(g,i)} = x^{(g,r_0)} + F(x^{(g,r_1)} - x^{(g,r_2)}) \tag{6}$$
$$\forall i \in [1, N_{pop}]$$

where r_0, r_1 and r_3 are randomly chosen vectors, F is a positive real number that controls the rate at which the population evolves, and N_{pop} is the population size.

Since the current population of vectors already satisfies all boundary constraints, only contributions from mutant vectors may violate the parameter limits. Consequently, bounds need to be checked only when a mutant parameter is selected for the trial vector.

A resseting method known as bounce-back [19], replaces a vector that has exceeded one or more of its bounds by a valid vector that satisfies all boundary constraints. The bounce-back strategy takes the progress toward the optimum into account by selecting a parameter value that lies between the base parameter value and the bound being violated.

When a mutant vector violates the parameter limits, Equations (7) and (8) replace those parameters to satisfy both upper and lower parameter bounds

$$v_j^{(g,i)} = x_j^{(g,r_0)} + w(x_j^L - x_j^{(g,r_0)}) \tag{7}$$

$$v_j^{(g,i)} = x_j^{(g,r_0)} + w(x_j^U - x_j^{(g,r_0)}) \tag{8}$$

where $w \sim U(0,1)$.

As the population moves towards its bounds, the bounce-back method generates vectors that will be located even closer to the bounds.

4 Results

This section describes the experimental results and performance evaluation of the proposed framework. For every experiment, each time series is divided into training and validation sets. The optimization model scheme described in Section 3 is used on the training set to obtain the best kNN parameter combination for every dataset. Once this parameters are obtained, we use the kNN forecasting methods described in Section 2 to produce 50 forecasts.

A comparison is made against AutoRegressive Integrated Moving Average (ARIMA) [6], using the same conditions. Comparisons with ARIMA models used to be problematic because some authors did not have sufficient expertise to fit a good ARIMA model, and so comparisons were sometimes made, for example, against a non-seasonal AR model when the data were obviously seasonal.

Table 1. ARIMA models and kNN parameters of the synthetic chaotic time series

Time series	Length	ARIMA model (p,d,q)	kNN-Parameters (m,τ,ϵ)
Logistic map	50000	$[0,0,0]$	$[1,1,3.55 \times 10^{-6}]$
Henon map	50000	$[4,0,5]$	$[2,1,3.12 \times 10^{-4}]$
Rossler attractor	50000	$[0,0,0]$	$[2,1,5.38 \times 10^{-4}]$
Lorenz attractor	50000	$[4,1,4]$	$[2,1,4.87 \times 10^{-4}]$
Mackey Glass	50000	$[1,0,4]$	$[3,1,9.47 \times 10^{-4}]$

Table 2. MAPE results for the synthetic chaotic time series

Time series	ARIMA One-step-ahead	kNN One-step-ahead	ARIMA	kNN Iterative	kNN Simultaneous
Logistic map	1426.5830	0.0138	1426.5830	280.6294	197.7657
Henon map	88.6130	0.0726	90.3512	111.0744	109.6362
Rossler	141.2604	5.4727	141.2604	75.3095	75.3095
Lorenz attractor	0.0007	0.3161	18.4772	1.9910	1.9910
Mackey Glass	0.0621	0.0711	17.4304	0.4734	0.1233

This should no longer be a problem as there are now good automatic ARIMA algorithms such as auto.arima() in the forecast package for the R language [2].

The experiments were performed in several datasets divided in two categories: Synthetic chaotic functions and the Santa Fe competition [23]. NNDEF has been tested with about twenty time series; we are reporting only ten of them in this paper for conciseness.

4.1 Synthetic Chaotic Time Series

Five synthetic chaotic time series were assessed, including the logistic map, the Henon map, the Rossler attractor, the Lorenz attractor, and the Mackey-Glass

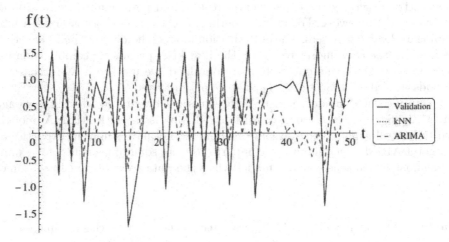

Fig. 1. Henon map time series. Real data and forecast data using one-step-ahead kNN and ARIMA

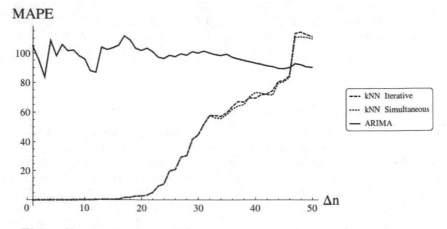

Fig. 2. Henon map time series. Prediction error versus prediction horizon

Table 3. ARIMA models and kNN parameters of the Santa Fe competition

Time series	Length	ARIMA model (p,d,q)	kNN-Parameters (m,τ,ϵ)
Laser	1000	$[4, 0, 2]$	$[8, 1, 8.49 \times 10^{-4}]$
Blood Oxigen	17000	$[4, 1, 4]$	$[1, 6, 3.42 \times 10^{-5}]$
Exchange Rate	15000	$[1, 1, 0]$	$[3, 2, 2.72 \times 10^{-4}]$
Particle	50000	$[5, 0, 4]$	$[4, 1, 5.64 \times 10^{-4}]$
Astrophysical	27204	$[4, 0, 5]$	$[1, 3, 2.11 \times 10^{-4}]$

Table 4. MAPE results of the Santa Fe competition

Time series	ARIMA One-step-ahead	kNN One-step-ahead	ARIMA Iterative	kNN Iterative	kNN Simultaneous
Laser	15.6203	6.3895	46.8827	18.1955	18.1955
Blood Oxigen	0.4903	0.5587	3.8206	3.6817	3.2346
Exchange rate	0.0298	0.0319	0.1065	0.0751	0.2293
Particle	6.4407	7.6367	38.8431	49.9560	49.9560
Astrophysical	176.7445	159.6290	137.5924	134.2523	117.2364

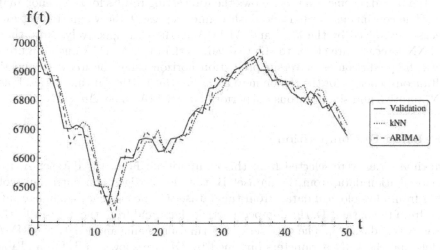

Fig. 3. Blood oxigen time series. Real data and forecast data using one-step-ahead kNN and ARIMA

delay differential equation [8,10,11,17]. The time series information (name and length), the ARIMA models and the kNN parameters obtained by DE are shown in Table 1. The results for one-step-ahead, iterative and simultaneous using ARIMA and kNN are shown in Table 2, where the lowest MAPE has been highlighted in bold. As expected, the deterministic structures found in the syntethic chaotic time series can be exploited by kNN, obtaining better results than

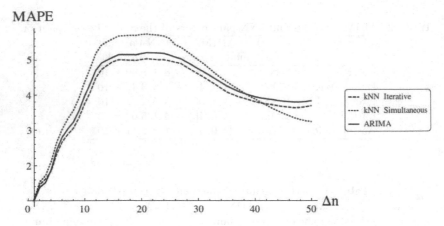

Fig. 4. Blood oxigen time series. Prediction error versus prediction horizon

ARIMA in three out of five time series for the one-step-ahead scheme and in four out of five time series for the iterative and simultaneous schemes. Finally, due to space constraints, we only present the real and forecasted values using the one-step-ahead scheme. Figure 1 shows the forecasting results for the Henon map data. The continuous, dotted and dashed lines represent the validation set and forecasts produced by the kNN and ARIMA methods, respectively. Note that, the kNN forecasts are closer to the real values than the ARIMA ones. Figure 2 shows the prediction error versus prediction horizon using the iterative and simultaneous schemes for the Henon map data. For this particular time series, both kNN iterative and simultaneous outperformed ARIMA when $\Delta n = 1, \ldots, 48$.

4.2   Santa Fe Competition

Five time series were selected from this competition: From the dataset A, the laser oscillation data, from the dataset B, the blood oxygen concentration (collected from physiological data), from the dataset C, the currency exchange rate data, from the dataset D, the damped particle data, and from the dataset E, the astrophysical data [23]. The time series information (name and length), ARIMA models and the kNN parameters obtained by DE are shown in Table 3. Table 4 shows the results for one-step-ahead, iterative, and simultaneous forecasting using kNN and ARIMA, where the lowest MAPE has been highlighted in bold. Although ARIMA performed better in three of five time series for the one-step-ahead scheme, the difference between those errors are insignificant. On the other hand, for the iterative and simultaneous schemes, kNN outperformed ARIMA in four out of five time series. Figure 3 shows the real and forecasted values using the one-step-ahead scheme. The continuous, dotted and dashed lines represent the validation set and forecasts produced by the kNN and ARIMA methods, respectively. Figure 4 shows the prediction error versus prediction horizon using the iterative and simultaneous schemes for the blood oxygen concentration data.

For this particular time series, kNN performs as good as ARIMA in the one-step-ahead, iterative and simultaneous schemes. It wins more time than looses although the difference is not as much as for synthetic time series.

5 Conclusions

Time series forecasting is useful in many research areas. In this paper, we presented the solution to three time series forecasting problems: one-step-ahead, iterative, and simultaneous forecasting. The proposed methods to deal with these forecasting problems are based on a combination between kNN and DE. kNN is used to forecast values and DE is used to optimize kNN's parameters. The results in all three problems proved our approach to be more accurate when implemented with DE, because we found the best parameter combination for every time series.

All the time series used were large datasets with complex data that it becomes dificult to process using traditional methods, however, the kNN forecasting methods proved to be efficient and consistent in their predictions, furthermore, they only need data to work with and do not require the selection of a proper model.

The experiments results showed that for the one-step-ahead forecasting problem, kNN is more reliable than ARIMA because for some instances of time series, ARIMA was not even capable of producing a model. On the other hand, for the iterative and simultaneous forecasting problem, kNN outperforms ARIMA in most cases. kNN can be very effective, especially when the prediction horizon ranges from short to moderate.

References

1. Baldi, P., Brunak, S.: Bioinformatics: the machine learning approach. MIT press (2001)
2. Barker, T.: Pro Data Visualization Using R and JavaScript. Apress (2013)
3. Brookwell, P.J., Davis, R.A.: Introduction to Time Series and Forecasting. Springer (2002)
4. Casdagli, M.: Nonlinear prediction of chaotic time series. Physica D: Nonlinear Phenomena 35(3), 335–356 (1989)
5. Cowpertwait, P.S., Metcalfe, A.V.: Introductory Time Series with R. Springer (2009)
6. Douglas, C., Montgomery, C.L.J., Kulahci, M.: Introduction To Time Series Analysis and Forecasting. Wiley-Interscience (2008)
7. Dragomir Yankov, D.D., Keogh, E.: Ensembles of nearest neighbor forecasts. ECMIL 1, 545–556 (2006)
8. Farmer, J.D., Sidorowich, J.J.: Predicting chaotic time series. Physical Review Letters 59(8), 845 (1987)
9. Gebhard Kirchgssner, J.W., Hassler, U.: Introduction To Modern Time Series Analysis. Springer (2013)
10. Grassberger, P., Procaccia, I.: Characterization of strange attractors. Physical Review Letters 50(5), 346 (1983)

11. Guckenheimer, J., Williams, R.F.: Structural stability of lorenz attractors. Publications Mathématiques de l'IHÉS 50(1), 59–72 (1979)
12. Lampinen, J., Zelinka, I.: Mixed integer-discrete-continuous optimization by differential evolution-part 1: the optimization method. In: Czech Republic. Brno University of Technology. Citeseer (1999)
13. Leven, R., Koch, B.: Chaotic behaviour of a parametrically excited damped pendulum. Physics Letters A 86(2), 71–74 (1981)
14. Troncoso Lora, A., Riquelme, J.C., Martínez Ramos, J.L., Riquelme Santos, J.M., Gómez Expósito, A.: Influence of kNN-based load forecasting errors on optimal energy production. In: Pires, F.M., Abreu, S.P. (eds.) EPIA 2003. LNCS (LNAI), vol. 2902, pp. 189–203. Springer, Heidelberg (2003)
15. Maguire, L.P., Roche, B., McGinnity, T.M., McDaid, L.: Predicting a chaotic time series using a fuzzy neural network. Information Sciences 112(1), 125–136 (1998)
16. Palit, A.K., Popovic, D.: Computational Intelligence in Time Series Forecasting. Springer (2005)
17. Pecora, L.M., Carroll, T.L.: Synchronization in chaotic systems. Physical Review Letters 64(8), 821 (1990)
18. Rabiner, L.R., Gold, B.: Theory and application of digital signal processing, vol. 777, p. 1. Prentice-Hall, Inc., Englewood Cliffs (1975)
19. Rainer Storn, K.P., Lampinen, J.: Differential Evolution A Practical Aproach to Global Optimization. Springer, Berlin (2005)
20. Shumway, R.H., Stoffer, D.S.: Time Series Analysis and its Applications. Springer (2011)
21. Sorjamaa, A., Lendsasse, A.: Time series prediction using dir-rec strategy. In: ESANN Proceedings-European Symposium on ANN's (2006)
22. Storn, R., Price, K.: Differential evolution- a simple and efficient heuristic for global optimization over continuous spaces. Global Optimization 11, 341–359 (1995)
23. Weigend, A.S., Gershenfeld, N.A.: Results of the time series prediction competition at the santa fe institute. In: IEEE International Conference on Neural Networks, pp. 1786–1793. IEEE (1993)

A Binary Differential Evolution with Adaptive Parameters Applied to the Multiple Knapsack Problem

Leanderson André and Rafael Stubs Parpinelli

Graduate Program in Applied Computing
Department of Computer Science,
State University of Santa Catarina, Joinville, Brazil
leanderson.andre@gmail.com, rafael.parpinelli@udesc.br
http://www.cct.udesc.br

Abstract. This paper introduces an adaptive Binary Differential Evolution (aBDE) that self adjusts two parameters of the algorithm: perturbation and mutation rates. The well-known 0-1 Multiple Knapsack Problem (MKP) is addressed to validate the performance of the method. The MKP is a NP-hard optimization problem and the aim is to maximize the total profit subjected to the total weight in each knapsack that must be less than or equal to a given limit. Results were obtained using 11 instances of the problem with different degrees of complexity. The results were compared using aBDE, BDE, a standard Genetic Algorithm (GA), and its adaptive version (aGA). The results show that aBDE obtained better results than the other algorithms. This indicates that the proposed approach is an interesting and promising strategy for control of parameters and for optimization of complex problems.

Keywords: Adaptive Parameter Control, Binary Differential Evolution, Multiple Knapsack Problem, Evolutionary Computation.

1 Introduction

The optimization of resource allocation is one major concern in several areas of logistics, transportation and production [8]. A well-known problem of this class is the 0-1 Multiple Knapsack Problem (MKP). The MKP is a binary NP-hard combinatorial optimization problem that consists in given a set of items and a set of knapsacks, each item with a mass and a value, determine which item to include in which knapsack. The aim is to maximize the total profit subjected to the total weight in each knapsack that must be less than or equal to a given limit.

Different variants of the MKP can be easily adapted to real problems, such as, capital budgeting, cargo loading and others [15]. Hence, the search for efficient methods to achieve such optimization aims to increase profits and reduce the use of raw materials.

A. Gelbukh et al. (Eds.): MICAI 2014, Part II, LNAI 8857, pp. 61–71, 2014.

According to the size of an instance (number of items and number of knapsacks) of the MKP, the search space can become too large to apply exact methods. Hence, a large number of heuristics and metaheuristics have been applied to the MKP. Some examples are the modified binary particle swarm optimization [4], the binary artificial fish swarm algorithm [3], and the binary fruit fly optimization algorithm [16]. In this work, is investigated the performance of a Differential Evolution algorithm designed for binary problems with adaptive parameters.

The Differential Evolution (DE) algorithm is an Evolutionary Algorithm which is inspired by the laws of Darwin where stronger and adapted individuals have greater chances to survive and evolve [13]. In this analogy, the individuals are candidate solutions to optimize a given problem and the environment is the search space. Evolutionary Algorithms simulate the evolution of individuals through the selection, reproduction, crossover and mutation methods, stochastically producing better solutions at each generation [5]. It is well documented in the literature that DE has a huge ability to perform well in continuous-valued search spaces [17]. However, for discrete or binary search spaces some adaptations are required [11]. Hence, this paper applies a Binary Differential Evolution (BDE) algorithm that is able to handle binary problems, in particular the 0-1 MKP. The BDE algorithm was first applied in [12] for the 0-1 MKP and the results obtained were promising. BDE consists in applying simple operators (crossover and bit-flip mutation) in candidate solutions represented as binary strings. In this work several different instances are approached.

As most metaheuristic algorithms, DE also has some control parameters to be adjusted. It is known that the optimum values of the control parameters can change over the optimization process, directly influencing the efficiency of the method [6]. The parameters of an algorithm can be adjusted using one of two approaches: on-line or off-line. The off-line control, or parameter tuning, is performed prior to the execution of the algorithm. In this approach several tests are performed with different parameter settings in order to find good configurations for the parameters. In the on-line control, or parameter control, the values for the parameters change throughout the execution of the algorithm. The control of parameters during the optimization process has been used consistently by several optimization algorithms and applied in different problem domains [2] [14] [7] [1] [10]. In this way, a method to adapt the control parameters (crossover and mutation rates) of DE is applied. The aim is to explore how effective the on-line control strategy is in solving the MKP.

This paper is structured as follows. Section 2 provides an overview of the Multiple Knapsack Problem. The Binary Differential Evolution algorithm is presented in Section 3. The adaptive control parameter mechanism is presented in Section 3.1. The experiments and results are presented in Sections 4 and 5, respectively. Section 6 concludes the paper with final remarks and future research.

2   Multiple Knapsack Problem

The 0-1 Multiple Knapsack Problem (MKP) is a well-known NP-hard combinatorial optimisation problem and its goal is to maximize the profit of items chosen to fulfil a set of knapsacks, subjected to constraints of capacity [8]. The MKP consists of m knapsacks of capacities $C_1, C_2, ...C_m$, and a set of n items $I = \{I_1, I_2, ...I_n\}$. The binary variables $X_i(i = 1, ..., n)$ represent selected items to be carried in m knapsacks. The X_i assumes 1 if item i is in the knapsack and 0 otherwise. Each item I_i has an associated profit $P_i \geq 0$ and weight $W_{ij} \geq 0$ for each knapsack j. The goal is to find the best combination of n items by maximizing the sum of profits P_i multiplied by the binary variable X_i, mathematically represented by Equation 1. Their constraints are the capacity $C_j \geq 0$ of each knapsack. Therefore, the sum of the values of X_i multiplied by W_{ij} must be less than or equal to C_j, represented mathematically by Equation 2.

$$\max \left(\sum_{i=1}^{n} (P_i \times X_i) \right) \tag{1}$$

$$\sum_{j=1}^{m} (W_{ij} \times X_i) \leq C_j \tag{2}$$

The MKP search space depends directly on the values of n and m. A binary exponential function with exponent n assembles all possibilities for n items respecting the capacity of each knapsack m. Therefore, to find the optimal solution should be tested all 2^n possibilities for each knapsack m, i.e., $m \times 2^n$ possibilities. Thus, depending on the instance, the search space can become intractable by exact methods. In such cases, metaheuristic algorithms are indicated. Hence, the Binary Differential Evolution is an interesting algorithm to be applied to solve the MKP. The algorithm was designed for binary optimization and is shown in next section.

3   Binary Differential Evolution

The Binary Differential Evolution (BDE) [12] is a population-based metaheuristic inspired by the canonical Differential Evolution (DE) [13] and is adapted to handle binary problems. Specifically, the BDE approach is a modification of the DE/rand/1/bin variant.

In BDE, a population of binary encoded candidate solutions with size POP interact with each other. Each binary vector $\vec{x}_i = [x_{i1}, x_{i2}...x_{iDIM},]$ of dimension DIM is a candidate solution of the problem and is evaluated by an objective function $f(\vec{x}_i)$ with $i = [1, ..., POP]$. As well as the canonical DE, BDE combines each solution of the current population with a randomly chosen solution through the crossover operator. However, the main modification to the canonical DE, besides the binary representation, is the insertion of a bit-flip mutation operator. This modification adds to the algorithm the capacity to improve its global search ability, enabling diversity.

The pseudo-code of BDE is presented in Algorithm 1. The control parameters: the number of dimensions (DIM), the population size (POP), the maximum number of generations or iterations $(ITER)$, the perturbation rate (PR) and the mutation rate (MUT)(line 1). The algorithm begins creating a random initial population (line 2) where each individual represents a point in the search space and is a possible solution to the problem. The individuals are binary vectors that are evaluated by a fitness function (line 3). An evolutive loop is performed until a termination criteria is met (line 4). The termination criteria can be to reach the maximum number of iterations $ITER$. The evolutive loop consists in creating new individuals through the processes of perturbation (mutation and crossover) (lines 6-17), evaluation of the objective function (line 18), and a greedy selection (lines 19-21).

Algorithm 1. Binary Differential Evolution (BDE)

1: Parameters : $DIM, POP, ITER, PR, MUT$
2: Generate initial population randomly: $\vec{x}_i \in \{0,1\}^{DIM}$
3: Evaluate initial population with the fitness function $f(\vec{x}_i)$
4: **while** termination criteria not met **do**
5:   **for** i = 1 **to** POP **do**
6:     Select a random individual: $k \leftarrow random\_integer(1, POP)$, with $k \neq i$
7:     Select a random dimension: $j_{rand} \leftarrow random\_integer(1, DIM)$
8:     $\vec{y} \leftarrow \vec{x}_i$
9:     **for** j = 1 **to** DIM **do**
10:       **if** $(random\_double(0, 100) < PR)$ **or** $(j == j_{rand})$ **then**
11:         **if** $(random\_double(0, 100) < MUT$) **then**
12:           BitFlip(y_j) {Mutation}
13:         **else**
14:           $y_j \leftarrow x_{kj}$ {Crossover}
15:         **end if**
16:       **end if**
17:     **end for**
18:     Evaluate $f(\vec{y})$
19:     **if** $(f(\vec{y}) > f(\vec{x}_i))$ **then** {Greedy Selection}
20:       $\vec{x}_i \leftarrow \vec{y}$
21:     **end if**
22:   **end for**
23:   Find current best solution $\vec{x}^*$
24: **end while**
25: Report results

Inside the evolutive loop, two random indexes k and j_{rand} are selected at each generation. k represents the index of an individual in the population and must be different from the current index of individual i (line 6). j_{rand} represents the index of any dimension of the problem (line 7).

In line 8, the individual $\vec{x}_i$ is copied to a trial individual $\vec{y}$. Each dimension of the trial individual is perturbed (or modified) accordingly to the perturbation rate or if the index j is equal to index j_{rand} (line 10). The equality ensures that at least one dimension will be perturbed. The perturbation is carried out by the bit-flip mutation using its probability (line 11-12) or by the crossover operator (line 14).

From the new population of individuals the best solution $\vec{x}^*$ is found (line 23) and a new generation starts. Algorithm 1 terminates reporting the best solution obtained $\vec{x}^*$ (line 25).

3.1   Adaptive Binary Differential Evolution

The Adaptive Binary Differential Evolution (aBDE) algorithm aims to control two parameters: perturbation (PR) and mutation (MUT) rates. To achieve that, a set of discrete values is introduced for each of parameter. Once defined a set of values for each parameter, a single value is chosen at each generation through a roulette wheel selection strategy. The probability of choosing a value is initially defined equally which is subsequently adapted based on a criteria of success. If a selected value for a parameter yielded at least one individual in generation $t+1$ better than the best fitted individual from generation t, then the parameter value has a mark of success. Hence, if at the end of generation $t+1$ the parameter value was successful, its probability is increased with an α value, otherwise, it remains the same. The α is calculated by a linear increase as shows Equation 3.

$$\alpha = min + \left(\frac{max - min}{ITER} \times i \right) \tag{3}$$

Where $ITER$ is the number of iterations, i is the current iteration, max is the maximum value of α and min is the minimum value of α. After adjusting the probabilities, the values are normalized between 0 and 1. To ensure a minimum of chance for each value of parameters, a β value is established.

4   Computational Experiments

The algorithms were developed using ANSI C language and the experiments were run on a AMD Phenom II X4 (2.80GHz) with 4GB RAM, under Linux operating system. For the experiments, 11 instances for the MKP were used[1]. Table 1 shows the optimum value, the number of knapsacks, and the number of items (or dimensions), respectively, for each instance.

For each instance, 100 independent runs were performed with randomly initialized populations. The parameters used for the BDE algorithm are: population size $(POP = 100)$, number of iterations $(ITER = 1,000)$, perturbation rate $(PR = 50\%)$, mutation rate $(MUT = 5\%)$.

A simple Genetic Algorithm (GA) was also developed for the sake of comparison [5]. It uses tournament selection, uniform crossover and elitism of one

---

[1] Available at: www.cs.nott.ac.uk/~jqd/mkp/index.html

Table 1. Benchmark Instances for the MKP

Instance	Optimum Value	Knapsacks	Items
PB1	3090	4	27
PB2	3186	4	34
PB4	95168	2	29
PB5	2139	10	20
PB6	776	30	40
PB7	1035	30	37
PET7	16537	5	50
SENTO1	7772	30	60
SENTO2	8722	30	60
WEING8	624319	2	105
WEISHI30	11191	5	90

individual. The parameters for the GA are: population size ($POP = 100$), number of iterations ($ITER = 1,000$), tournament size ($T = 3$), crossover rate ($CR = 80\%$), mutation rate ($MUT = 5\%$), and elitism of one individual.

The strategy to adapt parameters is applied in both algorithms, BDE and GA, leading to its adaptive versions aBDE and aGA, respectively. The parameters adjusted are PR and MUT for aBDE, and CR and MUT for aGA. Thus, the set of values for PR was defined as $\{20, 30, 40, 50, 60\}$ to aBDE, and the set of values for CR was defined as $\{50, 60, 70, 80, 90\}$ to aGA. MUT was defined as $\{1, 3, 5, 10, 15\}$ in both algorithms. A range of $[0.01, 0.1]$ was chosen for α and the β parameter was set to 0.01. The number of function evaluations is the same in all algorithms, resulting in a maximum of 100,000 function evaluations. All choices for the values of parameters were made empirically.

In all approaches, infeasible individuals in the population are fixed by dropping random items from the knapsack until feasibility is obtained. Feasibility of individual is verified inside the objective function as proposed in [9].

5   Results and Analysis

Table 2 presents the average and the standard deviation of the best result ($Avg \pm Std$) obtained in all runs for each algorithm, the average number of objective function evaluations ($Eval$) required to achieve the optimum value, the success rate ($Success$) calculated as the percentage that the algorithm reached the optimum value, and the dominance information (P) indicating which algorithms are better than the others concerning both the average best result and the average number of function evaluations. If more than one algorithm is marked in the same benchmark means that they are non-dominated (neither of them are better than the other in both criteria). Also, for each algorithm, the last line ($Average$) shows the average of evaluations and the average of success rate for all benchmarks. Best results are highlighted in bold.

Analyzing the results obtained by BDE and GA we can notice that BDE achieved better results (success rate) in all instances, except for $PB2$ and $PB5$.

Table 2. Results obtained by all algorithms for each instance

Benchmark	GA			aGA		
	Avg±Std	Eval	Success P	Avg±Std	Eval	Success P
PB1	3085.26±10.78	34995.18	82.00%	3086.98±8.17	45491.35	86.00%
PB2	3131.08±40.44	89051.75	17.00%	3142.10±32.96	91786.79	15.00%
PB4	95071.01±551.51	9251.30	97.00%	94956.92±769.63	21115.21	91.00%
PB5	2138.15±3.71	29852.48	**95.00%** x	2136.62±5.90	33728.52	86.00%
PB6	769.57±10.49	51759.22	68.00%	770.64±10.04	46877.06	72.00%
PB7	1026.34±6.92	92079.76	17.00%	1024.34±7.98	92400.93	12.00%
PET7	16428.88±47.93	100100.00	0.00%	16451.34±50.91	98634.27	6.00%
SENTO1	7640.90±50.75	100100.00	0.00%	7678.39±80.06	95481.81	14.00%
SENTO2	8620.05±37.74	100100.00	0.00%	8649.13±50.80	99942.68	1.00%
WEING8	566282.95±12678.93	100100.00	0.00%	583830.05±20597.21	100100.00	0.00%
WEISHI30	10824.70±92.10	100100.00	0.00%	10962.33±189.93	99851.97	3.00%
Average		73408.15	34.18%		75037.32	35.09%

Benchmark	BDE			aBDE		
	Avg±Std	Eval	Sucess P	Avg±Std	Eval	Sucess P
PB1	3089.07±4.96	14104.50	96.00%	3089.54±3.52	13074.74	**98.00%** x
PB2	3144.55±28.43	91164.94	14.00%	3165.17±24.20	78323.80	**40.00%** x
PB4	95168.00±0.00	4672.21	**100.00%** x	95168.00±0.00	5584.56	**100.00%** x
PB5	2135.60±6.80	32052.98	80.00%	2136.79±5.72	26676.96	**87.00%** x
PB6	775.86±1.39	7200.84	99.00%	776.00±0.00	6865.16	**100.00%** x
PB7	1034.12±2.57	35502.17	77.00%	1034.47±1.89	33620.13	**82.00%** x
PET7	16524.58±19.07	65795.81	56.00%	16529.52±15.30	64335.20	**71.00%** x
SENTO1	7771.44±3.53	17091.08	**97.00%** x	7770.66±4.61	25110.83	91.00%
SENTO2	8720.37±3.49	50493.94	67.00%	8721.17±2.37	42285.83	**78.00%** x
WEING8	624062.37±770.56	55705.08	86.00%	624241.30±457.11	34517.30	**95.00%** x
WEISHI30	11191.00±0.00	33645.37	**100.00%** x	11190.84±0.78	26192.99	96.00% x
Average		37038.99	79.27%		**32417.04**	**85.27%**

In fact, the average success rate of BDE is more than two times better than the average success rate of GA. This relation is almost the same for the average number of function evaluations. This can be explained by the diversification power that BDE employs in its operators.

Comparing the results obtained by BDE and its adaptive version, aBDE, we can notice that the results (success rate) were even better when using the adaptive parameter control strategy for almost all instances except for $SENTO1$ and $WEISHI30$ and equal for $PB4$. Also, the average number of function evaluations decreased when using the parameter control strategy. This improvement can be explained by the adaptive choices for the values of parameters during the optimization process.

Analyzing the effectiveness of the adaptive parameter control strategy, it is possible to notice that aBDE and aGA obtained better success rates for the majority of the instances when compared to its non-adaptive versions. The improvement is boosted in aBDE which has a differentiated diversification mechanism.

Using the dominance information (P) from Table 2, it is possible to notice that the Differential Evolution algorithm with adaptive parameter control, aBDE, is present in the non-dominated set in 10 out of 11 instances. This indicates that aBDE is robust concerning both criteria. The aBDE algorithm is dominated in only one instance ($SENTO1$) by BDE algorithm.

In order to illustrate the behavior of the adaptive control strategy, Figures 1 and 2 show the adaptation of values for the mutation and perturbation rates,

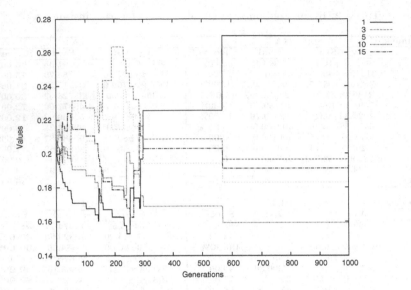

Fig. 1. Adaptive probabilities for mutation rate

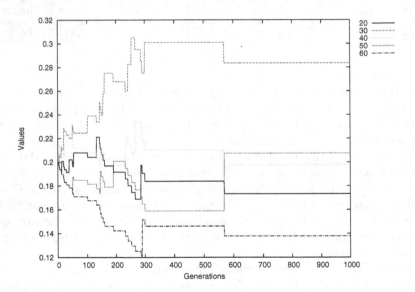

Fig. 2. Adaptive probabilities for perturbation rate

respectively. Also, a convergence plot is show in Figure 3. All three figures were acquired during a successful run of aBDE algorithm using instance $PET7$. For other instances, the behavior observed was similar.

In the first generation of the algorithm, all possibilities for the values of parameters have the same probabilities to be chosen. Through generations, these probabilities can change according to their success of creating better solutions,

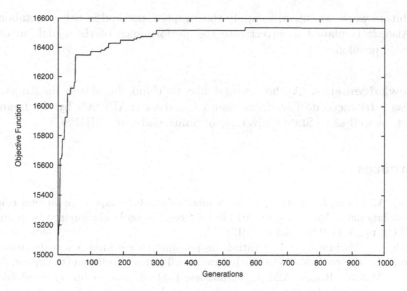

Fig. 3. Convergence graph for instance $PET7$

as explained in Section 3.1. From Figures 1 and 2 it is possible to notice that, in earlier generations, the probabilities of the values for each parameter change most often than in latter generations. This is explained by the diversity loss that occurs during the optimization process, as can be seen in the convergence plot (Figure 3). The adaptive method is able to better explore the values of parameters in the beginning of the optimization process, favoring the best values until its end.

6 Conclusion

In this work, a Binary Differential Evolution algorithm with adaptive parameters was applied to the well-known 0-1 MKP. The Adaptive Binary Differential Evolution (aBDE) algorithm aims to control two parameters: perturbation (PR) and mutation (MUT) rates. To achieve that, a set of discrete values is introduced for each of parameter and it is updated based on a criteria of success. If a selected value for a parameter yielded at least one individual in generation $t+1$ better than the best fitted individual from generation t, then the parameter value has a mark of success. Hence, if at the end of generation $t+1$ the parameter value was successful, its probability is increased, otherwise, it remains the same.

Results obtained using 11 instances of the problem strongly suggest that the adaptive selection strategy has advantages when compared with fixed values. This advantages can be seen in the results (average success rate and average number of function evaluations) when comparing aBDE with the other algorithms. This indicates that the proposed approach is an interesting and promising strategy for optimization of complex problems.

As future work, we intend to apply the adaptive method in other metaheuristics. Also, it is planed to investigate the performance of the aBDE in other real-world problems.

Acknowledgements. Authors would like to thank Fundação de Amparo a Pesquisa e Inovação do Estado de Santa Catarina (FAPESC) by the financial support, as well as to State University of Santa Catarina (UDESC).

References

1. Aleti, A., Moser, I.: Studying feedback mechanisms for adaptive parameter control in evolutionary algorithms. In: 2013 IEEE Congress on Evolutionary Computation (CEC), pp. 3117–3124. IEEE (2013)
2. André, L., Parpinelli, R.S.: Controle de parâmetros em inteligência de enxame e computação evolutiva. Revista de Informática Teórica e Aplicada (to appear, 2014)
3. Azad, M.A.K., Rocha, A.M.A., Fernandes, E.M.: Improved binary artificial fish swarm algorithm for the 0–1 multidimensional knapsack problems. Swarm and Evolutionary Computation 14, 66–75 (2014)
4. Bansal, J.C., Deep, K.: A modified binary particle swarm optimization for knapsack problems. Applied Mathematics and Computation 218(22), 11042–11061 (2012)
5. De Jong, K.: Evolutionary Computation: A Unified Approach. Bradford Book, Mit Press (2006)
6. Eiben, A., Hinterding, R., Michalewicz, Z.: Parameter control in evolutionary algorithms. IEEE Transactions on Evolutionary Computation 3(2), 124–141 (1999)
7. Fialho, Á., Da Costa, L., Schoenauer, M., Sebag, M.: Extreme value based adaptive operator selection. In: Rudolph, G., Jansen, T., Lucas, S., Poloni, C., Beume, N. (eds.) PPSN X. LNCS, vol. 5199, pp. 175–184. Springer, Heidelberg (2008)
8. Freville, A.: The multidimensional 0-1 knapsack problem: An overview. European Journal of Operational Research 155(1), 1–21 (2004)
9. Hoff, A., Løkketangen, A., Mittet, I.: Genetic algorithms for 0/1 multidimensional knapsack problems. In: Proceedings Norsk Informatikk Konferanse, pp. 291–301. Citeseer (1996)
10. Kramer, O.: Evolutionary self-adaptation: a survey of operators and strategy parameters. Evolutionary Intelligence 3(2), 51–65 (2010)
11. Krause, J., Cordeiro, J., Parpinelli, R.S., Lopes, H.S.: A survey of swarm algorithms applied to discrete optimization problems. In: Swarm Intelligence and Bio-inspired Computation: Theory and Applications. Elsevier Science & Technology Books, pp. 169–191 (2013)
12. Krause, J., Parpinelli, R.S., Lopes, H.S.: Proposta de um algoritmo inspirado em evolução diferencial aplicado ao problema multidimensional da mochila. In: Anais do IX Encontro Nacional de Inteligência Artificial–ENIA. SBC, Curitiba (2012)
13. Storn, R., Price, K.: Differential evolution: A simple and efficient heuristic for global optimization over continuous spaces. J. of Global Optimization 11(4), 341–359 (1997)
14. Thierens, D.: An adaptive pursuit strategy for allocating operator probabilities. In: Proceedings of the 2005 Conference on Genetic and Evolutionary Computation, pp. 1539–1546. ACM (2005)

15. Vasquez, M., Hao, J.K., et al.: A hybrid approach for the 0-1 multidimensional knapsack problem. In: IJCAI, pp. 328–333 (2001)
16. Wang, L., Long Zheng, X., Yao Wang, S.: A novel binary fruit fly optimization algorithm for solving the multidimensional knapsack problem. Knowledge-Based Systems 48(0), 17–23 (2013)
17. Yang, X.-S.: Chapter 6 - differential evolution. In: Nature-Inspired Optimization Algorithms, p. 89. Elsevier, Oxford (2014)

The Best Neural Network Architecture

Angel Fernando Kuri-Morales

Instituto Tecnológico Autónomo de México
Río Hondo No. 1
México 01000, D.F.
México
akuri@itam.mx

Abstract. When designing neural networks (NNs) one has to consider the ease to determine the best architecture under the selected paradigm. One possible choice is the so-called multi-layer perceptron network (MLP). MLPs have been theoretically proven to be universal approximators. However, a central issue is that the architecture of the MLPs, in general, is not known and has to be determined heuristically. In the past, several such approaches have been taken but none has been shown to be applicable in general, while others depend on complex parameter selection and fine-tuning. In this paper we present a method which allows us to determine the said architecture from basic theoretical considerations: namely, the information content of the sample and the number of variables. From these we derive a closed analytic formulation. We discuss the theory behind our formula and illustrate its application by solving a set of problems (both for classification and regression) from the University of California at Irvine (UCI) data base repository.

Keywords: Neural Networks, Perceptrons, Information Theory, Genetic Algorithms.

1   Introduction

In the original formulation of a NN a neuron gave rise to a simple analogy corresponding to a perceptron, shown in Figure 1. In this perceptron $y_i = \varphi\left(\sum_{j=0}^{m_0} w_{ij} x_j\right)$; where $x_0 = 1$; $w_{i0} = b_i$. The weights (w_{ij}) employed here define the coupling strength of the respective connections and are established via a learning process, in the course of which they are modified according to given patterns and a learning rule. Originally, the process of learning was attempted by applying individual perceptrons but it was shown [1] that, as individual units, they may only classify linearly separable sets. It was later shown [2] that a feed-forward network of strongly interconnected perceptrons may arbitrarily approximate any continuous function.

In view of this, training the neuron ensemble becomes a major issue regarding the practical implementation of NNs. Much of the success or failure of a particular

A. Gelbukh et al. (Eds.): MICAI 2014, Part II, LNAI 8857, pp. 72–84, 2014.
© Springer International Publishing Switzerland 2014

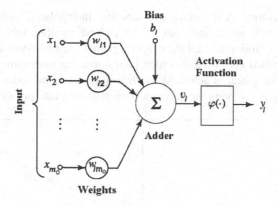

Fig. 1. A Perceptron

sort of NN depends on the training algorithm. In the case of MLPs its popularity was boosted by the discovery of the back-propagation learning rule [3]. It is a simple and efficient iterative algorithm which, by requiring a differentiable activation function, radically speeds up and simplifies the training process. The theoretical formalization of these basic concepts may be traced back to the original proof [4] of the Universal Approximation Theorem (UAT) which may be stated as follows:

"Let $\varphi(\cdot)$ be a nonconstant, bounded, and monotonically-increasing continuous function. Let Im_o denote the m_O-dimensional unit hypercube $[0,1]^{mO}$. The space of continuous functions on Im_o is denoted by $C(Im_o)$. Then, given any function and $f \in (Im_o)$ and $\varepsilon > 0$, there exist an integer M and sets of real constants $\alpha_i, \beta_i, w_{ij}$, where $i=1,2,...,m_I$ and $j=1,2,...,m_O$ such that we may define:

$$F(x_1,...,x_{m_O}) = \sum_{i=1}^{m_I}\left[\alpha_i \cdot \varphi\left(\sum_{j=0}^{m_O} w_{ij}x_j\right)\right] \tag{1}$$

as an approximate realization of the function $f(\ )$, that is,

$$| F(x_1,...,x_{m_O}) - f(x_1,...,x_{m_O}) | < \varepsilon \tag{2}$$

for all $x_1,...,x_{mO}$ in the input space."   □

The UAT is directly applicable to multilayer perceptron networks [5] and states that *a single hidden layer is sufficient for a multilayer perceptron to compute a uniform ε approximation to a given training set of pairs represented by a) The set of inputs $x_1,...,x_{mO}$ and b) A desired (target) output $f(x_1,...,x_{mO})$.*

To take practical advantage of the UAT, data must be mapped into the [0,1] interval. If the data set does not represent a continuous function, though, the UAT does not generally hold. This is the main reason to include a second hidden layer. This second layer has the purpose of mapping the original discontinuous data to a higher dimensional space where the discontinuities are no longer present [6].

However, it is always possible to replace the original discontinuous data by a continuous approximation with the use of a natural spline (NS) [7]. By properly using a NS, the user may get rid of the necessity of a second hidden layer and the UAT becomes truly universal. A discontinuous function interpolated with NS is shown in figure 2. On the left, an original set of 16 points; on the right 100 equi-distant interpolated points. Notice that all the original points are preserved and the unknown interval has been filled up with data which guarantees the minimum curvature for the ensemble. A similar effect is achieved by including a second hidden layer in a NN. What we are doing is relieving the network from this tacit interpolating task.

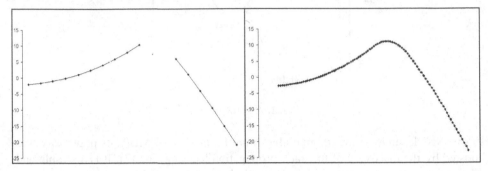

Fig. 2. Use of a Natural Spline to avoid discontinuities

Later studies led to alternative approaches where the architecture is rendered by the paradigm. Among them we find the Radial-Basis Function Networks (RBFN) [8] and the Support Vector Machines (SVM) [9]. Graphical representations of both paradigms are shown in Figure 3. Notice that MLPs may have several output neurons.

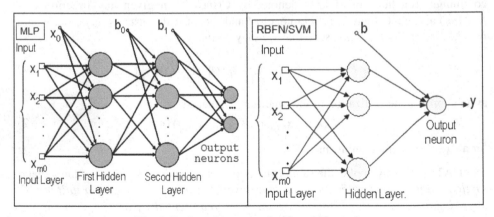

Fig. 3. Basic architecture of a Neural Network

RBFNs and SVMs are well understood and have been applied in a large number of cases. They, nonetheless, exhibit some practical limitations [10]. For example, as opposed to MLPs, RBFNs need unsupervised training of the centers; while SVMs are unable to directly find more than two classes. For this reason, among others, MLPs continue to be frequently used and reported in the literature.

The architecture of a MLP is completely determined by a) m_O (the input neurons), b) m_I (the hidden neurons), c) $\varphi(\cdot)$ (the activation function) and d) the w_{ij}'s. With the exception of m_I, all the values of the architecture may be readily found. m_I remains to be determined in every case and is not, in general, simple to assess. It determines 1) The complexity of the network and, more importantly, 2) Its learning capability. The proper and closed determination of m_I is the central topic of this work. The rest of the paper is organized as follows. In part 2 we derive a closed formulation for the lower bound on the value of m_I. In part 3 we present some experimental results. In part 4 we present our conclusions.

2   Determination of a Lower Bound on m_I

There have been several previous approaches to determine the value of m_I. A dynamic node creation algorithm for MLPs is proposed by Ash in [11], which is different from some deterministic process. In this algorithm, a critical value is chosen arbitrarily first. The final structure is built up through the iteration in which a new node is created in the hidden layer when the training error is below a critical value. On the other hand, Hirose et al in [12] propose an approach which is similar to Ash [11] but removes nodes when small error values are reached. In [13], a model selection procedure for neural networks based on least squares estimation and statistical tests is developed. In [14] Yao suggests an evolutionary programming approach where the architecture of a MLP is evolved and the actual connections may be optimized along with the number of hidden neurons. The Bayesian Ying-Yang learning criteria [15, 16] put forward an approach for selecting the best number of hidden units. Their experimental studies show that the approach is able to determine its best number with minimized generalization error, and that it outperforms the cross validation approach in selecting the appropriate number for both clustering and function approximation. In [17] an algorithm is developed to optimize the number of hidden nodes by minimizing the mean-squared errors over noisy training data. In [18] Fahlmann proposes a method dynamically increasing the number of neurons in the hidden layer while Reed [19] reduces the number of the connections between the neurons from a large a network and removes such connections which seem to have no significant effect on the network's functioning. In [20] Xu and Chen propose an approach for determining an optimal number of the hidden layer neurons for MLPs starting from previous work by Barron [21], who reports that, using MLPs for function approximation, the rooted mean squared (RMS) error between the well-trained neural network and a target function f is bounded by

$$O\left(C_f^2 / m_I\right) + O\left((m_I m_O / N) log\, N\right) \tag{3}$$

where N is the number of training pairs, and C_f is the first absolute moment of the Fourier-magnitude distribution of the target function f. Barron then mathematically proves that, with $m_I \sim C_f (N/(m_O\, log\, N))^{1/2}$ nodes, the order of the bound on the RMS error is optimized to be $O(C_f ((m_O /N)\, log\, N)^{1/2})$. We can then conclude that if the target function f is known then the best (leading to a minimum RMS error) value of m_I is

$$m_I = C_f (N/(m_O\, log\, N))^{1/2} \tag{4}$$

However, even though f were assumed unknown, from the UAT, we know it may be approached with ⟶ 0. In this case, Xu and Chen [20] use a complexity regularization approach to determine the constant C in

$$m_I = C \, (N/(m_O \log N))^{1/2} \tag{5}$$

by trying an increasing sequence of C to obtain different values of m_I, train a MLP for each m_I and then observe the m_I which generates the smallest RMS error (and note the value of the C). Notice that C_f depends on an unknown target function f, whereas C is a constant which does not.

2.1   Statistical Estimation of m_I's Lower Value

Instead of performing a costly series of case-by-case trial and error tests to target on the value of m_I as in [20] our aim is to obtain an algebraic expression yielding m_I's lower bound from

$$m_I = \sum_{i=0}^{d1} \sum_{j=0}^{d2} K_{ij} m_O^i N^j \tag{6}$$

where d_1 and d_2 are selected a priori and the K_{ij} are to be adequately determined for a predefined range of values of m_O and N. That is, we aim at having a simple algebraic expression which will allow us to establish the minimum architecture of a NN given the number of input variables and the number of training pairs. The values of m_I depend on N, m_O and C. Even though are several possible values of C for every pair (m_O, N) an appropriate value of the lower bound value of C may be set by considering values for C in a plausible range and calculating the mean (μ_C) and standard deviation (σ_C) for every pair (m_O, N). The upper value of the range of interest is given by the fact that the maximum of m_I is N/m_O; the lower value of the range is, simply, 1. Thus, we may find a statistically significant lower value of C (denoted by C_{min}) and the corresponding lower value of m_I from Chebyshev's theorem [22] which says that

$$P(\mu_C - k \, \sigma_C \leq C \leq \mu_C + k \, \sigma_C) > 1 - 1/k^2 \tag{7}$$

and makes no assumption on the form of the *pdf* of C. If, however, we consider that C's *pdf* is symmetric we have that $P(C > \mu_C - \sqrt{5} \, \sigma_C) \geq 0.9$. A very reliable and general value of C_{min} is, therefore, given by

$$C_{min} = \mu_C - \sqrt{5} \, \sigma_C \tag{8}$$

Now we propose to analyze all combinations of m_O and N in a range of interest and obtain the best regressive polynomial from these combinations. We considered the range of m_O between 2 and 82 (i.e. up to 82 input variables); likewise, we considered N between 100 and 25,000. That is we consider up to 25,000 *effective* objects in the training set. By *effective* we mean that they correspond to a sample devoid of unnecessarily redundant data, as will be discussed in the sequel. The number of combinations in this range is 81 x 25,000 (or 2,025,000 triples), which would have demanded us to find an algebraic expression for these many objects. To reduce the data set to more manageable proportions we sampled the combinations of m_O and N by increasing the values of m_O in steps of 5, while increasing those of N in steps of 100. The number of objects in the sample reduced to 4,250. The general procedure is as follows:

(a) Select lower and upper experimental values of m_O and N which we denote with m_L, N_L, m_H and N_H. These are set to 2, 100, 82 and 25,000, respectively.

(b) Define step sizes D_m and D_N (these were set to 5 and 100, respectively) which determine the values between two consecutive (m_O, N) pairs. That is, m_O will take consecutive values m_L, m_L+D_m, , . . . , m_H. Likewise, N will take consecutive values N_L, N_L+D_N,..., N_H.

(c) Obtain the values for all combinations of m_O and N in the range between (m_L, N_L) and (m_H, N_H), i.e. (m_L, N_L), (m_L, N_L+D_N),...,(m_H, N_H).

(d) For every pair (m_O, N) calculate μ_C and σ_C. Then obtain C_{min} from equation (8).

(e) For every pair (m_O, N) obtain $m_I = C_{min}(N/(m_O \log N))^{1/2}$.

The maximum and minimum values for (m_O, N, m_I) are shown in Table 1.

Table 1. Values of (m_O, N, m_I) in the range of interest

	m_O	N	m_I
Max	82	25,000	549
Min	2	100	0

(f) Store every triple (m_O, N, m_I) in a table T.

Once steps (c) to (f) have been taken, we have spanned the combinations of all triples (m_O, N, m_I) in the interval of interest.

(f) From T get a numerical approximation as per equation (6), which will be described in what follows.

The triples (m_O, N, m_I) were mapped into the interval [0,1]. The corresponding scaled values are denoted with $(m_O*, N*, m_I*)$.

Therefore,

$m_O*=(m_O-m_L)/(m_H-m_L)$ $\rightarrow m* = (m_O -2)/80$

$N* =(N-N_L)/(N_H-N_L)$ $\rightarrow N* = (N - 100)/24900$

$m_I* = (m_I-m_{min})/(m_{max}-m_{min})$ $\rightarrow m_I*=m_I /549$

From the 4,250 scaled vectors we obtained the purported polynomial expression $m_I*=f(m_O*,N*)$ with $d_1=d_2=7$, thus:

$$m_I* = \sum_{i=0}^{7} \sum_{j=0}^{7} \vartheta_{ij} K_{ij} (m_O*)^i (N*)^j \qquad (9)$$

$$|\vartheta| = 12 \qquad (10)$$

Where K_{ij} denotes a coefficient and ϑ_{ij} is an associated constant which can take only the values 0 or 1. Only 12 of the possible 64 combinations of (i, j) are allowed. This number was arrived at by trying several different values and calculating the associated RMS error, as shown in table 2.

Table 2. Best values of RMS for different number of terms

Terms	7	8	9	10	11	12	13
RMS	0.07104	0.03898	0.06574	0.05889	0.04618	0.03410	0.03885

Terms	14	15	16	17	18	19	20
RMS	0.03190	0.03712	0.02718	0.02500	0.01405	0.03068	0.02345

The best RMS error corresponds to $|\vartheta| = 18$; however, the simpler approximation when $|\vartheta| = 12$ is only marginally inferior (2%) and, for simplicity, we decided to remain with it. The final 12 coefficients are shown in table 3.

Table 3. Coefficients for $|\vartheta| = 12$

K01	K12	K13	K15	K22	K24	K32	K35	K42	K45	K52	K63
0.9307	-33.6966	24.5008	-3.4958	107.4970	-41.0848	-209.3930	52.8180	205.6786	-32.6766	-80.8771	9.7786

The subindices denote the powers of the associated variables. Therefore, we have that

$$m_I^* = K_{01}N^* + K_{12}mO^*(N^*)^2 + K_{13}mO^*(N^*)^3 + K_{15}mO^*(N^*)^5 + K_{22}(mO^*)^2(N^*)^2 + K_{24}(mO^*)^2(N^*)^4 + K_{32}(mO^*)^3(N^*)^2 + K_{35}(mO^*)^3(N^*)^5 + K_{42}(mO^*)^4(N^*)^2 + K_{45}(mO^*)^4(N^*)^5 + K_{52}(mO^*)^5(N^*)^2 + K_{63}(mO^*)^6(N^*)^3 \quad (12)$$

Finally,

$$m_I = (m_L - m_H)/m_I^* + m_L \quad \rightarrow \quad m_I = 549m_I^* \quad (13)$$

According to these results $K_{ij} = 0$ except for the combinations of (i,j) shown in table 3. Two views of equation (12) are shown in Figure 4.

How were the coefficients of (12) found? As follows: we define a priori the number $|\vartheta|$ of desired monomials of the approximant and then select which of the p possible ones these will be. There are $C(p, |\vartheta|)$ combinations of monomials and

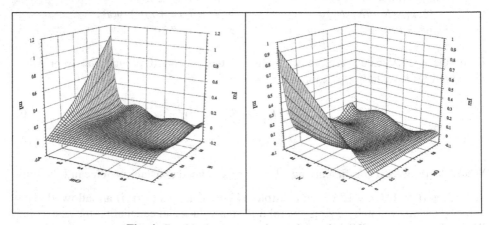

Fig. 4. Graphical representations of equation (13)

even for modest values of p and $| \vartheta |$ an exhaustive search is out of the question. This is an optimization problem which we tackled using the genetic algorithm (EGA) discussed in [23] [24].

2.1.1 Determination of the Coefficients of the Approximant
Consider an approximant of the form

$$f(v_1, ... v_n) = \sum_{i_1=0}^{d_1} ... \sum_{i_n=0}^{d_n} C_{i_1...i_n} v_1^{i_1} ... v_n^{i_n} \qquad (14)$$

There are $p = (d_1+1)x...x(d_n+1)$ possible monomials. We associate to this polynomial a chromosome which is a binary string of size p. Every bit represents a monomial ordered as per the sequence of the consecutive powers of the variables. If the bit is '1' it means that the corresponding monomial is retained while if it is a '0' it is discarded. One has to ensure that the number of 1's is equal to $| \vartheta |$. Because of this, the population of the EGA consists of a set of binary strings of length p having only $| \vartheta |$ 1's. For example, if $y=f(v_1, v_2, v_3)$ and $d_1=1$, $d_2=d_3=2$ the powers assigned to the $2 \times 3 \times 3 = 18$ positions of the genome are 000, 001, 002, 010, 011, 012, 020, 021, 022, 100, 101, 102, 110, 111, 112, 120, 121, 122. Taking $| \vartheta |=6$ the chromosome 110000101010000001 would correspond to $P(v_1,v_2,v_3) = k_{000} + k_{001}v_3 + k_{020}v_2^2 + k_{022}v_2^2v_3^2 + k_{101}v_1v_3 + k_{122}v_1v_2^2v_3^2$. For every genome the monomials (corresponding to the 1's) are determined by EGA. Then the so-called Ascent Algorithm ("AA"; discussed at length in [25]) is applied to every individual's polynomial's form and yields the set of $| \vartheta |$ coefficients which minimize $\varepsilon_{MAX} = max(| f_i - y_i |) \; \forall i$. For this set of coefficients the mean squared error ε_{RMS} is calculated. This is the fitness function of EGA. The EGA's 25 individuals are selected, crossed over and mutated for 200 generations. In the end, we retain the individual whose coefficients minimize ε_{RMS} out of those which best minimize ε_{MAX} (from the AA). From this procedure we derived the coefficients of table 3.

2.2   Considerations on the Size of the Training Data

We have successfully derived an algebraic formulation of the most probable lower bound of m_1 as a function of m_0 and N. The issue we want to discuss here is how to determine the effective size of the training data N so as to find the best architecture.

Intuitively, the patterns that are present in the data and which the MLP "remembers" once it has been trained are stored in the connections. In principle we would like to have enough connections for the MLP to have sufficient storage space for the discovered patterns; but not too much lest the network "memorize" the data and lose its generalization capability. It is for this obvious relation between the learning capability of the MLP and the size of the training data that equation (13) was formulated. A formalization of these concepts was developed by Vapnik and co-workers [26] and forms the basis of what is now known as statistical learning theory.

Here we wish to stress the fact that the formula of (13) tacitly (but now we make it explicit) assumes that the data is rich in information. By this we mean that it has been expressed in the most possible compact form.

Interestingly, none of the references we surveyed ([11], [12], [13], [14], [15, 16], [17], [18], [19], [20], [21]) makes an explicit consideration of the role that the information in the data plays when determining m_I. In the SVM paradigm, for example, this issue is considered when determining the number of support vectors and the so-called regularization parameter which reflects a tradeoff between the performance of the trained SVM and its allowed level of misclassification [10]. We know that the number of weights (connections) $|w|$ in the MLP directly depends on the number of hidden neurons, thus

$$|w| = m_O m_I + 2m_I + 1 \tag{15}$$

But it is easy to see that even large amounts of data may be poor in information. The true amount of information in a data set is exactly expressible by the Kolmogorov Complexity (KC) which corresponds to the most compact representation of the set under scrutiny. Unfortunately, the KC is known to be incomputable [27]. Given this we have chosen the PPM (Prediction by Partial Matching) algorithm [28] as our compression standard because it is considered to be the state of the art in lossless data compression; i.e. the best practical approximation to KC. Therefore, we will assume that the training data has been properly expressed by first finding its most compact form. Once having done so, we are able to estimate the effective value of N. Otherwise, (13) may yield unnecessarily high values for m_I.

To illustrate this fact consider the file F1 comprised of 5,000 equal records consisting of the next three values: "3.14159 <tab> 2.71828 <tab> 1.61803" separated by the ASCII codes for <cr><lf>. That is, $m_O=3$; $N=5,000$. This yields 125,000 bytes in 5,000 objects. A naïve approach would lead us to solve equation (13) yielding $m_I = 97$. However, when compressed with the PPM2 (PPM algorithm of order 2) the same data may be expressed with 49 bytes, for a compression ratio of 2,551:1. That is, every bit in the original file conveys less than 1/2,551 (i.e. $\approx.00039$) bits of information. Thus the true value of N is, roughly, 2; for which $m_I=1$. On the other hand, a file F2 consisting of 5,000 lines of randomly generated bytes (the same number of bytes as the preceding example), when compressed with the same PPM2 algorithm yields a compressed file of 123,038 bytes; a 1:1.02 ratio. Hence, from (13), $m_I = 97$. Therefore, for (13) to be applied it is important to, first, estimate the effective (in the sense that it is rich in information) size of N.

3   Experiments

Now we want to ascertain that the values obtained from (13) do indeed correspond to the lowest number of needed neurons in the hidden layer of a MLP. To exemplify this we analyze three data sets. Two of them are from UCI's repository. The third regards the determination of a MLP approximating the data of Figure 3. For every one we determine the value of m_I and show that it is the one resulting in the most efficient architecture.

Problem 1 [29] is a regression problem with $m_O=6$, $N=209$. In Figure 5 we show the learning curves using $m_I=2$ and $m_I=3$. The value of m_I from eq. (13) is 3. If we use a smaller m_I the RMS error is 4 times larger and the maximum absolute error is 6 times larger.

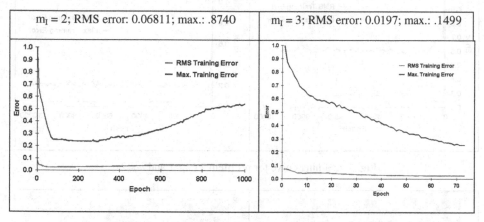

$m_I = 2$; RMS error: 0.06811; max.: .8740	$m_I = 3$; RMS error: 0.0197; max.: .1499

Fig. 5. Learning curve for problem 1 ($m_I=2$ and $m_I=3$)

Problem 2 [30] is a classification problem with $m_O=13$, $N=168$. The learning curves using $m_I=1$ and $m_I=2$ are shown in Figure 6. It is trivial to transform a classification problem into a regression one by assigning like values of the dependent variable to every class. In this case the classes 1, 2 and 3 were identified by the scaled values 0, 0.5 and 1. Therefore, a maximum absolute error (MAE) smaller than 0.25 is enough to guarantee that all classes will be successfully identified. The value of m_I from eq. (13) is 2. If we use a smaller m_I the MAE is 0.6154. If we use $m_I=2$ the MAE is 0.2289. The case where MAE>0.25 ($m_I=1$) and MAE<0.25 ($m_I=2$) are illustrated in Figure 7, where horizontal lines correspond to the 3 classes. As shown, these were poorly identified when $m_I=1$. The case $m_I=2$ leads to correct identification of the classes and 100% classification accuracy.

Problem 3 has to do with the approximation of the 4,250 triples (m_O, N, m_I) from which equation (12) was derived (see Figure 4). We used it to determine the architecture of the best MLP which approximates these data. PPM2 compression finds a 4:1 ratio between raw and compressed data. Hence, the effective value of N is 1,060, for which $m_I = 20$. Training the MLP for 20 hidden neurons (HN) yields a maximum absolute error of 0.02943 and an RMS error of 0.002163; doing it for 19 HNs yields larger corresponding errors of 0.03975 and 0.002493. If we go on to 21 HNs we get 0.03527 and 0.002488. In other words, "20" corresponds to the lowest effective number of HNs for this problem.

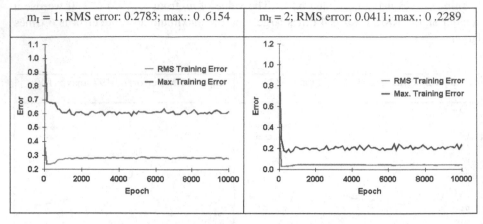

Fig. 6. Learning curve for problem 2 (m_I=1 and m_I=2)

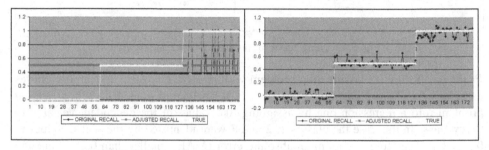

Fig. 7. Effective classification in problem 2 (m_I=1 and m_I=2)

4   Conclusions

We discussed the problem of finding the adequate number of neurons (m_I) in the hidden layer of a MLP network. We argued that MLPs offer advantages over alternative paradigms if data is continuous and scaled into [0, 1]. We have seen that approximate continuity of the training data is enough to render more than one hidden layer unnecessary and that such characteristic may be attained in practice by using natural splines to enrich the data. Hence, the conclusions derived from the UAT are directly applicable to any MLP network. Furthermore, we pointed out that the correct assessment of m_I depends on the determination of the effective size of the training data (N). The actual algorithmic information of N is incomputable but it may be approximated by considering the data after PPM2 compaction. Thus, we have shown that it is possible to determine a lower practical bound on the number of neurons in the hidden layer (m_I) of a MLP with only one such layer. We also showed how to obtain a closed and compact algebraic expression from the partial enumeration of the possible values of (m_O, N and m_I) based on the theoretical work of Barron [21]. To do this, we used a GA which selects the elements of an approximation polynomial. From experimental runs we determined that no more than 12 terms are needed for an adequate RMS error ($\approx 3.40\%$). The approximation polynomial directly delivers the smallest expected value of m_I with 90% reliability in the range ($2 \leq m_O \leq 82$) and ($100 \leq N \leq 25,000$). Finally, we offered a few experimental examples in which the correctness of the lower bound on m_I is clearly exhibited. The purpose of the experiments was to offer a practical illustration of the conclusions drawn from theoretical considerations. Similar results will be obtained for any data set which complies with the stipulated pre-conditioning. We finish our conclusions by pointing out that the purported algebraic expression $m_I = f(m_O, N)$ might have been replaced (as shown in experiment 3) by a properly trained MLP. The corresponding minimum MLP has 81 connections as opposed to only 12 coefficients of equation (12). An explicit algebraic expression is to be preferred if, as shown, it is accurate enough. As opposed to the "black box" nature of a MLP, it allows us to explore the relation between the input variables (m_O and N) and the dependent variable m_I. For instance, a combination of variables m_O*, $N*$ of degree 9 $[(mO*)^6(N*)^3]$ is enough for our approximation. Therefore, by allowing a direct determination of m_I the only practical inconvenience of the MLP paradigm has been superseded and the best architecture is reachable without the need to resort to heuristics.

References

[1] Minsky, M.L., Seymour, A.: Papert. Perceptrons - Expanded Edition: An Introduction to Computational Geometry. MIT press, Boston (1987)

[2] Hornik, K., Stinchcombe, M., White, H.: Multilayer feedforward networks are universal approximators. Neural Networks 2(5), 359–366 (1989)

[3] Hecht-Nielsen, R.: Theory of the backpropagation neural network. In: International Joint Conference on Neural Networks, IJCNN. IEEE (1989)

[4] Cybenko, G.: Approximation by superpositions of a sigmoidal function. Mathematics of Control, Signals and Systems 2(4), 303–314 (1989)

[5] Neural Networks, A Comprehensive Foundation, 2nd edn., ch. 4, p. 294, Notes and References 8. Prentice Hall International (1999)

[6] Huang, G.-B.: Learning capability and storage capacity of two-hidden-layer feedforward networks. IEEE Trans. on Neural Networks 14(2), 274–281 (2003)

[7] Shampine, L.F., Allen, R.C.: Numerical computing: an introduction, ch. 1.3, pp. 54–62. Harcourt Brace College Publishers (1973)

[8] Buhmann, M.D.: Radial basis functions. Acta Numerica 2000(9), 1–38 (2000)

[9] Hearst, M.A., Dumais, S.T., Osman, E., Platt, J., Scholkopf, B.: Support vector machines. IEEE Intelligent Systems and their Applications 13(4), 18–28 (1998)

[10] Haykin, S.S., et al.: Neural networks and learning machines, vol. 3. Pearson Education, Upper Saddle River (2009)

[11] Ash, T.: Dynamic Node Creation In Backpropagation Networks. Connection Science 1(4), 365–375 (1989)

[12] Hirose, Y., Yamashita, I.C., Hijiya, S.: Back-Propagation Algorithm Which Varies the number of hidden units. Neural Networks 1(4) (1991)

[13] Rivals, I., Personnaz, L.: A statistical procedure for determining the optimal number of hidden neurons of a neural model. In: Second International Symposium on Neural Computation (NC 2000), Berlin, May 23-26 (2000)

[14] Yao, X.: Evolving Artificial neural networks. Proceedings of the IEEE 87(9), 1423–1447 (1999)

[15] Xu, L.: Ying-Yang Machine: A Bayesian- Kullback scheme for unified learnings and new results on vector quantization. In: Keynote Talk, Proceedings of International Conference on Neural Information Processing (ICONIP 1995), October 30 - November 3, pp. 977–988 (1995)

[16] Xu, L.: Bayesian Ying-Yang System and Theory as A Unified Statistical Learning Approach (III) Models and Algorithms for Dependence Reduction, Data Dimension Reduction, ICA and Supervised Learning. In: Proc. Of International Workshop on Theoretical Aspects of Neural Computation, Hong Kong, May 26-28. LNCS, pp. 43–60. Springer (1997)

[17] Fletcher, L., Katkovnik, V., Steffens, F.E., Engelbrecht, A.P.: Optimizing The Number Of Hidden Nodes Of A Feedforward Artificial Neural Network. In: Proc. of the IEEE International Joint Conference on Neural Networks, vol. 2, pp. 1608–1612 (1998)

[18] Fahlman, S.E.: An empirical study of learning speed in back propagation networks. In: Proceedings of the 1988 Connectionist Models Summer School. Morgan Kaufman (1988)

[19] Reed, R.: Pruning Algorithms A Survey. IEEE Trans. on Neural Networks 4(5), 707–740 (1993)

[20] Xu, S., Chen, L.: A novel approach for determining the optimal number of hidden layer neurons for FNN's and its application in data mining. In: International Conference on Information Technology and Applications: iCITA, pp. 683–686 (2008)

[21] Barron, A.R.: Approximation and Estimation Bounds for Artificial Neural Networks. Machine Learning (14), 115–133 (1994)

[22] Saw, J.G., Yang, M.C., Mo, T.C.: Chebyshev inequality with estimated mean and variance. The American Statistician 38(2), 130–132 (1984)

[23] Kuri-Morales, A., Aldana-Bobadilla, E.: The best genetic algorithm I. In: Castro, F., Gelbukh, A., González, M. (eds.) MICAI 2013, Part II. LNCS, vol. 8266, pp. 1–15. Springer, Heidelberg (2013)

[24] Kuri-Morales, A.F., Aldana-Bobadilla, E., López-Peña, I.: The best genetic algorithm II. In: Castro, F., Gelbukh, A., González, M. (eds.) MICAI 2013, Part II. LNCS, vol. 8266, pp. 16–29. Springer, Heidelberg (2013)

[25] Cheney, E.W.: Introduction to approximation theory, ch. 2, pp. 45–51 (1966)

[26] Vapnik, V.: The nature of statistical learning theory. Springer (2000)

[27] Li, M., Vitányi, P.: An introduction to Kolmogorov complexity and its applications, 2nd edn. Springer, New York (1997)

[28] Teahan, W.J.: Probability estimation for PPM. In: Proceedings NZCSRSC 1995 (1995), http://www.cs.waikato.ac.nz/wjt

[29] Ein-Dor, P., Jacob Feldmesser, E.-D.: Computer Hardware Data Set: Faculty of Management, Ramat-Aviv, https://archive.ics.uci.edu/ml/datasets/Computer+Hardware

[30] Forina, M., et al.: Wine Data Set, PARVUS, Via Brigata Salerno, https://archive.ics.uci.edu/ml/datasets/Wine

On the Connection Weight Space Structure
of a Two-Neuron Discrete Neural Network: Bifurcations
of the Fixed Point at the Origin

Jorge Cervantes-Ojeda and María del Carmen Gómez-Fuentes

Universidad Autónoma Metropolitana - Cuajimalpa
{jcervantes,mcgomez}@correo.cua.uam.mx

Abstract. The dynamics of a two neuron artificial recurrent neural network depends on six parameters: four synaptic weights and two external inputs. There are complicated relationships between these parameters and the behavior of the system. The full parameter space has not been studied yet and has been limited to detect behaviors for specific configurations, i.e., when some parameters are pre-set, either for two or three neurons. In this study we analyze the nature of the fixed point at the origin in a two-neuron discrete recurrent neural network by plotting the bifurcation manifolds in the *full* weights space which is a 4-dimensinal one that gives a clear view of what the dynamics of the system can be around this fixed point, which is a very influent point in the global dynamics of the system. The possible bifurcations at the origin are *Saddle*, *Period Doubling* and *Neimark-Sacker*. We found, among other results, that the Neimark-Sacker bifurcation is only possible when the synaptic connections between neurons are one excitatory and one inhibitory.

Keywords: Discrete-time recurrent neural network dynamics, Bifurcation diagrams, Weight Space Structure.

1   Introduction

There is not yet a theory that fully explains the behavior of recurrent neural networks. A general theory of neural networks dynamics would allow the classification of the different network configurations so that it would not be necessary to make a comprehensive dynamic behavior analysis for each of the networks [Beer, 2006]. The dynamic analysis of Recurrent Neural Networks (RNN) helps in this general theory construction because it allows determining the network behavior for each of the regions in the parameter space (the connection weights and external inputs). Even small RNN may present all kinds of dynamic behaviors with a complexity that is accentuated as the number of neurons grows [Haschke & Steil, 2005].

Assuming that the same dynamical properties (and possibly more) will be present in more complex neural networks, we analyzed the dynamic behavior of a discrete-time RNN with two neurons. The two-neuron RNN dynamics is quite complex, and to our best knowledge, its entire parameter space structure has not yet been determined.

A. Gelbukh et al. (Eds.): MICAI 2014, Part II, LNAI 8857, pp. 85–94, 2014.

Up to date, the analysis has been limited to detect behaviors for specific configurations, in which some parameters are set (see section 2).

The study of the stability and bifurcations in the space of the connection weights is an important approach for the understanding of the complex dynamical behavior of an RNN. "The knowledge of the bifurcation manifolds on the one hand deepens the understanding of RNNs and on the other hand allows to directly choose parameter sets which cause a specific dynamical behavior" [Haschke & Steil, 2005]. This is why in this study we analyze all the existing bifurcations for one fixed point (at the origin) in a discrete-time RNN with two neurons for the full weights space. Knowing how the weights' variations affect the system, we can determine exactly how the neural network will behave (locally) when the weights vary slightly in any direction. This is valuable information for the configuration and training of RNN by means of evolutionary algorithms for instance. This can be linked to the study of the existence of multiple local optima in the search space of evolutionary algorithms when used to train an RNN.

It is worth mentioning that while the system dynamics do depend on the nature of the fixed point at the origin studied here, it also depends on the existence of other fixed points somewhere else. The scope of this study does not include this analysis and is left for future research.

The rest of this paper is organized as follows: Section 2 resumes related work showing how this work contributes to the existing literature. Section 3 provides the main bifurcation analysis. Section 4 has our conclusions.

2   Background

A considerable number of mathematical analyses have been done by examining various aspects of RNN dynamics. He & Cao (2007), Haschke & Steil (2005) and Haji-hosseini et al. (2011) made a detailed reference to these investigations. In none of these works has yet been done an analysis in which the nature of the fixed points is displayed throughout the full connection weights space.

Beer (2006) made a study of the local and global bifurcation manifolds in *Continuous*-Time Recurrent Neural Networks (CTRNN). This study was conducted in a three-neuron CTRNN completely interconnected using a symmetric weights matrix in order to analyze the input space bifurcations. This analysis found that the effective dimension of the system dynamics depends on the number of neurons that are saturated, and that these saturation states almost completely dominate the input space. When the number of neurons increases, the probability of finding circuits of saturated neurons is much greater than the probability of finding circuits where all neurons are dynamically active. It is also intuitive from there that the bifurcation manifolds shift and bend as the weight matrix becomes less regular. This study was carried out in the inputs domain, with a fixed symmetric weights matrix and with a slightly modified one. CTRNN are commonly used in neuroscience for the modeling of biological neurons. Neurons commonly used in artificial intelligence work in discrete time. In this paper we study a discrete-time RNN in the weights space and fixing external inputs to zero.

Haschke & Steil (2005) derived analytical expressions for bifurcation manifolds in a Discrete-Time Recurrent Neural Network (DTRNN) using three neurons fully connected in the inputs space. They obtained analytical expressions of the varieties in which bifurcations occur at fixed points in codimension-1. These varieties divide the input space into intricate regions and, each region has a different dynamic behaviour. The complex partitioning that was obtained makes its practical interpretation difficult. By practical we mean to translate this knowledge into an intuitive guide for the creation of learning algorithms for artificial RNNs. However this gave information that lets them choose the input values so that they can control the frequency and amplitude of the universal oscillator set by these three neurons. As in [Beer, 2006], the analysis was made on the input space and not on the interconnection weights space.

Passeman (2002) studied *chaotic neuromodules* which consist of two or three neurons with feedback, in discrete time. He analysed some sections of the parameter space in order to display areas where chaotic behaviour is present. In these sections some parameters were fixed with constant values, for example, the self connection weight of one neuron is set to zero. The full weight space was not covered.

Hajihosseini et al. (2011) proposed a two-neuron RNN in continuous time and showed that for a given weights configuration, there are codimension-2 bifurcations which make the network able to learn a wider range of periodic signals. They left for future work the study of the different qualitative system behaviours in the regions of the full parameter space.

Haschke & Steil (2005) proposed to investigate how the bifurcation curves of the input space are related to the weight matrix. In this direction, Cervantes et al. (2013) analysed the behaviour of a single neuron according to its feedback weight and its external input. They derived an analytic function of the values of the external input range for which the system exhibits hysteresis or oscillations, depending on the feedback weight. The next step would be the analysis of a two-neuron RNN, for wich this function would have 4 weights and 2 inputs, i.e., a space of dimension 6 which is impossible to plot. If the inputs are set to zero, the bifurcation manifolds in the weights space for each fixed point have dimension 4, so some strategy is needed to visualize and understand the structure of bifurcations in each fixed point. In this paper we provide part of this analysis by studying the full weight space bifurcation manifolds for the fixed point that exists in the origin whenever the inputs are zero. The influence of the inputs is left for further study.

3   Weight Space Bifurcations for the Fixed Point at the Origin

We did the dynamic analysis of a discrete-time RNN with two neurons configured in the following way (see Fig. 1): the output x_1 of neuron 1 is connected to itself with a weight a, and also to neuron 2 with a weight c. The output x_2 of neuron 2 is connected to itself with a weight d, and also to neuron 1 with a weight b, u_1 and u_2 are the external inputs of each neuron respectively. So, for two neurons, the evolution equation is then given by:

$$\begin{bmatrix} x_1(t+1) \\ x_2(t+1) \end{bmatrix} = \begin{bmatrix} \tanh(ax_1(t) + bx_2(t) + u_1) \\ \tanh(cx_1(t) + dx_2(t) + u_2) \end{bmatrix} \tag{1}$$

The use of *tanh* as the activation function has the advantage that whenever $\vec{u} = (0,0)$ the state $\vec{x} = (0,0)$ is always a fixed point. This fact allows studying the effects that changes in the connection weights have on the system dynamics without having to solve the fixed point equation for every set of weight values and, more importantly, allows us to study such effects independently of the effects from changing the external inputs.

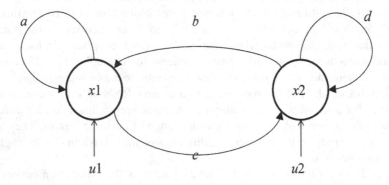

Fig. 1. The network configuration: $x1$ and $x2$ are the corresponding neuron outputs; a,b,c,d are the connection weights and $u1$ and $u2$ are the external inputs

3.1   Conditions for Bifurcations

The system behavior in the vicinity of a fixed point depends on the nature of that point. Furthermore, the nature of the fixed point changes when a curve crosses a bifurcation manifold. We call f to the right hand side of system (1). In order to calculate the bifurcation manifolds, we obtain the Jacobian of f and evaluate it for the fixed point at $x = \bar{x} = (0,0)$ with $\vec{u} = \vec{u}_0 = (0,0)$

$$J_0 = Jacobian(f(\bar{x}, \vec{u}_0)) = \begin{pmatrix} a & b \\ c & d \end{pmatrix} \tag{2}$$

So the fixed point $\bar{x} = (0,0)$ presents bifurcations as the 4 parameters a,b,c,d change. With the eigenvalues of this matrix we can know if the fixed point is an attractor, a saddle point, or repulsor and if it produces or not rotation around itself. Bifurcations from one of these to another are present for specific conditions on these values [Kuznetsov, 2004]. The conditions for bifurcations are given by the following expressions:

1.- For *Saddle bifurcation*: $\det(J_0 - 1) = 0$, at least one eigenvalue is 1. And the equation for the bifurcation manifold is:

$$1 - a - d + ad - bc = 0 \tag{3}$$

2.- For *Period Doubling*: $\det(J_0 + 1) = 0$, at least one eigenvalue is -1. And the equation for the bifurcation manifold is:

$$1 + a + d + ad - bc = 0 \tag{4}$$

3.- For *Neimark-Sacker*: $\det(J_0) - 1 = 0$ the product of the eigenvalues is 1. And the equation for the bifurcation manifold is:

$$ad - bc - 1 = 0 \tag{5}$$

3.2   Bifurcations at the Origin

As it is shown in equations (3), (4) and (5) the bifurcation manifolds at the origin depend on a, d and the products ad and bc. Since the weights b and c do not act independently, we can plot the bifurcation manifolds in three dimensions (a, d, bc). Fig. 2, shows the *Saddle* bifurcation in red, the *Period Doubling* in blue and the *Neimark-Sacker* bifurcation in green. All of them have the form of a hyperbolic paraboloid with different coordinates of its vertex. The first one has its vertex at (1, 1, 0), the second one at (-1, -1, 0) and the third one at (0, 0, -1). All of them have the same scale, i.e., if they are transported towards the same vertex they coincide in all their points.

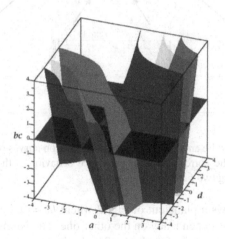

Fig. 2. Bifurcation manifolds for the fixed point $(x^*, y^*) = (0,0)$ in the space (a,d,bc): Saddle (red), Period Doubling (blue) and Neimark-Sacker (green). The plane $bc=0$ is in transparent dark grey.

In order to start analyzing these bifurcations we begin with the simplest case, where $b = c = 0$. This is the case in which both neurons work independently. In this case, the system behavior is simply the superposition of the individual behaviors of each neuron.

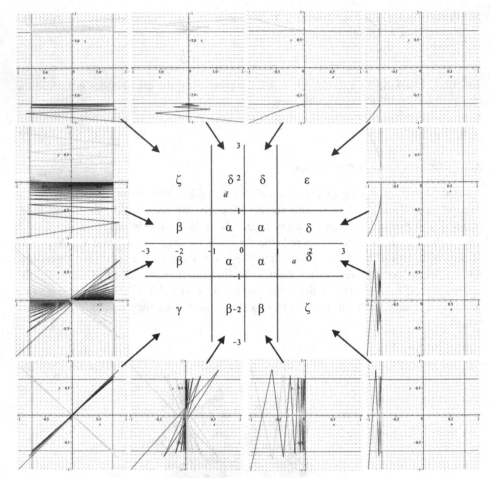

Fig. 3. Section of the Saddle and Period Doubling bifurcation curves of the fixed point (x*, y*) = (0,0) at $bc = 0$ and the corresponding phase space behavior of the system for each of the different regions showing two particular trajectories

Fig. 3 (center) shows a plane cut of Fig. 2 where $bc = 0$, i.e., when at least one of the two neurons has no dependency on the other one. The Neimark-Sacker bifurcation manifold is not displayed here for clarity. The horizontal axis a, represents the feedback weight form neuron 1 to itself, and the vertical axis d, is the feedback weight from neuron 2 to itself. Fig. 3 also shows examples of phase diagrams for each region in the central graph (except region α), each with the following parts: two trajectories (green/grey and red/black) one starting at the top left and the other at the bottom left; two null-change lines one for neuron x_1 (red) and one for neuron x_2 (blue); and the field of state differences of period 2 (grey arrows). In this case, the Jacobian of the evolution function at the origin is a diagonal matrix whose eigenvalues λ_1 and λ_2 match the values of a and d respectively.

In the central region (α), the fixed point at the origin presents stability since both eigenvalues of J_0 are between -1 and 1. This means that the origin is attractive in both directions of the eigenvectors of J_0. In region β, one of the eigenvalues of J_0 is less than -1, and the other is between -1 and 1, so the origin is attractive in one direction and (period-2) repulsive in the other. In region γ both eigenvalues are less than -1 so the origin is (period-2) repulsive in both directions. Fig 2 shows that in γ both neurons remain oscillating, either in phase (red / black) or out of phase (green / grey) while in β only one of the neurons remains oscillating.

In region δ, one of the eigenvalues is greater than 1 while the other is between -1 and 1 which means the fixed point at the origin is (period-1) repulsive in one direction and attractive in the other, i.e., an unstable fixed point. In this case one of the neurons converges to zero and the other exhibits hysteresis with respect to its external input, that is, it presents two (period-1) attractive fixed points when the external input is close to zero and one of these points disappears for sufficiently positive input and the other one disappears for sufficiently negative input. In region ε both eigenvalues are greater than 1, so both neurons present hysteresis and there are four stable fixed points of period 1 (for null inputs) in the phase space while the origin is repulsive in both directions of the eigenvectors of J_0. Finally in region ζ, one eigenvalue is greater than 1 while the other is below -1. In ζ there is a combination of hysteresis in one neuron and oscillation in the other. The information above is summarized in Table 1.

Table 1. Behavior around the origin when $bc = 0$

Region	a	b	Behavior
A	-1 < a < 1	-1 < b < 1	Stability
B	-1 < a < 1	b < -1	Oscillations
	a < -1	-1 < b < 1	
Γ	a < -1	b < -1	Double Oscillations
Δ	-1 < a < 1	1 < b	Hysteresis
	1 < a	-1 < b < 1	
E	1 < a	1 < b	Double Hysteresis
Z	1 < a	b < -1	Hysteresis and Oscillations
	a < -1	1 < b	

Now we turn our attention to the next case where only one of the neurons is connected with the other one with a synaptic weight different from zero. For example, if $b = 0$ and $c \neq 0$, then x_1 is independent of x_2 and *neuron* 2 receives as external input the output of *neuron* 1 with weight c. This external input may be constant or oscillatory depending on the configuration of the independent neuron taking into account its current external input, and it can be of any magnitude depending on the weight c. If this input is constant and large enough (see Cervantes et al (2013)) the dependent neuron can enter in a regime in which there is only one stable fixed point even when the neuron's self-feedback weight is set to oscillations or hysteresis. If the input is oscillatory the dependent neuron will also oscillate even when it is not configured to oscillate. In any case, this kind of configurations can be seen as a chain of single neurons receiving an external input, so the system's behaviour is similar to the case where neurons are independent. The complexity of the system starts when both neurons are interconnected which we analyze next.

3.3   Bifurcations When bc is Not Zero

The product bc can be seen as a measure of the weight for the period-2 feedback that a neuron receives via its influence on the other neuron combined with the influence from the other neuron. So the sign of this feedback weight determines the nature of the influence it has on both neurons either excitatory or inhibitory. Now we will see what happens when the product bc is close to zero meaning that its influence is minimal, first when it is positive and then negative.

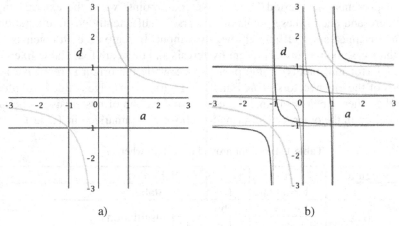

a)   b)

Fig. 4. Bifurcations in the space (a,d) with a) $bc = 0$ and b) $bc = 0.1$

Fig. 4a) shows the same graph section of Figure 2 (center) at $bc = 0$ (but including the Neimark-Sacker bifurcation manifold in green) just as a reference to be compared with Fig. 4b) that shows how these curves change when $bc > 0$ but close to zero ($bc=0.1$). The existing regions in the case $bc = 0$ are still there but now their boundaries have moved a little. As one can see, the α region (see Fig. 2 for reference) is now smaller. Now, if a and d are smaller than, but close, to 1, it is possible to reach region δ, where hysteresis is present. Similarly, if a and d are greater than but close to -1 it is possible to reach region β, where oscillations are present. This makes the stability of the fixed point at the origin be less probable than when $bc= 0$. It can also be seen that although a and d are greater than 1, if they are close to 1, one may still be in region δ. This means that, in order to reach region ε, it is necessary for a and d to take greater values than when $bc = 0$. Something similar happens when a and d are close but lower than -1 with β and γ regions respectively.

If the value of bc becomes even greater, the distance between the vertices of the hyperbolas seen in Figure 4b) is even greater. When bc is greater than 1, the α region disappears completely, which implies that the origin is always unstable.

Fig. 5a) shows bifurcations in the space (a,d) when bc is negative and close to zero ($bc = -0.1$). In this case there are the same regions that for the case $bc = 0$ plus a new region enclosed by two gray diagonal lines. In this region the eigenvalues of the Jacobian of f at the origin are complex conjugates and therefore the state of the system follows a rotational path around the fixed point at the origin. In turn, this region is cut by the green curves, which show the Neimark-Sacker bifurcation, dividing it in three parts. In the part that includes the origin $(a, d) = (0,0)$, the rotational path is a spiral towards the fixed point which is an attractor. in the other two parts the rotational path gets away from the fixed point which is a repulsor.

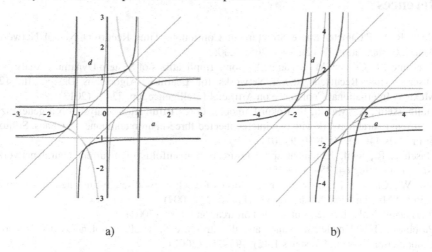

a)   b)

Fig. 5. Bifurcations in the (a,d) space a) with $bc = -0.1$ and b) with $bc = -1.1$

In Figure 5b) we have the case where $bc = -1.1$. The difference with the previous case is that the lines defining the region of the complex conjugate eigenvalues are further apart from each other and that the green curves are in quadrants II and IV. In this case the origin $(a, d) = (0,0)$ is in the region where the fixed point is a repulsor. The region where the fixed point is attractor is separated here into two regions (delimited by the red, blue and green curves) in quadrants II and IV. As the value of bc becomes more negative, this stability regions of the fixed point at origin are further apart from the origin and are smaller but never disappear.

4   Conclusions

It is clear from the results presented in this work that the behaviour of two discrete time neurons is affected whenever they are interconnected. The higher the weight of these interconnections is the higher the influence they have. The origin is a fixed point whenever the external input of the neurons is null. This fixed point can be rotationally attractive or repulsive for specific conditions of the neuron's interconnection weights. Precisely, these conditions are that one of the connection weights between the neurons is positive (excitatory) and the other negative (inhibitory). The nature of this fixed point determines the local behaviour of the system around it but it is also very influent on the global behaviour of the system. In the next phase of this analysis, we will work on the analysis of entire phase space to find the existing bifurcations for all fixed points of a DTRNN with two neurons and thus be able to characterize the global behaviour of the system in the full weight space. This study should show how a variation in the connection weights in a particular direction affects the system dynamics, which would be very useful for the design of learning algorithms.

References

1. Beer, R.D.: Parameter Space Structure of Continuous-Time Recurrent Neural Networks. Neural Computation 18(12), 3009–3051 (2006)
2. Cervantes, J., Gómez, M., Schaum, A.: Some Implications of System Dynamics Analysis of Discrete-Time Recurrent Neural Networks for Learning Algorithms Design. In: 12th Mexican International Conference on Artificial Intelligence, pp. 73–79 (2013)
3. Hajihosseini, A., Maleki, F., Rokni Lamooki, G.R.: Bifurcation analysis on a generalized recurrent neural network with two interconnected three-neuron components. Chaos, Solitons & Fractals 44(11), 1004–1019 (2011)
4. Haschke, R., Steil, J.J.: Input space bifurcation manifolds of recurrent neural networks. Neurocomputing 64, 25–38 (2005)
5. He, W., Cao, J.: Stability and bifurcation of a class of discrete-time neural networks. Applied Mathematical Modelling 31, 2111–2122 (2007)
6. Kuznetsov, Y.A.: Elements of applied bifurcation theory (2004)
7. Pasemann, F.: Complex dynamics and the structure of small neural networks. Network: Computation in Neural Systems 13(2), 195–216 (2002)

Stability of Modular Recurrent Trainable Neural Networks

Sergio Miguel Hernández Manzano and Ieroham Baruch

Department of Automatic Control, CINVESTAV-IPN, Mexico City, Mexico
{shernandez,baruch}@ctrl.cinvestav.mx

Abstract. This article presents the theorems and lemmas of stability, based on Lyapunov stability theory, for Modular Recurrent Trainable Neural Networks that have been widely used by the authors for the identification and control of mechanical systems.

Keywords: Modular Recurrent Neural Networks, System Identification, Stability of Recurrent Neural Networks, Mechanical Systems.

1 Introduction

In the last decade, the Computational Intelligence tools (CI), including Artificial Neural Networks (ANN), became universal means for many applications. Because of their approximation and learning capabilities, [1], the ANNs have been widely employed for dynamic process modeling, identification, prediction and control [2]. Among several possible neural network architectures the ones most widely used are the Feedforward NN (FFNN) and the Recurrent NN (RNN).The main NN property namely the ability to approximate complex non-linear relationships without prior knowledge of the model structure makes them a very attractive alternative to the classical modeling and control techniques. This property has been proved for both types of NNs by the universal approximation theorem, [1].

The authors have proposed a novel recurrent neural network topology, called Modular Recurrent Trainable Neural Network (MRTNN), consisting of a modular network which has two modules: The first module identifies the exponential part of the unknown plant and the second one identifies the oscillatory part of the plant. The correct operation of this topology has been successfully tested in the identification and control (direct [3] and indirect [4]), of several oscillatory plants.

Nevertheless the application of the MRTNN were successful, there is no formal proof of stability of this MRTNN topology. This paper introduces the theorems and lemmas of MRTNN's stability, and performs an identification of an oscillatory plant to show the effectiveness of this topology and its BP learning.

A. Gelbukh et al. (Eds.): MICAI 2014, Part II, LNAI 8857, pp. 95–104, 2014.

2   Recurrent Trainable Neural Networks

The Recurrent Trainable Neural Network (RTNN) topology, depicted on Fig. 1, is a hybrid one. It has one recurrent hidden layer and one feedforward output layer. This topology is inspired from the Jordan canonical form of the state-space representation of linear dynamic systems adding activation functions to the state and the output variables, [5].

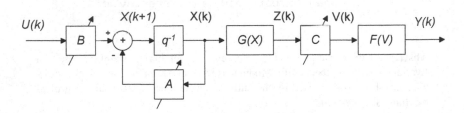

Fig. 1. Block-diagram of RTNN

The RTNN topology and its Backpropagation (BP) learning algorithm are described in vector-matrix form as:

$$X(k+1) = A(k)X(k) + B(k)U(k); \quad Z(k) = G[X(k)] \tag{1}$$

$$V(k) = C(k)Z(k); \quad Y(k) = F[V(k)] \tag{2}$$

$$A(k)=\begin{bmatrix} a_1(k) & 0 & \dots & 0 & 0 \\ 0 & \ddots & & & 0 \\ \vdots & & a_j(k) & & \vdots \\ 0 & & & \ddots & 0 \\ 0 & 0 & \dots & 0 & a_n(k) \end{bmatrix}; \quad |a_j(k)|<1; \quad j=1,2,\dots N; \tag{3}$$

$$W(k+1) = W(k) + \eta\Delta W(k) + \alpha\Delta W(k-1) \tag{4}$$

$$E(k) = T(k)-Y(k); E_1(k) = F'[Y(k)]E(k) \tag{5}$$

$$\Delta C(k) = E_1(k)Z^T(k) \tag{6}$$

$$E_3(k) = G'[Z(k)]E_2(k); \quad E_2(k) = C^T(k)E_1(k) \tag{7}$$

$$\Delta B(k) = E_3(k) U^T(k) \tag{8}$$

$$\Delta A(k) = E_3(k)X^T(k) \tag{9}$$

$$\Delta A(k) = diag(E_3(k)X^T(k)) \tag{10}$$

where X, Y, U are state, output, and input vectors with dimensions N, L, M, respectively; Z is N-dimensional output of the hidden layer; V is L-dimensional post-synaptic activity of the output layer; T is L-dimensional target vector, considered as a reference for identification; A is (NxN) state weight matrix; B and C are (NXM) and (LXN) input and output weight matrices; $F[.]$, $G[.]$ are vector-valued activation functions; $F'[.]$, $G'[.]$ are the derivatives of these functions. The matrix W is a general weight, denoting each weight matrix (C, A, B) to be updated; ΔW (ΔC, ΔA, ΔB), is the weight correction of W; η and α are learning rate parameters; for the update ΔA, there exists two possible cases, one in which A is complete matrix, given by (9), and the other in which A is diagonal matrix (10).

3   Modular Recurrent Trainable Neural Networks

The RTNN topology is completely parallel with respect to its states and completely interconnected with respect to its inputs and outputs. This feature reflects on its state feedback weight matrix which was defined as block- diagonal, having some peculiarity in the case of exponential and oscillatory reaction of the RTNN output, which permits to separate both parts.

The modular RTNN topology is depicted in Fig. 2. The first module represents the real (exponential) part of the RTNN through a diagonal state weight matrix A_1. The second module represents the complex (oscillatory) part of the RTNN through a complete state weight matrix A_2.

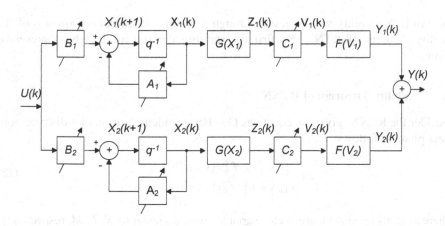

Fig. 2. Block-diagram of the MRTNN

The equations of the MRTNN and its BP learning algorithm include the equations (1) - (10) plus the following equations:

$$X(k) = [X_1(k)\ X_2(k)]^T\ ;\ Z(k) = [Z_1(k)\ Z_2(k)]^T;\ V(k) = [V_1(k)\ V_2(k)]^T \tag{11}$$

$$Y(k) = [Y_1(k)\ Y_2(k)]^T\ ;\ B(k) = [B_1(k)\ B_2(k)]^T;\ C(k) = [C_1(k)\ C_2(k)] \tag{12}$$

$$A(k) = \begin{bmatrix} A_1(k) & 0 \\ 0 & A_2(k) \end{bmatrix} \tag{13}$$

$$A_1(k) = \begin{bmatrix} a_{11}(k) & 0 & 0 \\ 0 & \ddots & 0 \\ 0 & 0 & a_{1j}(k) \end{bmatrix}; \quad |a_{1j}(k)| < 1; \quad j = 1,2,...n-2; \tag{14}$$

$$A_2(k) = \begin{bmatrix} a_{21}(k) & a_{22}(k) \\ a_{23}(k) & a_{24}(k) \end{bmatrix} \tag{15}$$

$$E_1(k) = [E_{11}(k) \quad E_{12}(k)]^T; \quad E_2(k) = [E_{21}(k) \quad E_{22}(k)]^T \tag{16}$$

$$E_3(k) = [E_{31}(k) \quad E_{32}(k)]^T \tag{17}$$

The diagonal blocks of the state matrix A corresponds to the exponential (A_1) and the oscillatory (A_2) modules of the RTNN. The state dimensions of both exponential and oscillatory RTNN modules are N-2 for A_1 and 2 for A_2. The vectors X, Y, Z, V, have two sub-vectors with appropriate dimensions, corresponding to the of the exponential and oscillatory RTNN modules. In the same way also the A, B, C, matrices are composed of sub matrices associated with the oscillatory and exponential modules. The error vectors E, $E1$, $E2$, $E3$, have appropriate dimensions.

4   Stability of MRTNN

The MRTNN stability will be tested through a lemma which is consequence of the stability theorem of RTNN. So first the stability theorem of RTNN is presented below.

4.1   Stability Theorem of RTNN

Consider the RTNN, given by equations (1)-(10), for identification of a discrete nonlinear plant, as follows

$$x(k+1) = f[x(k),u(k)] \tag{18}$$
$$y(k) = h[x(k)]$$

Where $x(k)$, $y(k)$ and $u(k)$, are vector variables with dimensions N, L, M, respectively; $f(.)$ and $h(.)$ are nonlinear vector functions with suitable dimensions. This plant's model provided the input–output data for identification. Now consider a Lyapunov function candidate as follows

$$V(k) = V_E(k) + V_1(k) \tag{19}$$

where

$$V_E(k) = \frac{1}{2} E(k)^2 \tag{20}$$

$$V_1(k) = \text{tr}\left[\tilde{A}(k)\tilde{A}(k)^{\text{T}}\right] + \text{tr}\left[\tilde{B}(k)\tilde{B}(k)^{\text{T}}\right] + \text{tr}\left[\tilde{C}(k)\tilde{C}(k)^{\text{T}}\right] \tag{21}$$

Where $E(k)$ is the instantaneous identification error between the plant's output and the RTNN´s output. Also are considered the parametric identification errors of the weights of RTNN.

$$\tilde{A}(k) = \hat{A}(k) - A^*$$
$$\tilde{B}(k) = \hat{B}(k) - B^* \tag{22}$$
$$\tilde{C}(k) = \hat{C}(k) - C^*$$

Where (A^*, B^*, C^*) are the ideal weights of RTNN identifier; ($\hat{A}(k), \hat{B}(k), \hat{C}(k)$) and are the weight estimation of RTNN at k instant. Then, deriving in discrete time the Lyapunov function candidate (19), is obtained

$$\Delta V(k+1) = V(k+1) - V(k) \tag{23}$$

$$\Delta V(k+1) = \Delta V_E(k+1) + \Delta V_1(k+1) \tag{24}$$

Where the condition for $\Delta V_E(k+1) < 0$ is that:

$$\frac{\left(1 - \frac{1}{\sqrt{2}}\right)}{\psi_{max}^2} < \eta_{max} < \frac{\left(1 + \frac{1}{\sqrt{2}}\right)}{\psi_{max}^2} \tag{25}$$

and for $\Delta V_1(k+1)$ it result:

$$\Delta V_1(k+1) < -\eta_{max} \left|E(k+1)\right|^2 - \alpha_{max} \left|E(k)\right|^2 + \beta_1(k+1) \tag{26}$$

Where all the unmodelled dynamics, the approximation errors and the perturbations, are represented by the term $\beta_1(k+1)$. For more details, the complete proof of this theorem is given in [6].

4.2 Stability Lemma of MRTNN

Given the above theorem, the MRTNN can be seen as two RTNN, one associated to exponential behaviour (A_1, B_1, C_1) and the other associated to oscillatory behavior(A_2, B_2, C_2). In the same way as the RTNN, consider the Modular-RTNN for identification of the discrete nonlinear plant (18). Now consider a Lyapunov function candidate as follow:

$$V(k) = V_E(k) + V_1(k) + V_2(k) \tag{27}$$

Where

$$V_E(k) = \frac{1}{2} E(k)^2 \tag{28}$$

$$V_1(k) = \mathrm{tr}\left[\tilde{A}_1(k)\tilde{A}_1(k)^\mathrm{T}\right] + \mathrm{tr}\left[\tilde{B}_1(k)\tilde{B}_1(k)^\mathrm{T}\right] + \mathrm{tr}\left[\tilde{C}_1(k)\tilde{C}_1(k)^\mathrm{T}\right] \tag{29}$$

$$V_2(k) = \mathrm{tr}\left[\tilde{A}_2(k)\tilde{A}_2(k)^\mathrm{T}\right] + \mathrm{tr}\left[\tilde{B}_2(k)\tilde{B}_2(k)^\mathrm{T}\right] + \mathrm{tr}\left[\tilde{C}_2(k)\tilde{C}_2(k)^\mathrm{T}\right] \tag{30}$$

Where $E(k)$ is the instantaneous identification error between the plant's output and the M-RTNN's output. Also are considered the parametric identification error of the weights of MRTNN.

$$\begin{aligned}
\tilde{A}_1(k) &= \hat{A}_1(k) - A_1^* & \tilde{A}_2(k) &= \hat{A}_2(k) - A_2^* \\
\tilde{B}_1(k) &= \hat{B}_1(k) - B_1^* & \tilde{B}_2(k) &= \hat{B}_2(k) - B_2^* \\
\tilde{C}_1(k) &= \hat{C}_1(k) - C_1^* & \tilde{C}_2(k) &= \hat{C}_2(k) - C_2^*
\end{aligned} \tag{31}$$

Where (A_1^*, B_1^*, C_1^*) and (A_2^*, B_2^*, C_2^*) are the ideal weights of M-RTNN identifier; $(\hat{A}_1(k), \hat{B}_1(k), \hat{C}_1(k))$ and $(\hat{A}_2(k), \hat{B}_2(k), \hat{C}_2(k))$ are the weight estimation of MRTNN at k instant. Then, deriving in discrete time, the Lyapunov function candidate is obtained

$$\Delta V(k+1) = V(k+1) - V(k) \tag{32}$$

$$\Delta V(k+1) = \Delta V_E(k+1) + \Delta V_1(k+1) + \Delta V_2(k+1) \tag{33}$$

Where the condition for $\Delta V_E(k+1)<0$ is that:

$$\frac{\left(1 - \frac{1}{\sqrt{2}}\right)}{\psi_{max}^2} < \eta_{max} < \frac{\left(1 + \frac{1}{\sqrt{2}}\right)}{\psi_{max}^2} \tag{34}$$

and for $\Delta V_1(k+1)$, $\Delta V_2(k+1)$ result:

$$\begin{aligned}
\Delta V_1(k+1) &< -\eta_{max}\left|E(k+1)\right|^2 - \alpha_{max}\left|E(k)\right|^2 + \beta_1(k+1) \\
\Delta V_2(k+1) &< -\eta_{max}\left|E(k+1)\right|^2 - \alpha_{max}\left|E(k)\right|^2 + \beta_2(k+1)
\end{aligned} \tag{35}$$

Where $\beta_1(k+1)$ and $\beta_2(k+1)$ represent unmodelled dynamics, approximation errors and perturbations of A_1, B_1, C_1 and A_2, B_2, C_2 respectively, in the same way as the previous theorem.

5   Simulation Results

In this section some identification results of an oscillatory plant with MRTNN are presented. The purpose here is to show the good performance of the MRTNN and its BP algorithm. So, first the input-output model of the plant for identification is presented below.

5.1   Analytical Model of an Nonlinear Oscillatory Plant

An oscillatory plant, known as Flexible Joint Mechanism-FJM [7], was used as nonlinear plant for system identification. This plant is shown in Fig.3 with parameters given on Table 1. It consists of an actuator connected to a load through a torsional spring, which represents the joint flexibility.

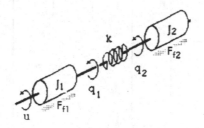

Fig. 3. Sketch of the flexible joint mechanism

This mechanical system is modeled by the next equations:

$$J_1\ddot{q}_1 + F_{f1} + k\left(q_1 - q_2\right) = u$$
$$J_2\ddot{q}_2 + F_{f2} - k\left(q_1 - q_2\right) = 0$$
(36)

$$F_{fi} = f_c\,\mathrm{sign}(\dot{q}_i) + f_v\dot{q} + f_s\,\mathrm{sign}(\dot{q}_i)e^{-(\dot{q}_i/\eta_s)} \quad i = 1, 2$$
(37)

Where q_1 is the actuator rotor angle, q_2 is the load angle; J_1, J_2 are the rotor and the load inertia; F_{f1} y F_{f2} are the load friction composed of coulomb friction and viscose friction static friction; and u is the input torque applied to the motor shaft.

Table 1. Summary of constants in the plant model

Parameter	Units	Value
J_2, J_2	Nms^2/rad	0.016
f_c	Nm	0.006
f_v	Nms/rad	0.003
f_s	Nm	0.002
η_s	rad/s	0.005
k	Nm/rad	5

5.2   System Identification Results

The system identification was performed by a MRTNN. The topology of the MRTNN is (1, 2, 1) and (1, 2, 1) for the first and the second module, respectively. The activation functions are tanh(.) for both layers and both modules. The learning rate parameters for the BP algorithm of learning are $\alpha=0$, $\eta=0.01$. The input excitation signal was a train pulses as shown in Fig. 4. The angular velocity of load inertia, $\dot{q}_2 = \omega_2$ from (36), was used as plant's output.

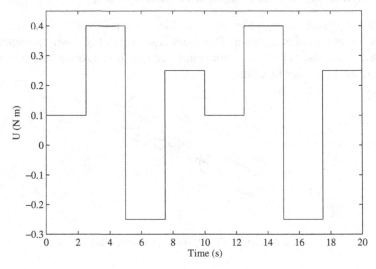

Fig. 4. Input excitation signal

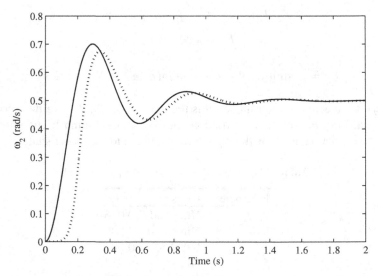

Fig. 5. Graphical results for the first moments of the plant identification. The solid line correspond to plant's output and the dotted line corresponds to MTRNN's output.

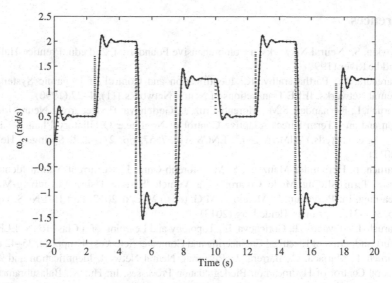

Fig. 6. Graphical results for the complete identification. The solid line correspond to plant's output and the dotted line corresponds to MTRNN's output.

The first moments of identification and the complete identification, during 20 s, are shown in Fig. 5 and Fig. 6, respectively. In these figures can be seen that the output of MRTNN follows the plant's output. The final Means Square Error MSE after 20 sec. of identification using the MRTNN is 0.0037.

6   Conclusion

This article presents the theorem and lemma for stability of Modular Recurrent Trainable Neural Networks. This is presented as an extension of the theorem of stability of RTNN. Also some simulation results for the identification of an oscillating mechanical plant are presented. The obtained MSE of identification is 0.0037, which is very small, confirms the good BP learning of the MRTNN. The obtained good graphical results support the effectiveness of MRTNN architecture and the BP learning algorithm for identification of nonlinear systems.

Acknowledgements. The author Sergio Hernández is grateful to CONACYT, Mexico for the fellowship received during his study at DCA, CINVESTAV-IPN, Mexico City, MEXICO.

References

1. Haykin, S.: Neural Networks, a Comprehensive Foundation, 2nd edn. Prentice-Hall, Upper Saddle River (1999)
2. Narendra, K., Parthasarathy, K.: Identification and Control of Dynamic Systems using Neural Networks. IEEE Transactions of Neural Networks 1(1), 4–27 (1990)
3. Baruch, I., Hernandez, S.M., Moreno-Cruz, J., Gortcheva, E.: Recurrent Neural Identification and an I-Term Direct Adaptive Control of Nonlinear Oscillatory Plant. In: Ramsay, A., Agre, G. (eds.) AIMSA 2012. LNCS, vol. 7557, pp. 212–222. Springer, Heidelberg (2012)
4. Baruch, I., Hernandez-Manzano, S.-M., Moreno-Cruz, J.: Recurrent Neural Identification and I-Term Sliding Mode Control of a Vehicle System Using Levenberg-Marquardt Learning. In: Batyrshin, I., Mendoza, M.G. (eds.) MICAI 2012, Part II. LNCS, vol. 7630, pp. 304–316. Springer, Heidelberg (2013)
5. Baruch, I., Stoyanov, I., Gortcheva, E.: Topology and Learning of a Class RNN. ELEKTRIK (Turkish Journal of Electrical Engineering and Computer Sciences) 4(suppl.1), 35–42 (1996)
6. Baruch, I., Mariaca, C., Barrera, J.: Recurrent Neural Network Identification and Adaptive Neural Control of Hydrocarbon Biodegradation Processes. In: Hu, X., Balasubramaniam, P. (eds.) Recurrent Neural Networks, pp. 61–88. I-Tech/ARS Press, Vienna Austria (2008)
7. Spong, M., Vidyasagar, M.: Robot Dynamics and Control. John Wiley & Sons Inc., USA (1989)

Intelligent Control of Induction Motor
Based Comparative Study: Analysis of Two Topologies

Moulay Rachid Douiri, El Batoul Mabrouki, Ouissam Belghazi, Mohamed Ferfra,
and Mohamed Cherkaoui

Mohammadia Engineering School, Department of Electrical Engineering,
Ibn Sina Avenue, 765, Agdal-Rabat, Morocco
douirirachid@hotmail.com

Abstract. In this paper, two intelligent direct torque control strategies are compared with the classical direct torque control (C-DTC) scheme, namely neural network control (NNC) and neuro-fuzzy control (NFC) are introduced to replace the hysteresis comparators and lookup table of the C-DTC for pulse width-modulation-inverter-fed induction motor drive, to solve the problems of torque ripple and inconstant switch frequency of inverter in the conventional direct torque control. These intelligent approaches are characterized by very fast torque and flux response, very-low-speed operation, the switching frequency of the inverter is constant and simple tuning capability. The proposed techniques are verified by simulation study of the whole drive system and results are compared with conventional direct torque control method.

Keywords: Neural network controller, neuro-fuzzy controller, direct torque control, induction motor.

1   Introduction

The C-DTC employs two hysteresis controllers to regulate stator flux and developed torque respectively, to obtain approximately decoupling of the flux and torque control. The key issue of design of the C-DTC is the strategy of how to select the proper stator voltage vector to force stator flux and developed torque into their prescribed band. The hysteresis controller is usually a two-value bang-bang controller, which results in taking the same action for the big torque error and small torque error. So it may produce big torque ripple [1], [2]. To improve the performance of the C-DTC it is natural to divide torque error into several intervals, on which different control action is; taken. As the C-DTC control strategy is not based on a motor mathematical model, it is not easy to give an apparent boundary to the division of torque error [3], [4], [5]. The above explained C-DTC limitations involve plenty of nonlinear functions Therefore, Artificial Intelligence is suggested to overcome the C-DTC limitations.

An artificial neural network (ANN) is essentially a way to learn the relationship between a set of input data and the corresponding output data [6]. That is, it can memorize data, generalize this information when given new input data, and adjust when the relationship changes. The training is normally done with input-output examples.

A. Gelbukh et al. (Eds.): MICAI 2014, Part II, LNAI 8857, pp. 105–115, 2014.

After training, ANNs have the capability of generalization [7]. That is, given previously unseen input data, they can interpolate from the previous training data [7], [8]. Inspired by the functioning of biological neurons, ANN became popular in the research community when architectures were found to enable the learning of nonlinear functions and patterns [6], [9].

The concept of a NFC has emerged in recent years, as researchers have tried to combine the advantages of both FLC and artificial neural networks (ANNs). The NFC utilizes the transparent linguistic representation of a fuzzy system with the learning ability of ANNs [10], [13]. In [11], [12], a large number of membership functions and rules are used for designing the controller; these cause high computational burden for the conventional NFC, which is the major limitation for practical industrial applications.

This paper is organized as follows: The principle of C-DTC is presented in the second part, the NN-DTC is developed in the third section, section four presents a NF-DTC, and the fifth part is devoted to illustrate the simulation performance of this control strategy, a conclusion and reference list at the end.

2   Classical Direct Torque Control (C-DTC)

In a C-DTC motor drive, the machine torque and flux linkage are controlled directly without a current control. The vector expressions of the machine in the frame of reference linked to the stator were used:

$$\begin{cases} \bar{v}_s = R_s \bar{i}_s + \dfrac{d\bar{\lambda}_s}{dt}, \\ \dfrac{L_m}{L_s} \bar{\lambda}_s = \sigma \tau_r \dfrac{d\bar{\lambda}_r}{dt} + (1 - j\omega_r \sigma \tau_r)\bar{\lambda}_r, \end{cases} \quad \text{where} \quad \sigma = 1 - \frac{L_m^2}{L_s L_r} \tag{1}$$

The electromagnetic torque is proportional to the vectorial product between the stator and rotor flux vector:

$$T_e = \frac{3}{2} n_p \frac{L_m}{\sigma L_s L_r} \left| \vec{\lambda}_s \right| \left| \vec{\lambda}_r \right| \sin \alpha \tag{2}$$

where α is the angle between the stator and rotor flux linkage vectors. The derivative of (2) can be represented approximately as:

$$\frac{dT_e}{dt} = \frac{3}{2} n_p \frac{L_m}{\sigma L_s L_r} \left| \vec{\lambda}_s \right| \left| \vec{\lambda}_r \right| \frac{d\alpha}{dt} \cos \alpha \tag{3}$$

The machine voltage equation can be represented and approximated in a short interval of Δt as:

$$\frac{d\vec{\lambda}_s}{dt} = \vec{v}_s - R_s \vec{i}_s \approx \vec{v}_s \quad \text{implying} \quad \Delta \vec{\lambda}_s = \vec{v}_s \Delta t \tag{4}$$

The magnitude of stator flux can be estimated by

$$\lambda_{ds} = \int_0^t (v_{ds} - R_s i_{ds})\mathrm{d}t \quad \text{and} \quad \lambda_{qs} = \int_0^t (v_{qs} - R_s i_{qs})\mathrm{d}t. \tag{5}$$

The torque can be calculated using the components of the estimated flux and measured currents:

$$T_e = n_p (\lambda_{ds} i_{qs} - \lambda_{qs} i_{ds}). \tag{6}$$

List of Symbols

R_s, R_r	stator and rotor resistance [Ω]
i_{sd}, i_{sq}	stator current dq axis [A]
v_{sd}, v_{sq}	stator voltage dq axis [V]
L_s, L_r	stator and rotor self inductance [H]
L_m	mutual inductance [H]
λ_{sd}, λ_{sq}	dq stator flux [Wb]
λ_{rd}, λ_{rq}	dq rotor flux [Wb]
T_e	electromagnetic torque [N.m]
E_{Te}	electromagnetic torque error [N.m]
$E_{\lambda s}$	stator flux error [Wb]
φ_s	stator flux angle [rad]
ω_r	rotor speed [rad/sec]
J	inertia moment [Kg.m^2]
n_p	pole pairs
σ	leakage coefficient

3   Neural Network Based Direct Torque Control

This section presents the outline of neural networks to emulate the table of inverter switching states of DTC. The input signals of the table are the errors of electromagnetic torque, stator flux and the position vector of flux. The output signals are the inverter switching states n_a, n_b and n_c. As the switching table depends only on the electromagnetic torque error, stator flux angle and sector where the flux is located, and induction motor parameters, this neural network can be trained independently of the set. With the changes in the switching table reduces the training patterns and increases the execution speed of training process. This has been achieved by reducing the table to convert input analog signals to a digital bit for the flux error, two bits for the torque error and three bits for the flux position, which has a total of six inputs and three outputs, and only sixty-four training patterns. With these modifications, the network used to simulate has the advantage that it is independent of parameter variation of induction motor. This allows applying to any induction motor irrespective of its power.

From the flux space vectors λ_{ds} and λ_{qs} we can calculate the flux angle φ and flux magnitude λ_s. The coding of the flux angle is given by ξ_1, ξ_2 and ξ_3 according to following equations:

$$\lambda_s = \sqrt{\lambda_{ds}^2 + \lambda_{qs}^2} \,, \quad \varphi_s = \tan^{-1}\frac{\lambda_{ds}}{\lambda_{qs}}, \quad \xi_1\xi_2\xi_3 = encoder(\varphi_s) \tag{7}$$

$$\xi_1 = \begin{cases} 1 & \lambda_{qs} \geq 0 \\ 0 & otherwise \end{cases} \tag{8}$$

$$\xi_2 = \begin{cases} 1 & \left(\frac{\lambda_{qs}}{\lambda_{ds}} \geq -\tan(\frac{\pi}{3}) \quad and \quad \lambda_{ds} \prec 0\right) or \left(\frac{\lambda_{qs}}{\lambda_{ds}} \prec -\tan(\frac{\pi}{3}) \quad and \quad \lambda_{qs} \prec 0\right) \\ 0 & otherwise \end{cases} \tag{9}$$

$$\xi_3 = \begin{cases} 1 & \left(\frac{\lambda_{qs}}{\lambda_{ds}} \prec \tan(\frac{\pi}{3}) \quad and \quad \lambda_{ds} \geq 0\right) or \left(\frac{\lambda_{qs}}{\lambda_{ds}} \geq \tan(\frac{\pi}{3}) \quad and \quad \lambda_{qs} \prec 0\right) \\ 0 & otherwise \end{cases} \tag{10}$$

The network structure used, as shown in Fig. 1 has an input layer with five neurons, a first hidden layer with six neurons, a second hidden layer with five neurons and an output layer with three neurons. After training satisfactory, taking the weights and thresholds calculated and placed into the neural network prototype replacing the switching table. This network is incorporated as a part of the DTC.

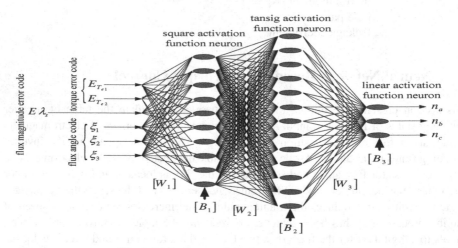

Fig. 1. Neural-network implementation of DTC

4   Neuro-Fuzzy Direct Torque Control

In this section, the Neuro-Fuzzy (NF) model is built using the multilayer fuzzy neural network shown in Fig.2. The controller has a total of five layers as proposed by *Lin and Lee* [13], with two inputs (stator flux error $E_{\psi s}$, electromagnetic torque error E_{Te}) and a single output (voltage space vector) is considered here for convenience. Consequently, there are two nodes in layer 1 and one node in layer 5. Nodes in layer 1 are input nodes that directly transmit input signals to the next layer. The layer 5 is the output layer. The nodes in layers 2 and 4 are "term nodes" and they act as membership functions to express the input/output fuzzy linguistic variables. A bell-shaped function is adopted to represent a membership function, in which the mean value p and the variance χ are adjusted through the learning process. The two fuzzy sets of the first and the second input variables consist of k_1 and k_2 linguistic terms, respectively. The linguistic terms are numbered in descending order in the term nodes; hence, k_1+k_2 nodes and n_3 nodes are included in layers 2 and 4, respectively, to indicate the input/output Linguistic variables.

Layer 1. Each node in this layer performs a MF:

$$y_i^1 = \mu_{Ai}(x_i) = \exp\left\{-\left[\left(\frac{x_i - c_i}{a_i}\right)^2\right]^{b_i}\right\}$$ (11)

where x_i is the input of node i, A_i is linguistic label associated with this node and (a_i, b_i, c_i) is the parameter set of the bell-shaped MF. y_i^1 specifies the degree to which the given input belongs to the linguistic label A_i, with maximum equal 1 and minimum equal to 0. As the values of these parameters change, the bell-shaped function varies accordingly, thus exhibiting various forms of membership functions. In fact, any continuous and piecewise differentiable functions, such as trapezoidal or triangular membership functions, are also qualified candidates for node functions in this layer.

Layer 2. Every node in this layer represents the firing strength of the rule. Hence, the nodes perform the fuzzy AND operation:

$$y_i^2 = w_i = \min\left(\mu_{A\lambda_s}(E_{\lambda_s}), \mu_{BT_e}(E_{T_e}), \mu_{C\varphi_s}(\varphi_s)\right)$$ (12)

Layer 3. The nodes of this layer calculate the normalized firing strength of each rule:

$$y_i^3 = \overline{w}_i = \frac{w_i}{\sum_{i=1}^n w_i}$$ (13)

Layer 4. Output of each node in this layer is the weighted consequent part of the rule table:

$$y_i^4 = \overline{w}_i f_i = \overline{w}_i\left(p_i E_{\lambda_s} + q_i E_{T_e} + m_i \varphi_s + n_i\right)$$ (14)

where $\overline{w}_i$ is the output of layer 3, and $\{p_i, q_i, m_i, n_i\}$ is the parameter set. Which determine the ith component of vector desired voltage. By multiplying weight y_i by voltage continuous V side of the inverter according to (15):

$$V^* = y_i V \qquad (15)$$

Layer 5. The single node in this layer computes the overall output as the summation of all incoming signals:

$$y_i^5 = \sum_{i=1}^{n} \overline{w}_i f_i \qquad (16)$$

Which determine the vector reference voltage v_s^* (see Fig. 4), from (17):

$$v_s^* = \sum_{i=1}^{9} y_i V e^{j\xi_i^*} \qquad (17)$$

The angle ξ is obtained from the actual angle of stator flux φ_s and angle increment $d\varphi_i$ given by this (18):

$$\xi_i = \varphi_s + d\varphi_i \qquad (18)$$

y_i ($i = 1..9$) are the output signals order i of the third layer respectively.

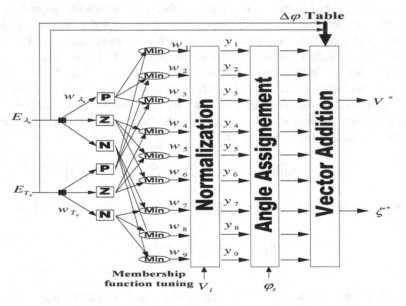

Fig. 2. Topology of the neuro-fuzzy model used

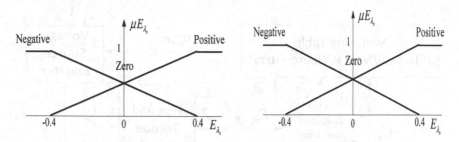

Fig. 3. Triangular membership function sets

Table 1 represents the angle increment λ_i of reference voltage vector, where the torque and flux errors are represented by three subsystems: value, positive (P), zero (Z), negative (N) (Fig. 3).

Table 1. Angle increment of the reference voltage vector

				$E_{\lambda s}$					
		P			Z			N	
E_{Te}	P	Z	N	P	Z	N	P	Z	N
$\Delta\lambda$	$\pi/3$	0	$-\pi/3$	$\pi/2$	$\pi/2$	$-\pi/2$	$2\pi/3$	π	$2\pi/3$

The model setting is listed in Table 2.

Table 2. Parameters setting for ANFIS model

ANFIS Setting	Details
Input variables	Electromagnetic torque error, and stator flux error
Output response	Space voltage vector
Type of input MFs	Generalized Bell MF
Number of MFs	2,3, 4 and 5
Type of output MFs	Linear and constant
Type inference	Linear Sugeno
Optimization Method	Hybrid of the least-squares and the back propagation gradient descent method.
Number of data	520
Epochs	1000

To compare and verify the proposed techniques in this paper, a digital simulation based on Matlab/Simulink program with a Neural Network Toolbox and ANFIS Toolbox is used to simulate the NN-DTC and NF-DTC, as shown in Fig. 5 and Fig. 6. The block diagram of a C-DTC/FL-DTC/NN-DTC controlled induction motor drive fed by a 2-level inverter is shown in Fig. 4.

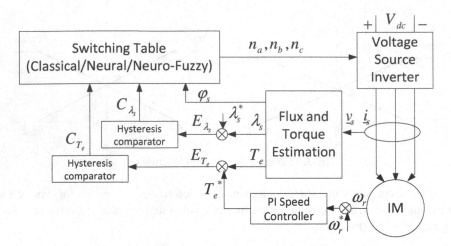

Fig. 4. General configuration of C-DTC/NN-DTC/NF-DTC scheme

The induction motor used for the simulation studies has the following parameters:

Rated power = 7.5kW, Rated voltage = 220V, Rated frequency = 60Hz, R_r = 0.17Ω, R_s = 0.15Ω, L_r = 0.035H, L_s = 0.035H, L_m = 0.0338H, J = 0.14kg.m^2.

Fig. 5 shows the starting transient performance response of electromagnetic torque for the four control strategies: C-DTC, NN-DTC and NF-DTC. The NF-DTC has the best transient response where the motor torque is approximately built up in less than 0.0074 s.

Figs. 6(a), 6(b) and 6(c) show the torque response of the C-DTC, NN-DTC and NF-DTC respectively with a torque reference of [20-10-15]Nm. While Figs. 6(a'), 6(b') and 6(c') show the flux response of the C-DTC, NN-DTC and NF-DTC respectively with a stator flux reference of 1Wb.

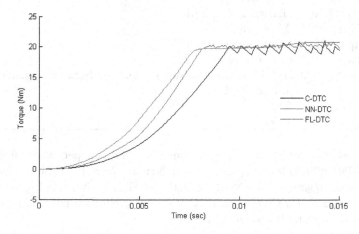

Fig. 5. Starting transient performance of electromagnetic torque according different control strategies

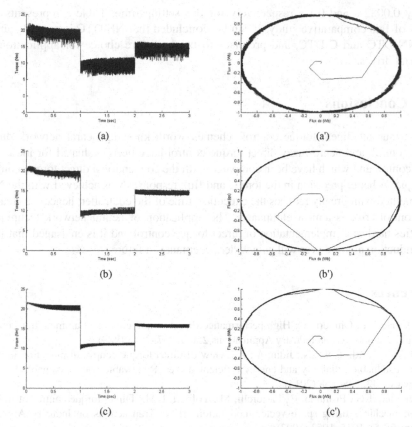

Fig. 6. (a), (b) and (c) torque response of C-DTC, NN-DTC and NF-DTC respectively, (a'), (b') and (c') Stator flux trajectory response of C-DTC, NN-DTC and NF-DTC respectively

Table 3. Comparative study of C-DTC, FL-DTC and NF-DTC

Control strategies	Torque ripple (%)	Flux ripple (%)	Rise time (sec)	Setting time (sec)
C-DTC	10.6	2.3	0.009	0.01
NN-DTC	2.9	1.6	0.006	0.0082
NF-DTC	2.4	1.3	0.004	0.0074

The minimum ripple for both electromagnetic torque and stator flux is obtained using NF-DTC, where the torque ripple percentage is approximately 2.4%, and 1.3% for the flux ripple percentage, while the NN-DTC and C-DTC have a relatively large ripple, where the torque ripple percentage was approximately 2.9%, and 10.6% respectively, and approximately 1.6% and 2.3% respectively for the flux ripple percentage. Further, the NF-DTC has the best transient response for the torque, where the rise time is 0.004 s, and the setting time 0.0074 s, faster than NN-DTC and C-DTC, where the rise time is approximately 0.006 s and 0.009 s respectively, and approximately 0.0082 s and 0.1 s respectively for the setting time. Table 3 represents the results of this comparative study. It can be concluded that NF-DTC is more accurate than NN-DTC and C-DTC, and promises to be the future choice for application in industrial drives.

5   Conclusions

Two various intelligent torque control schemes worth knowing neural network direct torque control, and neuro-fuzzy direct torque control have been evaluated for induction motor control and which have been compared with the conventional direct torque control technique. A better precision in the torque and flux responses was achieved with the NF-DTC method with greatly reduces the execution time of the controller; hence the steady-state control error is almost eliminated. The application of neural network techniques simplifies hardware implementation of direct torque control and it is envisaged that NF-DTC induction motor drives will gain wider acceptance in future.

References

1. Takahashi, I., Ohmori, Y.: High-performance direct torque control of an induction motor. IEEE Transactions on Industry Applications 25(2), 257–264 (1989)
2. Sutikno, T., Idris, N.R.N., Jidin, A.: A review of direct torque control of induction motors for sustainable reliability and energy efficient drives. Renewable and Sustainable Energy Reviews 32, 548–558 (2014)
3. Habetler, T.G., Profumo, F., Pastorelli, M., Tolbert, L.M.: Direct torque control of induction machines using space vector modulation. IEEE Transactions on Industry Applications 28(5), 1045–1053 (1992)
4. Kazmierkowski, M.P., Kasprowicz, A.B.: Improved direct torque and flux vector control of PWM inverter-fed induction motor drives. IEEE Transactions on Industrial Electronics 42(4), 344–350 (1995)
5. Tiitinen, P., Surandra, M.: Next generation motor control method, DTC direct torque control. In: Proceedings of the IEEE International Conference on Power Electronics, Drives and Energy Systems for Industrial Growth, PEDES, vol. 1, pp. 37–43 (1996)
6. Livingstone, D.J.: Artificial Neural Networks: Methods and Applications. Humana Press Inc. (2009)
7. Dai, S., Wang, C., Wang, M.: Dynamic learning from adaptive neural network control of a class of nonaffine nonlinear systems. IEEE Transactions on Neural Networks and Learning Systems 25(1), 111–123 (2014)
8. Chow, T.W.S., Cho, S.-Y.: Neural Networks and Computing: Learning Algorithms and Applications. Imperial College Press, Har/Cdr (2007)
9. Cong, W., Hill, D.J.: Learning From Neural Control. IEEE Transactions on Neural Networks 17(1), 130–146 (2006)
10. Rutkowski, L.: Flexible Neuro-Fuzzy Systems: Structures, Learning and Performance Evaluation. The Springer International Series in Engineering and Computer Science. Springer (2004)

11. Grabowski, P.Z., Kazmierkowski, M.P., Böse, B.K., Blaabjerg, F.A.: Simple direct-torque neuro-fuzzy control of pwm-inverter-fed induction motor drive. IEEE Transactions on Industrial Electronics 47(4), 863–870 (2000)
12. Grabowski, P.Z., Blaabjerg, F.: Direct torque neuro-fuzzy control of induction motor drive DSP implementation. In: IECON Proceedings (Industrial Electronics Conference), vol. 2, pp. 657–662 (1998)
13. Lin, C.-T., Lee, C.S.G.: Neural-Network-Based Fuzzy Logic Control and Decision System. IEEE Transactions on Computers 40(12), 1320–1336 (1991)
14. Kar, S., Das, S., Ghosh, P.K.: Applications of neuro fuzzy systems: A brief review and future outline. Applied Soft Computing Journal 15, 243–259 (2014)

Auto-Adaptive Neuro-Fuzzy Parameter Regulator for Motor Drive

Moulay Rachid Douiri, Mohamed Ferfra, Ouissam Belghazi,
and Mohamed Cherkaoui

Mohammadia Engineering School, Department of Electrical Engineering,
Ibn Sina Avenue, 765, Agdal-Rabat, Morocco
douirirachid@hotmail.com

Abstract. In this paper, a new adaptive network based fuzzy-inference system (ANFIS) architecture is proposed for rotor position and speed estimation over wide range of speed operation for indirect field orientation controlled induction motor drive. This intelligent approach controller incorporates Sugeno model based fuzzy logic laws with a five-layer artificial neural networks (ANNs) scheme. Moreover, for the proposed neuro-fuzzy controller (NFC) an improved self-tuning method is developed based on the induction motor theory and its high performance requirements. The principal task of the tuning method is to adjust the parameters of the fuzzy logic controller (FLC) in order to minimize the square of the error between actual and reference output. The convergence/divergence of the weights is discussed and investigated by simulation.

Keywords: Adaptive network based fuzzy-inference system, indirect field oriented control, induction motor, self-tuning, speed control.

1 Introduction

The continuous information of rotor position and speed is essentially required for vector control of induction motor to have optimal torque control. For this purpose, generally shaft mounted speed sensors are used, resulting into additional cost and complexity of the system. To avoid the additional sensor cost, complexity and the other associated problems, there has been significant interest in the sensorless control of IM [1], [2]. Moreover, the elimination of these sensors and their connecting leads increases the mechanical robustness and reliability of overall system. All these factors have made the sensorless control of IM more attractive. But the rotor speed and position estimation typically requires the accurate knowledge of motor parameters, which may not be easily available or difficult to obtain, especially under varying operating conditions [3], [4]. This method works satisfactorily at higher speeds. However, the speed estimation becomes very difficult at lower speeds. Some state observer methods based on Extended Kalman Filter (EKF) [5], [6], Extended Luenberger Observer (ELO) [7], [8], and Sliding Mode Observer (SMO) [9] etc., have also been reported. Most of them suffer due to complex computation, sensitivity to parameter variation

A. Gelbukh et al. (Eds.): MICAI 2014, Part II, LNAI 8857, pp. 116–127, 2014.

and need of accurate initial conditions. However, the EKF has the advantage of estimating the parameters and speed simultaneously by considering them as state, but at
the increased cost of computational burden. The sliding mode observer is simple and
offers a limited robustness against the parameter variation. However, sliding mode,
being a discontinuous control with variable switching characteristics, has chattering
problems, which may affect the control accuracy. Recently, some more advanced
adaptive estimation techniques based on Artificial Neural Network (ANN) [10], [11],
[12] and Fuzzy Logic Control (FLC) [13], [14] have also been reported. However, the
estimation accuracy depends on number of neurons and number of fuzzy membership
functions used for rule base.

To overcome these problems, a novel ANFIS based rotor speed estimator of indirect vector controlled induction motor has been proposed for wide range of speed
operation. The ANFIS architecture has well known advantages of modeling a highly
non-linear system, as it combines the capability of fuzzy reasoning in handling uncertainties and capability of ANN in learning from processes. Thus, the ANFIS is used to
develop an adaptive model of variable speed IM under highly uncertain operating
conditions, which also automatically compensates any variation in parameters such as
inductance, resistance etc. An error gradient based dynamic back-propagation [15],
[16] method has been used for the online tuning of ANFIS architecture.

Nomenclature

d,q	direct and quadrature components
Rs , R_r	stator and rotor resistance [Ω]
i_{ds} , i_{qs}	stator current d-q axis [A]
i_{dr} , i_{qr}	rotor current d-q axis [A]
L_s, L_r, L_m	stator, rotor and mutual inductance [H]
$\lambda dr, \lambda qr$	d-q rotor fluxes [Wb]
T_{em}	electromagnetic torque [N.m]
$\omega_r, \omega_e, \omega_{sl}$	rotor speed, synchronous and slip frequency [rad/s]
τ_r	rotor time constant [s]
J	inertia moment [Kg.m^2]
n_p	motor pole number

2   Induction Motor Model for Indirect Field Oriented Control

Field oriented control provides a method of decoupling the two components of stator
currents; one producing the air gap flux and the other producing the torque. Therefore,
independent control of torque and flux, which is similar to a separately excited direct
current motor, can be achieved. The magnitude and phase of the stator currents are
controlled in such a way that flux and torque components of current remain decoupled
during transient and steady-state conditions. Since the d-q frame has been defined as
rotating with the same angular velocity as the vector quantities of the motor, any one
of these vectors can be used as a reference with which the d-q frame is to be aligned

in order to further simplify the torque. In classical approach the d-q frame is aligned with rotor flux vector λ_r. This leads to:

$$\lambda_{qr} = 0. \tag{1}$$

Then the torque equation becomes:

$$T_{em} = \frac{2n_p}{3R_r}\frac{L_m}{\tau_r}i_{qs}\lambda_{dr} = C_T\lambda_{dr}i_{qs} \quad \text{where} \quad C_T = \frac{2n_p}{3R_r}\frac{L_m}{\tau_r}. \tag{2}$$

Hence, when λ_{qr} = Constant there is a linear relationship between current i_{qs} and torque. Indirect field oriented control avoids the requirement of flux estimation by computing the appropriate motor slip frequency ω_{sl} to obtain the desired flux position θ_e:

$$\theta_e = \int(\omega_r + \omega_{sl})dt \quad \text{where} \quad \omega_{sl} = \frac{L_m}{|\lambda_r|_{command}}\frac{R_r}{L_r}i_{qs}. \tag{3}$$

The rotor flux magnitude is related to the direct axis stator current by a first-order differential equation; thus, it can be controlled by controlling the direct axis stator current:

$$\lambda_r = L_m i_{ds}. \tag{4}$$

Indirect vector control can be calculated as follow:

$$i_{ds}^* = \frac{\lambda_r^*}{L_m}. \tag{5}$$

$$i_{qs}^* = \frac{2L_r T_e^*}{3n_p L_m \lambda_r^*}. \tag{6}$$

$$\omega_{sl}^* = \frac{R_r L_m i_{qs}^*}{L_r \lambda_r^*}. \tag{7}$$

$$\theta_e^* = \int\omega_e^* dt = \int(\omega_r + \omega_{sl}^*)dt. \tag{8}$$

3   Self-adaptive ANFIS Speed Controller for Induction Motor

3.1   Design of the ANFIS Speed Controller

In this paper, the neuro-fuzzy (NF) model is built using the multilayer fuzzy neural network. The system has a total of five layers. A model with one input and a single output is considered here for convenience. Accordingly, there are one node in layer 1 and one node in layer 5. Node in layer 1 is input node that directly transmits input signals to the next layer. Nodes in layers 2 and 4 are "term nodes" and they act as membership functions to express the input/output fuzzy linguistic variables. The two fuzzy sets of the first and the second input variables consist of n_1 and n_2 linguistic terms, respectively. The linguistic terms, such as positive big (PB), positive medium (PM), positive small (PS), approximate zero (AZ), negative small (NS), negative medium (NM), negative big (NB), are numbered in descending order in the term nodes, Hence, n_1+n_2 nodes and n_3 nodes are included in layers 2 and 4, respectively, to indicate the input/output Linguistic variables [17].

Each node of layer 3 is a "rule node" and represents a single fuzzy control rule. In total, there are $n_1 \times n_2$ nodes in layer 3 to form a fuzzy rule base for two linguistic input variables. The links of layers 3 and 4 define the preconditions and consequences of the rule nodes, respectively [17]. For each rule node, there are two fixed links from the input term nodes. Layer 4 links, are adjusted in response to varying control situations. By contrast, the links of layers 2 and 5 remain fixed between the input/output nodes and their corresponding tem nodes. The NF model can adjust the fuzzy rules and their membership functions by modifying layer 4 links and the parameters that represent the membership functions for each node in layers 2 and 4.

An ANFIS based on Takagi-Sugeno-Kang (TSK) [18] method having $1 \rightarrow 6 \rightarrow 3 \rightarrow 3 \rightarrow 1$ architecture with one input (difference between reference speed ω_r^* and actual speed ωr) and one outputs (T_{em}^*) is used to develop the dynamic model of induction motor. The errors between the reference and actual speed $e = \omega_r^* - \omega_r$ are used to tune the precondition and consequent parameters.

The node functions of each layer in ANFIS architecture are as described below:

Layer 1: This layer is also known as fuzzification layer where each node is represented by square. Here, three membership functions are assigned to each input. The trapezoidal and triangular membership functions are used to reduce the computation burden, and their corresponding node equations are as given below [19]:

$$\mu_{A_1}(e) = \begin{cases} 1 & e \leq b_1 \\ \dfrac{e-a_1}{b_1-a_1} & b_1 \prec e \prec a_1 \\ 0 & e \geq a_1 \end{cases} \tag{9}$$

$$\mu_{A_2}(e) = \begin{cases} 1 - \dfrac{e-a_2}{0.5b_2} & |e-a_2| \leq 0.5b_2 \\ 0 & |e-a_2| \geq 0.5b_2 \end{cases} \tag{10}$$

$$\mu_{A_3}(e) = \begin{cases} 0 & e \le a_3 \\ \dfrac{e - a_3}{b_3 - a_3} & a_3 \prec e \prec b_3 \\ 1 & e \ge b_3 \end{cases} \tag{11}$$

where the value of parameters (a_i, b_i) changes with the change in error and accordingly generates the linguistic value of each membership function. Parameters in this layer are referred as premise parameters or precondition parameters.

Layer 2: Every node in this layer is a circle labeled as Π which multiplies the incoming signals and forwards it to next layer [19].

$$\mu_i = \mu_{A_i}(e_1).\mu_{A_i}(e_2)..., \quad i = 1, 2, 3. \tag{12}$$

But in our case there is only one input, so this layer can be ignored and the output of first layer will directly pass to the third layer. Here, the output of each node represents the firing strength of a rule.

Layer 3: Every node in this layer is represented as circle. This layer calculates the normalized firing strength of each rule as given below [19]:

$$\bar{\mu}_i = \frac{\mu_i}{\mu_1 + \mu_2 + \mu_3} \quad i = 1, 2, 3. \tag{13}$$

Layer 4: Every node in this layer is a square node with a node function [19]:

$$O_i = \bar{\mu}_i.f_i = \bar{\mu}_i \left(a_0^i + a_1^i e \right) \quad i = 1, 2, 3. \tag{14}$$

where the parameters $\left(a_0^i, a_1^i \right)$ are tuned as the function of input (e). The parameters in this layer are also referred as consequent parameters.

Layer 5: This layer is also called output layer which computes the output as given below [19]:

$$Y = \bar{\mu}_1.f_1 + \bar{\mu}_2.f_2 + \bar{\mu}_3.f_3. \tag{15}$$

The output from this layer is multiplied with the normalizing factor to obtain the reference electromagnetic torque (T_{em}^*).

4   Training of ANFIS Architecture

To minimize the error, the ANFIS structure is tuned with gradient descent technique (usually a cost function given by the squared error) where the weights are iterated by propagating the error from output layer to input layer. The "back-propagation" [16] is qualified for such a calculation. The on-line training algorithm is completed in two stages, known as precondition parameter tuning and consequent parameter tuning, where the objective function to be minimized is defined as:

$$e^2 = \left(\omega_r^* - \omega_r \right)^2. \tag{16}$$

The fuzzy membership functions are required to update by the precondition parameters as discussed in previous section for layer 1. The change in each precondition parameter must be proportional to the rate of change of the error function with respect to that particular precondition parameter to minimize the error function by gradient descent method, *i.e.*:

$$\Delta a_{A_i} = -\eta \frac{\partial e^2}{\partial a_{A_i}} \quad i = 1, 2, 3. \tag{17}$$

η is the constant of proportionality defined as the learning rate. Therefore, the new value of the consequent parameter is given as:

$$a_{A_i}(p+1) = a_{A_i}(p) + \Delta a_{A_i} \quad i = 1, 2, 3. \tag{18}$$

or

$$a_{A_i}(p+1) = a_{A_i}(p) - \eta \frac{\partial e^2}{\partial a_{A_i}} \quad i = 1, 2, 3. \tag{19}$$

Now the partial derivative term in (19) can be found by the chain rule of differentiation as follows:

$$\frac{\partial e^2}{\partial a_{A_i}} = \frac{\partial e^2}{\partial \omega_r} \cdot \frac{\partial \omega_r}{\partial T_{em}^*} \cdot \frac{\partial T_{em}^*}{\partial \bar{\mu}_1} \cdot \frac{\partial \bar{\mu}_1}{\partial \mu_{A_i}} \cdot \frac{\partial \mu_{A_i}}{\partial a_{A_i}}. \tag{20}$$

where

$$\frac{\partial e^2}{\partial \omega_r} = -2\left(\omega_r^* - \omega_r \right) = -2e. \tag{21}$$

$$\frac{\partial \omega_r}{\partial T_{em}^*} = J_m. \tag{22}$$

$$T_{em}^* = \bar{\mu}_1 . f_1 + \bar{\mu}_2 . f_2 + \bar{\mu}_3 . f_3 \Rightarrow \frac{\partial T_{em}^*}{\bar{\mu}_1} = f_1. \tag{23}$$

$$\bar{\mu}_1 = \frac{\mu_{A_1}}{\mu_{A_1} + \mu_{A_2} + \mu_{A_3}} \Rightarrow \frac{\partial \bar{\mu}_1}{\mu_{A_1}} = \frac{(\bar{\mu}_2 + \bar{\mu}_3)}{\mu_{A_1} + \mu_{A_2} + \mu_{A_3}}. \tag{24}$$

$$\mu_{A_1} = \frac{e - a_{A_1}}{b_{A_1} - a_{A_1}} \Rightarrow \frac{\partial \mu_{A_1}}{\partial a_{A_1}} = \frac{\mu_{A_1} - 1}{b_{A_1} - a_{A_1}}. \tag{25}$$

J is Jacobean matrix, which can be taken as constant being single input single output ANFIS architecture and can be included in learning rate. On computing all the terms of (20) and putting in (21), we can find the updated value of parameter a_{A_1} as follows:

$$a_{A_1}(p+1) = a_{A_1}(p) + 2.\eta.e(p).f_1(p). \frac{\bar{\mu}_2(p) + \bar{\mu}_3(p)}{\mu_{A_1}(p) + \mu_{A_2}(p) + \mu_{A_3}(p)} \cdot \frac{\mu_{A_1}(p) - 1}{b_{A_1}(p) - a_{A_1}(p)}. \tag{26}$$

Similarly

$$b_{A_1}(p+1) = b_{A_1}(p) + 2.\eta.e(p).f_1(p). \frac{\bar{\mu}_2(p) + \bar{\mu}_3(p)}{\mu_{A_1}(p) + \mu_{A_2}(p) + \mu_{A_3}(p)} \cdot \frac{\mu_{A_1}(p)}{b_{A_1}(p) - a_{A_1}(p)}. \tag{27}$$

In the same manner, the precondition parameters for the remaining fuzzy membership functions can be derived as follows:

$$b_{A_2}(p+1) = b_{A_2}(p) + 2.\eta.e(p).f_2(p). \frac{\bar{\mu}_1(p) + \bar{\mu}_3(p)}{\mu_{A_1}(p) + \mu_{A_2}(p) + \mu_{A_3}(p)} : \frac{1 - \mu_{A_2}(p)}{b_{A_2}(p)}. \tag{28}$$

$$a_{A_3}(p+1) = a_{A_3}(p) + 2.\eta.e(p).f_3(p). \frac{\bar{\mu}_1(p) + \bar{\mu}_2(p)}{\mu_{A_1}(p) + \mu_{A_2}(p) + \mu_{A_3}(p)} \cdot \frac{\mu_{A_2}(p) - 1}{b_{A_2}(p) - a_{A_3}(p)}. \tag{29}$$

$$b_{A_3}(p+1) = b_{A_3}(p) - 2.\eta.e(p).f_3(p). \frac{\bar{\mu}_1(p) + \bar{\mu}_1(p)}{\mu_{A_1}(p) + \mu_{A_2}(p) + \mu_{A_3}(p)} \cdot \frac{\mu_{A_3}(p)}{b_{A_3}(p) - a_{A_3}(p)}. \tag{30}$$

To tune the consequent parameters as discussed in layer 4, the following updated laws are developed:

$$a_{0_i}(p+1) = a_{0_i}(p) - \eta_c. \frac{\partial e^2}{\partial a_{0_i}} \quad i = 1, 2, 3. \tag{31}$$

$$a_{1_i}(p+1) = a_{1_i}(p) - \eta_c \cdot \frac{\partial e^2}{\partial a_{1_i}} \quad i=1,2,3. \tag{32}$$

η_c is the learning rate for consequent parameters. The derivative terms in (31) and (32) can be found by the chain rule as already discussed in case of precondition parameters as follows:

$$\frac{\partial e^2}{\partial a_{0_i}} = \frac{\partial e^2}{\partial \omega_r} \cdot \frac{\partial \omega_r}{\partial T^*_{em}} \cdot \frac{\partial T^*_{em}}{\partial f_i} \cdot \frac{\partial f_i}{\partial a_{0_i}} \quad i=1,2,3. \tag{33}$$

$$\frac{\partial e^2}{\partial a_{1_i}} = \frac{\partial e^2}{\partial \omega_r} \cdot \frac{\partial \omega_r}{\partial T^*_{em}} \cdot \frac{\partial T^*_{em}}{\partial f_i} \cdot \frac{\partial f_i}{\partial a_{1_i}} \quad i=1,2,3. \tag{34}$$

In the above (33) and (34), the first two terms are already known and the last two terms can be derived as:

$$\frac{\partial T^*_{em}}{\partial f_i} = \frac{\mu_i}{\mu_{A_1} + \mu_{A_2} + \mu_{A_3}} \quad i=1,2,3. \tag{35}$$

$$\frac{\partial f_i}{\partial a_{i_0}} = 1 \quad i=1,2,3. \tag{36}$$

$$\frac{\partial f_i}{\partial a_{i_1}} = e \quad i=1,2,3. \tag{37}$$

On substituting the terms derived in (35) and (37) in to the (33) and (34), the updated value of consequent parameters can be derived as follows:

$$a_{0_i}(p+1) = a_{0_i}(p) + 2.\eta_c.e \frac{\mu_i}{\mu_{A_1} + \mu_{A_2} + \mu_{A_3}} \quad i=1,2,3. \tag{38}$$

$$a_{1_i}(p+1) = a_{1_i}(p) + 2.\eta_c.e \frac{\mu_i}{\mu_{A_1} + \mu_{A_2} + \mu_{A_3}}.e \quad i=1,2,3. \tag{39}$$

The effectiveness of the proposed simplified ANFIS based IM drive is investigated extensively at first in simulation. The initial values of precondition and consequent parameters used in the simulation model are $a_1=0$, $a_3=0$, $b_1=0.1$, $b_2=0.007$, $b_3=0.5$, and $a_0^1 = 0$, $a_1^1 = 3$, $a_0^2 = 0$, $a_0^2 = 0$, $a_0^3 = 0$, $a_1^3 = 3$. The values of tuning rate of precondition and consequent parameters are $2e^{-8}$ and 0.09 respectively.

The performance of the proposed ANFIS is compared to conventional tuned PI controller. The proportional gain k_p is set as 0.9303, and the integral gain ki is set as 0.04. The parameters of the IM utilized for simulations are listed as follows:

P_n=3Kw, V_n=230V, R_s=2.89Ω, R_r=2.39Ω, L_s=0.225H, L_r=0.220H, L_m=0.214H, J=0.2Kg.m², n_p=2.

Figure 1 shows the simulated rotor speed of the proposed ANFIS and conventional PI controller for IM drive, which are verified on loading and unloading. The drive is accelerated to 200rad/s and full load is applied at 0.2s; then, the load completely at 0.4s. Later, after speed reversal, full load is applied at 0.8s, and, the load is fully removed at 1s. It is shown from this figure that the performance for the proposed ANFIS controller is fast and smooth, the drive can follow the command speed without overshoot or undershoot and less settling time compared to PI controller.

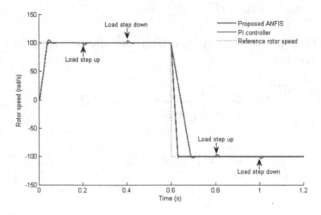

Fig. 1. Acceleration and reversal rotor speed for proposed ANFIS compared to PI controller

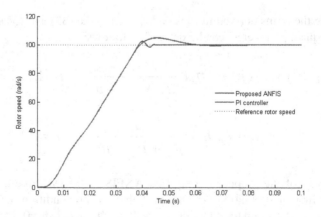

Fig. 2. Speed starting transient performance for proposed ANFIS compared to PI controller

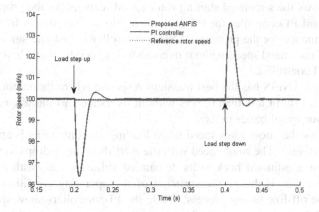

Fig. 3. Speed disturbance rejection property for proposed ANFIS compared to PI controller

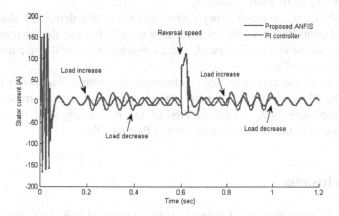

Fig. 4. Single-phase stator current i_a for proposed ANFIS compared to PI controller

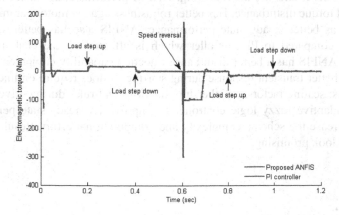

Fig. 5. Electromagnetic torque for proposed ANFIS strategy compared to PI controller

Figure 2 shows the simulated starting rotor speed response of the proposed ANFIS and conventional PI controller for IM drive at full load. It is shown from this figure that the performance for the proposed ANFIS controller is fast and smooth, the drive can follow the command speed without overshoot or undershoot and less settling time compared to PI controller.

The proposed ANFIS has the best transient response where the motor speed is approximately built up in less than 0.045s without overshoot. PI has a speed overshoot of 5% and motor speed builds in 0.6s.

Figure 3 show the zoom rotor speed when loading and unloading is applied at 0.2s and 0.4s respectively. The rotor speed with the ANFIS strategy drops to 99.95rad/s at 0.1ms and then is adjusted back to its demanded value in 0.2s, with a steady state error of 0.01%. This is due to the variation of the operating conditions from those used during the off-line tuning process. While the PI controllers show speed drops to 96.36rad/s at 0.2s, and rises to 103.65rad/s at   0.4 s, but is corrected back after 0.1s, with a steady state error of 0.03%. Due to their adaptive features, the ANFIS control strategy show fast disturbance rejection.

Figure 4 shows the corresponding stator currents of the drive, the starting stator current for PI controller is higher as compared to ANFIS, and the current responses for ANFIS are sinusoidal and balanced, and its distortion is small compared with that obtained by PI controller.

Figure 5 shows the corresponding electromagnetic torque responses of the drive. Obviously, the PI controller needs more torque and hence more current to start the motor. The electromagnetic torque of ANFIS reaches steady-state in a very short amount of time (less than 0.03ms) compared to PI controller.

5   Conclusions

A novel ANFIS controller based indirect vector controlled induction motor drive has been presented in this paper, and compared to a conventional well-tuned PI controller. The comparisons results are the following: ANFIS performs better than PI controller during a load torque disturbance. Has better robustness against motor parameter variation as well as better steady state performance. ANFIS also has better steady-state performance compared to PI controller which is affected by the chattering in the steady state. ANFIS has a better disturbance rejection capability compared to PI controller and a better transient response during starting. It does require on-line tuning of its parameters: scaling factors, membership functions and rules during drive operation to form an adaptive fuzzy logic controller to improve its steady-state performance. This will increase the scheme complexity and computational effort. Results obtained from ANFIS look promising.

References

1. Harnefors, L., Nee, H.-P.: A general algorithm for speed and position estimation of AC motors. IEEE Transactions on Industrial Electronics 47(1), 77–83 (2000)
2. Holtz, J.: Sensorless speed and position control of induction motors. In: IECON Proceedings (Industrial Electronics Conference), vol. 1, pp. 1547–1562 (2001)
3. Montanari, M., Peresada, S., Tilli, A., Tonielli, A.: Speed sensorless control of induction motor based on indirect field-orientation. In: Conference Record - IAS Annual Meeting (IEEE Industry Applications Society), vol. 3, pp. 1858–1865 (2000)
4. Sivakumar, A., Muthamizhan, T., Gunasekhar, N.O., Ramesh, R.: A novel sensorless speed control strategy of induction motor based on vector control. International Review of Electrical Engineering 8(4), 1211–1217 (2013)
5. Alonge, F., D'Ippolito, F., Sferlazza, A.: Sensorless control of induction-motor drive based on robust kalman filter and adaptive speed estimation. IEEE Transactions on Industrial Electronics 61(3), art. no. 6494615, 1444–1453 (2014)
6. Barut, M., Bogosyan, S., Gokasan, M.: Speed-sensorless estimation for induction motors sing extended Kalman filters. Transactions on Industrial Electronics 54(1), 272–280 (2007)
7. Yongchang, Z., Zhengming, Z.: Speed sensorless control for three-level inverter-fed induction motors using an extended Luenberger observer. In: IEEE Vehicle Power and Propulsion Conference, art. no. 4677412 (2008)
8. Jouili, M., Jarray, K., Koubaa, Y., Boussak, M.: Luenberger state observer for speed sensorless ISFOC induction motor drives. Electric Power Systems Research 89, 139–147 (2012)
9. Li, J., Xu, L., Zhang, Z.: An adaptive sliding-mode observer for induction motor sensorless speed control. IEEE Transactions on Industry Applications 41(4), 1039–1046 (2005)
10. Ren, T.-J., Chen, T.-C.: Robust speed-controlled induction motor drive based on recurrent neural network. Electric Power Systems Research 76(12), 1064–1074 (2006)
11. Oguz, Y., Dede, M.: Speed estimation of vector controlled squirrel cage asynchronous motor with artificial neural networks. Energy Conversion and Management 52(1), 675–686 (2011)
12. Kim, S.-H., Park, T.-S., Yoo, J.-N., Park, G.-T.: Speed-sensorless vector control of an induction motor using neural network speed estimation. IEEE Transactions on Industrial Electronics 48(3), 609–614 (2001)
13. Choi, H.H., Jung, J.-W.: Takagi-Sugeno fuzzy speed controller design for a permanent magnet synchronous motor. Mechatronics 21(8), 1317–1328 (2011)
14. Masiala, M., Vafakhah, B., Salmon, J., Knight, A.M.: Fuzzy self-tuning speed control of an indirect field-oriented control induction motor drive. IEEE Transactions on Industry Applications 44(6), 1732–1740 (2008)
15. Matsuoka, K.: Approach to the generalization problem in the backpropagation method. Systems and Computers in Japan 22(2), 97–106 (1991)
16. Hecht-Nielsen, R.: Theory of the backpropagation neural network. In: International Joint Conference on Neural Networks, vol. 1, pp. 593–605 (1989)
17. Kwak, K.-C.: An incremental adaptive neuro-fuzzy networks. In: International Conference on Control, Automation and Systems, pp. 1407–1410 (2008)
18. Sugeno, M., Takagi, T.: Multi-dimensional fuzzy reasoning. Fuzzy Sets and Systems 9(1-3), 313–325 (1983)
19. Fuller, R.: Introduction to Neuro-Fuzzy Systems. Advances in Intelligent and Soft Computing. Physica-Verlag GmbH & Co., Collection (1999)

Voting Algorithms Model with a Support Sets System by Class

Dalia Rodríguez-Salas[1], Manuel S. Lazo-Cortés[2], Ramón A. Mollineda[3],
J. Arturo Olvera-López[4], Jorge de la Calleja[1], and Antonio Benitez[1]

[1] Systems and Intelligent Computing Post-Graduate Department, Polytechnic
University of Puebla, Mexico
{dalia.rodriguez,jorge.delacalleja,antonio.benitez}@uppuebla.edu.mx
[2] Computer Science Department, National Institute of Astrophysics, Optic and
Electronics, Puebla, Mexico*
mlazo@inaoep.mx
[3] Institute of New Imaging Technologies, University Jaume I, Castellón, Spain**
mollined@uji.es
[4] Computer Science Department, Autonomous University of Puebla, Mexico
aolvera@cs.buap.mx

Abstract. The voting algorithms model (AlVot) allows building supervised classification methods based in partial analogies. These algorithms
use a collection of features subsets as support to classify a new object,
which is called support set system. Each support set consists of selected
features that are intended to discriminate the class of each object in the
learning matrix. In this paper, a new model called AlVot By Class (AlVot
BC) is proposed. It is aimed to build a support set system by class, so
that each class-specific support set provides evidence of the membership
of an object to the class represented by that support set. The classification performance of the proposed algorithm is evaluated on seven
databases from the UCI Machine Learning Repository. The results show
a clear improvement over its analogous algorithm based on AlVot.

1 Introduction

In a supervised classification environment, AlVot [1] is a model to build classifiers where a collection of support sets votes on the membership of a new object
in each class. Votes are then summarized and the object class is predicted. The
features of each support set are selected in a way that they are able to differentiate objects of different classes in the learning matrix (LM). Thus, this support
set is expected to provide helpful evidence on the class to which a new object
belongs. However, this general criterion could select unnecessary features to distinguish objects from a specific class. For example, Fig. 1(a) shows a LM with

* This work was partly supported by the National Council of Science and Technology
of Mexico (CONACyT) through the project grant CB2008-106366.
** This work has been partially funded by the Spanish University Jaume I through the
grant P1-1B2012-22.

six objects, each one of them belonging to a particular class. They are described by 25 features (see Fig. 1(b)), which should be able to separate objects of different classes. But, to distinguish the object Φ from the rest, features x_3 and x_8 are sufficient (see Fig. 1(d)), as it is illustrated in Fig. 1(c).

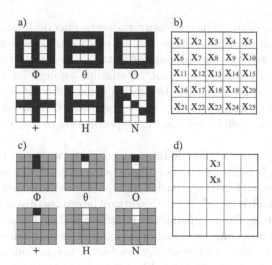

Fig. 1. a) Learning matrix of characters. b) Features that describe the characters in (a). c) Learning matrix of characters using features to discriminate the character Φ. d) Features that describe the characters in (c).

The idea of working with class-specific features has been present since the 90's decade. In [2,3] the use of class-specific features to estimate probability density functions in a Bayesian classifier is proposed. The class-specific feature selection can be strongly linked to a particular classifier. For example, in [4] the authors presented a method for class-specific feature selection in a hyperspher net. Nevertheless, in [5] a framework to use any traditional feature selector to obtain class-specific features is proposed, disregarding the classifier used.

AlVot, as known so far, builds a support set system using a traditional feature selection method. In this paper we propose a modification of AlVot considering a class-specific feature selection scheme to generate support set systems. From now on, the original method will also be referred to as the classic AlVot, while the modified version proposed in this paper will be called AlVot By Class (AlVot BC). AlVot BC is based on class-dependent collections of feature subsets used as support set systems by class. Experiments show a clear improvement in the classification performance yielded by AlVot BC over that produced by the classic AlVot.

The rest of the paper is organized as follows. Section 2 summarizes the related work, in particular the proposal presented in [5]. In Section 3, classic AlVot as primary background is presented, Section 4 defines rigorously AlVot BC, while Section 5 describes a proposed algorithm based on AlVot BC. Section 6 shows and discusses classification results. Finally, conclusions and promising directions for future research are given in Section 7.

2 Related Work

A classification problem requires features able to encode low intra-class difference, but also high inter-class difference. In this regard, most known classifiers assume that features can discriminate objects in any class. However, a feature useful to a particular class could not be suitable enough for another class. It thus makes sense to build models by classes using different sets of features for different classes. For instance, a method to estimate class-conditional probability density functions (pdf) based on class-specific sets of features is proposed in [2,3].

Another related work is the one introduced in [4], where a classifier based on a hypersphere net is built, each hypersphere being defined on a particular feature subspace. The selected features in each hypersphere are those that maximize a *separability* index, which is calculated as the ratio of inter-class distances to intra-class distances. The radius of each hypersphere is determined as the distance between its center and the farthest training object of the same class that belongs to this hypersphere. The classification of a new object involves its projection on all hypersphere subspaces, and to check whether the object lies within any hypersphere. If so, the object is assigned to the class associated to the "winning" hypersphere. Otherwise, the nearest neighbor rule is used with respect to the hypersphere centers.

Class-specific feature sets were also obtained in [5], by a framework based on applying any traditional feature selector separately on each one-against-all binary problem. This framework consists of the following four stages:

Class binarization. A classification problem of m classes is divided into m one-against-all binary problems [6]. Figure 2 illustrates this practice.

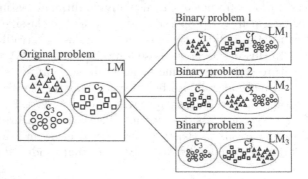

Fig. 2. Example of the one-against-all binarization strategy in a three-class problem

Class Balancing. In case of unbalanced binary problems, where the isolated class is the minority one, authors proposed to oversample it by repeating its objects until the balance is achieved.

Class-specific Feature Selection. It consists in eliciting features for each binary problem, by using any traditional feature selector. Then, features selected from a particular binary problem determined by the class c_i are attached to this class.

Classification. Once features of the class c_i are selected, a class-dependent classifier e_i performs on the LM corresponding to the original m-class problem, but only considering those features associated to the i-th class. To predict a class label for a given new object O_{new}, each classifier e_i produces a classification hypothesis. Authors propose a decision rule based on the following criteria, which are listed in order of use:

1. If only one classifier e_i supports its associated class c_i, then c_i is given as the predicted class.
2. If two or more classifiers e_i support their associated classes c_i, then the class most voted by the rest of classifiers, among those supported, is given as the predicted class.
3. When no classifier e_i supports its associated class, the class most voted by all classifiers is given as the predicted class.
4. When there is no winning class according to the above criteria (a tie), the majority class is given as the predicted class.

3   AlVot

This section presents the classic AlVot, which is the primary foundation of the method proposed in this paper (AlVot By Class).

The classic AlVot can be defined in terms of the six stages explained below. However, to ease the method definition, a number of notations should be previously stated:

- A, algorithm based in classic AlVot.
- Ω^A, support set system to A.
- n, number of features for objects in LM.
- $R = \{x_1, x_2, ..., x_n\}$, feature set to describe objects in the LM.
- $\Omega_k = \{x_{p_1}, x_{p_2}, ..., x_{p_{s_k}}\}$, k-th support set, $s_k \leq n$, $\Omega_k \subseteq R$ and $\Omega_k \in \Omega^A$.
- X_j, full description vector of the object O_j, according to R.
- X_j^k, partial description vector of the object O_j, according to Ω_k.
- x_p^j, value of the feature x_p in the object O_j.
- m, number of classes in LM.
- $C = \{c_1, ..., c_m\}$, set of class labels.
- y_j, class value of the object O_j, $y_j \in C$.

AlVot's stages can be summarized as follows:

1. **Support Set System.** The first stage consists in building each support set Ω_k. It is expected that features in each support set can be able to discriminate to which class each object in LM belongs.

2. **Partial Similarity Function.** This function allows comparing object pairs based on partial description vectors. An example could be:
   - $\beta(X_i^k, X_j^k) = |\{x_t \in \Omega_k | x_t^i = x_t^j\}|$. This function computes the number of features where the compared objects O_i and O_j agree.

3. **Partial Evaluation Function for a Fixed Support Set at Object Level.** Each support set is used to compute similarities between the new object O_{new} and the objects in LM. These values may be considered as the primary votes. Each object in LM votes as many times as there are support sets. Each vote is obtained considering only features in the current support set. An example could be:
   - $\Gamma_k(X_i^k, X_{new}^k) = \rho(\Omega_k)\beta(X_i^k, X_{new}^k)$, where $\rho(\Omega_k)$ weights the relevance of the support set Ω_k.

4. **Partial Evaluation Function for a Fixed Support Set at Class Level.** This function summarizes the votes given to a new object O_{new} by the objects of some class, given a particular support set. An example could be:
   - $\Gamma_k^j(O_{new}) = \frac{1}{n_j} \sum_{t=1}^{n_j} \Gamma_k(X_t^k, X_{new}^k)$, where n_j denotes the amount of objects in the class c_j.

5. **Total Evaluation Function for all Support Sets at Class Level.** This function summarizes the votes given to a new object O_{new} by the objects of some class, considering all support sets. An example could be:
   - $\Phi_j(O_{new}) = \frac{1}{|\Omega^A|} \sum_{\Omega_k \in \Omega^A} \Gamma_k^j(O_{new})$.

6. **Decision Rule.** This rule determines to which class O_{new} belongs. For instance, O_{new} can be classified in the class c_i if
   - $\Phi_i(O_{new}) > \Phi_j(O_{new})$ $\forall j = 1, ..., m$, $j \neq i$.

Figure 3 depicts an example of classifying a new object O_{new} by a method A based on AlVot in a context of a three-class problem. The example shows four support sets, $\Omega^A = \{\Omega_1, \Omega_2, \Omega_3, \Omega_4\}$, while $\Gamma_k^j(O_{new})$ denotes the average similarity between O_{new} and all objects in the class c_j, given the support set Ω_k. Finally, $\Phi_j(O_{new})$ summarizes the votes given to O_{new} by the class c_j over the whole support set system.

4   AlVot By Class

This section introduces the main contribution of this paper, which consists in an AlVot scheme based on class-specific support sets (AlVot By Class).

Unlike the classic AlVot, the new model considers a support set system where each support set is intended to discriminate objects of a particular class. To this end, we propose to turn the original m-class problem into m one-against-all binary problems, and to build an independent support set system for each binary problem. To better describe the new strategy, the notations introduced in the previous section need to be suited as follows:

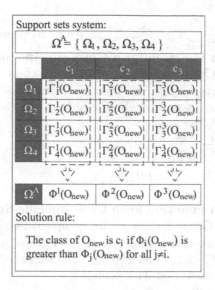

Fig. 3. Example of classifying a new object O_{new} in a problem of 3 classes with an algorithm A based in classic AlVot

- A, algorithm based in AlVot BC.
- Ω_i^A, support set system corresponding to the i-th class.
- $\Omega_k^i = \{x_{p_1}, x_{p_2}, ..., x_{p_{s_{ik}}}\}$, k-th support set linked to the i-th class, $s_{ik} \leq n$, $\Omega_k^i \subseteq R$ and $\Omega_k^i \in \Omega_i^A$.
- X_j^{ik}, partial description vector of the object O_j, according to Ω_k^i.
- $C' = \{c_1', ..., c_m'\}$, complementary class labels obtained from the one-against-all transformation, where c_i' represents the union of all classes except c_i.

The methodology of the classic AlVot also needs to be tailored to fit the requirements of AlVot BC. As a result, a procedure based on seven stages is shown below:

1. **Support Set Systems by Classes.** An independent support set system Ω_i^A is built for each class c_i. It is expected that each support set in Ω_i^A be able to discriminate objects of c_i from objects of c_i'.
2. **Partial Similarity Function.** No change with regard to the classic AlVot.
3. **Partial Evaluation Function for a Fixed Support Set at Object Level.** No change with regard to the classic AlVot.
4. **Partial Evaluation Function for a Fixed Support Set at Class Level and at its Complement Level.** Given a class c_j, its complement c_j', and a class-specific support set Ω_k^j, this function summarizes the votes given to a new object O_{new} by the objects in c_j, as well as by the objects in c_j' according to Ω_k^j. For example:

    - $\Gamma_k^j(O_{new}) = \frac{1}{n_j} \sum_{i=1}^{n_j} \Gamma_{jk}(X_i^{jk}, X_{new}^{jk})$, where n_j denotes the size of c_j.

- $\Gamma'^j_k(O_{new}) = \frac{1}{n'_j} \sum_{i=1}^{n'_j} \Gamma_{jk}(X_i^{jk}, X_{new}^{jk})$, where n'_j denotes the size of c'_j.

5. **Total Evaluation Function for a Class-specific Support Set System at Class and its Complement Level.** Given a class c_j, its complement c'_j, and a support set system Ω_j^A, this function summarizes the total votes given to a new object O_{new} separately by the objects in c_j and c'_j, considering all support sets in Ω_j^A. For example:
   - $\Phi_j(O_{new}) = \frac{1}{|\Omega_j^A|} \sum_{\Omega_k^j \in \Omega_j^A} \Gamma_k^j(O_{new})$.
   - $\Phi'_j(O_{new}) = \frac{1}{|\Omega_j^A|} \sum_{\Omega_k^j \in \Omega_j^A} \Gamma'^j_k(O_{new})$.

6. **Total Evaluation Function for a Class-specific Support Set System at Class Level.** Given a class c_j, its complement c'_j, and a support set system Ω_j^A, this function combines the total votes given to a new object O_{new} in terms of $\Phi_j(O_{new})$ and $\Phi'_j(O_{new})$, so that the belonging of O_{new} to c_j can be suitably measured. For example:
   - $\lambda_j(O_{new}) = \Phi_j(O_{new}) - \Phi'_j(O_{new})$

7. **Decision Rule.** No change with regard to the classic AlVot.

This process is illustrated in Fig. 4. Note that an independent support set system Ω_j^A is available for each class c_j, and that the complement c'_j is also added. All things considered, $\Gamma_k^j(O_{new})$ and $\Gamma'^j_k(O_{new})$ denote the partial similarities over Ω_k^j between O_{new} and objects in c_j and c'_j, respectively, while $\Phi_j(O_{new})$ and $\Phi'_j(O_{new})$ summarize the total votes given to O_{new} by c_j and c'_j, respectively, over the class-condicional Ω_j^A. Finally, $\lambda_j(O_{new})$ estimates the overall membership degree of O_{new} to the class c_j.

5 Algorithm Based in AlVot BC with Typical Testors as Support Sets Systems

In this section, an algorithm based on AlVot BC is presented, with the main characteristic being the use of *testors* as support sets. The testor concept first appeared in works on electrical circuits [7], but since the 60's decade it was related to classification problems and, specifically, to feature selection tasks [8]. The simplest way of defining a testor is as a subset of features that are able to distinguish any pair of objects from different classes in a *LM*. A *LM* can have one or more testors. A testor T for *LM* is called *typical* if there is no $T' \subset T$, such that T' is also a testor.

The algorithm described in this section uses class-specific typical testors as support sets, which are drawn from the binary problems built from the one-against-all decomposition of the original problem. The algorithm is based on the seven steps defined for AlVot BC, as it is described next:

Support sets systems:

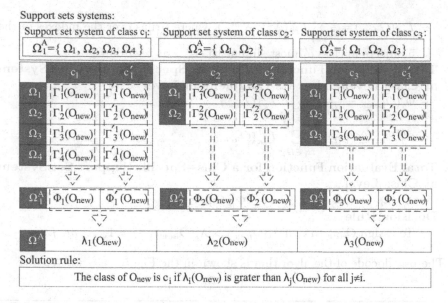

Fig. 4. Example of classifying a new object O_{new} in a problem of 3 classes with an algorithm A based in AlVot BC.

1. **Support Set System by Classes**
   - Ω_j^A contains the typical testors elicited from LM_j.
2. **Partial Similarity Function**
   - $\beta(X_i^{jk}, X_{new}^{jk}) = 1 - HEOM(X_i^{jk}, X_{new}^{jk})$
   where:
   - $HEOM(X_i^{jk}, X_{new}^{jk}) = \sqrt{\sum_{x_p \in \Omega_k^j} d(x_p^i, x_p^{new})^2}$
   - $d(x_p^i, x_p^{new}) = \begin{cases} 1 & if \quad x_p^i \vee x_p^{new} \quad is \; missing \\ overlap(x_p^i, x_p^{new}) & if \quad x_p \quad is \; nominal \\ rn\_diff(x_p^i, x_p^{new}) & if \quad x_p \quad is \; numerical \end{cases}$
   - $overlap(x_p^i, x_p^{new}) = \begin{cases} 0 & if \quad x_p^i = x_p^{new} \\ 1 & in \; other \; case. \end{cases}$
   - $rn\_diff(x_p^i, x_p^{new}) = \frac{|x_p^i - x_p^{new}|}{range(x_p)}$
   - $range(x_p) = max(x_p) - min(x_p)$
3. **Partial Evaluation Function for a Fixed Support Set at Object Level**
   - $\Gamma_{jk}(X_i^{jk}, X_{new}^{jk}) = \beta(X_i^{jk}, X_{new}^{jk})$
4. **Partial Evaluation Function for a Fixed Support Set at Class Level and at its Complement Level**
   - $\Gamma_k^j(O_{new}) = \frac{1}{5} \sum_{i=1}^{5} \Gamma_{jk}(X_i^{jk}, X_{new}^{jk})$, where i runs over the indexes of the 5 objects in class c_j most similar to O_{new} as regards Ω_k^j.

- $\Gamma'^j_k(O_{new}) = \frac{1}{5} \sum_{i=1}^{5} \Gamma_{jk}(X_i^{jk}, X_{new}^{jk})$, where i runs over the indexes of the 5 objects in class c'_j most similar to O_{new} as regards Ω_k^j.

5. **Total Evaluation Function for a Class-Specific Support Set System at Class Level and at Its Complement Level**
   - $\Phi_j(O_{new}) = \frac{1}{|\Omega_j^A|} \sum_{\Omega_k^j \in \Omega_j^A} \Gamma_k^j(O_{new})$.
   - $\Phi'_j(O_{new}) = \frac{1}{|\Omega_j^A|} \sum_{\Omega_k^j \in \Omega_j^A} \Gamma'^j_k(O_{new})$.

6. **Total Evaluation Function for a Class-Specific Support Set System at Class Level**
   - $\lambda_j(O_{new}) = \Phi_j(O_{new}) + (1 - \Phi'_j(O_{new}))$

7. **Decision Rule**
   - To assign O_{new} to c_i if $\lambda_i(O_{new}) > \lambda_j(O_{new})$, $\forall j = 1, \ldots, m$, $j \neq i$.

The pseudocode of the algorithm is shown in the Fig. 5.

Algorithm 1. Pseudocode of the proposed algorithm based on AlVot BC

Ensure: O_{new}, MA
1: **for all** c_i in MA **do**
2:      $\Phi_i(O_{new}) = \Phi'_i(O_{new}) = 0$
3:      $MA_i = \text{getBinaryProblem}(i)$
4:      $\Omega_i^A = \text{getTypicalTestors}(MA_i)$
5:      **for all** Ω_j^i in Ω_i^A **do**
6:          **for all** O_k in MA_i **do**
7:              **if** $y_k = c_i$ **then**
8:                  $vote(i)(j)(k) = 1 - HOEM(Onew, O_k)$
9:              **else**
10:                 $vote'(i)(j)(k) = 1 - HOEM(Onew, O_k)$
11:              **end if**
12:          **end for**
13:          $\Gamma_j^i(O_{new}) = \text{getAverageOfBiggest5}(vote(i)(j))$
14:          $\Gamma'^i_j(O_{new}) = \text{getAverageOfBiggest5}(vote'(i)(j))$
15:          $\Phi_i(O_{new}) = \Phi_i(O_{new}) + \Gamma_j^i(O_{new})$
16:          $\Phi'_i(O_{new}) = \Phi'_i(O_{new}) + \Gamma'^i_j(O_{new})$
17:      **end for**
18:      $\Phi_i(O_{new}) = \Phi_i(O_{new})/|\Omega_i^A|$
19:      $\Phi'_i(O_{new}) = \Phi'_i(O_{new})/|\Omega_i^A|$
20:      $\lambda_i(O_{new}) = \Phi_i(O_{new}) + (1 - \Phi'_i(O_{new}))$
21: **end for**
22: $win = \arg\max_i \lambda_i(O_{new})$, $\forall i = 1, \ldots, m$
23: **return** c_{win}

Fig. 5. Classification algorithm based on AlVot BC that uses typical testors by class as class-dependent support sets

6   Results

In this section, we present experiments to compare the classification performance and the number of features used by the proposed algorithm, with regard to those from its base algorithm (classic AlVot) and also from other methods frequently used in the literature.

Experiments involve several data sets from the well-known UCI Machine Learning repository [9]. They are briefly described in the Tab. 1.

Table 1. UCI data sets used in the experiments

Data set	Number of features	Number of classes	Number of objects	Features type	Missing values
Zoo	16	7	101	Nominal	No
Wine	13	3	178	Numerical	No
Iris	4	3	150	Numerical	No
Yeast	8	10	1484	Numerical	No
Glass	9	6	214	Numerical	No
Vehicle	18	4	846	Numerical	No
Anneal	38	5	898	Mixed	Yes

6.1   Classification Performance

Table 2 shows the average performances achieved by the proposed algorithm and by the classic AlVot over all data sets, using a 5×10-fold cross-validation process. The best result for each data set (row) is indicated by a '*'.

Table 2. Classification performances of the algorithms based on AlVot BC and classic AlVot, by averaging independent results from a 5×10-fold CV

Data set	Classic AlVot	AlVot BC
Zoo	93.86	94.06*
Wine	97.30	97.86*
Iris	95.47	95.73*
Yeast	59.58*	59.07
Glass	69.09	70.36*
Vehicle	70.50	70.97*
Anneal	97.88	98.02*

To get insight into the generalization capabilities of the proposed algorithm, it was also compared to three widely-used classifiers: k-Nearest Neighbors (k-NN, with $k = 3$ and $k = 5$), C4.5 and Naive Bayes (NB), using their implementations available in the WEKA library [10]. Table 3 shows the average performances achieved by the proposed algorithm and by the three aforementioned classifiers over all data sets, using the same performance estimation technique. The best result for each data set (row) is indicated by a '*'.

Table 3. Classification performances of the algorithm based on AlVot BC and three well-known classifiers, by averaging independent results from a 5×10-fold CV

Data sets	3-NN (%)	5-NN (%)	C4.5 (%)	NB (%)	AlVot BC (%)
Zoo	92.47	94.65	92.28	95.05*	94.06
Wine	96.07	96.07	92.81	97.19	97.86*
Iris	95.33	95.73*	94.67	95.60	95.73*
Yeast	55.43	56.97	56.23	57.91	59.07*
Glass	70.47*	66.73	68.50	48.13	70.36
Vehicle	70.21	70.31	72.91	44.85	70.97*
Anneal	97.30	97.37	98.71*	86.55	98.02

6.2   Number of Features

Figure 6 shows the mode of the number of features obtained for each classifier in each data set, using a 10-fold cross-validation scheme. It is important to note that classic AlVot has the same mode value in all the classes, because it has a single support set system which is common to all classes.

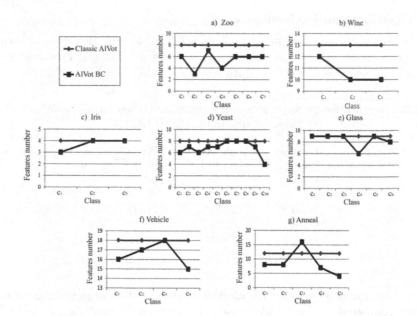

Fig. 6. Mode of the number of features in the support sets for each class, obtained by the algorithms based on the classic AlVot and AlVot BC

7   Conclusions

Experimental results show that the algorithm based on AlVot By Class is able to achieve high classification accuracies with a small number of features by class. According to these two criteria, this method clearly overcomes the algorithm determined by the classic AlVot and three well-known classifiers in most data sets. Therefore, the proposed algorithm empirically proved to be competitive against methods that can be considered as *de facto* standards to deal with classification problems. This suggests that global features could be unsuitable for some classes, thus they might introduce noise in the classification process.

It is worth noting that this paper proposes and assesses a particular algorithm designed to fit AlVot BC, which can be considered a general voting model based on class-conditional feature subsets. As suggested above, future work may comprehend new ways of developing the seven stages of AlVot BC. For example, the support set systems could be built by using different feature selectors, while the similarity functions could admit feature weighting. In addition, it could also be possible to learn how to weight the relevance of each support set within a voting scheme. In summary, the main focus would be to learn how to get the model as close as possible to reality.

References

1. Zhuravlev, Y., Nikiforov, V.: Algorithms for recognition based on calculation of evaluations. Kibernetilca, 1–11 (1971) (in Russian)
2. Baggenstoss, P.M.: Class-specific feature sets in classification. In: ISIC/CIRA/ISAS Joint Conference, pp. 413–416 (1998)
3. Baggenstoss, P.: Class-specific feature sets in classification. IEEE Transactions on Signal Processing 47, 3428–3432 (1999)
4. Roy, A., Mackin, P., Mukhopadhyay, S.: Methods for pattern selection, class-specific feature selection and classification for automated learning, 41, 113–129 (2013)
5. Pineda-Bautista, B., Carrasco-Ochoa, J., Martínez-Trinidad, J.: General framework for class-specific feature selection. Expert Systems with Applications 38, 10018–10024 (2011)
6. Fürnkranz, J.: Round robin classification. The Journal of Machine Learning Research 2, 721–747 (2002)
7. Chegis, I., Yablonsky, S.: Logical methods for controlling electrical circuits. Trudy Matematicheskogo Instituta Steklova 51, 270–360 (1958)
8. Lazo-Cortes, M., Ruiz-Shulcloper, J., Alba-Cabrera, E.: An overview of the evolution of the concept of testor. Pattern Recognition 34, 753–762 (2001)
9. Bache, K., Lichman, M.: UCI machine learning repository (2013)
10. Hall, M., Frank, E., Holmes, G., Pfahringer, B., Reutemann, P., Witten, I.H.: The weka data mining software: an update. ACM SIGKDD Explorations Newsletter 11, 10–18 (2009)

A Meta Classifier by Clustering of Classifiers

Mohammad Iman Jamnejad, Sajad Parvin, Ali Heidarzadegan, and Mohsen Moshki

Department of Computer Engineering, Beyza Branch, Islamic Azad University, Beyza, Iran
parvin@iust.ac.ir

Abstract. To learn any problem, many classifiers have been introduced so far. Each of these classifiers has many strengths (positive aspects) and weaknesses (negative aspects) that make it suitable for some specific problems. But there is no powerful solution to indicate which classifier is the best classifier (or at least a good one) for a special problem. Fortunately the ensemble learning provides us with a powerful approach to prepare a near-to-optimum classifying system for any given problem. How to create a suitable ensemble of base classifiers is the most challenging problem in classifier ensemble. An ensemble vitally needs diversity. It means that if a pool of classifiers wants to be successful as an ensemble, they must be diverse enough to cover the errors of each other. So during creation of an ensemble, we need a mechanism to guarantee the ensemble classifiers are diversity. Sometimes this mechanism is to select/remove a subset of the produced base classifiers with the aim of maintaining the diversity among the ensemble. This paper proposes an innovative ensemble creation named the Classifier Selection Based on Clustering (CSBC). The CSBC guarantees the necessary diversity among ensemble classifiers, using the clustering of classifiers technique. It uses bagging as generator of the base classifiers. After producing a large number of the base classifiers, CSBC partitions them using a clustering algorithm. After that by selecting one classifier from each cluster, CSBC produces the final ensemble. The weighted majority vote method is taken as aggregator function of the ensemble. Here it is probed how the cluster number affects the performance of the CSBC method and how we can choose a good approximate value for cluster number in any dataset adaptively. We expand our studies on a large number of real datasets of UCI repository to reach a decisive conclusion.

Keywords: Classifier Ensembles, Bagging, AdaBoosting.

1 Introduction

In general, it is an ever-true sentence that combining diverse classifiers usually results in a better classification [6]. The diversity is essentially important for an ensemble to be succeeded. The diversity among the base classifiers of an ensemble assures the undependability of those base classifiers; it means that the misclassifications of the classifiers don't occur simultaneously. It has been shown that the ensemble of a number of base classifiers can always reach a better performance (even can reach a perfect accuracy) as the number of classifiers becomes greater, provided that they are independent (diverse) [7], [14]. It has been shown that the ensemble philosophy is also successfully applicable to Bayesian Networks [15].

A. Gelbukh et al. (Eds.): MICAI 2014, Part II, LNAI 8857, pp. 140–151, 2014.
© Springer International Publishing Switzerland 2014

The only challenge in the creation of a classifier ensemble is to provide a general approach to guarantee the diversity that is vital and necessary for an ensemble, can be achieved. It means that if a pool of classifiers wants to be successful as an ensemble, they should be diverse enough to cover the errors of each other. This is a challenging problem how to create a number of classifiers diverse enough to be suitable to participate in an ensemble. To reach a satisfactory diversity in an ensemble there are a very large variety of approaches. Kuncheva proposes an approach based on the metrics that represents the amount of similarities or differences of classifier outputs. He has proposed a series of methods for creation of an ensemble based on the mentioned metrics [18].

Clustering is the task of assigning a set of objects into groups (also called clusters) so that the objects in the same group are more similar (in some sense) to each other than to those in other groups. It has widely employed in data mining applications such as information retrieval, text categorization and text ranking [10-13].

Giacinto and Roli propose a clustering and selection method to present a method that produces a host of classifiers with a high degree of diversity [5]. They first produce a large number of artificial neural network classifiers [16-17] by different initializations of their parameters. After that they select a subset of them according to their distances in their output space.

Parvin et al. inspired from the clustering and selection method propose a new clustering and selection method to deal with the drawbacks of the simple ensemble methods in generating diversity [9]. In spite of Giacinto and Roli's method they take into consideration how the base classifiers are created. In their work it is explored that usage of Bagging [2] and Boosting [4] as the sources of generators of diversity how can affect on Giacinto and Roli's method. They first train a large number of classifiers using Bagging and Boosting methods, after that they partition the classifiers using their outputs over the training set. Finally a random classifier from each cluster is selected and is inserted into the ensemble. The weighted majority voting mechanism is taken as the consensus function of the ensemble.

Decision Tree (DT) is one of the most versatile classifiers in the machine learning field. DT is considered as one of the unstable classifiers that can produce different results in its successive trainings on the same condition. It uses a tree-like graph or model of decisions. The kind of representation is appropriate for experts to understand what classifier does [10]. Its intrinsic instability can be employed as a source of diversity in classifier ensemble. The ensemble of a number of DTs is a well-known algorithm called Random Forest (RF) which is one of the most powerful ensemble algorithms. The algorithm of Random Forest was first developed by Breiman [2]. In this paper, DT is totally used as one of the base classifiers.

2   Related Work

Generally, there are two important challenging approaches to combine a number of classifiers that use different training sets. They are Bagging and Boosting. Both of them are considered as two methods that are sources of diversity generation. Indeed they are considered as the best ensemble methods and still the most challenging meta-learners to any new classifier ensemble method.

First assume that training set is denoted by TS. Also let's denote the ith dataitem in *TS* by o_i. Let's m be the number of dataitems in *TS*. Fig. 1 generally depicts the training phase of CSBC by the modified Bagging method as the generator of the base classifiers in the ensemble.

The term Bagging is first used by Breiman [2] abbreviating for Bootstrap AGGregatING. The idea of Bagging is simple and interesting: the ensemble is made of classifiers built on bootstrap copies of the training set. Using different training sets, the necessary diversity for ensemble is obtained. It is worthy to be mentioned that Bagging does not assure that the necessary diversity is met.

Breiman [3] proposes a variant of Bagging that it is called Random Forest. Random Forest is a general class of ensemble building methods using a decision tree as the base classifier. To be labeled a "Random Forest", an ensemble of decision trees should be built by generating independent identically distributed random vectors and should use each vector to grow a decision tree. Like Bagging, Random Forest also does not assure that the ensemble classifiers are sufficiently diverse.

In this paper Random Forest algorithm that is one of the most well-known versions of Bagging classifier [7] is implemented and compared with the proposed method. It is worthy to be mentioned that Random Forest is first modified a little before usage.

Boosting is inspired by an online learning algorithm called Hedge(β) [4]. This algorithm allocates weights to a set of strategies used to predict the outcome of a certain event. At this point we shall relate Hedge(β) to the classifier combination problem. Boosting is defined in [4] as related to the "general problem of producing a very accurate prediction rule by combining rough and moderately inaccurate rules of thumb." The main boosting idea is to develop the classifier team D incrementally, adding one classifier at a time. The classifier that joins the ensemble at step k is trained on a dataset selectively sampled from the train dataset Z. The sampling distribution starts from uniform, and progresses towards increasing the likelihood of "difficult" data points. Thus the distribution is updated at each step, increasing the likelihood of the objects misclassified at step k-1. Here the correspondence with Hedge(β) is transposed. The classifiers in D are the trials or events, and the data points in Z are the strategies whose probability distribution we update at each step. The algorithm is called AdaBoost which comes from ADAptive BOOSTing. Another version of these algorithms is arc-x4 which performs as another version of recently ADAboost [7].

Giacinto and Roli propose a clustering and selection method [5]. They first produce a large number of MLP classifiers with different initializations. After that they partition them by a clustering method over their outputs. They select one classifier from each cluster of the classifiers. Finally they consider the selected classifiers as an ensemble. Majority voting is considered as their aggregator.

Parvin et al. propose a framework for development of combinational classifiers. In their framework, a number of train data-bags are first bootstrapped from train dataset. Then a pool of weak base classifiers is created; each classifier is trained on one distinct data-bag. After that to get rid of similar base classifiers in the ensemble and select a diverse subset of classifiers, the classifiers are partitioned using a clustering algorithm. The partitioning is done considering the outputs of classifiers on training dataset as new feature space. In each cluster, one random classifier is selected to participate in final ensemble. Then, to produce consensus vote, different votes (or outputs) are gathered out of ensemble. After that the weighted majority voting mechanism is applied as their aggregator. The weights are determined using the accuracies of the base classifiers on training dataset [9].

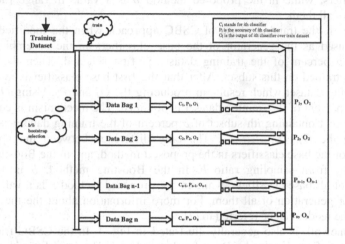

Fig. 1. Training phase of CSBC by modified Bagging method as generator of base classifiers

3   Classifier Selection by Clustering

The main idea behind the CSBS approach is to use the most diverse subset of the base classifiers obtained by Bagging or Boosting methods. Indeed a number of base classifiers are first generated by the two well-known ensemble creation mechanisms: Bagging or Boosting. After that the produced classifiers are partitioned according their outputs over training set. Then a random base classifier is selected from each cluster. Since each cluster is produced according to classifiers' outputs, it is highly likely that selecting one classifier from each cluster, and considering them as an ensemble can produce a diverse ensemble that outperforms the traditional Bagging and Boosting, i.e. usage of all base classifiers as an ensemble without selection phase. It is also more likely that selecting the nearest classifier to the head of each produced cluster produces an ensemble with a higher diversity than the ensemble of those classifiers any of that is randomly extracted out of each cluster. The algorithm for training phase of CSBC approach by the modified Bagging method as the generator of the base classifiers for the ensemble is depicted in Fig. 1 schematically.

As it is obvious from Fig. 1, n subsets of TS are firstly bootstrapped with b percent of the training dataset. The ith dataset (subset) that is bootstrapped with b percent of the training dataset is named ith data bag; it is denoted by DB_i. It is clear that the cardinality of DB_i is $m*b/100$. Then a base classifier is trained on each of DB_i. Let's denote the base classifier trained on DB_i by C_i. After that the classifier C_i is tested over the whole of training dataset and its accuracy is calculated. The output of ith classifier over jth dataitem in TS will be a vector denoted by O_{ij}. It means $O_{ij}^{\ k}$ stands for the ith base classifier confidence in belonging dataitem o_j to class k. The output of ith classifier over total training dataset is also denoted by O_i and its accuracy is denoted by P_i. The only difference between the approach of generation of the base classifiers in the proposed method (depicted by Fig. 1), and in the Bagging method comes from sampling ratio b. In the Bagging method, b is 100 during generation of all base classifiers, while in the proposed method b is a value in range [30-100] for generation of all them.

Like Fig. 1, the training phase of CSBC approach when the modified Boosting method is used as the generator of the base classifiers in the ensemble, a subset containing b percent of the training dataset is first selected. Then the first base classifier is trained on this subset. After that the first base classifier is tested on the whole training dataset which results in producing the O_1 and P_1. Using O_1, the next subset of b percent of the training dataset is obtained. The mechanism is continued in such a way that obtaining ith subset of b percent of the training dataset is produced considering the O_1, O_2, ..., O_{i-1}. The only difference between the approach of generation of the base classifiers in the proposed method, and in the Boosting method again comes from sampling ratio b. In the Boosting method, b is 100 during generation of all base classifiers, while in the proposed method b is a value in range [30-100] for generation of all them. For more information about the mechanism of Boosting, the reader can be referred to [7].

This framework is also generally illustrated in Fig. 3. In the CSBC framework a dataset of classifiers denoted by DC is firstly produced. The DC whose ith dataitem is denoted by X_i has f features. pth feature of ith dataitem in DC denoted by X_{ip} is obtained by equation 1.

$$X_{ip} = O_{ij}^k \tag{1}$$

where j and k are obtained by equation 2 and 3 respectively.

$$j = \lceil p/c \rceil \tag{2}$$

where c is the number of classes.

$$k = p - j*c \tag{3}$$

Features of the DC dataset are opinions of different base classifiers C_i over real data items of under-leaning dataset. So a new dataset having n dataitems, where any of them stands for a base classifier, and f features, where $f=m*c$, is available. Parameter n is a predefined value showing the number of classifiers produced by Bagging or Boosting. To better clarify the DC dataset consider Fig. 2.

O_{11}^1	O_{11}^2	O_{12}^1	O_{12}^2	.	O_{1m}^1	O_{1m}^2
O_{21}^1	O_{21}^2	O_{22}^1	O_{22}^2	.	O_{2m}^1	O_{2m}^2
...	...	...	...	.	...	...
O_{n1}^1	O_{n1}^2	O_{n2}^1	O_{n2}^2	.	O_{nm}^1	O_{nm}^2

Fig. 2. The Classifier Selection Based on Clustering framework

In Fig. 2, we assume that there are two classes, i.e. $m=2$. After producing the mentioned DC dataset, it is partitioned by use of a clustering algorithm that results in producing some clusters of classifiers. We denote the number of clusters by r. Each of the classifiers falling into a cluster has similar outputs on the train dataset; it means these classifiers have low diversities, so it is better to use one of them in the final ensemble rather than all of them. For escaping from outlier classifiers, the clusters which contain number of classifiers smaller than a predefined threshold are ignored.

```
Input:
    E: Ensemble of Classifiers
    P: Accuracies of Classifiers
    O: Outputs of Classifiers
    th: Threshold of Selectin a Classifier
Output:
    SC: Ensemble of Classifiers
    SP: Accuracies of Classifiers
[n m] = size (O)
C = K-means (O, r)
Cluster_of_Classifiers (1 : r) = { }
For i = 1 : n
    CC (i) = CC (i)∪{C(i)}
    Acc_C(i) = Acc_C (i)∪{P(i)}
End
j=0
For i = 1 : r
    SizeOfCluster = | CC (i) |
    If (SizeOfCluster > th)
        j=j+1
        tmp = RandomSelect (1 : SizeOfCluster)
        SC (j) = CC (tmp)
        SP (j) = Acc_C (tmp)
    End
End
```

Fig. 3. Pseudo-code of the Classifier Selection Based on Clustering framework

Let us assume that E is the ensemble of n classifiers $\{C_1, C_2, C_3 ... C_n\}$. Also assume that there are c classes in the case. Next, assume applying the ensemble over data sample o_j results in a D^j matrix like equation 4.

$$D^j = \begin{bmatrix} O^1_{1j} & O^1_{2j} & . & O^1_{nj} \\ . & & . & . \\ O^{c-1}_{1j} & O^{c-1}_{2j} & . & O^{c-1}_{nj} \\ O^c_{1j} & O^c_{2j} & . & O^c_{nj} \end{bmatrix} \tag{4}$$

Now the ensemble decides the data sample o_j to belong to class q according to equation 5.

$$q = \arg\max_{i=1}^{c} \left| \sum_{k=1}^{n} w_k * D^j_i{}_k \right| \tag{5}$$

where w_j is the effect weight of classifier j which is obtained optimally [7] according to equation 6.

$$w_j = \log \frac{p_j}{1 - p_j} \tag{6}$$

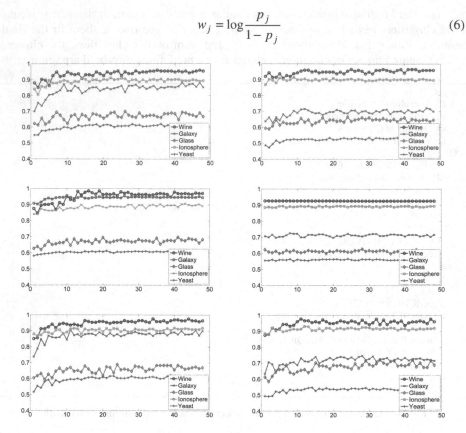

Fig. 4. The performance of CSBC by the modified boosting (UP) and the Gianito's method (MIDDLE) the modified bagging (DOWN) ensemble over some datasets with n=151 and different r and MLP (LEFT) and DT (RIGHT) as base classifier

where p_j is accuracy of classifier j over total TS. Note that a tie breaks randomly in equation 5. For dataitem o_j consider a vector L^j. L^j_q is one if dataitem o_j belongs to class q otherwise it is zero. Now the accuracy of classifier C_k over TS is obtained using equation 7.

$$p_k = \frac{\sum\limits_{j=1}^{m} \sum\limits_{i=1}^{c} |L_i^j - o_{kj}^i|}{c \times m} \tag{7}$$

4   Experimental Study

The accuracy is taken as the evaluation metric throughout all the paper. All the experiments are done using 4-fold cross validation. The results obtained by 4-fold cross validation are also repeated as many as 10 independent runs. It means that to reach the accuracy of any method on a dataset ,e.g. *Iris*, the accuracy of the method is computed by 4-fold cross validation and it is denoted by acc_1. Repeating the same scenario again we reach acc_2. After repeating the scenario as many as 10 times, we reach acc_i where $i \in \{1,2,...,10\}$. The averaged accuracies acc_i over the 10 independent runs are reported as the accuracy of the method over *Iris* dataset.

The proposed method is examined over 13 different standard datasets and also one artificial one. It is tried for datasets to be diverse in their number of true classes, features and samples. A large variety in used datasets can more validate the obtained results and makes the conclusions more decisive. These real datasets are available at UCI repository [1]. The details of HalfRing dataset can be available in [8].

The measure of decision for each employed decision tree is taken as Gini measure. The threshold of pruning is also set to 2. Also the classifiers' parameters are fixed in all of their usages. All MLPs which are used in the experiments have two hidden layers including 10 and 5 neurons respectively in the first and second hidden layers. All them are permitted to be trained in 100 epochs. In all experiments the default value for parameters n, b and threshold of accepting a cluster are set to 151, 30 and 2 (i.e. only the clusters with one classifier is dropped down) respectively. All the experiments are done using 4-fold cross validation. Clustering is done by k-means clustering algorithm with different k parameters.

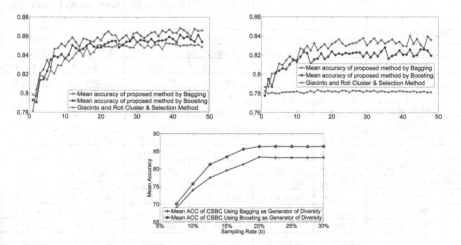

Fig. 5. The performance of CSBC methods averaged over 14 used datasets with n=151 and different r and MLP (UP LEFT), DT (UP RIGHT) as base classifier. The performance of proposed CSBC methods averaged over 14 used datasets with $n=151$ and different $r=33$ and different b (DOWN).

To see how the parameter r affects over the performance of classification over CSBC methods (by bagging, boosting and Gianito [18]) with two base classifiers (MLP, DT [2,10]), take a look at Fig. 4.

These figures depict the accuracies of different methods by 4-fold cross validation on some benchmarks. As it can be inferred from these figures, increasing the cluster number parameter r is not always resulted in the improvement in the performance.

Indeed an $r=15$ is a well choice for all of the datasets. It means that if the classifier number parameter, n, is 151 then $r=15$ is a good value for the cluster number parameter. In other words, using 10 percent of the base classifiers in the final ensemble can be considered as a good option. Indeed in this option, a classifier is selected from each cluster of classifiers that contains about 10 classifiers, so it gives the method the ability to select each classifier from a good coverage of classifiers.

The performances of CSC by boosting over some dataset with $n=151$ and different r are depicted in Fig 5 while MLP and DT are used as base classifier. The same results are depicted in the same figure for CSC by Gianito's method respectively while the same classifiers are used as base classifier. Fig 5 also represents the performances of CSC by bagging method respectively while the same classifiers are used as base classifier.

Table 1. Comparison between the results obtained by applying different ensemble methods considering DT and MLP as the base classifiers. * indicates the dataset is normalized. 4 fold cross validation` is taken for performance evaluation. ** indicates that the train and test sets are predefined and averaged over 10 independent runs is reported. Note that X-Y indicates X is accuracy of DT as the base classifiers and Y is accuracy of MLP as the base classifiers.

	AdaBoost	Arc-X4	Random Forest	Classifier Selection By RF	Classifier Selection By Arc-X4	Cluster and Selection
Breast Cancer*	96.19-96.49	95.74-97.06	96.32-96.91	96.47-96.91	95.05-96.47	93.68-96.19
Balance Scale*	91.52-93.12	94.44-93.27	93.6-91.99	94.72-91.35	94.24-92.95	94.44-95.75
Bupa*	66.96-68.41	70.64-70.06	72.09-71.22	72.97-72.09	66.28-68.02	64.53-71.98
Glass*	70.09-66.36	65.04-66.04	70.28-66.98	70.28-67.45	62.26-66.04	60.85-67.05
Galaxy*	71.83-85.14	70.59-87	73.07-85.62	72.45-85.62	70.28-84.52	70.94-87
Half-Ring*	97.25-97.25	97.25-97.25	95.75-95.75	97.25-97.25	95.75-97.25	95.75-97.25
SAHeart*	67.32-69.48	70-73.04	71.3-72.39	72.61-71.52	69.7-71.09	68.04-70.18
Ionosphere*	91.17-89.17	90.31-90.03	92.31-88.51	91.45-90.31	89.74-87.64	87.64-88.51
Iris*	94.67-94.67	96.62-96.62	95.27-96.62	96.62-97.97	95.95-97.33	94.59-93.33
Monk problem1**	98.03-98.99	98.11-98.06	97.49-92.23	98.76-98.43	97.37-97.87	98.34-98.34
Monk problem2**	91.65-87.48	97.01-87.35	86.64-85.68	97.62-87.41	86.73-87.23	97.14-87.21
Monk problem3**	95.51-96.84	87.29-97.09	96.92-95.87	96.97-97.33	96.34-96.99	87.31-96.77
Wine*	96.63-94.38	96.07-96.59	97.19-96.06	97.19-97.19	95.51-95.51	92.61-95.23
Yeast*	54.78-59.5	53.17-60.85	53.98-61.19	53.98-61.19	52.09-60.85	54.51-60.56
Average	84.54-85.52	84.45-86.45	85.16-85.5	86.38-86.57	83.38-85.7	82.88-86.1

Fig. 5 depicts averaged accuracies over all 14 different datasets. Fig. 5 reports performances of the proposed framework by using MLP as base classifier. As it is illustrated in Fig. 5, the usage of bagging as generator of base classifiers for CSBC method is better than Boosting and Giacinto and Roli's ensemble methods. Also it is concluded that using $r=33$ instead of $r=15$ is a better choice for all of 14 datasets. In other words, using 22 percent of the base classifiers in the final ensemble can be a better option. Comparing figures of Fig. 5 one can find out that the usage of decision tree as base classifier increases the gap between the three approaches in generating an ensemble of the base classifiers. It is due to special feature of the decision tree. Because it is very sensitive to its training set, the usage of decision tree as the base classifier is very consistent with the Bagging mechanism. Fig. 5 also shows the effect of sampling rate over the performance of two different proposed methods. The base classifier used to reach the results reported in the figure is decision tree. As it is obvious if a very low value is chosen for b, the performance is very weak. Also the higher values for b in the proposed method can't monotonically improve the performance. It even causes to decrease the performance for values after 40%.

Table 1 shows the accuracies obtained by applying different ensemble methods considering DT as the base classifiers. Table 1 also shows the accuracies obtained by applying the same ensemble methods presented in Table 1 considering MLP as the base classifiers. The parameter r is set to 33 to reach the results of Table 1.

While we choose only at most 22 percent of the base classifiers produced by modified Bagging, the accuracy of their ensemble outperforms their full ensemble, i.e. Bagging Method. Also it outperforms Boosting method and proposed method based on Boosting method.

Because the classifiers selected in this manner (by Bagging along with clustering), have different outputs, i.e. they are as diverse as possible, they are more suitable than ensemble of all them. It is worthy to mention that the Boosting is inherently diverse enough to be an ensemble totally; and the reduction of ensemble size by clustering destructs their Boosting effect. Take it in the consideration that in Boosting ensemble, each member covers the drawbacks of the previous ones.

Table 2. Effect of usage of the new methods based on that a classifier is selected from a cluster. RS stands for "random selection"; TMAS stands for "the most accurate selection"; TNTCCS stands for "the nearest-to-cluster-center selection".

	CSBC By Bagging and RS	CSBC By Bagging and TMAS	CSBC By Bagging and TNTCCS
Breast Cancer*	96.91	95.73	**97.36**
Balance Scale*	91.35	91.51	**91.98**
Bupa*	**72.09**	71.87	71.21
Glass*	67.45	65.98	**68.67**
Galaxy*	**85.62**	85.34	84.51
Half-Ring*	97.25	**97.72**	97.18
SAHeart*	71.52	71.49	**72.13**
Ionosphere*	90.31	**91.07**	90.01
Iris*	97.97	96.06	**98.21**
Monk problem1**	98.43	**100.00**	**100.00**
Monk problem2**	87.41	86.83	**87.89**
Monk problem3**	97.33	98.10	**98.18**
Wine*	97.19	98.21	**98.55**
Yeast*	61.19	60.91	**61.62**
Average	86.57	86.49	**86.96**

The method based on that a classifier is selected from a cluster in CSBC framework has been based on random selection so far. It means a random classifier is selected from each partition. Table 2 depicts the performance for three methods for selecting a representative classifier from any partition. The three methods for selecting a representative classifier from any partition are RS, TMAS and TNTCCS. RS stands for "random selection". TMAS stands for "the most accurate selection". In TMAS the most accurate classifier in any cluster is selected as the representative classifier of the cluster; it means that in any cluster, the most accurate classifier is selected for the representative classifier of the cluster. The accuracy of the classifier is achieved by testing the classifier over all training dataset. TNTCCS stands for "the nearest-to-cluster-center selection". In TNTCCS the nearest classifier to cluster center in any cluster is selected as the representative classifier of the cluster. The measure of distance is the same measure used for partitioning algorithm.

As it is completely understandable from Table 2, the method TNTCCS for classifier selection method is the most dominant one among the three methods. The RS is surprisingly the second one. Although it may be expected that TMAS is the best one among the three methods at first, the experimentations show it is the worst one.

5   Conclusions

In this paper, we have proposed a new approach to improve the performance of classification. The proposed method uses a modified version of bagging ensemble as the generator of the base classifiers of the ensemble. After that using k-means we partition the base classifiers. Then a random classifier is selected from each cluster. The selected classifiers are jointly considered as the proposed ensemble. Since each cluster is produced according to classifiers' outputs, it is highly likely that selecting one classifier from each cluster, and using them as an ensemble can produce a diverse ensemble that outperforms the traditional Bagging and Boosting, i.e. usage of all classifiers as an ensemble. It is also more likely that selecting the nearest classifier to the head of each produced cluster produces an ensemble with a higher diversity than the ensemble of those classifiers any of that is randomly extracted out of each cluster. This can also be worked as another investigation.

. There is a clear difference between our method and bagging and boosting, since they are classifier generation procedures but ours involves in both classifier generation and classifier selection. Our method, only in the first phase (i.e. classifier generation phase) uses bagging (or boosting) procedure. But due to the lack of flexibility in the original bagging (or boosting) procedure, it uses a modified version.

Using the decision tree as base classifier increases the gap between the three approaches in generating an ensemble of the base classifiers. It is due to special feature of the decision tree. Because it is very sensitive to its train set, the use of decision tree as base classifier is very consistent with the Bagging mechanism.

While we choose only at most 22 percent of the base classifiers of Bagging, the accuracy of their ensemble outperforms their full ensemble. Also it outperforms Boosting. Therefore it is concluded that using 22 percent of the base classifiers in the final ensemble can be a well option generally.

Although tuning parameters is also an aim of the paper, mostly paper says that (1) clustering of classifier is better to be done on an ensemble produced by bagging or boosting and (2) clustering classifier works well by bagging, not boosting.

As a future work, one can turn to research on the variance of the method. Since it is said about Bagging can reduce variance and Boosting can simultaneously reduce variance and error rate.

References

1. Blake, C.L., Merz, C.J.: UCI Repository of machine learning databases (1998), http://www.ics.uci.edu/~mlearn/MLRepository.html
2. Breiman, L.: Bagging Predictors. Journal of Machine Learning 24(2), 123–140 (1996)
3. Breiman, L.: Random Forests. Machine Learning 45(1), 5–32 (2001)
4. Freund, Y., Schapire, R.E.: A Decision-Theoretic Generalization of On-Line Learning and an Application to Boosting. Journal Computer Syst. Sci. 55(1), 119–139 (1997)
5. Giacinto, G., Roli, F.: An approach to the automatic design of multiple classifier systems. Pattern Recognition Letters 22, 25–33 (2001)
6. Günter, S., Bunke, H.: Creation of Classifier Ensembles for Handwritten Word Recognition Using Feature Selection Algorithms. In: Proceedings of the Eighth International Workshop on Frontiers in Handwriting Recognition, p. 183 (2002)
7. Kuncheva, L.I.: Combining Pattern Classifiers, Methods and Algorithms. Wiley, New York (2005)
8. Minaei-Bidgoli, B., Parvin, H., Alinejad-Rokny, H., Alizadeh, H., Punch, W.F.: Effects of resampling method and adaptation on clustering ensemble efficacy. AIR 41(1), 27–48 (2014)
9. Parvin, H., Minaei-Bidgoli, B., Shahpar, H.: Classifier Selection by Clustering. In: Martínez-Trinidad, J.F., Carrasco-Ochoa, J.A., Ben-Youssef Brants, C., Hancock, E.R. (eds.) MCPR 2011. LNCS, vol. 6718, pp. 60–66. Springer, Heidelberg (2011)
10. Parvin, H., Alinejad-Rokny, H., Minaei-Bidgoli, B., Parvin, S.: A new classifier ensemble methodology based on subspace learning. JETAI 25(2), 227–250 (2013)
11. Parvin, H., Minaei-Bidgoli, B., Alinejad-Rokny, H., Punch, W.F.: Data weighing mechanisms for clustering ensembles. CEE 39(5), 1433–1450 (2013)
12. Parvin, H., Minaei-Bidgoli, B.: A clustering ensemble framework based on elite selection of weighted clusters. Adv. Data Analysis and Classification 7(2), 181–208 (2013)
13. Parvin, H., Beigi, A., Mozayani, N.: A Clustering Ensemble Learning Method Based on the Ant Colony Clustering Algorithm. An International Journal of Applied and Computational Mathematics 11, 286–302 (2012)
14. Parvin, H., MirnabiBaboli, M., Alinejad, H.: Proposing a Classifier Ensemble Framework based on Classifier Selection and Decision Tree. In: Engineering Applications of Artificial Intelligence, EAAI, pp. 34–42 (2014)
15. Peña, J.M.: Finding Consensus Bayesian Network Structures. Journal of Artificial Intelligence Research 42, 661–687 (2011)
16. Khashei, M., Bijari, M.: An Artificial Neural Network (p, d, q) Model for Timeseries Forecasting. Expert Systems with Applications 37, 479–489 (2010)
17. Pazos, A.B.P., Gonzalez, A.A., Pazos, F.M.: Artificial NeuroGlial Networks. In: Encyclopedia of Artificial Intelligence, New York, pp. 167–171 (2009)
18. Kuncheva, L.I., Whitaker, C.: Measures of diversity in classifier ensembles and their relationship with ensemble accuracy. Machine Learning, 181–207 (2003)

Multiple Kernel Support Vector Machine Problem Is NP-Complete

Luis Carlos Padierna[1], Juan Martín Carpio[1,*], María del Rosario Baltazar[1],
Héctor José Puga[1], and Héctor Joaquín Fraire[2]

[1] Tecnológico Nacional de México-Instituto Tecnológico de León, León, México
{luiscarlos.padierna,juanmartin.carpio}@itleon.edu.mx
{charobalmx,pugahector}@yahoo.com
[2] Tecnológico Nacional de México-Instituto Tecnológico de Cd. Madero, Cd. Madero, México
automatas2002@yahoo.com.mx

Abstract. In this work a polynomial-time reduction to the NP-complete subset sum problem is followed in order to prove the complexity of Multiple Kernel Support Vector Machine decision problem. The Lagrangian function of the standard Support Vector Machine in its dual form was considered to derive the proof. Results of this derivation allow researchers to properly justify the use of approximate methods, such as heuristics and metaheuristics, when working with multiple kernel learning algorithms.

Keywords: Support Vector Machine, Complexity, Multiple Kernels, Subset sum Problem, NP-completeness.

1 Introduction

Support Vector Machines (**SVMs**) have been widely studied. Key design aspects for achieving high performance rates involve: selection of the quadratic programming solver, kernel selection and kernel parameter tuning [1,2].

Selection of the quadratic programming (QP) solver is essential when working with large datasets. In this case, the density of the Gram matrix becomes a technical obstacle. To solve this issue, a whole family of algorithms called decomposition methods has been developed. Some representative algorithms of this family are the Sequential Minimal Optimization (SMO) type methods [4].

Basically, decomposition methods partition the original problem into subproblems which are iteratively improved. In each iteration, the variable indices are split into two parts, a *working set* and a set with remaining variables. The objective is to find a working set that best approximates the original one. The decision problem of determining if such a working set exists has been proved to be **NP–complete** [10].

The NP-completeness of the working set selection problem allows researchers to justify the use of approximate methods in order to find the best possible solution,

---

* Corresponding author.

A. Gelbukh et al. (Eds.): MICAI 2014, Part II, LNAI 8857, pp. 152–159, 2014.

since a NP-complete problem indicates that there not exists a deterministic (exact) algorithm that can solve it in polynomial time.

On the other hand, kernel selection has been traditionally done by trial-and-error method. This is because there is not an efficient way of finding the best kernel for a specific application [3]. Using more than one single kernel in order to improve performance in learning tasks is a recent approach known as Multiple Kernel Learning (**MKL**).

MKL algorithms are proposed to combine kernels in order to obtain a better similarity measure or to integrate feature representations coming from different data sources. Several MKL methods of different nature, together with its algorithmic complexity, have been surveyed and classified in [6].

Combining kernels has been done by a wide range of techniques, from linear combinations to evolutionary methods [7]. A taxonomy of methods for evolving multiple kernels is provided in [2]. The objective of these techniques is to find a multiple kernel that helps to reach better performance than single kernels.

In contrast with working set selection, the multiple-kernel selection problem remains unclassified into a complexity category. In consequence, the use of approximate methods, such as evolutionary ones, is not formal justified. Our objective is to demonstrate the complexity of MK-SVM to fill this technical gap.

A brief introduction to SVM and the concept of multiple kernels are provided in section 2. The process of proving the complexity of MK-SVM is derived in section 3. A discussion of the implications on the result of the proof is on section 4.

2 Support Vector Machines and Multiple Kernels

SVMs are non-probabilistic binary classifiers that can be used to construct a hyperplane to separate data into one of two classes. Its formulation is as follows [9][12]:

Given a training dataset $D = \{x_i, y_i\}_{i=1}^m$ where $x_i \in \mathfrak{R}^d$, $y_i \in \{+1, -1\}$, SVM classifies with an optimal separating hyperplane, which is given by:

$$D(x) = w^\mathrm{T}x + b \tag{1}$$

When working with data non-linearly separable, this hyperplane is obtained by solving the following quadratic programming problem:

$$\mathrm{Min} \frac{1}{2}w^\mathrm{T}w + C \sum_{i=1}^m \xi_i$$
$$\mathrm{s.t.}\ y_i(w^\mathrm{T}x_i + b) \geq 1 - \xi_i,\ \xi_i > 0\ for\ i = 1, ..., \mathrm{m} \tag{2}$$

Introducing the nonnegative Lagrange multipliers α and β and following the KKT conditions:

$$\nabla_w L = w - \sum_{i=1}^m \alpha_i y_i x_i = 0$$

$$\nabla_b L = -\sum_{i=1}^m \alpha_i y_i = 0$$

$$\nabla_{\xi_n} L = C - \alpha_i - \beta_i = 0 \tag{3}$$

The problem (2) is equivalent to the following dual problem

$$\text{Max } L(\alpha) = \sum_{i=1}^{M} \alpha_i - \frac{1}{2}\sum_{i=1}^{m}\sum_{j=1}^{m} y_i y_j \alpha_i \alpha_j k(x_i, x_j)$$
$$\text{s. t. } C \geq \alpha_i \geq 0 \; \forall i = 1, \dots, m$$
$$\text{and } \sum_{i=1}^{m} \alpha_i y_i = 0 \qquad (4)$$

This expression is considered the standard C-SVM. Nowadays there exist several variants of this classifiers, namely, nu-SMV, least-squares SMV, linear programming SVM, among others [9]. However, for the sake of our proof it is enough to consider the function $L(\alpha)$ as expressed in (4).

A kernel is generally a non-linear function that maps the original input space into a high-dimensional dot-product feature space in order to enhance linear separability. Table 1 illustrates some common kernel functions [1].

Table 1. Some common kernel functions

Kernel	$K(x, x_j) =$	Kernel	$K(x, x_j) =$
Lineal	$x^T x_j$	Powered	$-\|x - x_j\|^\beta \; 0 < \beta \leq 1$
Polynomial	$(a \times x^T x_j + b)^d$	Log	$-log\left(1 + \|x - x_j\|^\beta\right) \; 0 < \beta \leq 1$
RBF	$e^{\left(-\frac{\|x-x_j\|^2}{\sigma^2}\right)}$	Generalized Gaussian	$e^{-(x-x_j)^T A(x-x_j)}$ where A is a symmetric PD matrix
Sigmoid	$\tanh(\sigma x^T x_j + r)$	Hybrid	$e^{-\frac{\|x-x_j\|^2}{\sigma^2}} \times (\tau + x^T x_j)^d$

To implement a multiple kernel in a SVM, the requirement is that this kernel fulfills the Mercer condition [1]:

$$K(x, x_j) = \sum_{i}^{\infty} a_i \varphi_i(x)\varphi_i(x_j), \; a_i > 0$$
$$\iint K(x, x_j) g(x)g(x_j)dx dx_j > 0 \qquad (5)$$

Linear combinations of kernels also satisfy Mercer's condition. Let $K_1(x, x_j)$ and $K_2(x, x_j)$ be Mercer kernels, and $c_1, c_2 \geq 0$, then:

$$K(x, x_j) = c_1 K_1(x, x_j) + c_2 K_2(x, x_j) \qquad (6)$$

is also a Mercer kernel. This property of linear combinations will be fundamental in proving the complexity of Multiple Kernel Learning.

3   Multiple Kernel Support Vector Problem and Its Complexity

In this section, a four-step process is followed in order to prove the complexity of MK-SVM problem. This problem will be denoted by π. The four steps are: (1)

Showing that π is in NP. (2) Selecting a known NP-complete problem π'. (3) Constructing a transformation f from π' to π and (4) Proving that f is a polynomial transformation [5].

3.1   MK-SVM Problem (π)

Given a finite set of Mercer kernels $A = \{k_1, \ldots, k_n\}$, a dataset of labeled input patterns $D \subset X \times Y$, such that $X \subset \mathfrak{R}^d$, $Y = \{+1, -1\}$; a set of Lagrange Multipliers $V = \{\alpha_1, \ldots, \alpha_m\}$ and an optimal objective function value in terms of a kernel in A expressed as a positive integer B; find the subset $A' \subseteq A$ of maximum size q that minimizes the cost:

$$C(A') = \left[\sum_{k \in A'} \left(\frac{1}{q} \left[\sum_{i=1}^m \alpha_i - \frac{1}{2q^2} \sum_{i=1}^m \sum_{j=1}^m y_i y_j k(x_i, x_j) \alpha_i \alpha_j \right] \right)^2 - B \right]^2 \qquad (7)$$

Seen as a decision problem, the question is if there exists such a subset A'.

The cost function $C(A')$ depends upon the objective function to be maximized in the dual form of a standard SVM (4). Function cost basically expresses the idea of reaching a bound B by means of a set of kernels, a fixed dataset and a SVM represented by its support vectors.

3.2   MK–SVM is in NP

For MK–SMV to be in NP it is enough to show that an instance (A') of the problem can be guessed and that this instance can be verified to solve or not to solve the problem in polynomial time.

Let R be a random function that accepts $q \in \mathbb{Z}^+$ and returns the q indexes of the Mercer kernels selected from a list with $n \in \mathbb{Z}^+$ kernels, $R: \mathfrak{R} \to A'$, then the instance A' can be easily generated by R.

To show that the instance A' can be verified in polynomial time, the equation (7) should be analyzed. As V, D, q and B are *a priori* known, the only computations in the verification stage lies in evaluating $m \times m$ kernels. And due to the fact that all kernel evaluations mainly consists in dot products or differences among d-dimensional vectors, the $m \times m$ evaluations of the kernels remains polynomial in time, thus, MK-SVM is in NP.

3.3   Selecting a Known NP-Complete Problem

The known problem (π') selected for this proof is the subset sum, whose definition is as follows [5]:

Given a finite set A, a size $s(a) \in \mathbb{Z}^+$ for each $a \in A$ and a positive integer B. Is there an $A' \subseteq A$ such that the sum of the sizes of the elements in A' is exactly B?

3.4   Constructing a Transformation f from π' to π

The transformation f should map every instance (I) in π' to π in such a way that every instance with answer "yes" in π is an instance with answer "yes" in π', and analogously with instances with answer "no". For doing this mapping its necessary to show how the form of $A, A', s(a)$, and B will be transform from MK-SVM to Subset sum.

First, A stands for any finite set, so we consider a finite set of n Mercer kernels $A = \{k_1, ..., k_n\}$. A' is simply a subset of A.

Then, to compute B the following procedure should be followed:

1. Solve a standard SVM for each $k \in A$ and with the same input dataset D
2. Take the kernel $k^*(x_i, x_j)$ and the Lagrange multipliers $V = \{\alpha_1, ..., \alpha_m\}$ of the SVM that reaches the best classification performance in step 1. For example, by using cross-fold validation and taking the accuracy index. Denote $M^* = (V^*, k^*)$ as the optimal SVM.
3. Calculate

$$B = \left[\sum_{i=1}^{m} \alpha_i - \frac{1}{2} \sum_{i=1}^{m} \sum_{j=1}^{m} y_i y_j k^*(x_i, x_j) \alpha_i \alpha_j \right]^2 \tag{8}$$

That represents the maximum value of the dual-form objective function for the optimal SVM.

Finally, the size $s(a) = s(k \in A)$ will be computed using V^* and the dataset D to calculate

$$s(k) = \left[\left(\frac{1}{q} \sum_{i=1}^{m} \alpha_i - \frac{1}{2q^2} \sum_{i=1}^{m} \sum_{j=1}^{m} y_i y_j k(x_i, x_j) \alpha_i \alpha_j \right) \right]^2 \tag{9}$$

Where $q = |A'|$ is added to eliminate bias in the measurement by distributing the weight of α's among the number of kernels to combine. The $s(k)$ measurement represents the value of the objective function for the dual form of the optimal SMV, which works with a kernel not necessarily being $k^*(x_i, x_j)$.

Now it is proved that using the measurement $s(k)$ and the bound B above defined, the sum $\sum_{k \in A'} s(k) = B$ only when $k^*(x_i, x_j) = \frac{1}{q^2} \sum_{k \in A'} k(x_i, x_j)$.

First, $\sum_{k \in A'} s(k) = B$ is expressed in its extended form

$$\left[\sum_{k \in A'} \left(\frac{1}{q} \sum_{i=1}^{m} \alpha_i - \frac{1}{2q^2} \sum_{i=1}^{m} \sum_{j=1}^{m} y_i y_j k(x_i, x_j) \alpha_i \alpha_j \right) \right]^2 =$$
$$\left[\sum_{i=1}^{m} \alpha_i - \frac{1}{2} \sum_{i=1}^{m} \sum_{j=1}^{m} y_i y_j k^*(x_i, x_j) \alpha_i \alpha_j \right]^2 \tag{10}$$

Taking the root squared of both members

$$\sum_{k \in A'} \left(\frac{1}{q} \sum_{i=1}^{m} \alpha_i - \frac{1}{2q^2} \sum_{i=1}^{m} \sum_{j=1}^{m} y_i y_j k(x_i, x_j) \alpha_i \alpha_j \right) =$$
$$\sum_{i=1}^{m} \alpha_i - \frac{1}{2} \sum_{i=1}^{m} \sum_{j=1}^{m} y_i y_j k^*(x_i, x_j) \alpha_i \alpha_j \tag{11}$$

Applying summation properties to the left member

$$\Sigma_{k \in A'} \left(\frac{1}{q} \Sigma_{i=1}^m \alpha_i\right) + \Sigma_{k \in A'} \left[-\frac{1}{2q^2} \Sigma_{i=1}^m \Sigma_{j=1}^m y_i y_j k(x_i, x_j)\alpha_i\alpha_j\right] =$$
$$\Sigma_{i=1}^m \alpha_i - \frac{1}{2}\Sigma_{i=1}^m \Sigma_{j=1}^m y_i y_j k^*(x_i, x_j)\alpha_i\alpha_j \qquad (12)$$

Simplifying terms

$$\Sigma_{k \in A'} \left[-\frac{1}{2q^2} \Sigma_{i=1}^m \Sigma_{j=1}^m y_i y_j k(x_i, x_j)\alpha_i\alpha_j\right] = -\frac{1}{2}\Sigma_{i=1}^m \Sigma_{j=1}^m y_i y_j k^*(x_i, x_j)\alpha_i\alpha_j \qquad (13)$$

Multiplying by (-2) both members

$$\Sigma_{k \in A'} \left[\frac{1}{q^2} \Sigma_{i=1}^m \Sigma_{j=1}^m y_i y_j k(x_i, x_j)\alpha_i\alpha_j\right] = \Sigma_{i=1}^m \Sigma_{j=1}^m y_i y_j k^*(x_i, x_j)\alpha_i\alpha_j \qquad (14)$$

Making $\Delta_{i,j} = y_i y_j \alpha_i \alpha_j$ to simplify notation

$$\Sigma_{k \in A'} \left[\frac{1}{q^2} \Sigma_{i=1}^m \Sigma_{j=1}^m \Delta_{i,j} k(x_i, x_j)\right] = \Sigma_{i=1}^m \Sigma_{j=1}^m \Delta_{i,j} k^*(x_i, x_j) \qquad (15)$$

Taking an equivalent form of the left member in (15)

$$\Sigma_{i=1}^m \Sigma_{j=1}^m \Delta_{i,j} \frac{1}{q^2} \Sigma_{k \in A'} k(x_i, x_j) = \Sigma_{i=1}^m \Sigma_{j=1}^m \Delta_{i,j} k^*(x_i, x_j) \qquad (16)$$

Which indicates that

$$\frac{1}{q^2} \Sigma_{k \in A'} k(x_i, x_j) = k^*(x_i, x_j) \qquad (17)$$

And thus

$$\Sigma_{k \in A'} s(k) = B \leftrightarrow k^*(x_i, x_j) = \frac{1}{q^2} \Sigma_{k \in A'} k(x_i, x_j) \qquad (18)$$

This implies that the problem of finding a subset of measurements such that the sum is equals to a positive integer could be transformed to the problem of finding a subset of kernels which, in combination, are equivalent to an optimal kernel. Therefore, every instance (I) of the subset sum problem whose answer is "yes" can be mapped into an instance (I') of the MK-SMV whose answer is also "yes". In summary, Subset Sum problem can be transformed into MK-SVM problem.

3.5   Proving that f is a Polynomial Transformation

The last part of this proof consists in showing f is polynomial. To prove this, consider the most expensive step in computational terms that the function f does, computing B, i.e., solving n Support Vector Machines for a given dataset D.

The problem of training a SVM reduces to solve a quadratic programming problem (QP). When QP is viewed as a decision problem, it is *NP-complete* by itself. However, when working with SVM, QP is convex. And there exist methods like Ellipsoid or Interior Point algorithms that solve convex QP in polynomial time [13].

Not only the convex QP is solvable in polynomial time, but also it is known that training a standard SVM has a complexity of $O(m^3)$ where m is the number of input vectors. [11].

Furthermore, it is m what determines the required algorithm to solve the SVM. According to [8], for small and moderately sized problems (less than 5000 examples), interior point algorithms are reliable and accurate methods to choose. And that for large-scale problems, methods that exploit the sparsity of the dual variables must be adopted; furthermore, if limitations on the storage is required, compact representation should be considered, for example, using an approximation to the kernel matrix.

In conclusion, solving a standard SVM is done in polynomial time, and thus, subsequent operations in f remains polynomial. Consequently, f is a polynomial transformation.

4   Discussion

In this paper it was shown that MK-SVM is in **NP** and that it is possible to make a polynomial reduction to the NP-complete subset sum problem. Therefore, MK-SVM viewed as a decision problem is NP-complete.

This result has an impact in the Multiple Kernel Learning area because the complexity of the problem justifies the use of approximate methods when trying to find an optimal solution.

To our knowledge, this is the first work that put the focus on the complexity of Multiple Kernel Learning as a decision problem. Previous reviews such as that of [6] are concerned to computational complexity and talks about heuristic methods for combining kernels; however, omit the essential proof that makes the use of this approach justifiable, the NP-completeness of MK-SVM.

Recently, studies have been done by using metaheuristics for evolving multiple kernels, see for example, [2] or [7]. These proposals establish frameworks for obtaining kernel expressions automatically. However, they also assume, without any reference, that the Genetic Programming techniques are properly justified for that commitment.

This proof is then a fundamental and complementary building block for those works dealing with Multiple Kernels. As future work it is visualized to include the result of this proof as a reference to justify the application of metaheuristics in multiple kernel learning tasks.

Acknowledgments. Luis Carlos Padierna García wishes to acknowledge the financial support of the Consejo Nacional de Ciencia y Tecnología (CONACYT grant 375524). The authors also wish to acknowledge the motivation and technical support provided by the Tecnológico Nacional de México.

References

1. Boolchandani, D., Sahula, V.: Exploring Efficient Kernel Functions for Support Vector Machines Based Feasibility Models for Analog Circuits. International Journal on Design, Analysis and Tools for Circuits and Systems, 1–8 (2011)
2. Diosan, L., Rogozan, A., Pecuchet, J.: Learning SVM with complex multiple kernels evolved by genetic programming. International Journal on Artificial Intelligence Tools 19, 647–677 (2010)
3. Essam, A.D., Hamza, T.: New empirical nonparametric kernels for support vector machines classification. Applied Soft Computing 13, 1759–1765 (2013)
4. Fan, R.-E., Chen, P.-H., Lin, C.-J.: Working Set Selection Using Second Order Information for Training Support Vector Machines. Journal of Machine Learning Research, 1889–1918 (2005)
5. Garey, M., Johnson, D.: Computers and Intractability a guide to the theory of NP-Completeness. Freeman and Company, New York (1979)
6. Gönen, M., Alpaydin, E.: Multiple Kernel Learning Algorithms. Journal of Machine Learning Research, 2211–2268 (2011)
7. Koch, P., Bischl, B., Flasch, O., Bartz-Beielstein, T., Weihs, C., Konen, W.: Tuning and Evolution of Least-Squares Support Vector Machines. Evolutionary Intelligence, 1–30 (2011)
8. Shawe-Taylor, J., Sun, S.: A review of optimization methodologies in support vector machines. Neurocomputing, 3609–3618 (2011)
9. Shigeo, A.: Support Vector Machines for Pattern Classification. Springer, New York (2010)
10. Simon, H.: On the complexity of working set selection. Theoretical Computer Science, 262–279 (2007)
11. Tsang, I., Kwok, J., Cheung, P.-M.: Core Vector Machines: Fast SVM Training on Very Large Data Sets. Journal of Machine Learning Research, 363–392 (2005)
12. Vapnik, V.: Statistical Learning Theory. John Wiley and Sons, New York (1998)
13. Vavasis, S.A.: Complexity issues in global optimization: a survey. In: Horst, R., Pardalos, P. (eds.) Handbook of Global Optimization, pp. 27–41. Springer (1995)

Feature Analysis for the Classification of Volcanic Seismic Events Using Support Vector Machines

Millaray Curilem, Fernando Huenupan, Cesar San Martin, Gustavo Fuentealba,
Carlos Cardona, Luis Franco, Gonzalo Acuña, and Max Chacón

Departamento de Ingeniería Eléctrica, Universidad de La Frontera, Francisco Salazar 01145,
Temuco, Chile
{millaray.curilem, fernando.huenupan,
cesar.sanmartin}@ufrontera.cl
Departamento de Ciencias Físicas, Universidad de La Frontera, Salazar 01145, Temuco, Chile
gustavo.fuentealba@ufrontera.cl
Observatorio Vulcanológico de los Andes Sur, Temuco, Chile, Rudecindo Ortega 03850,
Temuco, Chile
{carlos.cardona, luis.franco}@sernageomin.cl
Departamento de Ingeniería Informática, Universidad de Santiago de Chile,
Avenida Ecuador #3659, Estación Central, Santiago de Chile
{gonzalo.acuna, max.chacon}@usach.cl

Abstract. This paper shows a preliminary study to perform a pattern recognition process for seismic events of the Llaima volcano, one of the most active volcanoes in South America. 1622 classified events registered from the Llaima volcano were considered in this study, taken from 2009 to 2011. The events were divided in four classes: TREMOR (TR), LONG-PERIOD (LP), VOLCANO-TECTONICS (VT) and OTHERS (OT). All of them correspond to specific activities. TR and LP events, are related to magmatic fluid through the ducts: continuous flux correspond to TR and discrete flux to LP. VT events occurs when excess of the magmatic pressure provides enough energy for rock failure. The group of OT contains events not related to the three first volcanic classes. Many features extracted from de amplitude, the frequency and the phase of the events were used to characterize the different classes. A classifier step based on Support Vector Machines was implemented to evaluate the contribution of each feature to the classification. The paper shows the results of this process and gives insights for future works.

Keywords: Volcanic Seismicity, Pattern Recognition, SVM.

1 Volcanic Seismology and Pattern Recognition

Because of its geographical location, Chile has about one hundred volcanoes considered active. At latitude of 38.4 S is the volcano Llaima, located in the Araucanía Region (38 ° 41'S - 71 ° 44'W). The "Observatorio Vulcanológico de los Andes Sur" (OVDAS) is the state agency responsible for establishing systems to continuously

A. Gelbukh et al. (Eds.): MICAI 2014, Part II, LNAI 8857, pp. 160–171, 2014.
© Springer International Publishing Switzerland 2014

monitor and record over forty active Chilean volcanoes. This monitoring is mainly of seismological type. Volcanic seismicity has a prominent role in monitoring volcanoes [1]. Today Llaima volcano is monitored through twelve seismic stations, located at different parts of its external structure. The seismic signals suggest internal processes that are occurring inside the volcano structure [2, 3]. The challenge of monitoring volcanoes includes the need to incorporate tools that automate the identification of its activity. Tools from the area of signal processing and pattern recognition are used. Within seismic signal processing, the problem is generally tackled in two stages, feature extraction and classification. The feature extraction stage defines what information (i.e., features) will be used for facilitating the classification. The classification stage performs the discrimination of the events. Literature tackles these two stages with many different tools.

From the perspective of the features, Langer et al. [4] used autocorrelation functions, obtained by the fast Fourier transform (FFT) to represent the spectral content of the seismic signals. They applied an amplitude ratio to distinguish between signal peaks and long duration, with similar frequency content. Other widely used methods are the wavelet transform [5, 6, 7] and cross-correlation methods [8] to denoise the seismic events. In [9] the feature vector is composed of a set of data related to the statistical distribution of the spectral characteristics of the signal, 13 cepstral coefficients and their time evolution along the signal. In [10], short-time Fourier transform (STFT) was applied to identify changes in the activity of Etna volcano tremor through the variations in its features. In [11], the authors used amplitude statistics (mean, standard deviation, skewness and kurtosis), and incorporated statistical wavelet decomposition phase and power to detect seismic events in southern India. They proposed a system to detect small earthquakes, distinguishing between seismic and non-seismic sources. Volcanoes of the Araucanía Region of Chile have also been studied, in particular the Villarrica and Llaima volcanoes [12]. In [13] a feature selection process showed that the mean, median, maximum amplitude, the energy in the frequency band [1.5625 – 3.125] Hz, and the peak frequency were dominant signal descriptors. In [14], 893 signals were used to classify different events of the Llaima volcano, considering three classes on segmented windows of one minute length. This work applied circular statistics, specifically the first circular moment was used together with the wavelet energy in the [1.5625 – 3.125] Hz sub-band. All these works reached classifying performances superior to 80%.

The classification step was also implemented using many tools for the design of the classifier. In [9] the authors worked with Hidden Markov Models to model and identify different patterns online. In [13] a multilayer Perceptron was used to classify different events from the Villarrica Volcano, in Chile. In [14] a linear discriminator was used with a very high performance to discriminate between the three considered classes. In [11] the authors compared various types of classifiers and reported that support vector machine (SVM) provided the best performance with an accuracy of 94%. This conclusion supported the results of [15] and [16] that also reached the best results with a SVM classifier. In [17] the authors presented a comparative study of two supervised methods, which are SVM and Radial Basis Analysis (RBA), and two unsupervised methods which are cluster analysis and self-organizing maps. The SVM gave superior results (>90%) compared to the RBA (> 80%). The clustering methods allowed identifying the characteristics of the tremor changes over time.

The literature shows that the application of pattern recognition tools to seismic signals analysis of volcanoes has led to an intense research effort. This paper focuses on the automatic classification of events of the Llaima volcano and its aim is to investigate which are the most useful features to discriminate the seismic events of this volcano. Thus, the main motivation of the paper is to improve the discrimination capacity of the classifying step. This is why a wide feature extraction was performed to evaluate which are the best descriptors per class.

2   Material and Methods

2.1   Data Description

OVDAS analysts defined three stations to provide the seismic signals for the study. Their different distances from the crater ensures an adequate variability of the records. Only the Z component is considered in this work. The records belong to the posteruptive period from 2009 to 2011. The analysts classified all the events and stored them in files with variable length, according to the duration of the events. The events considered were of type LP, TR and VT. A fourth group was created, termed as "other" type (OT) that contains the signals which do not correspond to any of the three listed above (like tectonic earthquakes, noise, ice breakdown, etc.). The purpose of creating the OT class of signals is to be enable the classifier recognizing signals that do not correspond to any of the others. It is important to highlight that the length of the events stored in the database is variable. The whole database was divided into three sets, defining the training, validation and test sets that will be used for the implementation of the classifiers. Table 1 gives the breakdown of signals used in this work.

Table 1. Seismic events used to train and validate the classifier.

Class	Training set	Validation set	Test set	Complete Data set
TR	176	163	161	500
VT	57	42	49	148
LP	156	182	161	499
OT	156	158	161	475
TOTAL	545	545	532	1622

2.2   Feature Extraction

Signals prior to 2011 were sampled at 50 Hz and after that at 100Hz. Since the interesting information lies below 25Hz [3], signals of 100Hz were down-sampled to 50Hz. All the signals were then filtered with a band-pass filter of type Butterworth with order 8 between [0.5-15] Hz.

The feature extraction step considered many features obtained from literature. Unlike most of previous works, in this work the features are calculated from variable length windows that covers the entire events. However, the segments do not exactly match the events, because some background signals remained at the beginning and the end. This arbitrary segmentation error was considered to simulate the error of an automatic segmentation algorithm that detects the beginning and the end of the events. This algorithm is being developed in another work, and presumably, it will imply that the segmentation of the signals will not be as exact as the segmentation performed by an expert, manually. Therefore, the classifiers have to be adapted to these situations. All the extracted features were linearly normalized between [-1, 1] and stored in a matrix of 1622 rows (all the events) and 22 columns, each one is a specific feature, according to the order presented in table 2. Each feature is explained next.

Table 2. Overview of the features extracted from each volcano's event

Column	Feature	Name	Column	Feature	Name
1	Moment 1	M1	12	Energy 0-50 Hz	Es
2	Moment 2	M2	13	5 bands energy sum	Ex
3	Moment 3	M3	14	Max, amplitude	AMAX
4	Variance	var	15	Mean	MEAN
5	Asymmetry	y1	16	Median	MDN
6	Elevation	y2	17	5 freq. peaks mean	Propf
7	Energy 0.1-1,5 Hz	Ea4	18	LTA/STA	LTA/STA
8	Energy 1,5-3,1 Hz	Ed4	19	Log of the variance	Lvar
9	Energy 3,1-6,3 Hz	Ed3	20	Skewness	SKW
10	Energy 6,3-15,5 Hz	Ed2	21	Kurtosis	KURT
11	Energy 12,5-25 Hz	Ed1	22	Pitch	PITCH

Circular Moment Statistics

The circular moments reflects the behavior of the phase part of the volcanic signals. The phase is obtained using the Hilbert transform in the range of $[0\ 2\pi)$. Afterwards, circular statistics are applied to obtain the statistical properties of this phase. As in the case of statistical linear dispersion measures, and sharpness symmetry, underlying probability distribution can be defined from trigonometric moments. Several circular statistics were analyzed i.e. mean, variance, skewness and kurtosis. The pth order of the circular moment is obtained using equation 1:

$$\mu_p = \frac{1}{N}\sum_{n=1}^{N} \exp\left(jp\theta_p\right) \tag{1}$$

where $n=1,\ldots$, N is the number of samples and $\theta=\{\theta_p\}$ is the set of values in the circular range $[0\ 2\pi)$ of the instantaneous phase of a random variable. This complex number can be interpreted as the vector resulting from the sum of n unit vectors with angles given by θ. The resulting vector has magnitude $\|\mu_p\| = 1$ and angle $\angle\mu_p$, called direction, in the complex plane.

Variance

The circular variance quantifies the data dispersion, obtained from the first order circular moment, as shown in equation 2:

$$\sigma^2 = 1 - |\mu_1| \tag{2}$$

where σ^2 is the variance, and $|\mu_1|$ is the first circular moment obtained from equation 1.

Asymmetry and Elevation

These features are obtained from the circular statistics of the signals. The asymmetry is obtained by equation 3 and Elevation by equation 4.

$$y_1 = \frac{|\mu_2|sin(\angle(\mu_2) - 2\angle(\mu_1))}{(\sigma)^{\frac{3}{2}}} \tag{3}$$

$$y_2 = \frac{|\mu_2|cos(\angle(\mu_2) - 2\angle(\mu_1) - |\mu_2|^2)}{(\sigma)^2} \tag{4}$$

Energy of the Wavelet Band

To obtain the relative energy per band the signal is decomposed using the wavelet transform. A Daubechies mother wavelet type five with a decomposition level equal to four was used. The percentage of energy was calculated using the following formula

$$EX_n = \frac{E_w}{E_x} * 100 \tag{5}$$

where E_w is the sum of the components of one wavelet band (ED1..ED4, EA4), and E_x is the sum of all bands wavelet components. Relative energy of all bands was tested.

Maximum Amplitude, Mean and Median

Some characteristics are extracted from the amplitude of the signal, like maximum amplitude that identifies the maximum value of the segmented event. The mean value performs the mean of all the signals of the event. The median calculates the median of the samples of the event.

Mean of the 5 Frequency Peaks

The signals are transformed using the FFT and the 5 highest peaks are detected and their mean is calculated to obtain this feature.

LTA/STA Ratio

The short-time-average/long-time-average (STA/LTA) continuously calculates the average values of the absolute amplitude of the seismic signal in two consecutive moving-time windows: a short time window (STA) and a long time window (LTA). Usually when the ratio of both times exceeds a predefined value, an event is detected. In this work, the ratio is used to discriminate the 3 kind of events to classify. The equation 6 and 7 show how it is calculated.

$$STA = \frac{1}{ns}\Sigma_{j=i-ns}^{i} CF_j \tag{6}$$

$$LTA = \frac{1}{nl}\Sigma_{j=i-nl}^{i} CF_j \tag{7}$$

where: ns and nl represent the number of samples used by each STA and LTA window, and CFj are the values of the samples.

Variance, Skewness and Kurtosis

The Lvar feature is computed as the logarithm of the statistical variance of the samples of the seismic event.

Skewness is a statistical parameter that measures the assimetry of a distribution, in this case, the seismic event, thus measures the shape of the event. This feature is calculated using equation 8:

$$C = \frac{1}{N}\Sigma_{i=1}^{N}\left(\frac{X(i)-\bar{X}}{\sigma}\right)^{3} \tag{8}$$

where $\bar{X}$, σ and N are the mean, the standard deviation and the number of samples of the event, respectively.

Kurtosis is a statistical parameter that measures the sharpness of a distribution, in this case the seismic event, this is why it is also a shape attribute of the signal. It can be calculated using equation 9:

$$D = \frac{1}{N}\Sigma_{i=1}^{N}\left(\frac{X(i)-\bar{X}}{\sigma}\right)^{4} - 3 \tag{9}$$

where $\bar{X}$, σ and N are the mean, the standard deviation and the number of samples of the event, respectively.

Pitch

This feature is mainly used in speech processing and is related to the fundamental frequency of a signal. In this work pitch has been defined by the auto correlation of the signal. The expression for its calculation is shown in equation 10:

$$R(m) = \frac{1}{N}\Sigma_{n=0}^{N-1-m} x(n)x(n+m), \ 0 \le m \le M_0 \tag{10}$$

where $x(n)$ are the samples of the signal, m is the delay of the auto-correlation. The pitch is the delay value that maximizes the function presented in equation 10.

2.3   Classification

Support vector machine tackles classification problems by nonlinearly mapping input data into high-dimensional feature spaces, wherein a linear decision hyperplane separates two classes, as described in figure 1 (a and b) [18].

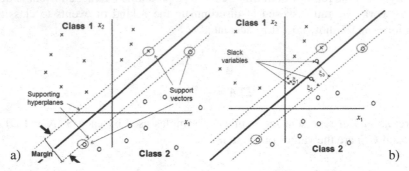

Fig. 1. Linear decision hyperplane of two classes: a) maximum margin b) soft margin

The decision hyperplane parameters (w,b) are obtained by an optimization algorithm that finds the largest distance (margin) to the nearest training data points of any class, called the support vectors [19, 20]. They define the supporting hyperplanes shown in figure 1a). Meanwhile, figure 1b) shows the soft margin situation, when some points are allowed to cross the supporting hyperplanes. Slack variables ξ are error terms that measure how far a particular point lies on the wrong side of its respective supporting hyperplane. To solve nonlinear problems it is necessary to transform the input space where the data is not linearly separable into a higher-dimensional space called a feature space where the data is linearly separable. The transformation function φ maps the input space into the feature space, as shown in figure 2.

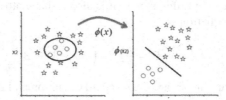

Fig. 2. Effect of mapping the input space into a higher dimensional feature space, where a linear separation plane is possible

Some of these functions called kernels allow computing the inner product between two independent original variables $\vec{x}_i \cdot \vec{x}_j$ in the input space as if it was in the feature space, making it unnecessary to fully evaluate the transformation. Equation 11 shows the most generally used RBF Kernel.

$$k(\vec{x}_i, \vec{x}_j) = \vec{x}_i \cdot \vec{x}_j = \varphi(\vec{x}_i) \cdot \varphi(\vec{x}_j) = \frac{e^{-\left\| \vec{x}_i - \vec{x}_j \right\|^2}}{2\sigma^2} \tag{11}$$

The optimization problem is then expressed as shown in equation 12.

$$\min_{w,b,\xi} \left(\frac{1}{2}w^T w + c \sum_{k=1}^{N} \xi_k\right) \; s.t. \; \begin{matrix} y_k[w^T x_k + b] \geq 1 - \xi_k \\ \xi_k \geq 0, \; k = 1,..,N \end{matrix} \tag{12}$$

where c is a hyperparameter determining the trade-off between the complexity of the model, expressed by $\bar{w}$, and the points that remain in the wrong side of the decision hyperplane, expressed by the slack variablesξ. The solution of this minimization problem for obtaining the weight vectors is found by the standard optimization procedure for a problem with inequality restrictions when applying the conditions of Karush-Kuhn-Tucker to the dual problem.

In classification tasks with RBK kernel, SVM has two hyperparameters to adjust: the RBF parameter (σ) and the penalty parameter (c).

2.4   Performance Indices

To evaluate the performance of each classifier in the classifying structure, the contingency table was built considering the "one versus all" structure, which is considering the events of one class as positive and all the others as negative. Four statistical indices measure the performance of the individual classifiers: sensitivity (Se), specificity (Sp), exactitude (Ex) and error (Er), as calculated in the following relations.

$$Se = \frac{TP}{TP+FN} \; (13); \quad Sp = \frac{TN}{TN+FP} \; (14); \quad Ex = \frac{TP+TN}{n}(15); \quad 15Er = \frac{FP+FN}{n} \; (16)$$

where TP (true positives) is the number of events correctly classified as being of the positive class; TN (true negatives) is the number of events correctly classified as being of the negative class; FP (false positives) and FN (false negatives) is the number of events classified erroneously and n is the total number of events.TP, TN, FP and FN were extracted from the contingency table. The statistical indices are calculated for each model in all simulations.

3   Simulation and Results

The simulations were carried out with Matlab of Mathworks, in an Intel Core™ i5 CPU with 3 GHz and 8 GB RAM. As SVM perform two-class classification a "one versus all" configuration was necessary. The same single input was presented to all the classifiers. For each feature, four classifiers had to be trained, each one for TR, VT, LP and OT events. For each feature the resulting classifying structure is shown in figure 3. The output of the whole classification system was coded as shown in table 3.

The results are presented in the next tables. Table 4 shows the performance of the best classifiers for each class. All the indices were calculated on the test set. Table 5 presents the best sigma and c values of the classifiers, for each situation presented in table 4. Table 6 presents the whole simulating process, with the performance of the best classifiers, designed with a single variable. The best values shown in table 6 are underlined in dark gray and light gray. It can be seen that some classes reach the best performance (test exactitude) with different features (e.g. Ed3 and Propf, for TR class). Table 6 presents the features that better described each class, thus they are the best candidates to be studied, as will be discussed in the 4th section.

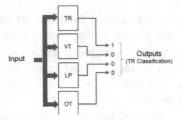

Fig. 3. Classifying Structure: "one versus all" structure of the classifiers

Table 3. Codification of the outputs

	Classifier			
Class	**1**	**2**	**3**	**4**
TR	1	0	0	0
VT	0	1	0	0
LP	0	0	1	0
OT	0	0	0	1

Table 4. Performance Indices for the best classifiers of each class

Class	Feature	Sensitivity	Specificity	Exactitude	Error
TR	**MDN**	0.75	0.84	0.81	0.19
	Ed2	0.63	0.89	0.81	0.19
VT	**Lvar**	0.73	1.00	0.97	0.03
	MDN	0.67	1.00	0.97	0.03
	MEAN	0.67	1.00	0.97	0.03
	AMAX	0.71	1.00	0.97	0.03
LP	**Propf**	0.88	0.56	0.65	0.35
OT	**Ed3**	0.63	0.90	0.82	0.18

Table 5. Best values of c and sigma for the best classifiers of each class

Class	c	sigma
TR	-3	-3
	-3	1
VT	1	1
	-2	0
	5	-2
	-3	-3
LP	-2	-3
OT	0	-1

Table 6. Exactitude for the test set for all the classifiers of each class. The best values are in dark gray while other interesting performance values are underlined in light gray.

	Feature	TR	VT	LP	OT
1	M1	0.68	0.94	0.69	0.69
2	M2	0.53	0.86	0.65	0.71
3	M3	0.6	0.86	0.68	0.71
4	var	0.65	0.8	0.65	0.69
5	y1	0.57	0.92	0.68	0.69
6	y2	0.57	0.9	0.68	0.7
7	Ea4	0.74	0.94	0.66	0.68
8	Ed4	0.77	0.72	0.87	0.73
9	Ed3	0.81	0.94	0.75	0.73
10	Ed2	0.77	0.9	0.89	0.74
11	Ed1	0.6	0.87	0.65	0.77
12	Es	0.61	0.91	0.63	0.77
13	Ex	0.64	0.72	0.67	0.5
14	AMAX	0.78	0.97	0.85	0.81
15	MEAN	0.77	0.97	0.85	0.81
16	MDN	0.76	0.97	0.85	0.82
17	Propf	0.81	0.96	0.87	0.79
18	LTA/STA	0.74	0.91	0.77	0.71
19	Lvar	0.77	0.97	0.86	0.81
20	SKW	0.63	0.92	0.67	0.7
21	KURT	0.65	0.89	0.69	0.76
22	PITCH	0.7	0.91	0.86	0.65

4   Discussion and Conclusions

In a previous work [21], the authors demonstrated that the features selected for the classification of the seismic events of the Villarrica volcano, also performed well for the Llaima volcano. These are neighbor volcanoes with similar composition. However, the mean of the exactitude was superior to 90% for the Villarrica volcano, while it was superior to 80% for the Llaima volcano. One possible reason for this exactitude decrease is that other features of the Llaima events are needed to improve classification. This is why this paper shows a preliminary study on new characteristics extracted from literature that may improve the discrimination performance of a classifying structure.

One of the most important results is included in table 4 where the exactitude of the identification of each class with only one feature is high. However, sensitivity for TR, VT and OT is low. For all classes, there are less true positives than true negatives, due to the "one vs. all" configuration. This is critical for the VT class, for which there are only 49 true positives against 483 true negatives (see table 1). This makes the error very low, even with a low sensitivity. In addition LP class is also difficult to classify because its specificity is very low. In conclusion, even with good exactitude, the individual features are not good discriminators for the four classes.

Table 6 shows that some features like those extracted from the amplitude (AMAX, MEAN, MDN), the one extracted from its spectrum (Propf) and Lvar are the best discriminators for all classes. This is an interesting result as all of them, with the exception of Lvar, were considered in previous works [13, 21] as good discriminators.

The SVM technique used to design the classification step gave robustness to the feature analysis process. Artificial Neural Networks are difficult to train most of all, because of the high number of weights' initialization needed to find the best model, avoiding over fitting. SVM are better when the number of models is high -like in this work- as one model for each class and for each feature had to be trained.

The main contribution of this paper is to quantify how well each feature performs for each class. As shown in table 6, the exactitude may be high for one class but not for another. Thus, in future works, combinations of these features will be tested and their impact in the classification performance will be evaluated.

Acknowledgements. This study is being supported by the projects FONDEF IDeA CA13I10273, Fondecyt 11110391 and the ANILLO project of CONICYT ACT 1120.

References

1. Zobin, V.M.: Seismic Monitoring of Volcanic Activity and Forecasting of Volcanic Eruptions. Introduction to Volcanic Seismology, pp. 407–431. Elsevier (2012)
2. Chouet, B.: A Seismic Model for the Source of Long-Period Events and Harmonic Tremor, Volcanic Seismology, pp. 133–156. Springer, Heidelberg (1992)
3. Lahr, J.C., Chouet, B.A., Stephens, C.D., Power, J.A., Page, R.A.: Earthquake classification, location and error analysis in a volcanic environment: implications for the magmatic system of the 1989-1990 eruptions at Redoubt Volcano, Alaska. Journal of Volcanology and Geothermal Research 62(1-4), 137–151 (1994)
4. Langer, H., Falsaperla, S., Powell, T., Thompson, G.: Automatic classification and a-posteriori analysis of seismic event identification at Soufriere Hills volcano, Montserrat. Journal of Volcanology and Geothermal Research 153, 1–10 (2006)
5. Dowla, F.U.: Neural networks in seismic discrimination. In: Husebye, E.S., Dainty, A.M. (eds.) NATO ASI (Advanced Science Institutes) – Series E, vol. 303, pp. 777–789. Kluwer, Dordrecht (1995)
6. Erlebacher, G., Yuen, D.A.: A wavelet toolkit for visualization and analysis of large data sets in Earthquake Research. Pure and Applied Geophysics 161, 2215–2229 (2004)

7. Gendron, P., Nandram, B.: An empirical Bayes estimator of seismic events using wavelet packet bases. Journal of Agricultural, Biological, and Environmental Statistics 6(3), 379–402 (2001)
8. Lesage, P., Glangeaud, F., Mars, J.: Applications of autoregressive models and time-frequency analysis to the study of volcanic tremor and long-period events. Journal of Volcanology and Geothermal Research 114, 391–417 (2002)
9. Ibáñez, J.M., Benítez, C., Gutiérrez, L.A., Cortés, G., García-Yeguas, A., Alguacil, G.: The classification of seismo-volcanic signals using Hidden Markov Models as applied to the Stromboli and Etna volcanoes. Journal of Volcanology and Geothermal Research 187, 218–226 (2009)
10. Messina, A., Langer, H.: Pattern recognition of volcanic tremor data on Mt. Etna (Italy) with KKAnalysis - A software program for unsupervised classification. Computers & Geosciences 37, 953–961 (2011)
11. Joevivek, V., Chandrasekar, N., Srinivas, Y.: Improving Seismic Monitoring System for Small to Intermediate Earthquake Detection. International Journal of Computer Science and Security (IJCSS) 4(3), 308–315 (2010)
12. Mora-Stock, C., Thorwart, M., Wunderlich, T., Bredemeyer, S., Hansteen, T.H., Rabbel, W.: Comparison of seismic activity for Llaima and Villarrica volcanoes prior to and after the Maule, earthquake. International Journal of Earth Sciences 1–14 (2012)
13. Curilem, G., Vergara, J., Fuentealba, G., Acuña, G., Chacón, M.: Classification of seismic signals at Villarrica volcano (Chile) using neural networks and genetic algorithms. Journal of Volcanology and Geothermal Research 180, 1–8 (2009)
14. San-Martin, C., Melgarejo, C., Gallegos, C., Soto, G., Curilem, M., Fuentealba, G.: Feature Extraction Using Circular Statistics Applied to Volcano Monitoring. In: Bloch, I., Cesar Jr., R.M. (eds.) CIARP 2010. LNCS, vol. 6419, pp. 458–466. Springer, Heidelberg (2010)
15. Giacco, F., Esposito, A.M., Scarpetta, S., Giudicepietro, F., Matinaro, M.: Support Vector Machines and MLP for automatic classification of seismic signals at Stromboli volcano. In: Proceedings of the 2009 Conference on Neural Nets, WIRN 2009, pp. 116–123 (2009)
16. Langer, H., Falsaperla, S., Masotti, M., Campanini, R., Spampinato, S., Messina, A.: Synopsis of supervised and unsupervised pattern classification techniques applied to volcanic tremor data at Mt Etna, Italy. Geophysical Journal International 178, 1132–1144 (2009)
17. Álvarez, I., García, L., Cortés, G., Benítez, C., De la Torre, Á.: Discriminative Feature Selection for Automatic Classification of Volcano-Seismic Signals. IEEE Geoscience And Remote Sensing Letters 9(2), 151–155 (2012)
18. Vapnik, V.: The Nature of Statistical Learning Theory. Springer (1995)
19. Burges, C.J.C.: A tutorial on support vector machines for pattern recognition. Data Mining and Knowledge Discovery 2, 121–167 (1998)
20. Hamel, L.: Knowledge Discovery with Support Vector Machines. John Wiley & Sons (2009)
21. Curilem, M., Vergara, J., San Martin, C., Fuentealba, G., Cardona, C., Huenupan, F., Chacón, M., Khan, S., Hussein, W., Becerra, N.: Pattern Recognition applied to Seismic Signals of the Llaima Volcano (Chile): An analysis of the events' features. Journal of Volcanology and Geothermal Research 282, 134–177 (2014)

A Hierarchical Reinforcement Learning Based Artificial Intelligence for Non-Player Characters in Video Games

Hiram Ponce[1,2] and Ricardo Padilla[3]

[1] Graduate School of Engineering, Tecnologico de Monterrey,
Campus Ciudad de Mexico, 14380 Mexico City, Mexico
[2] Faculty of Engineering, Universidad Panamericana, 03920 Mexico City, Mexico
[3] Department of Computer Science, Tecnologico de Monterrey,
Campus Ciudad de Mexico, 14380 Mexico City, Mexico
{hiram.ponce,A01211519}@itesm.mx

Abstract. Nowadays, video games conforms a huge industry that is always developing new technology. In particular, artificial intelligence techniques have been used broadly in the well-known non-player characters (NPC) given the opportunity to users to feel video games more real. This paper proposes the usage of the MaxQ-Q hierarchical reinforcement learning algorithm in non-player characters in order to increase the experience of the user in terms of naturalness. A case study of an NPC with the proposed artificial intelligence based algorithm in a first personal shooter video game was developed. Experimental results show that this implementation improves naturalness from the user's point of view. In addition, the proposed MaxQ-Q based algorithm in NPCs allow to programmers a robust way to give artificial intelligence to them.

Keywords: Hierarchical reinforcement learning, non-player characters, naturalness, human assessment, video games.

1 Introduction

Nowadays, video games conforms a huge industry that is always developing new technology. In particular, artificial intelligence techniques have been used broadly in the well-known non-player characters (NPC) given the opportunity to users to feel video games more real [1]. Specially for artificial intelligence scientists, video games have proved to be a test bed for different artificial intelligence (AI) techniques because they can be designed and manipulated in a computer framework, making it easy to measure and control them. Thus, a video game is an easy environment to access for any artificial intelligence technique [1,9,13].

Games can be used to simulate real situations with no risk and cost (the cost of experimenting with real environment), but they are mostly used to entertain the users. In that way, video games have been changing in order to create a more entertaining and realistic world, to make the users feel more immersed in the game [13,9,1]. This is mostly achieved by improving graphics and game

A. Gelbukh et al. (Eds.): MICAI 2014, Part II, LNAI 8857, pp. 172–183, 2014.

performance [13]. Improving the performance of the game requires to program NPCs to make the user feel connected by making the agents interact with their environment according to the current situation of a game. To implement the latter, artificial intelligence in video games is applied at NPC-level [1]; given to NPCs the look and feel of intelligent agents, and a more natural humanness assessment [8]. It is remarkable to say that, in this work, natural humanness assessment is related to the ability of an agent to be unpredictable as possible, and to learn and adapt from changes of the environment.

The problem to improve an intelligent decision in NPCs is that the response of this decision has to be in real-time, such that, the performance of the game does not be affected. In that sense, the decision-making process of NPCs has been previously coded (reactive approach), resulting in an easier but non-intelligent agent performance [9,6]. For example, graph trees have been widely used as an AI technique of NPCs [6]. In time processing, this approach is excellent; but when NPCs are tried to be more natural and more human-like agents, then this approach fails [9]; for example, NPCs become more predictable for users. A deliberative approach has to be more effective; however, time consuming and memory consuming (data related to the training step) should be another problem.

To this end, reinforcement learning techniques should tackle the decision-making process with a trade-off between reactive and deliberative approaches. In that sense, the training step of reinforcement learning allows an agent to learn from the environment (e.g. a more natural humanness assessment) while the implementation step allows an agent to act reactively (e.g. reducing online time consuming) [3]. However, curse of dimensionality is a weakness of reinforcement learning; but, it can be improved by using hierarchical reinforcement learning, as shown in [3].

In that sense, this work proposes an alternative solution based on a hierarchical reinforcement learning approach in order to reduce predictability of NPCs, make them adapt from changes of the environment, and act as a human-like agent as possible, to provide a more enjoyable game experience for players.

The rest of the paper is organized as follows: Sect. 2 presents the related work of this approach, Sect. 3 briefly describes the MaxQ-Q hierarchical reinforcement learning algorithm used in this approach, Sect. 4 describes the proposal of the work, Sect. 5 presents results and discussion of the proposal, and Sect. 6 concludes the paper.

2   Related Work

Artificial intelligence in video games has pushed this industry farther because of the quality that provides to the games and how it affects users in their in-game decisions. The main purpose of artificial intelligence in video games is to control the behavior of NPCs in the game [9]. The latter makes the role of artificial intelligence in NPCs crucial for having a good gameplay and satisfying the player. The behavior of NPCs employs different techniques as described below, making them more deliberative and not a mere reactive agent in an environment.

2.1 AI-Based Video Games Techniques

One of the most famous AI-based video games techniques is finite state machines (FSM) that represents behavior in a very straightforward way. It is very easy to program and design. FSM has some drawbacks like less scalability and usability, lacking a dynamic way of sharing tasks or auto-generate decisions [13].

For instance, Halo brought the idea of behavioral trees within its NPC's artificial intelligence. Halo team generates decision-making processes for groups of NPCs that work together. In that sense, NPCs started at the top of the tree and headed down at the same time to fulfill the most important tasks of the moment [6]. Every task in the tree has constrains and a heuristic cost function, in order to achieve a good behavior. This technique allows the environment be scalable, making really easy to deal with, and tasks can be shared between NPCs with no problems. However, behavioral trees have to be completely designed and scripted, thus NPCs cannot evolve from the initial behavior established [6].

Another artificial intelligence based game is F. E. A. R. [13]. It uses a simple finite state machine that has only three states, but the transitions are not hard-coded. Instead, it decides when to move to other states, in real-time. The way the actions are accomplished is similar to STRIPS methodology [14]: according to some pre-conditions, actions are performed in a different way. According to the set of actions, an NPC tries to reach its goal. This behavior allows reacting differently to the environment, increasing the intelligence of the NPC. For planning purposes (i.e. choose the order of actions), the A* algorithm is used to get the lowest cost of a set of actions [13].

In addition, Forza Motorsport is a game that introduces machine learning to create avatars that learn adaptively from racers using supervised learning [5]. This avatar learns from the player and imitates its movements, that changes while the player continues playing and it evolves into the game. This technique actually imitates human behavior and arises more natural opponents in races because they will be other player's avatars, known as drivatars [5].

2.2 Reinforcement Learning Mechanisms

Indeed, machine learning gives to NPCs the ability of adaption to the environment by creating their own plans of action [13,14,8,5]. This characteristic produces more believable characters in the game (i.e. more natural humanness assessment) [8]. However, if NPCs are trained based on human behavior (e.g. drivatars), then it produces human behavior imitation; but quite predictable. To this end, this work uses reinforcement learning because its main source of knowledge is experience, not imitation. In addition, behavioral approaches of NPCs will be less dependant to the programmers who determine off-line planning actions of agents (e.g. at the implementation stage of the video game). However, an illness of reinforcement learning is the curse of dimensionality that can be explained as the exponential behavior of a learning algorithm when dealing with high dimensional states and a large set of actions. Moreover, reinforcement learning tends to consume large amounts of time and memory space [10].

To solve the above problems, hierarchical reinforcement learning (HRL) is proposed as a technique that divides the overall state of environment - modeled as a decision-making process based on Markov Decision Processes (MDP), or Semi-Markov Decision Processes (SMDP) when dealing with time - as a set of subtasks becoming in a set of SMDPs with their local policies [3,13]; and, each subtask is formed with an initiation set and a termination set. In fact, this approach allows HRL fighting against to dimensionality problems. In addition, some HRL techniques can abstract features from states in certain subtasks, making it even simpler [3]. There are several hierarchical reinforcement learning techniques, like: Options [12], hierarchical abstract machines (HAM) [11], and MaxQ [3].

3   MaxQ-Q Algorithm

MaxQ is a hierarchical reinforcement learning method that provides a hierarchical decomposition of the problem into a set of sub-problems [3]. Since, the main problem is divided into subtasks, the value function (a state reward) is also divided into a set of functions for each subtask, this also means each sub-problem has its own policy. Every subtask is independent, and if any other problem has a subtask identical to any other problem, it can be reused.

Since, each subtask is a little part of the overall problem, it only needs to use a subset of features to learn. Thus, MaxQ is a faster learning method than simple reinforcement learning. This reduction of features in a subtask is also known as state abstraction [3].

Formally, a subtask is defined as $\{T_i, A_i, \hat{R}_i\}$; where, T_i is a predicate that defines terminal states of the subtask, A_i is a set of actions that can be performed in the subtask to achieve the goal, and $\hat{R}_i$ is the pseudo-reward function that tells how well the terminal state is. In fact, when solving the decision-making process, the method has to return the set of actions that an agent must follow to end the subtask, also known as a policy $\pi_i(s)$ of subtask i in state s. The set of all policies in the graph is known as hierarchical policy [3].

At last, MaxQ requires a hierarchy of the problem defined with a set of nodes [3]: Max nodes (representing primitive actions or subtasks), and Q nodes (actions of subtasks). In particular, Max nodes store V values that represent state rewards, and Q nodes store completion functions $C^\pi(i, s, a)$ that represent the cumulative reward of completing subtask i after invoking action $a \in A_i$ in state s. The graphical representation of the hierarchy is called MaxQ-graph [3].

An implementation of MaxQ method is the so-called MaxQ-Q algorithm that works with arbitrary $\hat{R}_i$ functions. In [3], it is shown that $\hat{R}_i$ functions contaminate completion functions C^π. To solve this problem, MaxQ-Q uses two completion functions: the contaminated $\hat{C}_i$ function using $\hat{R}_i$, and the clean C_i function without using $\hat{R}_i$. Algorithm 1 shows MaxQ-Q originally introduced by Dieterich in [3].

Algorithm 1. MaxQ-Q algorithm [3]. $\gamma < 1$ represents the discount factor, and α is the learning rate that should be gradually decreased to zero in the limit.

---

function MaxQ-Q(MaxNode i, State s)

let $seq = 0$ sequence of states visited while executing i
if i is a primitive MaxNode
    execute i, receive r, observe result state s'
    $V_{t+1}(i, s) = (1 - \alpha_t(i)) \cdot V_t(i, s) + \alpha_t(i) \cdot r_t$
    push s onto the beginning of seq
else
    let $count = 0$
    while $T_i(s)$ is false **do**
        choose an action a according to the current exploration policy $\pi_x(i, s)$
        let $childSeq = $ MaxQ-Q(a, s)
        observe result state s'
        let $a^* = \arg\max_{a'}[\hat{C}_t(i, s', a') + V_t(a', s')]$
        let $N = 1$
        for each s in $childSeq$ **do**
            $\hat{C}_{t+1}(i, s, a) = (1 - \alpha_t(i)) \cdot \hat{C}_t(i, s, a) + \alpha_t(i) \cdot \gamma^N[\hat{R}_i(s') + \hat{C}_t(i, s', a^*) + V_t(a^*, s)]$
            $C_{t+1}(i, s, a) = (1 - \alpha_t(i)) \cdot C_t(i, s, a) + \alpha_t(i) \cdot \gamma^N[C_t(i, s', a^*) + V_t(a^*, s')]$
            $N = N + 1$
        end
        append $childSeq$ onto the front of seq
        $s = s'$
        end
    end
return seq
end MaxQ-Q

---

4   Description of the Proposal

In order to reduce predictability in NPCs, making them more adaptable to the environment, and improving their human-like behavior; this work proposes to use MaxQ-Q algorithm as a decision-making process in NPCs. In particular, MaxQ method meets three favorable characteristics [3] that this work exploits for improving natural humanness assessment in NPCs:

- temporal abstraction (it takes several steps to accomplish)
- state abstraction (relevant features are used for each subtask)
- task sharing (one task can be shared with several subtasks, if needed)

This section presents the proposal as follows: firstly, a description of the architecture of an NPC; then, the computational implementation of NPCs in a strategic game; later on, the experiment design, and lastly, the metrics of evaluation.

4.1   Architecture of an NPC

In order to implement the MaxQ-Q algorithm in NPCs for video games, the proposal defines two entities: agents and the environment.

On one hand, the environment is defined as the game with all its components included (other NPCs, players, obstacles, etc.). Note that the game changes every time agents act upon it. On the other hand, agents are defined as NPCs that perceive current states and perform actions over the environment. In fact, agents receive feedback (i.e. rewards) that tells them how good or bad the action was in contrast to their objectives. Figure 1 shows the interaction agent-environment and the proposed architecture of an NPC.

As shown in Fig. 1, the architecture of an NPC consists of two components: the knowledge base, and the deliberation procedure. The knowledge base stores information provided by the rewards obtained from the reinforcement procedure. In this particular case, an agent performs a MaxQ value decomposition in which the Max node, invoked by the action, updates its values. After this information is updated, the MaxQ-Q algorithm learns the policies of the hierarchy based on the knowledge base. Thus, these values help the MaxQ-Q algorithm to deliberate the next action to take and to perform it upon the environment. To this end, this cycle continues until an episode is over (e.g. each event game), and then it resets itself. It is remarkable to say that knowledge base has not be reset because it simulates human-like learning by experience.

In a nutshell, the NPC will receive rewards from the environment for every action it does. Then, this reward will be kept in a knowledge base (MaxQ) and the decision-making process (hierarchical policy) will be performed at the deliberative (MaxQ-Q) layer of the NPC.

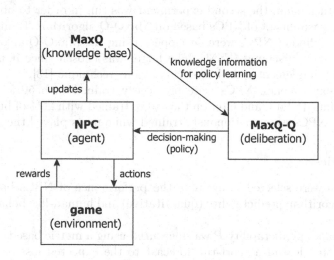

Fig. 1. Proposed architecture of an NPC

4.2 Implementation

A simple case study was designed to test and validate the proposal NPC based on MaxQ-Q algorithm. In particular, the case study consisted on a strategic game called Capture the Flag (CTF) with a first person shooter (FPS) player and an NPC enemy. The objective of CTF is to reach a flag and return to the base before the other player finds it first.

The NPC enemy was automated with the MaxQ-Q algorithm as its artificial intelligence decision-making process. For simplicity, the NPC was restricted in its movements, containing just five actions: move to the front, move back, move to the left, move to the right, and stay stopped. In addition, the implementation of the NPC based on MaxQ-Q algorithm was programmed in a middleware called *Pogamut* that allows interaction with the game "Unreal Tournament 2004" using Java in the IDE Netbeans [4]. Figure 2 shows a first person view of the game.

4.3   Experiment Design

In order to measure the performance of the NPC based on MaxQ-Q algorithm, two experiments were designed. The first experiment considered to expose the CTF strategic game to twelve[1] different young people (ages from 18 to 25 years old) randomly selected from a pool of people previously experienced in FPS games (at least two years of playing), in order to avoid inexperienced performance and time lagging, and to obtain high qualitative information. Then, the game was played seven times for each user, assuming that players understand well the overall game after these trials. In addition, a post-survey was applied to them.

On the other hand, the second experiment was run in order to obtain a predictability measurement of NPCs based on MaxQ-Q algorithm. To make a comparison, two different NPCs were developed: using the MaxQ-Q algorithm, and using finite state machines (FSM). The latter was chosen since it is the most preferred and implemented AI-based video game technique [13].

In both experiments, NPCs were previously trained with 50% of artificial (preprogrammed) data, and later on they were trained with 20% of human data. In addition, NPCs were continuously trained while users played the game.

4.4   Metrics

Two metrics were selected to evaluate the performance of NPCs based on the MaxQ-Q algorithm: predictability (quantitative) and human-like behavior (qualitative).

On one hand, predictability P was measured using a metric based on the ratio of the expected loss of a short-run forecast to the expected loss of a long-run forecast, reported in [2], and it is expressed as (1); where, L is a loss function, Ω is the data set used for the measurement, E represents the expected function over the loss function, j is the starting forecast boundary, k is the second forecast boundary with $k > j$, all at time t.

$$P\left(L, \Omega, j, k\right) = 1 - \frac{E\left(L_{t+j,t}\right)}{E\left(L_{t+k,t}\right)} \tag{1}$$

Translating (1) into the MaxQ-Q predictability measurement, the absolute value function V can be seen as the expected loss function $E(L_{t+j,t})$ because it considers the probability of an action to happen weighted by its own cost

---

[1] Sample size was selected using the methodology reported in [7].

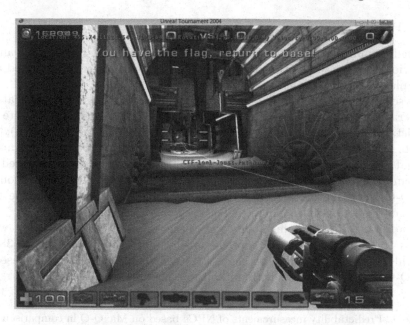

Fig. 2. Example of a first person view of the CTF strategic game for the case study

(reward). Similarly, the absolute value function V of taken actions in finite state machines can be seen as $E(L_{t+k,t})$. Then, the predictability of the selected hierarchical policy of an NPC based on MaxQ-Q algorithm will be measured from 0.0 (predictable) to 1.0 (unpredictable), in comparison to the selected policy of an NPC based on FSM. To this end, data series were obtained from the NPCs based on MaxQ-Q at the last user's trial, and from NPCs based on FSM at the first user's trial. Notice that the NPC based on FSM did not be displayed to the user.

On the other hand, human-like behavior was measured qualitatively using post-surveys applied to the users when finished seven trials of the game. This methodology was based on the work of [7]. For instance, surveys asked to the users in two dimensions: entertainment and naturalness. Entertainment dimension measured the user experience of the game in terms of: enjoyable, challenging and non-boring. Naturalness dimension measured the impression of the user over NPCs in terms of: subjective predictability, randomized actions, non-adaptation to users' gameplay, humanness assessment, and hardness of beating.

5   Results and Discussion

The case study about the CTF strategic game was run using the methodology presented above. Following, quantitative and qualitative results are reported, as well as the discussion about them.

5.1   Predictability

Unpredictability of an artificial agent is expected when simulating a human-like behavior. Table 1 summarizes the predictability measurements calculated after each player finished the game.

As seen in Table 1, NPCs based on MaxQ-Q algorithm are 47.5% predicatable, in average, in comparison with NPCs based on FSM. It is important to note that predictable values vary with a standard deviation of 29.61% ($47.5\pm29.61\%$); thus, results should be treated carefully and they do not have to be overestimated. In that sense, if assuming that finite state machines is the most preferred and implemented AI-based video game technique [13]; then, NPCs based on the MaxQ-Q algorithm are 52.5% more unpredictable, in average, than the most NPCs developed in video games, so far.

In addition, 75% of predictability values are concentrated below 61.4% which means that three-quarters of unpredictable values are enclosed under 38.6%. Roughly speaking, the latter represents a strong evidence that NPCs based on MaxQ-Q challenge to users with unthinkable actions.

Table 1. Predictability measurements of NPCs based on MaxQ-Q in comparison with NPCs based on FSM

Player	P
1	0.5910
2	0.5909
3	0.4090
4	0.6363
5	0.2413
6	0.5909
7	0.9091
8	0.5455
9	0.0909
10	0.9091
11	0.1851
12	0.0001
μ	0.4749

It is remarkable to say that predictability, empirically, is expected to be 50.0% in average because it has to reflect that an NPC maintains its AI-based ability to solve the game, but it also has to challenge to the user with this unpredictable capability. To this end, remember that unpredictability is measured relative to FSM-based actions. This means that, from the classical point of view of AI-based NPCs, MaxQ-Q algorithm adds a new feature to NPCs without devaluing intelligence.

5.2   Natural Humanness Assessment

As said, natural humanness assessment of NPCs was measured with surveys applied to users after the game finished. Figure 3 shows the survey questions and Fig. 4 shows the results obtained. Each question was presented in a Likert scale from -2 to 2 without a neutral option (0) in order to polarize results and make them more decisive at the final conclusion: -2 (*totally disagree*), -1 (*disagree*), 1 (*agree*), and 2 (*totally agree*). In addition, Fig. 4 presents the expected value representing a reference of comparison.

Entertainment:
Q1 - is the game enjoyable?
Q2 - the game does not prove to be challenging
Q3 - the game is boring

Naturalness:
Q4 - is the NPC predictable?
Q5 - NPC seems to have random actions
Q6 - NPC does not adapt to my gameplay
Q7 - NPC seems like a human
Q8 - NPC is hard to beat

Fig. 3. Survey questions about the natural humanness assessment perception of users in NPCs based on MaxQ-Q

For instance, the entertainment dimension was definetely accepted by users (see Fig. 4). It means that players perceive NPCs based on MaxQ-Q enjoyable, challenging and non-boring. These positive results motivates users to play the game and to keep them playing it.

In addition, the naturalness dimension was also positive (see Fig. 4). In terms of subjective predictability, users were disagreed that NPCs are predicatable, in average, 22% less than the expected answer. These qualitative result reinforces previous quantitative results of P. Notice that the expected answer is not totally disagree (-1.5 out of -2.0). In terms of randomness of actions, users thought that NPCs do not act randomly which means that users perceives that NPCs have plans (they differ 6% relative to the expected answer). On the other hand, users reported that NPCs did not adapt to their gameplays (1.5 out of 2.0 expected). However, users expected much more human-like behavior in NPCs (25% less than expected) than they actually do. Finally, users experienced that NPCs were too much hard to beat (2 out of 1 expected). The latter can be explained with the training level of NPCs.

To this end, the usage of the MaxQ-Q algorithm in NPCs shows that it improves the natural human-like behavior of them, giving unpredictable and humanness assessment characteristics, in contrast with the well-known performance of NPCs based on finite state machines.

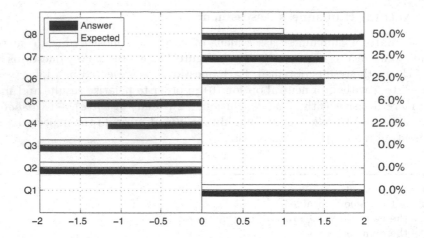

Fig. 4. Chart of results summarizing the natural humanness assessment perception of users in NPCs based on MaxQ-Q. Right numbers represent the relative error of an answer value in contrast with the expected value.

6 Conclusions

This work proposes the implementation of the hierarchical reinforcement learning MaxQ-Q algorithm in order to improve the natural humanness assessment of non-player characters in video games, because artificial intelligence algorithms used in the state-of-the-art are mostly reactive, and with scripted actions. The latter presents drawbacks in user experience, mainly on the perception of human-like behavior in NPCs that the current work improves.

Experimental results were done over a simple case study using an implementation of the Capture the Flag strategic game. In particular, quantitative predictability was measured between NPCs based on the MaxQ-Q algorithm and NPCs based on finite state machines. In fact, results revealed that NPCs based on MaxQ-Q are 52.5% more unpredictable, in average, than NPCs based on FSM. Moreover, qualitative results showed that users experimented this unpredictable behavior. Furthermore, user experience results showed that NPCs based on MaxQ-Q also fulfill non-randomization of actions (i.e. they use plans), non-adaptation to users' gameplay, and improve hardness of beating and humanness assessment.

Concluding, the usage of the MaxQ-Q algorithm as an artificial intelligence basis of decision-making process in NPCs improves their natural human-like behavior, giving unpredictable and natural humanness assessment characteristics, in contrast with the performance of NPCs based on finite state machines. In addition, this work formally introduces a measurement of predictability in NPCs of video games.

Future work considers enlarging the sample size in the case study, covering a wide range of gamers. Also, other quantitative metrics have to be evaluated in the case study, such as: online time processing, memory usage, and the Turing test. Additionally, incorporating automated generation of the state abstraction in MaxQ technique has been considering, too.

References

1. Botea, A., Herbrich, R., Graepel, T.: Video Games and Artificial Intelligence. Microsoft Research Cambridge, Sydney (2008)
2. Diebold, F.X., Kilia, L.: Measuring predictability: Theory and macroeconomic applications. Journal of Applied Econometrics, 16, 675–669 (2001)
3. Dietterich, T.: Hierarchical reinforcement learning with MAXQ value function decomposition. Journal of Artificial Intelligence Research 13, 227–303 (2000)
4. Gemrot, J., Kadlec, R., Bída, M., Burkert, O., Píbil, R., Havlíček, J., Zemčák, L., Šimlovič, J., Vansa, R., Štolba, M., Plch, T., Brom, C.: Pogamut 3 can assist developers in building AI (Not only) for their videogame agents. In: Dignum, F., Bradshaw, J., Silverman, B., van Doesburg, W. (eds.) Agents for Games and Simulations. LNCS, vol. 5920, pp. 1–15. Springer, Heidelberg (2009)
5. Herbich, R., Hatton, M., Tipping, M.: Mixture model for motion lines in a virtual reality environment. Technical Report US Patent 7358973 B2, Microsoft Corporation (2013)
6. Isla, D.: Building a better battle. In: Game Developers Conference, San Francisco (2008)
7. Kluwer, T., Xu, F., Adolphs, P., Uszkoreit, H.: Evaluation of the komparse conversational non-player characters in a commercial virtual world. In: International Conference on Language Resources and Evaluation, number 3535-3542, Istanbul (2012)
8. Llargues, J., Peralta, J., Arrabales, R., Gonzalez, M., Cortez, P., Lopez, A.: Artificial intelligence approaches for the generation and assessment of believable human-like behaviour in virtual characters. Expert Systems With Applications 41(15), 7281–7290 (2014)
9. Mikkulainen, R.: Creating intelligent agents in games. In: The Bridge, pp. 5–13 (2006)
10. Mitchell, T.: Machine Learning. McGraw Hill (1997)
11. Parr, R., Russell, S.: Reinforcement learning with hierarchies of machines. In: Proceedings of the 1997 Conference on Advances in Neural Information Processing Systems, pp. 1043–1049. MIT Press, Cambridge (1997)
12. Sutton, R., Precup, D., Singh, S.: Between MDPs and semi-MDPs: A framework for temporal abstraction in reinforcement learning. Artificial Intelligence 112, 181–211 (1999)
13. Taylor, A.: HQ-DoG: Hierarchical q-learning in domination games. Master's thesis, The University of Georgia (August. 2012)
14. Wooldridge, M.: An Introduction to Multi-Agent Systems. John Wiley & Sons (2009)

Wind Power Forecasting Using Dynamic Bayesian Models

Pablo H. Ibargüengoytia[1], Alberto Reyes[1], Inés Romero-Leon[1], David Pech[1], Uriel A. García[1], Luis Enrique Sucar[2], and Eduardo F. Morales[2]

[1] Instituto de Investigaciones Eléctricas, Cuernavaca, Morelos, México
{pibar,areyes,uriel.garcia}@iie.org.mx,
{senileon,davidpech_01}@hotmail.com
[2] Instituto Nacional de Astrofísica, Óptica y Electrónica, Tonantzintla, Puebla, México
{esucar,emorales}@ccc.inaoep.mx

Abstract. This paper presents the development of a novel dynamic Bayesian network (DBN) model devoted to wind forecasting. An original procedure was developed to approximate this model, based on historical information in the form of time series. The DBN structure and parameters are learned from historical data, and this methodology can be applied to any prediction problem. In contrast to previous approaches, the proposed model considers all the relevant variables in the domain and produces a probability distribution for the predictions; providing important additional information to the decision makers. The method was evaluated experimentally with real data from a wind farm in Mexico for a time horizon of 5 hours, showing superior performance to traditional time-series prediction techniques.

1 Introduction

Due to the cleanness and low-cost of wind energy, wind farms (an array of wind turbines) are designed to produce as much energy as possible. However, the production of electricity using such energy is affected by external atmospheric parameters such as wind speed and direction, temperature, humidity and pressure; and internal factors like maintenance schedules and design restrictions.

A wind turbine is designed according to the historical atmospheric conditions of the site and it is described by its nominal power. Intrinsically, the wind farm energy production can be expressed as a joint nominal power, which is a monotonic submodular function of the array of wind turbine's nominal power (typically around 0.6 to 3 MW). A typical prediction of the electric power produced by a wind farm is computed using a fixed weighted measure of the wind farm's nominal power [7], with the weight computed using historical data of atmospheric conditions. As a result, this approximation will not match with the actual farm production curves [2]. These (inaccurate) predictions will become a potential point of failure when scheduling generation units on/off cycles (i.e. what wind turbines to switch on/off and at what time) to satisfy a demand of energy.

A. Gelbukh et al. (Eds.): MICAI 2014, Part II, LNAI 8857, pp. 184–197, 2014.

Given this background, it is desirable to develop methods that allow adjusting the offer of a wind farm based on the prediction of wind conditions. These predictions should have such prediction horizon to help computing the power production that fits better with the real demand curves. The current wind forecasting models such as ALEASOFT, AEOLIS,CASANDRA, CENER, GARRAD HASSAN, METEOROLOGICA, METEOSIM or METEOTEMP [6], that are based on the predictions of atmospheric changes coming from certain numerical models, do not have enough precision to forecast wind speed for horizons of more than 5 hours. Alternative techniques based on statistical models or neural networks, usually do not taken into account other relevant variables and produce single value predictions.

The aim of this work is to develop novel techniques that allow predicting a wind farm electric power production based on wind forecasting with more than 5 hours in advance. We have developed a tool for learning Dynamic Bayesian Networks (DBNs) [15] from data, which identifies the relevant factors for wind forecasting.

We learned the prediction models for wind speed and direction using two year historical data from a wind power experimental station at La Ventosa in Oaxaca, Mexico. In order to evaluate the quality of our proposed solution, we used the mean absolute error of the wind speed. Compared with classical forecasting methods, the experiments show satisfactory results in the sense that, the average error is acceptable and better than using other techniques.

This paper is organized as follows. The next section reviews alternative forms to forecast wind power in the literature. Section 3 describes the application domain, namely the wind and power forecasting. Section 4 presents our proposed approach using dynamic Bayesian networks. In Section 5, we show some experiments performed and preliminary results. Finally, Section 6 concludes the paper and suggests future work.

2   Related Work

Among the most popular techniques for very short-time wind speed forecasting some authors report the use of Neural Networks (NN) and Time Series based on ARIMA models. Maqsood et al. [12] presented the idea of using more than one model to forecast three meteorological variables (including wind speed) for a 24-hour-ahead interval. Four different types of NNs are considered: the multilayer perceptron (MLP), the recurrent neural network of Elman, the radial basis function (RBF), and the Hopfield neural networks. A NN of each type was trained for each season of the year. The best result was the one obtained with the RBF neural network, but accuracy increases when all of the models are combined (i.e., into an ensemble of models). Kavasseri et al. [10] presented the fractional-ARIMA (f-ARIMA) model to forecast the wind speed day-ahead and two-days-ahead. The forecasted wind speed is then converted into wind power by using a manufacturers power curve. The main weaknesses of these methods are that they are deterministic, sometimes univariate, and predict a value per time step and not a probability distribution. One alternative to overcome these lacks is the usage of probabilistic methods which exhibit more flexibility.

Bossanyi [3] was one of the pioneers on using probabilistic methods for short-term wind prediction. In that work, a Kalman filter used the last six measured values as inputs to forecast wind speed for the following minutes. The results are good when compared with the persistence for time horizons below 10 minutes of averaged data. The improvement was poorer in longer averages and was nonexistent for 1-hour averages.

Miranda et. al. [13] focused on one-hour-ahead wind speed prediction using a Bayesian approach to characterize the wind resource. In that work, Markov Chain Monte Carlo (MCMC) simulation was used to estimate the model parameters, which can be used to predict wind speeds at future time-steps. The results obtained indicate that Bayesian inference can be a useful tool in wind speed/power prediction.

MingYang et. al. [20] showed a practical approach for probabilistic short-term generation forecast of a wind farm. The proposed approach is based on Sparse Bayesian Learning (SBL) algorithm. Since the wind generation time series exhibits strong non-stationary property, a componential forecast strategy was used to improve the forecast accuracy. According to the strategy, the wind generation series is decomposed into several more predictable series by discrete wavelet transform (DWT), and then the resulted series are forecasted using SBL algorithm respectively. To fulfill multi-look-ahead wind generation forecast, a multi-SBL forecast model is constructed in the context. Tests on a 74-MW wind farm located in southwest Oklahoma demonstrated the effectiveness of the proposed approach.

Jursa [9] compared different techniques for wind power forecasts, such as a classical MLP NN, mixture of experts [19], Support Vector Machine (SVM), and nearest neighbor search with a Particle Swarm Optimization (PSO) algorithm for feature selection of the input of several locations in a spread area [8]. The author additionally combines different models by averaging the model outputs. The results for 10 wind farms located in Germany were compared, and Numerical Weather Prediction (NWPs) were available for each wind farm. The best model was the ensemble with three different models (i.e., mixture of experts, nearest neighbor, and SVM), with a 15% improvement over an NN. The best individual model was the mixture-of-experts model, which achieved an 8.8% improvement over the NN. The results of the SVM are always better when compared with the neural network results. The nearest-neighbor model was better than the NN in some wind farms. However, in others, the NN performed better.

In this work the development of a dynamic Bayesian network (DBN) model devoted to wind forecasting is presented. Intrinsically, it profits the conditional dependence among meteorological variables to better deal with the uncertain nature of wind behavior. This method combines expert knowledge and knowledge discovery from data. The resulting model provides a probability distribution around a point-value. Throughout a learning algorithm the model considers conditional dependences among variables so that it automatically selects attributes.

3   Wind Power Forecasting

Weather conditions are different according to physical conditions like solar radiation, latitude, altitude, atmospheric pressure, and temperature. Any change on these conditions produces weather changes which result in air movement. These changes can exhibit some periodicity in days, months, seasons or years. Wind occurs on a range of scales, from thunderstorm flows lasting for few minutes to hurricane.

Wind is also a free renewable energy source that brings some electric power per unit of time. Wind energy is converted into mechanical- rotational energy by the wind turbine rotor. Unfortunately, according to Betz [2] the available wind energy cannot be extracted completely by a wind turbine. The theoretical maximum power that can be extracted from wind is 59%.

In order to forecast the power generation in wind power farms it is required to know the weather conditions that influence the wind and, in consequence, the power generation capability. The time horizon for prediction of wind speed and direction (minutes, hours, etc.) determines the prediction time horizon of energy generated.

The wind power is directly related to the wind speed and it is represented in a graph called "the power curve" [2] (shown in Fig. 1). The curve indicates the energy that will be generated for different wind speeds. It is obtained empirically and is delivered by the turbine manufacturer. The generation is null up to a boot speed (3 m/sec. in the figure) and from it grows rapidly to a nominal speed where control mechanisms act to maintain a constant power. If the wind reaches a stop speed (25 m/sec. in the figure), the power output decreases and the wind turbine protection mechanisms stops the turbine for protection.

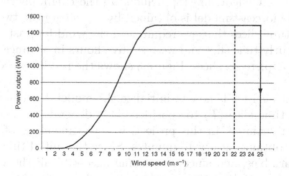

Fig. 1. Power wind curve: power against wind speed. The dotted line represents the speed of wind for re-start after stop for protection.

4   Dynamic Bayesian Network Model

Bayesian Networks [17] are directed acyclic graphs that provide a compact representation of a probability distribution, in which nodes represent propositional variables and arcs probabilistic dependencies. Dynamic Bayesian Networks [15] represent temporal process by replicating each variable for every time instant in the temporal range of interest, including dependency relations within and between temporal intervals (time is usually discretized according to fixed temporal intervals). In general, DBNs follow two basic assumptions:

Markovian process, so each variable only depends on variables from the previous and current time steps,

Stationary process, so the structure and parameters of the model remain the same for all time steps.

According to these assumptions, the dynamic Bayesian model developed considered in this project is inspired on the DBN definition presented by Murphy [15]. The DBN is formed by certain initial conditions and by a two-slice temporal Bayes net which defines $P(X_t \mid X_{t-1})$ for all t in the process. This is called the transition model.

For instance, the transition model of the wind prediction DBNs developed in this study is shown in Figure 2. The variables included in the model are defined in Section 5.

Notice that there exist relations between variables intra time slice and other relations inter time slices. For example, relative humidity (HR) influences the temperature (Temp) and solar radiation (RS) at certain time t, and it maintains an influence with these same variables at time $t + 1$ for all t. The model was learned using the PC algorithm[18] included in the Hugin package[1].

The complete forecast model is obtained by *unrolling* the two slice model in the number of time slices that are required in the wind forecast. For example, if we define an hourly time slice and we need five hours in advance, then the DBN is unrolled to complete six slices. Figure 3 shows the resultant six slices dynamic model.

An important decision is how to initialize the model. First, we need to define the size of the time slice (T) to consider. This depends on the data obtained and the forecast required. In this project, we use time slices of one hour, even if we have data obtained every 10 minutes. Since the initial time slice is formed by the same variables, and since we assume access to all the values, then the initial slice is only useful for entering the values of variables at time t. Thus, the propagation in the network shown in Fig. 3 produces a probability distribution of the forecasted value of wind velocity five hours ahead ($VelV_5$). This is the second parameter considered in this application, namely the forecast horizon (N). In the network shown in Fig. 3, $N = 5$.

Section 5 shows the results for wind forecasting in experiments conducted in the models described above.

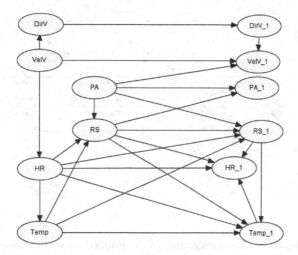

Fig. 2. An example of one of the transition model learned for wind forecasting. (See Section 5 for the nomenclature of the variables.)

Based on the previous considerations, the procedure for learning a DBN model, according to parameters T and N, can be summarized as follows:

1. Separate the database in a file for training and a file for testing. Notice that each file must be continuous in time, since that data are time series of the meteorological variables.
2. If the time between data registers in the data set are lower than T, then average the measures of all variables and obtain registers every T time.
3. Discretize the training set using a uniform partition.
4. Duplicate the training dataset with the double of columns to include the registers of (X_t, X_{t-1}). We use the PC learning algorithm [18] available in Hugin package [1] to construct the transition network as in Fig. 2.
5. Unroll the transition model to the required N time slices. This is, replicate the $t + 1$ slice of transition network, N times to form the dynamic network of Fig. 3.
6. Utilize EM algorithm [11] to learn the parameters of the complete unrolled model of Fig. 3.

We designed a software tool that automates the whole procedure for learning DBNs. The next section describes the experiments conducted to test the performance of the different tested models.

5   Experiments and Discussion

5.1   Wind Farm

The Regional Wind Technology Center (CERTE) of the Electric Research Institute (IIE) is located in the area of La Ventosa, in Oaxaca, Mexico. This infrastructure is sized to install up to 5 MW wind power, which can be integrated with wind turbines of different capacities and models.

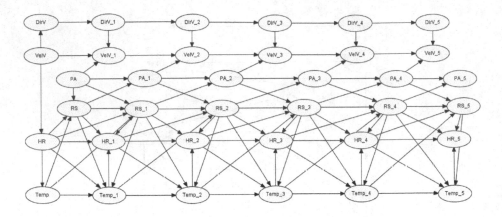

Fig. 3. A wind forecasting DBN unrolled for 5 time slices

The CERTE sells electric energy produced by the Japanese wind turbine Komai 300 kW that was donated to IIE by the Global Environment Facility (GEF), through the United Nations Development Program (UNDP).

The historical data of the wind and other meteorological variables obtained from this center, consists on time series with date and time stamp, during more than two years. The information collected includes the following data: ambient temperature (Temp), relative humidity (HR), solar radiation (RS), wind direction (DirV) and wind speed (VelV) in two heights and two different altitudes, date and time. The data registers were taken every ten minutes. We used data from 2012 and 2013 for training and the remaining January and February 2014 for testing.

5.2   Experiments

The wind power prediction system consists in a program that executes the following procedures:

1. Reads the model of Fig. 3,
2. Reads a data file with the testing values of the variables (January and February 2014 in this experiment),
3. Loads one by one, the hourly registers into the network, instantiating the nodes of the first slice,
4. Propagates probabilities in the dynamic network and obtains a posterior probability vector of the wind velocity (see Fig. 6),
5. Calculates the expected value in that vector for generating a point velocity value. We refer this value as *Forecast* in the graphs below,
6. Calculates the uncertainty of the forecast and the error obtained between the real and forecasted value,
7. Repeats for all data registers in the testing file.

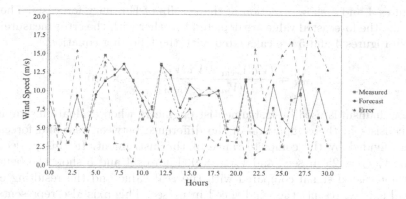

Fig. 4. Partial graph with the results of the experiments from 0 to 5 am. The *Measured* line represents the real value, the *Forecast* represents the forecasted and the *Error* line is the measured error. Vertical axis is in m/sec. for lines *Measured* and *Forecast*, and % of error for *Error* line.

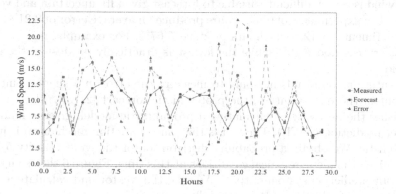

Fig. 5. Partial graph with the results of the experiments from 12 to 17 hours

As mentioned above, the model was learned using meteorological data from CERTE on the periods of January 2012 to December 2013. The model is shown in Fig. 3. The experiments were executed with hourly data from January-February 2014. In order to revise the performance of the forecast system according to specific meteorological conditions, we run experiments loading current conditions at specific hours. For example, we load evidence from 0:00 hours (midnight) and compare the forecast at 5:00 am. We analyze in this paper the experiments from 0 to 5 hours, and from 12 to 17 hours (midday). These two periods have important differences like solar radiation and temperature. Figures 4 and 5 show a portion of the results in the experiments. The *Measured* line represents the real value, the *Forecast* represents the forecasted and the *Error* line is the measured instrumentists error. This measure is explained below.

Notice that the horizontal axis represents the 5 am wind speed from all days of February and March 2014. It is not an every hour continuous forecast.

Figures 4 and 5 show a section of the results of February forecasts. The real value and the forecasted value are depicted together with the error measure. The error in Figures 4 and 5 are calculated with the following equation:

$$E_{Inst} = \frac{(VelV_{real} - VelV_{forecast})}{(V_{max} - V_{min})} \times 100 \qquad (1)$$

This mechanism is used by instrumentist engineers when evaluate instruments. This consists in the comparison of the difference between real and forecasted values, divided by the complete range of the instrument. In this project, we assume $V_{max} = 25$ m/sec., and $V_{min} = 0$. Figures 4 and 5 show the behavior of the forecasted signal compared with the real value and the resulting error. Vertical axis represents the wind speed in m/sec. This axis also represents the percentage of error in the *Error* line. The scales of both units coincide in this axis. The horizontal axis represents the instances of the experiments. One per one hour of each day.

According to the literature, the results obtained look promising. The velocity of the wind is a very difficult variable to forecast given its uncertain and volatile nature. The experiments of 0 to 5 hours produce an average error of 8.21%, while the experiments of 12 to 17 hours produce 5.67%. For example, in Fig. 4, the highest error is above 19% while the lowest is practically 0. Most of the errors are below 5%.

Literature recommends not only to measure the error in a single point forecast, but in the uncertainty of the probabilistic forecast [21,14]. These reports establishes the necessity of calculating a probabilistic model, given a numerical weather prediction (NWP). The fact is that our prediction mechanism is indeed probabilistic. We obtain a probability distribution of the wind velocity 5 hours ahead, given the meteorological conditions at this time. Figure 6 shows an example of our prediction system output. We take this vector and calculate a NWP using the expected value of the probability, i.e.,

$$V_{est} = \sum_n VelV_i P_i \qquad (2)$$

where $VelV_i$ is the central value of the interval i, and P_i is the corresponding probability of this interval. VelV = 3.84 m/sec. in the example in Fig. 6.

The uncertainty estimation of our wind forecast is calculated with the *quantiles* mechanism [5]. Given a probability distribution of the wind velocity P_{t+k}, where t is the current time and k is the forecast horizon (number of time steps ahead), the quantile q_{t+k}^{α} with proportion $\alpha \in [0, 1]$ is uniquely defined as the value x such that $prob(P_{t+k} < x) = \alpha$.

Figures 7 and 8 show the results of the same experiment that Figs. 4 and 5 with the two quantiles at 20% and 80%, forming a confidence interval with probability 60%.

This mechanism establishes that the expected power generation for a given horizon is between 1 and 1.6 MW for example, with 60% probability.

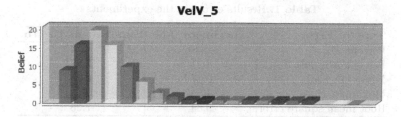

Fig. 6. Probability distribution of the forecast of wind velocity in 5 hours. The velocity variable has been discretized in 20 intervals.

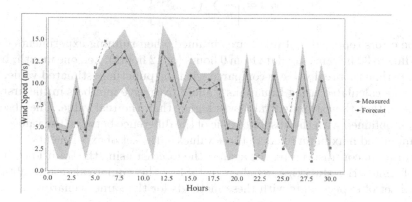

Fig. 7. Experimental results with defined uncertainty. The region shown represents 60% probability.

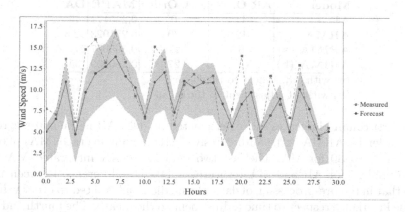

Fig. 8. Experimental results with defined uncertainty. The region shown represents 60% probability.

To complete the experiments evaluation, Table 1 shows different measures of errors [16] of the two experiments described above.

Table 1. Results errors in the experiments

Type of Error	Experiment 0-5h.	Experiment 12-17h.
Percent E_{Inst}	-4.40	-2.3
Percent Absolute E_{Inst}	8.21	5.67
Minimum E_{Inst}	0.17	0.18
Maximum E_{Inst}	19.4	17.36
Root mean square error	9.84	7.28

The root mean square error (rms) is defined as [16]:

$$rms = \left[\frac{1}{n} \sum_{i=1}^{n} (E_{Inst})^2 \right]^{\frac{1}{2}} \tag{3}$$

The errors reported in Table 1 are obtained when running experiments corresponding to 30 instances of data from 0 hours (or 12 hours), i.e., one month. In every experiment, a real value is compared with the punctual estimated value. The errors are calculated using Equations 1 and 3. Negative numbers in the first row represent that the estimated value was higher than the real value. The absolute E_{Inst} is obtained with the absolute value of the difference between the values. The minimum and maximum refers to those values in the set of experiments.

In order to contrast our results against the forecast using the traditional methods of time series statistics, we show in table 2 the numerical results obtained from a set of experiments with these methods for the same scenarios and same data sets.

Table 2. Resulted errors in experiments using traditional methods

Model	AR Order	MA Order	MAPE	DA
AR	44	0	0.235171	45
ARMA	12	30	0.271023	52.5
ARIMA (a)	6	27	0.365057	27.5
ARIMA (b)	6	27	0.280259	35

(a) with adjustment to the mean
(b) without adjustment to the mean

The first column indicates the experimented models. AR is the autorregresive model order 44. ARMA is the autoregresive (AR) moving average (MA) of order 12 for AR and 30 for MA. The last two models are AR integrated MA with order 6 and 27 for AR and MA respectively [4]. The difference between these two is that in the pre-processing of data, the media is subtracted to every value to provide invariance respect to time (adjustment to the mean). The fourth and fifth columns are the MAPE (Mean Absolute Percentage Error) y DA (Directional Accuracy). MAPE measures the precision or accuracy of the model to predict the future, and DA measures the model capability to predict changes in the direction of the predicted variable. Both metrics are expressed in percentage. Ideally, a model obtains a low MAPE and a high DA. Figure 9 shows a small section of the experiments results using time series statistics.

Comparing the results using DBN (Figures 4 and 5) with the results using time series methods (Figure 9), it can be noticed that the multivariable characteristic, and the dynamic representation of the Bayesian networks produces better results.

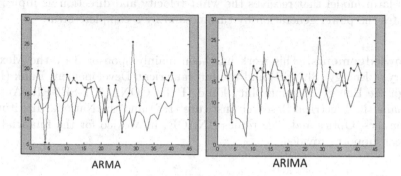

ARMA   ARIMA

Fig. 9. Partial graph with the results of the experiments using ARMA and ARIMA methods. The marked line represents the real value and the solid line represents the forecasted value.

6   Conclusions and Future Work

This paper describes a novel dynamic Bayesian models for wind velocity prediction. This new approach considers that all the variables are known at the initial step (so no special structure for the initial step is required), and considers that all time series are stationary (so the transition model is unrolled the steps that the horizon requires).

The time step and the forecast horizon can be combined to construct models for different forecasting needs. This paper has shown the initial experiments considering hourly steps and a short term forecast of five hours. Alternative techniques based on statistical models or neural networks, usually do not taken into account other relevant variables and produce single value predictions.

The experiments show promising results for wind velocity forecasting. However, the ultimate objective will be the power forecasting in one turbine or in a complete wind farm. Moreover, the final user of this forecast system will be the energy control centers that control the energy generation, and dispatched energy to consumers. Thus, uncertainty measures of the forecast are essential to take the proper decisions in the energy market.

Several additional developments are necessary to increase the performance of the wind forecasting. For example:

- Consider other meteorological variables like the difference of temperatures from yesterday to today.
- Investigate about semi-stationary characteristics of the time series. For example, to learn one model for day and other for night, or one for summer and other for winter.

- Identify the optimal number of intervals in the discretization of the meteo-rological variables, and trying different learning algorithms.

The next step in this project is the integration of our forecasting system with a wind farm model that receives the wind velocity and direction as input, and calculates the power generation by turbine and by a complete farm.

Acknowledgements. This work has been mainly sponsored by the Mexican Ministry of Energy (SENER) and the Interamerican Developement Bank (IDB) through the Energy Sustaintability Fund (FSE) CONACYT-SENER. Authors also thank the Electrical Research Institute (IIE) and the National Institute of Astrophysics, Optics and Electronics (INAOE) in Mexico for the financial and technical support provided.

References

1. Hugin expert, hugin expert A/S. aalborg, denmark (2000)
2. Ackermann, T.: Wind power in power systems. John Wiley & Sons Ltd., West Sussex (2005)
3. Bossanyi, E.A.: Short-term wind prediction using kalman filters. Wind Engineering 9(1), 1–8 (1985)
4. Box, G.E.P., Jenkins, G.M.: Time-Series Analysis, Forecasting and Control. Prentice Hall, Englewood Cliffs (1994)
5. Bremnes, J.B.: Probabilistic wind power forecasts using local quantile regression. Wind Energy 7(1), 47–54 (2004)
6. Enke, W., Spekat, A.: Downscaling climate model outputs into local and regional weather elements by classification and regression. Climate Research 8, 195–207 (1997)
7. Hollingsworth, Lonnberg, P.: The statistical structure of short-range forecast errors as determined from radiosonde data. Part I: the wind field. John Wiley & Sons Ltd. (1986)
8. Jursa, R.: Variable selection for wind power prediction using particle swarm optimization. In: Proceedings of the 9th Annual Conference on Genetic and Evolutionary Computation, London, England, pp. 2059–2065 (2007)
9. Jursa, R.: Wind power prediction with different artificial intelligence models. In: Proceedings of the European Wind Energy Conference EWEC 2007, Milan, Italy (2007)
10. Kavasseri, R.G., Seetharaman, K.: Day-ahead wind speed forecasting using f-arima models. Renewable Energy 34(5), 1388–1393 (2009)
11. Lauritzen, S.L.: The em algorithm for graphical association models with missing data. Computational Statistics & Data Analysis 19, 191–201 (1995)
12. Maqsood, I., Khan, M., Huang, G., Abdalla, R.: Application of soft computing models to hourly weather analysis in southern saskatchewan, canada. Engineering Applications of Artificial Intelligence 18(1), 115–125 (2005)
13. Miranda, M.S., Dunn, R.W.: One-hour-ahead wind speed prediction using a bayesian methodology. In: IEEE Power Engineering Society General Meeting, Montreal, Que, Canada (2006)

14. Monteiro, C., Bessa, R., Miranda, V., Botterud, A., Wang, J., Conzelmann, G.: Wind power forecasting: State-of-the-art-2009. Technical Report ANL/DIS-10-1, Argonne National Laboratory, Decision and Information Sciences Division, Porto, Portugal (2009)
15. Murphy, K.P.: Dynamic Bayesian Networks: Representation, Inference and Learning. Ph.d. thesis, University of California, Berkeley, Berkeley, CA, USA (2002)
16. Osman, E.A., Abdel-Wahhab, O.A., Al-Marhoun, M.A.: Prediction of oil pvt properties using neural networks. In: SPE Middle East Oil Show, Bahrain, March 17-20, p. 14. Society of Petroleum Engineers (SPE) (2001)
17. Pearl, J.: Probabilistic reasoning in intelligent systems: networks of plausible inference. Morgan Kaufmann, San Francisco (1988)
18. Spirtes, P., Glymour, C., Sheines, R.: Causation, Prediction and Search. MIT Press, Cambridge (2000)
19. Weigand, A.S., Mangeas, M., Srivastava, A.N.: Nonlinear gated experts for time series: discovering regimes and avoiding overfitting. International Journal of Neural Systems 6, 373–399 (1995)
20. Yang, M., Fan, S., Lee, W.-J.: Probabilistic short-term wind power forecast using componential sparse bayesian learning. In: 48th IEEE/IAS Industrial & Commercial Power Systems Technical Conference (I&CPS), Louisville, KY, U.S.A. (2012)
21. Zhang, Y., Wang, J., Wang, X.: Review on probabilistic forecasting of winf power generation. Renewable and Sustainable Energy Reviews 32, 255–270 (2014)

Predictive Models Applied to Heavy Duty Equipment Management

Gonzalo Acuña[1], Millaray Curilem[2], Beatriz Araya[3], Francisco Cubillos[1],
Rodrigo Miranda[1], and Fernanda Garrido[2]

[1] Universidad de Santiago de Chile (USACH), Facultad de Ingeniería, Santiago, Chile
gonzalo.acuna@usach.cl
[2] Universidad de La Frontera (UFRO), Departamento de Ingeniería Eléctrica, Temuco, Chile
milaray.curilem@ufrontera.cl
[3] DIRECTIC Soluciones Tecnológicas, Santiago, Chile

Abstract. In this work we present the development of nonlinear autoregressive
with exogenous inputs models to predict some relevant variables for asset management of heavy mining equipment, like Mean Time between Failures
(MTBF), Mean Time to Repair (MTTR) and Availability is presented.
The models were developed using support vector machine with historical data
obtained on a daily basis during 2013 from one heavy mining equipment of an
important copper mine site in Chile. One-step-ahead predictions of the
predicted variables confirmed good performance of the dynamic models.

Keywords: SVM, NARX, Mining Equipment, Asset Management, Availability, Mean Time between Failures, Mean Time to Repair, Predictive Models.

1 Introduction

The fleet of heavy mining equipment corresponds to the most important asset of
the mining industry. Maintenance budgets of these assets are relevant and contribute to a large part of the cost of production. One reason is the poor precision of
maintenance plans which today are based on a simple historical analysis. Having a
predictive tool to forecast availability and other variables may allow improving
those maintenance plans. Well known computing intelligence techniques, like artificial neural networks (ANN) and support vector machine (SVM), have been
extensively used as classifiers and also as regressive models for developing adequate dynamic models of complex systems. Concetti et al. [1] developed a system
for the management of plants in order to ensure full availability and zero failures.
It consists of a Management Model Results of Plant and a tele-maintenance smart
for predicting reliability and safety level of each plant and for the planning and
scheduling of maintenance operations. They show that tele-maintenance system,
which uses computational intelligence tools to predict the evolution of events and
signals-is capable of learning and improving their operational efficiency being
ANN more appropriate for these purposes. As inputs to the neural model they use

A. Gelbukh et al. (Eds.): MICAI 2014, Part II, LNAI 8857, pp. 198–205, 2014.
© Springer International Publishing Switzerland 2014

multiple electrical and physical variables. The outputs of the model are the index of plant safety and the plant reliability/plant availability index. Oladokun et al. [2] show the usefulness of ANN in maintenance planning and management. A model based on the multilayer perceptron with three hidden layers and four processing elements per layer was built to predict the expected downtime as a result of a fault or a maintenance activity. The model achieves an accuracy of over 70% in predicting. The use of SVM as a tool for the development of systems to support maintenance has also been reported in the literature. Zeng et al. [3] propose a method for improving SVM performance using a select feature subsets for training and parameter optimization of SVM based on fuzzy techniques and adaptive swarm of particles. Case analysis shows that this algorithm is efficient and adapts to predictive maintenance management for any complicated equipment. Ding et al. [4], investigated a methodology for application of SVM to predict the reliability of the computerized numerical control (CNC) machine tool manufacturing digital system. Actual reliability data were used for CNC training. The SVM can learn the historical relationship between reliability indices and corresponding goals allows the prediction of future reliability or failures. Experimental results show that the SVM prediction model has good potential for predicting the reliability and system failures.

In this work SVM is used as a regressive tool for developing dynamic models for predicting Mean Time between Failures (MTBF), Mean Time to Repair (MTTR) and Availability using the Use of Physical Availability (UPA) as an exogenous input for both dynamic models. Prediction of those variables is a valuable tool for asset management of heavy mining equipment.

2   Material and Methods

2.1   Data

Data correspond to historical information of 4 variables: Availability, MTBF, MTTR and UPA obtained in a daily basis during 2013 for one heavy mining equipment. The used methodology includes splitting the data into 3 sets: training data set (150 examples); validation data set (100 examples) and test data set (86 examples). All data were normalized between (0,1).

2.2   Dynamic Models

One commonly used dynamic model is the well known non-linear regressive model with exogenous input (NARX) given by equation (1) [5]:

$$y_{(t)} = f(y_{t-1}, \dots y_{t-n}, u_{t-1}, \dots u_{t-m}) + e_t \tag{1}$$

where e (k), is the prediction error at time k and is modeled as a Gaussian white noise zero mean process with variance σ. It represents the model uncertainty and the noise of the experimental data. The predictor associated with this type of models is given by equation (2) and is outlined in Figure 1, where $\hat{y}$ is the prediction of the autoregressive variable y from previous experimental data of itself and of the exogenous variable u in times t-1, t-2, ... considering the nonlinear function ψ [5].

$$\hat{y}_{(t)} = \psi(y_{t-1}, \; \ldots \; y_{t-n}, u_{t-1}, \ldots u_{t-m}) \tag{2}$$

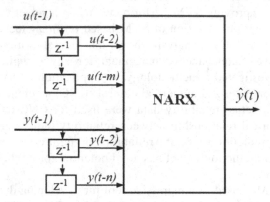

Fig. 1. Associated predictor for NARX-type models. u is the exogenous input and y the autoregressive variable. $\hat{y}$ corresponds to the prediction of the autoregressive variable.

From Figure 1 it can be seen that for identification of such models the simple series-parallel identification method can be used. Indeed, it is enough to provide the following to the chosen approximator of the prediction function -ANN or SVM in the case of this work.

As input:

• experimental data for the autoregressive variables from t-1 to t-n (n has to do with the order of the system model).
• experimental data of the exogenous variables from t-1 to t-m.

As output:

• experimental data of autoregressive variables at a later time, t.

In the case of ANN the required training algorithm consists of the well known back-propagation. In the case of SVM it is enough to provide adequate input and output to the optimization method used to train SVM for regression [6].

2.3   Support Vector Machine

In 1995 Vapnik proposed the classification technique called Support Vector Machine (SVM) [7]. The approach proposed for classification problems, can be adapted to regression. Regression is defined as the fitting of data into a hypertube of radius ε [8], as shown in figure 2. The radius defines the insensitive zone, which is the zone that contains the data. The optimization problem is expressed as shown in equation (3). The constant c determines the trade off between complexity and the amount up to which deviations larger than ε are tolerated [6]. The kernel trick allows the application of SVR to non linear problems.

The process that finds the optimal hypertube requires the tuning of some parameters, such as the regularization parameter c, the kernel parameter sigma and the radius of the hypertube ε. In this work the RBF kernel was used. The exponents of c and sigma parameters were increased by powers of 2. The exponents took values from -5 to 15, with step 1. Parameter ε varied between 0 and 0.5 with a step of 0.1. The performance of every combination was assessed calculating the validation error. The library of tools developed at INSA de Rouen, France [9] was used to implement the SVR models.

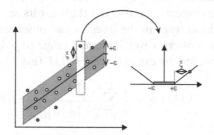

Fig. 2. Optimal hypertube fitting the data and the insensitive region

$$
\begin{cases}
\displaystyle \min_{w,b,\xi} \frac{1}{2}w^T w + c\frac{1}{2}\sum_{k=1}^{N}(\xi_k + \xi_k') \\[2mm]
s.t. \quad y_k - \left[w^T \varphi(x_k) + b\right] \le \varepsilon + \xi_k, \\[2mm]
\quad \left[w^T \varphi(x_k) + b\right] - y_k \le \varepsilon + \xi_k' \\[2mm]
\quad \xi_k, \xi_k' \ge 0, \quad k = 1,...,N
\end{cases}
\tag{3}
$$

2.4   Performance Indices

Two indices were used to quantify the prediction performance of the models.

The index of agreement (IA) developed by Willmott [10] as a standardized measure of the degree of model prediction error and varies between 0 and 1. A values of 1 indicates a perfect match, and 0 indicates no agreement at all. It is a dimensionless statics and its value should be evaluated based on (a) the phenomenon studied, (b)

measurement accuracy and (c) the model employed. IA becomes intuitively meaningful after repeated use in a variety of problems. (Eq. 4)

$$IA = 1 - \frac{\sum_{i=1}^{n} (y_i - \hat{y}_i)^2}{\sum_{i=1}^{n} (|y_i'| + |\hat{y}_i'|)^2} \tag{4}$$

with

$$y_i' = y_i - y_m$$

$$\hat{y}_i' = \hat{y}_i - y_m$$

The index is the symmetric mean absolute percentage error (SMAPE) which is an
average of the absolute percentage errors but these errors are computed using a deno-
minator representing the average of the forecast and observed values. SMAPE has an
upper limit of 200% and offers a well designed range to judge the level of accuracy
and should be influenced less by extreme values [11]. (Eq. 5).

$$SMAPE = \frac{1}{n} \sum_{i=1}^{n} \frac{|\hat{y}_i - y_i|}{(|\hat{y}_i| + |y_i|)/2} * 100 \tag{5}$$

3   Results

Three dynamic models using SVR were developed. They were built as NARX models
with MTBF (or MTTR or Availability) as the regressive variable while UPA was
used as the exogenous input. The training data set and the validation data set were
used for adapting SVR parameters while the test data set served for testing the elaborated models in a one-step-ahead (OSA) prediction scheme. The order of the models
was obtained in a trial and error basis. The final developed models are presented in
Figure 3.

All models were tested using the test data set. One Step Ahead (OSA) predictions
for MTBF, MTTR and Availability are shown in Figure 4 where yTEST is the experimental data and yOSA the predicted values. The time was normalized between 0
and 1. The best values for the MTBF model were obtained with two delays (2nd order
model), for the MTTR model with three delays (3d order) while for Availability only
one delay (1st order) was necessary. For MTBF and MTTR models the tuning process
lead to c=211, sigma=25, ε=0.1 while for Availability they were c=2-4, sigma=20,
ε=0.1.

The comparison between experimental data and the predicted values, as shown in
Figure 4 and Table 1, shows good performance of the developed models with a
SMAPE and IA indexes of 27.96 and 0.99   for MTBF, 151.85 and   0.96 for MTTR

and 33.25 and 0.95 for Availability. The developed models were able to predict with good accuracy the three variables even though they exhibit a rather rough behaviour.

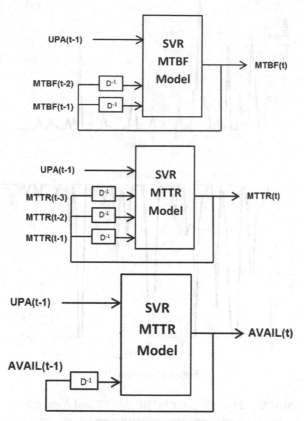

Fig. 3. NARX SVR models for MTBF, MTTR and AVAIL (availability) variables for the test set

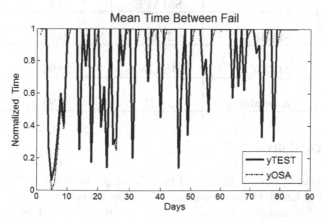

Fig. 4. Experimental and predicted data for MTBF, MTTR and Availability variables for the test set

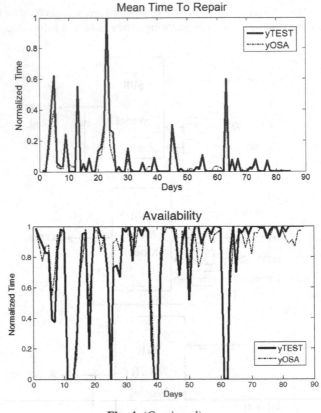

Fig. 4. *(Continued)*

Table 1. SMAPE and IA indices for MTBF, MTTR and Availability predictions

	SMAPE	IA
MTBF	27.96	0.99
MTTR	151.85	0.96
Availability	33.25	0.95

4   Conclusions

This paper presents three NARX SVM models for predicting variables used for asset management of heavy mining equipment. This can be very useful for asset management needs. For instance the operator can use the predicted MTBF and MTTR variables to classify in advance an equipment into "critical", "chronic", "critical&chronic" and "under control" categories. Both variables required a nonlinear model being MTTR more complex to model (3d order) than MTBF (2nd order). In the case of Availability a simpler model (1st order) was needed. Although results are promising this is a preliminary work that should be improved when more data and other relevant variables –like monitoring conditions, environmental variables, etc …- could be available. The goals are to improve OSA predictions and also to achieve good multiple step ahead predictions perhaps also exploring the use of another dynamic models like the nonlinear autoregressive with exogenous inputs (NARMAX) models.

Acknowledgements. The authors acknowledge partial financial support of Chilean Government under FONDEF-IDeA GRANT CA13I10121 and of the Research Direction of Universidad de La Frontera.

References

1. Concetti, M., Cuccioleta, R., Fedele, L., Mercuri, G.: Tele-maintenance intelligent system for technical plants result management. Reliability Enginnering and System Safety 94, 63–77 (2009)
2. Oladokun, V.O., Charles-Obawa, O.E., Nwaouzru, C.S.: An application of artificial neural network to maintenance management. Journal of Industrial Engineering International 2(3), 19–26 (2006)
3. Zeng, Y., Jiang, W., Zhu, C., Liu, J., Teng, W., Zhang, Y.: Prediction of equipment maintenance using optimized support vector machine. In: Huang, D.-S., Li, K., Irwin, G.W. (eds.) ICIC 2006. LNCS (LNAI), vol. 4114, pp. 570–579. Springer, Heidelberg (2006)
4. Ding, F., He, Z., Zi, Y., Chen, X., Tan, J., Cao, H., Chen, H.: Application of support vector machine for equipment reliability forecasting. In: Proceedings of the IEEE International Conference on Industrial Informatics, pp. 526–530 (2008)
5. Ljung, L.: System Identification, Theory for the user, 2nd edn. Prentice Hall PTR, Springer, NJ, USA (1999)
6. Schölkopf, B., Smola, A., Williamson, R.C., Bartlett, P.L.: New support vector algorithms. Neural Computation 12, 1083–1121 (2000)
7. Vapnik, V.: The Nature of Statistical Learning Theory. Springer (1995)
8. Drucker, H., Burges, C.J.C., Kaufman, L., Smola, A.: andVapnik, V., 1997, Support vector regression machines. In: Mozer, M., Jordan, M., Petsche, T. (eds.) Advances in Neural Information Processing Systems, vol. 9, pp. 155–161. MIT Press, Cambridge (1997)
9. Canu, S., Grandvalet, Y., Guigue, V., Rakotomamonjy, A.: SVM and Kernel Methods Matlab Toolbox. Perception Systèmeset Information, INSA de Rouen, Rouen, France (2005)
10. Willmott, C.J.: On the validation of models. Physical Geography 2, 184–194 (1981)
11. Swanson, E.A., Tayman, J., Bryan, T.M.: MAPE-R: A rescaled measure of accuracy for Cross-Sectional Forecasts. Journal of Population Research 28, 25–243 (2011)

Customer Churn Prediction in Telecommunication Industry: With and without Counter-Example

Adnan Amin, Changez Khan, Imtiaz Ali, and Sajid Anwar

Institute of Management Sciences, Hayatabad Phase VII Peshawar, Pakistan Zip Code: 25000
{geoamins,sajidanwar.2k}@gmail.com

Abstract. This study contributes to formalize customer churn prediction where rough set theory is used as one-class classifier and multi-class classifier to investigate the trade-off in the selection of an effective classification model for customer churn prediction. Experiments were performed to explore the performance of four different rule generation algorithms (i.e. exhaustive, genetic, covering and LEM2). It is observed that rough set as one-class classifier and multi-class classifier based on genetic algorithm yields more suitable performance as compared to the other three rule generation algorithms. Furthermore, by applying the proposed techniques (i.e. Rough sets as one-class and multi-class classifiers) on publicly available dataset, the results show that rough set as a multi - class classifier provides more accurate results for binary/multi-class classification problems.

Keywords: One-Class Classification, Multi-Class Classification, Churn Prediction, Rough Set theory.

1   Introduction

Customer churn- shifting from one service provider to next competitor in the market is a mounting issue for various service-based industries and particularly for telecommunication industry [1]. It is one of the greatest importance for project managers because losing a customer is a low cost opportunity for competitors to gain customer [2, 3]. It has been reported that the associated cost with the acquisition of new customer is often times more as compared to retaining the existing customers [4]. Retaining existing customers leads to significant increase in sales and reduced marketing cost. These facts ultimately focused on customer churn prediction as an indispensable part of telecom companies' strategic decision making and planning process that is the primary objective of customer relationship management (CRM) as well. The importance of this growing issue has also led to the development of several predictive tools that support some vital tasks in predictive modelling and classification process.

In recent decades, the explosion of data is a challenging task for extracting valuable information that is contained in this data. On the other hand, data mining entails the overall process of knowledge extraction from the data bank. There are many data mining applications which have been successfully applied to various knowledge

A. Gelbukh et al. (Eds.): MICAI 2014, Part II, LNAI 8857, pp. 206–218, 2014.

discovery techniques [1, 5–9] to extract hidden and meaningful relationships between entities and attributes. These facts led the competitive companies to invest in CRM to maintain customer information. Data is maintained in such CRM Systems can be converted into meaningful information to consider the mounting issue of customer churn in order to identify the customer's churn behavior before the customers are lost which increase the customer strength [2].

Although, customer churn prediction modeling has been extensively studied in various domains such as banking, online gaming, airlines, telecommunication, financial services and social network services [10] using multi-classification algorithms but one-class classification using rough set theory has not been widely applied in predicting customer churn in the telecom sector. Therefore, this study focuses over explore the powerful applications and trade-off in one-class and multi-class classifications using rough set theory in churn prediction by constructing predictive classifiers that achieve more performance to forecast churns, based on accumulated knowledge.

The remainder of this paper is organized as follows; In Section 2, the domain of customer churn and churn prediction modeling is briefly described by means of broad literature review. The primarily study about One-Class and Multi-Class classifications is thoroughly explained in Section 3. In Section 4 both techniques are evaluated to predict customer churn, and the experimental setup followed by results of a series of experiments are discussed. Finally, the conclusion of the paper has been presented in the last section of the paper.

2   Customer Churn and Churn Prediction Modeling

2.1   Customer Churn

Customer Churn is a key challenge in competitive markets and is highly observed in telecommunication section [8, 11]. Customer churns are those specific customers who have decided to leave the use of service, product, or even company and shifting to next competitor in the market. Literature reveals the following types of customer churns [12].

- Volunteer: When customers want to quit the contract and move to the next service provider.
- Non-Volunteer: When the company quit the service to a customer.
- Silent Churn: Those customers who discontinued the contract without prior knowledge of both parties (customer-company).

The first two types of churns can be predicted easily with the help of traditional approaches in term of Boolean class value, but the third type of churn may exist which is difficult to predict because there may have such type of customers who may possibly churns in the near future. It should be the goal of the decision maker and marketers to decrease the churn ratio because it is a well-known phenomenon that existing customers are the most valuable assets for companies as compared to acquiring new one [3].

2.2   Churn Prediction Modelling

Churn prediction has been widely studied in the past decade. Keaveney [13] in 1995 published an early and influential study about customer churn in the service provider sector by conducting a survey to find out the reasons why customers switch services. Various techniques, methodologies and approaches have been proposed which mainly leverage both static and dynamic analysis. The marketing strategy within competitive companies has been germinating from approaching product-oriented to customer-centric due to the advancement in the machine learning technology [3]. The database technologies not only provide useful information to the organization's decision makers about their past and current customer behavior but even also provide future prediction with the help of predictive modelling techniques.

Churn prediction has received a tremendous focus from both types of researchers (academia and industry). Similarly, the central theme of this study is also based on both theoretical and applied studies. The churn analysis problem is an equally high alarming issue for various domains such as Social Networks   [14], Banks & Financial Services [15], Credit cards accounts [2], Games [16], HRM [11] and Insurance & Subscription services [17]. Similarly, In a study [18] presented a ChurnVis system for visualizing the churn and subscriber actions over the time in telecommunication but the major attention given to social influence on churn behavior rather than the problem of predicting the churn.

Most of the previous studies have been strongly focused on a few specific factors (e.g., Customer satisfaction & dissatisfaction, loyalty, social influence) pertaining to customer churn instead of scientifically and empirical investigation and testing of prediction model which encompasses relationships between different constructs such as important churn related variables, service usage, switching reasons, behavior and costs. For instance, in a study [13] classified the customers switching of service with eight general categories. Furthermore, survey based studies [13, 19, 20] and have used a small sample of customer data that may undermine the threat validity and reliability of outcomes. On the other hand, a proprietary dataset was investigated   [15] of an in-house data-warehouse (DWH) in the European financial service market while the study [19] used survey and actual transaction data to analyze churn behavior in the service market. Similarly the study [21] indicated that the call quality factor is highly influenced on customer churn in the proprietary dataset of Korean mobile telecommunication service.

The literature reveals that various machine learning techniques have been used for churn prediction in the telecom industry such as SVM [22], neural network [5, 12, 22, 23],   decision tree [6, 22, 23], Regression analysis [23], Naïve Bayes and Bayesian Network [6] and Neuro-Fuzzy [24] but conflicts arise when studying results and comparing the conclusion of few of these published studies in the domain of churn prediction because it is also reported that most of the studies have only evaluated a limited number of traditional machine learning techniques on small sample sizes [13, 19, 20] and have used proprietary dataset. The most important problem of classification technique that could be used to approach the churn prediction in a more appropriate fashion still remains an open research problem. Some experts from research community have investigated that SVM is one the state-of-the-art approaches for classification in machine learning due to its ability of model nonlinearities [25]. On the other hands, a couple of studies [12, 26] have reported that artificial neural networks can outperform as compared to other traditional machine learning algorithms.

A benchmarking and empirical study is proposed with the aim to contribute further in customer churn prediction domain in term of not only achieving suitable accuracy and performance, but also investigating trade-off between one-class and multi-class classifiers for customer churn prediction and extraction of decision rules from hidden existing patterns. Based on extracted rules, decision maker can easily adopt new retention policies and improve the overall performance of the organization. In this study, we have used rough set theory which has many advantages such as [27]; (1) Mathematical power to extract hidden patterns from small to large datasets, (2) Finding minimal sets of reduction, (3) A straightforward generation and easy interpretation of decision rules. The primarily study about one-class, multi-class classification and rough set theory are explained in the next section.

3   Primarily Study

This section describes the primarily foundation about the following;

3.1   Rough Set Theory (RST)

RST was originally proposed by Pawlak [28] in 1982. The fundamental idea of rough set theory is to deal with the data analysis and classification of imprecise or uncertain information. A rough set theory has a precise concept of lower and upper approximation and the boundary region. The boundary region separates the lower approximation from upper approximation. Mathematically, all these concepts of rough set can be defined as; suppose set $X \subseteq U$ and B is an equivalence relation in information system IS= (U, B). Then BL= $\cup$ {Y $\in$ U/ B: Y $\subseteq$ X} is lower approximation and exact member of X while BU = $\cup$ {Y $\in$ U/ B: Y $\cap$ X $\neq \emptyset$} is upper approximation which is possibly a member of X. BR = BL - BU is the boundary region. The detailed study about RST can be found in [27, 28]. To extract the decision rules, the following classification algorithms (Exhaustive algorithm, Genetic Algorithm, Covering Algorithm & LEM2) can be used to produce sets of decision rules by matching the trainings instances against the set of generating reducts.

— *Exhaustive Algorithm:* It takes subsets of features incrementally and then returns the reducts of required one. It needs more concentration because it may lead to extensive computations in case of complex and large decision table. It is based on a Boolean reasoning approach [29].
— *Genetic Algorithm:* It is based on order-based GA coupled with heuristic and this evolutionary method is presented by [30], [31][31]. It is used to reduce the computational cost in large and complex decision table.

— *Covering Algorithm:* It is customized implementation of the LEM2 idea and implemented in the RSES covering method. It was introduced by Jerzy Grzymala [32].
— LEM2 Algorithm: It is a separate-&-conquer technique paired with lower and upper approximation of rough set theory and it is based on local covering determination of each object from the decision class [32]. It is implementation of LEM2 [33].

3.2   One-Class Classifier

The one-class classification (OCC) problem differs from the conventional multi-class classification (MCC) in that data from two or more classes are present in MCC while OCC is   concerned with information about one of the classes (target class) only [34, 35]. It means that the description of a particular class at OCC is called target class and a classifier is trained from target class patterns. New patterns are classified based on learnt description of the target class and if the new instance, or pattern does not belong to target class, it is labeled as outliers [35, 36]. Mathematically a one class classifier is expressed as in (1);

$$h(x)=\begin{cases} \text{Target if } f(x) \leq \theta \\ \text{Outlier if } f(x) > \theta \end{cases} \qquad (1)$$

Where θ is threshold that define a boundary region of the target class and accepts as much possible the target objects. On the other hand, it minimizes the chances of the accepting outlier instances [35, 36].

3.3   Multi-class Classifier

In MMC classification problem, the classifier learns from the training data set of multiple classes. The decision boundary is supported by the availability of data instances from each class. In such classification, most of the classes are facing the problems of imbalanced data and does not perform well on under sampled [34, 35]. On the other hand, OCC constructs the boundary of one class because it has no input from the outlier [36] or has very few of them. Such outliers will not be considered in the classifier performance evaluation [37].

3.4   Evaluation Measures

It is nearly impossible to build a perfect classifier or a model that could perfectly characterize all the instances of the test set [6]. To assess the classification results, we count the number of True Positive (TP), True Negative (TN), False Positive (FP) and False Negative (FN). The FN value actually belongs to Positive P (e.g. TP + FN = P) but wrongly classified as Negative N (e.g. TN + FP = N) while FP value actually part of N but wrongly classified as P. The detailed description about evaluation measures which are used later in this study can be found in study [38].

4   Evaluation Setup

In this section, an analytical environment is setup to perform the proposed technique using rough set explanation system (RSES) [39]. We have also evaluated four different rules generation algorithms (i.e. exhaustive, genetic, covering, LEM2). These experiments were carried out to fulfill the objectives of the proposed study and to address the following points also;

- **P1:** *Which features are more indicative for churn prediction in the telecom sector?*
- **P2:** *Can derived rules help the decision makers in strategic decision making and planning process?*
- **P3:** *Which algorithm (Exhaustive, Genetic, Covering, and LEM2) is more appropriate for calculating rules set for rough set as a one-class and multi-class classifier in telecommunication sector?*

5   Data Preparation and Feature Selection

Evaluation of existing data mining approaches on publicly available or open datasets has many benefits in term of comparability of results, ranking techniques, evaluating of existing methodologies with new one [40]. In this study, we have used publicly available dataset which can be obtained from URL [41]. Data preparation and feature selection are important steps in knowledge discovery process that identify those relevant variables or attributes from the large number of attributes in a dataset which are too relevant and reduce the computational cost [30]. To make sure that only relevant features are included in decision table that also reduce the computational cost and addressed to P1 (Which features are more indicative for churn prediction in telecom sector?), the selection of most appropriate attributes from the dataset in hands was carried out using feature ranking method titled as "Information Gain Attribute Evaluator", using WEKA toolkit [42]. It evaluates the attributes worth through the information gain measurement procedure as per the class value and diversifies the selection and ranking of attributes that significantly improves the computational efficiency and classification [43]. The dataset contains 19 conditional features, along with one unique identifier and a decision attribute about telecom/wireless operator. After feature ranking, it includes most relevant and ranked attributes in the decision table. The Table 1 describes the selected attributes.

5.1   Preparation of Decision Tables

The preparation of decision tables is an important stage of the proposed study for one-class and multi-class classifiers' training and validation sets. A decision system is any information system of the form $S = (U, C \cup \{d\})$, where C is conditional attribute and $d \notin C$ is the decision attribute. The Union of C and $\{d\}$ are elements of Set A. The decision table which consists of objects, conditional attributes and decision attribute are organized in Table 2.

Table 1. Description of attributes

Attributes	Description
Int'l Plan	Whether a customer subscribed international plan or not.
VMail Plan	Whether a customer subscribed Voice Mail plan or not.
Day Charges	A continuous variable that holds day time call charges.
Day Mins	No. of minutes that a customer has used in daytime.
CustSer Calls	Total No. of calls made a customer to customer service.
VMail Msg	Indicates number of voice mail messages
Int'l Calls	Total No. of calls that used as international calls.
Int'l Charges	A continuous variable that holds international call charges
Int'l Mins	No. of minutes that used during international calls.
Eve Charges	A continuous variable that holds evening time call charges.
Eve Mins	No. of minutes that a customer has used at evening time.
Churn?	The Class label whether a customer is churn or non-churn.

Table 2. Organization of attributes for decision table

Sets	Description
Objects	{ 3333 distinct objects}
Conditional Attributes	{Intl Phan, VMail_Plan, VMailMsg, Day_Mins, Day Charges, Eve_Mins, Eve_Charges, Intl_Mins, Intl_Calls, Intl_Charges, CustServ_Calls}
Decision Attribute	{Churn?}

After applying rough set theory technique to find out the lower bound, upper bound and boundary regions, the resultant information is presented as follows;

Table 3. Rough set approximation boundaries

Class	No. Of Objects	Lower Approximation	Upper Approximation	Accuracy
NC	2850	2850	2850	1.000
C	483	483	483	1.000

*NC=Non-Churn and C=Churn

The upper and lower approximations are equivalent in the given Table 3. Therefore, there is no uncertainty in classification of decision classes.

Decision Table for OCC. According to the concept of OCC, which is discussed in Section 3.2, we have selected the lower approximation (exactly churn instances) as target class and build a decision table from these instances as well as also included about 17 outliner samples because OCC constructs the boundary of one class and it has no input from the outlier [35] or has very few of them.

Decision Table for MCC. The combination of both classes NC and C instances are included in another decision table which is used for training the MCC classifier.

5.2   Cut and Discretization

Cut and Discretization is the plausible approach to handle the large data by reducing the data set horizontally. It is a common approach used in rough set where the variables which contains continuous values is partitioned into a finite number of intervals or groups [44]. The cut and discretization process is carefully performed on the prepared decision table using RSES toolkits. It adds cuts in subsequent loop one by one for a given attribute. It considers all the objects in decision table at every iteration and generate less number of cuts [33].

5.3   Training and Validation Set

In data mining, validation is an extremely important step to ensure that the prediction model is not only remembering the instances that were given during the training process, but it should also perform the same on unseen new instances [45]. One way to overcome this problem is not to use the entire dataset for classifier's learning process. Some of the data are excluded from the training process as it begins, and when it is completed and the classifier is trained, then the excluded data can be used to validate the performance of the learned classifier on new data. This overall idea of model evaluation or classifier evaluation is called cross validation.

In this study, hold-out cross validation (train-and-test) method [33] is used. We divide the data set into two sets: training set and test set. After multiple splitting attempts during the experiments, we concluded that the best performance is obtained if the split factor parameter is set to 0.7 using RSES toolkit that randomly splits the data into two disjoint sub-tables. The division of a dataset into training and validation set is performed multiple times irrespective of class label and noted the average performance of the classifier to minimize the biases in the data.

5.4   Reduct and Decision Rules Set Generation

The decision rules can be obtained by selecting either of methods i.e. global rules or local rules using RSES. In proposed study, the global rule method has been selected which scans the training set object-by-object and generates decision rules by matching objects with reduct set and selecting attributes from conditional attributes in reduct set. However, local method, slightly faster than the global method but, it is generating much more cuts as compared to global method. The decision rules specify rules in the form of *"if C then D"* where *C* is a condition and *D* refers to decision attribute. For example:

```
If Day_Mins=(108.8, 151.05) & Eve_Mins=(207.35, 227.15) &
   CustServ_Calls=(3.5, *) then Churn=(True).
```

To address P2, important decision rules can be induced from the decision table by generating rules using four different rules generation methods (i.e. exhaustive, genetic, covering and LEM2). Based on these simple and easy interpretable rules, the decision makers can easily understand the flow of customer churn behavior and they can adopt suitable strategic plan to retain their churn. All the generated decision rules cannot be shown here due to limitation of pages. Table 4 reflects that the statistical information about rules induced from both decision tables (with and without outlier class) which are prepared for OCC and MCC.

Table 4. Statistical Information Of Four Methods Applied on OCC and MCC To Induce Decision Rules

Classifiers	Methods for Calculating Rules							
	Exhaustive		Genetic		Covering		LEM2	
	MCC	OCC	MCC	OCC	MCC	OCC	MCC	OCC
Total No. of Rules	4184	81	9468	80	369	1	625	11
# of rules induced that classifying customer as churn	1221	67	2674	67	122	1	160	11
# of rules induced that classifying customers as non-churn	2963	14	6715	13	247	0	465	4

5.5   Predictive Performance of Classifiers

We have evaluated four different algorithms for rules calculation with rough set based classification approach using RSES toolkit on both decision tables.

In the first experiment, we have applied these algorithms on the decision table was prepared for MCC. The number of churns was much smaller than non-churns customers in the decision table which can provides tough time to churn prediction classifier during the learning process. The overall evaluation of the first experiment (MCC) is shown in Table 6.

In the next experiment, we have applied the same methods on the decision table which was organized for OCC. Finally, we have evaluated the overall performance of four methods on MCC and OCC classifiers which were used in both experiments. Table 7 reflects the performance of OCC classifier based on discussed evaluation measures in Section 3.4.

Table 5. Evaluation of Four Rules Calculating Mehtods Using Rough Set On Multi-Class Classification Approach

METHODS	TP	FP	FN	TN	COV	PRE	REC	ER	ACC	SPEFM
Exhaustive	98	39	35	828	1	0.72	0.74	0.074	0.926	0.960.726
Genetic	**118**	**19**	**0**	**863**	1	**0.86**	**1.00**	**0.019**	**0.981**	**0.980.925**
Covering	37	41	37	525	0.64	0.47	0.50	0.122	0.878	0.930.487
LEM2	52	26	19	571	0.668	0.67	0.73	0.067	0.993	0.960.698

Table 6. Evaluation of Four Rules Calculating Mehtods Using Rough Set On One-Class Classification Approach

METHODS	TP	FP	FN	TN	COV	PRE	REC	ER	ACC	SPE	FM
Exhaustive	142	1	3	0	1	0.979	0.99	0.023	0.973	0	0.986
Genetic	**142**	**1**	**3**	**0**	**1**	**0.979**	**0.993**	**0.027**	**0.973**	**0**	**0.986**
Covering	59	0	0	0	0.494	1	1	0.51	1	-	0
LEM2	122	0	1	0	0.836	0.992	1	0.51	1	0	0.995

6 Discussion

MCC Classifier: The maximum accuracy is obtained to LEM2 which is about 0.993 but it has 66.8% coverage of all instances (which means it has classified 66.8% customers only while 33.2% customers were not considered). The exhaustive method has achieved less accuracy (0.926) than LEM2. However, exhaustive algorithm has performed better as compared to LEM2 and Covering methods in term of coverage and overall evaluation measures given in Table 6. On the other hand, Genetic algorithm has shown more improved overall performance in the rough set classification process because it has not only covered all objects in classification process, but also obtained 98.1% accuracy which is indicating the best approach among these four algorithms.

OCC Classifier. The maximum accuracy is obtained using covering method which is about 100% but it has considered 49.4% objects only. Therefore, exhaustive and genetic algorithms performed almost similar and these two algorithms achieve much better performance.

MCC vs OCC. It is observed from experiments that the prediction of true churn customers based on genetic algorithm in MCC have classified 86% customers and misclassified 14% customers. On the other hand, genetic & exhaustive algorithms in OCC have shown much improved performance on prediction of true churn customers, which is about 96% and misclassification reduced from 14% to 4% only which also reporting to P3.

7 Conclusion

Customer churn prediction is an important practice in rapidly growing and competitive telecom industries. Due to the high cost associated with acquiring new customers, customer churn prediction has emerged as an indispensable part of strategic decision making and planning process in telecom sector. In this study, we have attempted to make use of rough set theory as one-class and multi-class classifiers and investigated the trade-off in the selection of an effective classification model for forecasting customer churn in telecommunication industry. A series of experiments were performed and explored the performance of four different rule generation algorithms. It is observed from the results shown in Table 6 and Table 7 that genetic algorithm base rules generation methods perform very well for multi-class classification while exhaustive and genetic gives almost similar results for One-class classification. Overall genetic algorithm base rules generation gives best performance. It is also investigated that the true churn prediction rate has also improved from 86% in MCC to 96% in OCC.

References

1. Verbeke, W., Martens, D., Mues, C., Baesens, B.: Building comprehensible customer churn prediction models with advanced rule induction techniques. Expert Syst. Appl. 38, 2354–2364 (2011)
2. Lin, C.-S., Tzeng, G.-H., Chin, Y.-C.: Combined rough set theory and flow network graph to predict customer churn in credit card accounts. Expert Syst. Appl. 38, 8–15 (2011)
3. Hadden, J., Tiwari, A., Roy, R., Ruta, D.: Computer assisted customer churn management: State-of-the-art and future trends. Comput. Oper. Res. 34, 2902–2917 (2007)
4. Khan, I., Tariq Usman, G.U.R.: Intelligent Churn prediction for Telecommunication Industry. Int. J. Innov. Appl. Stud. 4, 165–170 (2013)
5. Sharma, A.: A Neural Network based Approach for Predicting Customer Churn in Cellular Network Services. Int. J. Comput. Appl. 27, 26–31 (2011)
6. Kirui, C., Hong, L., Cheruiyot, W., Kirui, H.: Predicting Customer Churn in Mobile Telephony Industry Using Probabilistic Classifiers in Data Mining. IJCSI Int. J. Comput. Sci. Issues 10, 165–172 (2013)
7. Soeini, R.A., Rodpysh, K.V.: Applying Data Mining to Insurance Customer Churn Management 30, 82–92 (2012)
8. Hung, S.-Y., Yen, D.C., Wang, H.-Y.: Applying data mining to telecom churn management. Expert Syst. Appl. 31, 515–524 (2006)
9. Huang, B., Kechadi, M.T., Buckley, B.: Customer churn prediction in telecommunications. Expert Syst. Appl. 39, 1414–1425 (2012)
10. Wolniewicz, R.H., Dodier, R.: Predicting customer behavior in telecommunications. IEEE Intell. Syst. 19, 50–58 (2004)
11. Saradhi, V.V., Palshikar, G.K.: Employee churn prediction. Expert Syst. Appl. 38, 1999–2006 (2011)
12. Lazarov, V., Capota, M.: Churn Prediction. Bus. Anal. Course. TUM Comput. Sci.
13. Keaveney, S.M.: Customer switching behavior in service industries: An exploratory study. J. Mark. 59, 71–82
14. Verbeke, W., Martens, D., Baesens, B.: Social network analysis for customer churn prediction. Appl. Soft Comput. 14, 431–446 (2014)
15. Van den Poel, D., Larivière, B.: Customer attrition analysis for financial services using proportional hazard models. Eur. J. Oper. Res. 157, 196–217 (2004)
16. Suznjevic, M., Stupar, I., Matijasevic, M.: MMORPG Player Behavior Model based on Player Action Categories. IEEE (2011)
17. Burez, J., Van den Poel, D.: Handling class imbalance in customer churn prediction. Expert Syst. Appl. 36, 4626–4636 (2009)
18. Archambault, D., Hurley, N., Tu, C.T.: ChurnVis: Visualizing mobile telecommunications churn on a social network with attributes, 894–901
19. Bolton, R.N.: A Dynamic Model of the Duration of the Customer's Relationship with a Continuous Service Provider: The Role of Satisfaction. Mark. Sci. 17, 45–65 (1998)

20. Kim, M.-K., Park, M.-C., Jeong, D.-H.: The effects of customer satisfaction and switching barrier on customer loyalty in Korean mobile telecommunication services. Telecomm. Policy 28, 145–159 (2004)

21. Ahn, J.-H., Han, S.-P., Lee, Y.-S.: Customer churn analysis: Churn determinants and mediation effects of partial defection in the Korean mobile telecommunications service industry. Telecomm. Policy 30, 552–568 (2006)

22. Shaaban, E., Helmy, Y., Khedr, A., Nasr, M.: A Proposed Churn Prediction Model. Int. J. Eng. Res. Appl. 2, 693–697 (2012)

23. Qureshi, S.A., Rehman, A.S., Qamar, A.M., Kamal, A., Rehman, A.: Telecommunication subscribers' churn prediction model using machine learning. In: Eighth International Conference on Digital Information Management (ICDIM 2013), pp. 131–136. IEEE (2013)

24. Abbasimehr, H.: A Neuro-Fuzzy Classifier for Customer Churn Prediction. Int. J. Comput. Appl. 19, 35–41 (2011)

25. Farquad, M.A.H., Ravi, V., Raju, S.B.: Churn prediction using comprehensible support vector machine: An analytical CRM application. Appl. Soft Comput. 19, 31–40 (2014)

26. Mozer, M.C., Wolniewicz, R., Grimes, D.B., Johnson, E., Kaushansky, H.: Predicting subscriber dissatisfaction and improving retention in the wireless telecommunications industry. IEEE Trans. Neural Netw. 11, 690–696 (2000)

27. Pawlak, Z.: Rough Sets, Rough Relations and Rough Functions. Fundamenta Informaticae 27(2-3)   (1996),
    http://iospress.metapress.com/content/vr21hm11p17k3uh0/

28. Pawlak, Z.: Rough sets. Int. J. Comput. Inf. Sci. 11, 341–356 (1982)

29. Nguyen, S.H., Nguyen, H.S.: Analysis of STULONG Data by Rough Set Exploration System (RSES). In: Proc. ECML/PKDD Work, pp. 71–82 (2003)

30. Bazan, J.G., Nguyen, H.S., Nguyen, S.H., Synak, P., Wróblewski, J.: Rough set algorithms in classification problem, pp. 49–88 (2000)

31. Wróblewski, J.: Genetic Algorithms in Decomposition and Classification Problems. Rough Sets Knowl. Discov. 2(19), 471–487 (1998)

32. Grzymala-Busse, J.W.: A New Version of the Rule Induction System LERS. Fundam. Informaticae 31, 27–39 (1997)

33. Bazan, J., Szczuka, M.S.: The Rough Set Exploration System. In: Peters, J.F., Skowron, A. (eds.) Transactions on Rough Sets III. LNCS, vol. 3400, pp. 37–56. Springer, Heidelberg (2005)

34. Khan, S., Madden, M.: One-class classification: taxonomy of study and review of techniques. Knowl. Eng. Rev. 29, 345–374 (2014)

35. Tax, D.M.J.: One-Class Classification, Concept Learning in the Absence of Counter Examples. Ph.D. Thesis, Delft Univ. Technol. Delft, Netherl. (2001)

36. Khan, M.A., Jan, Z., Ishtiaq, M., Asif Khan, M., Mirza, A.M.: Selection of Accurate and Robust Classification Model for Binary Classification Problems. Signal Process. Image Process. Pattern Recognit. 61, 161–168 (2009)

37. Tax, D.M.J., Duin, R.P.W.: Uniform object generation for optimizing one-class classifiers. J. Mach. Learn. Res. 2, 155–173 (2002)

38. Amin, A., Shehzad, S., Khan, C., Ali, I., Anwar, S.: Churn Prediction in Telecommunication Industry Using Rough Set Approach. In: Camacho, D., Kim, S.-W., Trawiński, B. (eds.) New Research in Multimedia and Internet Systems. SCI, vol. 572, pp. 83–96. Springer, Heidelberg (2015)

39. Lee, K.C., Chung, N., Shin, K.: An artificial intelligence-based data mining approach to extracting strategies for reducing the churning rate in credit card industry. J. Intell. Inf. Syst. 8, 15–35 (2002)

40. Vandecruys, O., Martens, D., Baesens, B., Mues, C., De Backer, M., Haesen, R.: Mining software repositories for comprehensible software fault prediction models. J. Syst. Softw. 81, 823–839 (2008)
41. Dataset Source, http://www.sgi.com/tech/mlc/db/
42. Holmes, G., Donkin, A., Witten, I.H.: WEKA: a machine learning workbench. In: Proceedings of ANZIIS 1994 - Australian New Zealnd Intelligent Information Systems Conference, pp. 357–361. IEEE (1994)
43. Novakovic, J.: Using Information Gain Attribute Evaluation to Classify Sonar Targets. In: 17th Telecommun. forum TELFOR, pp. 1351–1354 (2009)
44. He, F., Wang, X., Liu, B.: Attack Detection by Rough Set Theory in Recommendation System. In: 2010 IEEE International Conference on Granular Computing, pp. 692–695. IEEE (2010)
45. Bellazzi, R., Zupan, B.: Predictive data mining in clinical medicine: current issues and guidelines. Int. J. Med. Inform. 77, 81–97 (2008)

Audio-to-Audio Alignment for Performances Tracking

Alain Manzo-Martínez[1,*] and Jose Antonia Camarena-Ibarrola[2]

[1] Instituto Tecnológico de Morelia, Morelia, Michoacán, México
`alainmama@gmail.com`
[2] Universidad Michoacana de San Nicolás de Hidalgo, Morelia, Michoacán, México
`camarena@umich.mx`

Abstract. On-line audio-to-audio alignment could be used for building intelligent systems that are able to follow incoming audio by content. Tracking of musical performances is a key concept to implement virtual teachers of musical instruments, automatic accompanying or virtual orchestras, and automatic special effects adding in live presentations. In this paper, we describe a new and efficient method for on-live tracking of polyphonic music. We use a Partially Observable Markov Process (POMP) to align sequences of feature vectors extracted from the audio signal. We compute the entropy per chroma of the audio signals of both musical renditions to extract the both sequences of feature vectors. In order to assess our proposal we make use of another tracking system that uses Hidden Markov Models (HMM). The results are encouraging, we managed to track live concert performances by on-line alignment with studio performances of the same songs.

Keywords: Audio-to-Audio Alignment, Belief State, Chroma, Entropy, Tracking.

1 Introduction

Tracking a song in real time consists of setting the position of every short segment of the song as it is played with respect to a target audio, which is another performance of the same song previously recorded. Considered two different performances of a musical piece or song, where the audio of one of them is completely known and the other is acquired as it is being played, aligning these performances in real time becomes a complex problem.

The renditions have slight variations in tempo, rhythm, volume, Etc., they may be played by different musicians and even with different musical instruments. In a musical performance, high level information such as structure and emotion is communicated by the performer through parameters such as tempo, dynamics, articulation and vibrato. These parameters vary within a musical piece, between musical pieces and between performers. Another inconvenient is the noise added to the audio signal of the performance played live. The noise can be formed by the reverberation of the place, an environmental sound, a direct sound since other instruments or simply the noise of the scenario (people). All these factors distort the audio signal captured by the microphones making difficult the matching between both performances. Finally, the tempo of the performance played live, the excitement of

A. Gelbukh et al. (Eds.): MICAI 2014, Part II, LNAI 8857, pp. 219–230, 2014.

the performer, the backing vocals, and possibly the incursion of new or different musical instruments to the used in the audio recorded in studio, they are factors that make both audios quite different.

We benefit from the robustness of *entropy* as a perceptual feature and perform an analysis of *eigen-values* applied at the study of audio signals. We perform *Audio tracking* using a *partially observable Markov process* (POMP). The ability of POMPs to update the *belief state* of the system by the perceived observations about the environment, was what motivated us to use them in music tracking.

2   Related Work

Real time *audio tracking* systems are characterized by two aspects; the features extracted from the audio signal, and the technique used to align the score (target audio) with the performance. The first aspect is important due to it is related to the efficient of a system to recognize the incoming audio stream. The second aspect establishes the correlation between the extracted features of both performances.

Normally a piece of music is represented or encoded in a symbolic score, as a matter of fact, *audio tracking*, may be accomplished by aligning the music with the symbolic score (usually referred as score following), a review of this approach can be found in [1], [2]. Another approach is the *audio-to-audio alignment* where a previously recorded performance of a song (i.e. played in studio) is preferred over the symbolic score.

In [3], *chroma-values* are extracted from the audio-signal of the song to be tracked. MIDI data is converted into a reference audio signal using a sequencer. By generating the reference audio signal, the *audio-to-MIDI* matching problem is simplified as an *audio-to-audio* matching problem. Next, both the performance and reference audio signals are transformed to *chromagrams*. Finally, the alignment is obtained by *Dynamic Time Warping* (DTW) between the *chromagrams*. In [4], a unified methodology for the real time alignment of audio to both a symbolic score and an audio reference by exploiting sequential *Montecarlo* inference techniques is presented. The tempo is the explicit parameter within the stochastic framework defined through musical motion equations. Thus, both symbolic and audio alignment problems are formulated within the same framework by exploiting a continuous representation of the reference media. In [5] and [6] a variation of DTW, an "*on-line time warping*" was proposed as an adaptation to allow for on-line music tracking, onsets of tones and increases in energy in frequency bins were used as features. The *on-line time warping* algorithm attempts to predict the optimal warping path by partially filling the matrix of costs with windows of a fixed size. In practice, the *on-line time warping* algorithm tends to deviate from the optimal path since the error is cumulative, this algorithm may completely loose track of the music. In [7] a local non-alignment scheme was introduced, this approach is based on searching short segments of audio taken from the musical performance to get the k-nearest audio segments using a proximity index for that purpose. The current audio segment of the play is paired with the nearest (in time) between the k previously selected audio segments of the target audio. This is the first algorithm able to start up from an arbitrary point in the audio end, for example, if the musical performance had already begun when the monitoring system just went on. This strategy is complemented through a simple heuristic of ignoring the candidates when they are all too far in time with respect to the last position reported by the system.

The rest of this paper is organized as follows: In the next section we explain our method to extract audio features which let us represent the audio signal of any performance in a straightforward way involving both *entropy* and *eigen-values* analysis. In Section 4 we describe POMPs theoretically, how we model music with it and the procedure to obtain the observations set to train the POMP used in the *audio-to-audio alignment* problem. In Section 5 we describe the database, the experiments and preliminaries results obtained using both *Viterbi* and *belief path* algorithms. Finally, we arrive to some conclusions written in Section 6 where we also propose some future extensions to this work.

3   Audio Feature Extraction Method

As we mentioned before in Section 2, any *audio tracking* system involves a stage to extract audio features from the audio signal. We will now explain how we process audio signals to determine our convenient audio features for the issue of this paper.

3.1   Entropy-per-Chroma Feature

In this subsection we present the *Entropy-per-Chroma* (EC) as we call this new feature, it is intended to be more robust the popular *chroma-values* based feature for audio following as was shown in [8]. EC is based on estimating the level of information content inside a *chroma* bin by using the *entropy* of a random process [10]. In order to extract it, *bag-of-frames* approach is used in [11]. EC consists of determining the spectrum from each frame, which is divided into octaves and, by using of the *equal-tempered* scale, lumping spectral components in *chroma* bins. Finally, we compute *entropy* in each *chroma* bin. The *entropy* in each *chroma* bin represents an *entropy-per-chroma value* (ECV). The general procedure to get these values is as follows: Given a number of values of *entropy-per-chroma*, b, a low frequency, f_0, a high frequency, f_{max}, and the sampling frequency, f_s, we need to determine the bounding frequencies by (1) and (2). Then, we determine N by (3), corresponding to the amount of samples to be extracted off the audio-signal.

$$f(k) = 2^{k/b} f_0, \quad \forall \, k = 0, 1, ..., K - 1 \tag{1}$$

$$K = b \times log_2 \left(\frac{f_{max}}{f_0} \right) \tag{2}$$

$$N = \frac{f_s}{f_0(2^{1/b} - 1)} \tag{3}$$

A Hann window $W(k)$ is applied to the audio samples denoted as $x(k)$, for $k = 0, 1, ..., N - 1$. The product $x(k)W(k)$ is zero, if $k \notin [0, N - 1]$, thus, a frame which is denoted as $y(n)$ is determined by (4).

$$y(n) = x\left(n + \frac{N}{2}\right)W\left(n + \frac{N}{2}\right) \tag{4}$$

for $n = -N, ..., N - 1$. According to (4), each frame has a length of $2N$ (i.e. N zeros were padded). Using this length, the DFT is computed by (5)

$$X_{DFT}(l) = \sum_{n=0}^{2N-1} y(n)e^{\frac{-2\pi nl}{2N}} \tag{5}$$

for $l = 0, 1, ..., 2N - 1$. The spectral components lumped in each *chroma* bin should be chosen accordingly to the next frequency relation,

$$f(i + md) \le \frac{lf_s}{2N} \le f(i + 1 + md)$$

for $i = 0, 1, ..., b - 1$ and $m = 0, 1, ..., M$, where $M = K/b$ and $b = d$. The term $\frac{lf_s}{2N}$ is referred to the frequency of the spectral components of $X_{DFT}(l)$ and $f(\cdot)$ are the bounding frequencies between each *chroma* bin. We assume that the spectral components distribute normally inside each *chroma* bin, so, for the 2-dimensional case, the *entropy* of a vector on a random process using a normal distribution with mean of zero can be computed by (6), where σ_x^2 and σ_y^2 are the variances of the real and imaginary parts of the spectral components respectively, and σ_{xy}^2 is covariance between real and imaginary parts.

$$H = \ln(2\pi e) + \frac{1}{2}\ln(\sigma_x^2\sigma_y^2 - \sigma_{xy}^2) \tag{6}$$

Finally, the *entropy-per-chroma values* are obtained by (7), where H_b denotes the *entropy* of the *bth chroma* bin.

$$ECV(b) = H_b \tag{7}$$

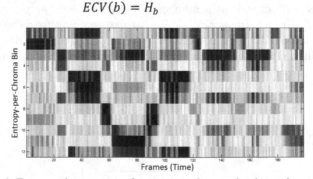

Fig. 1. Entropy-chromagram of a segment of monophonic music

For each frame, a vector with ECV is obtained. A $b \times t$ matrix, which we call *entropy-chromagram*, can be formed by a sequence of these vectors, where t denotes the number of frames analyzed. Fig. 1 shows the *entropy-chromagram* from an excerpt of monophonic music with length of 10s and twelve *chroma* bins.

An *entropy-chromagram* shows the harmonic and melodic content (the darkest regions) along this representation. For *entropy-chromagrams*, these regions are the places where the level of information content increases with respect to each *chroma* bin. We make a procedure to the signal before extracting EC. This procedure is described in the next steps:

1. Stereo signals are first converted to mono-aural by averaging both channels.
2. A pre-emphasis filter $h(i) = x(i) - ax(i - 1)$ is applied to the signal in order to highlight the energy in high frequencies. This process helps to identify better the harmonic and melodic content. The constant a is equal to 0.9.
3. Frames are of 100ms, namely, we need set $b = 20$ and $f_0 = 283.568$ Hz to get a length of $N = 4410$ audio samples, if the sampling frequency is 44.1 KHz.
4. The frames are overlapped 50%, therefore, in a second there are 20 frames.
5. The highest frequency considered is 8000Hz.

3.2   Eigenvalues Analysis

One of the goals to find *eigenvalues* from a matrix is to reduce the dimensionality of a high-dimensional data set consisting of a large number of interrelated variables and at the same time retain as much as possible of the variation present in the data set. The *eigen-values* are new variables that are uncorrelated and ordered such that the first few retain most of the variation present in all of the original variables. In the previous subsection, we proposed how to form a matrix by mean of vectors of ECV called *entropy-chromagram*. To make an *eigen-values* analysis, we need a square matrix. To extract the *eigen-values*, it is required that $b = t$, i.e., the number of ECV should be equal to the number of frames. This analysis considers *entropy-chromagrams* of audio segments with length of 1s. Using frames of 100ms overlapped 50%, then we obtain a matrix of 20 frames (i.e columns) every second. Taking into account this number of frames, we must consider 20 ECV to get a square matrix. Let C be a square matrix of order n. A non-zero vector $u \in \mathcal{R}^n$ is named an *eigen-vector* of C if, for some $\lambda \in \mathcal{R}$, it holds:

$$Cu = \lambda u$$

where λ is called *eigen-value* of C. The condition for λ, in order to belong to the *eigen-values* of C, is that the lineal and homogenous system of equations given by $(\lambda I - C)u = 0$ has a non-trivial solution, namely, $u \neq 0$, this is equivalent to $|(C - \lambda I)| = 0$. A real matrix has not necessarily real *eigen-values*. Any $n \times n$ matrix has exactly n *eigen-values* counting multiplicities. An *entropy-chromagram* has both real and complex *eigen-values*. Inside the *eigen-values* set of an *entropy-chromagram* we observed $\lambda_1 \gg \lambda_j$ for all $j > 1$. This *eigen-value* is known in the literature as the *dominant eigenvalue* (DE) and its module represents the spectral radius of the matrix [12]. It is important to notice that the module of this *eigen-value* is much larger than the module of the rest of them, therefore, this *eigen-value* and its associated *eigen-vector* provide the most valuable information from which the matrix came from. Fig. 2 shows the plot of the modules of the *eigen-values* set versus time obtained from a sequence of *entropy-chromagrams* with spacing of twenty frames between them. These *entropy-chromagrams* have been obtained from two different songs. Each plot shows up the existence of the DE along the whole song. It is important to notice that the rest of the *eigen-values* have modules so small in relation to DE it is barely appreciable over the axis of time. The components of the *eigen-vector* associated to DE represent a dominant fraction of the embedded information on the *entropy-chromagram*, in other words, the remaining *eigen-values* and their associated *eigen-vectors* do not provide meaningful information about the elements of the matrix and therefore they can be put aside.

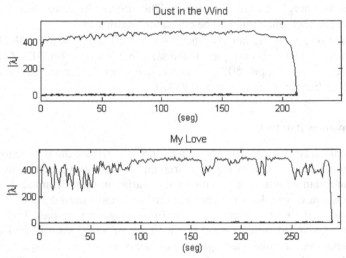

Fig. 2. Modules of the *eigen-values* of a sequence of *entropy-chromagrams* of songs interpreted by the Sarah Brightman and Beatles

To determine DE and its associated *eigen-vector*, we use the *Power Iteration* method [13] which starts with vector x_i and uses the recurrence (8) to converge to the *dominant eigen-vector,* this method requires $|\lambda_1| > |\lambda_2| \geq \cdots \geq |\lambda_n|$ to converge.

$$y_{k-1} = Cx_{k-1}, \qquad x_k = \frac{y_{k-1}}{\|y_{k-1}\|_\infty} \tag{8}$$

4   Partially Observable Markov Process

In this section, we explain the stochastic model to make live performances tracking in real time using the components of the *eigen-vector* associated to the DE. A POMP maintains the *belief state* to create the path in the *belief space*. The architecture of a POMP resembles that of a HMM. Both schemes have a finite set of states S, a matrix dictating the transition probabilities, P, and a matrix designating the probability distribution of the observations Ψ. In the training stage, an observation sequence, in our case one or more components of the *eigen-vector* associated to DE, is provided to the model to estimate the transition matrix P and the probability distributions of the observations. For this purpose the *Baum Welch* algorithm can be used. A POMP maintains a probability distribution about the *belief state* instead of maintaining the current state. The set of all the possible *belief states* forms the *belief space*. To update the value of the *belief state* $b_t(s)$ we use (9) where ρ is a constant of normalization and φ_{km} is the probability to observe $o_m \in \Omega$ when the process core changes to state s_k.

$$b_t(s_k) = \rho\varphi_{km} \sum_{s_j \in S} p_{jk} b_{t-1}(s_j) \tag{9}$$

Iterating over all possible states we get the *belief path* followed by the model through the time, we use the algorithm given in Table 1 for that purpose.

Table 1. Algorithm to compute the *belief path* followed by the model

$b_0(s) \leftarrow$ *Assign initial state*
$\forall\ o_m \in \Omega$
$\quad \forall\ s_k \in S$
$\qquad b_t(s_k) = \rho\varphi_{km} \sum_{s_j \in S} p_{jk} b_{t-1}(s_j)$
$\quad$ End
$\quad$ Path $= max\{b_t(s)\}$
End

4.1 Obtaining the Model

After extracting the *eigen-vector* associated to DE from a sequence of *entropy-chromagrams* spaced 100ms between them, we use the components of this vector to determine the observations sequence of the model. We use the absolute magnitudes of the components since it gives robustness to the observations sequence. Fig. 3 shows the plot of the first component of two sequences obtained from two performances of the song *all my loving* played by the Beatles. It is easy to see how both components are similar in behavior through time despite the different dynamic variations (tempo) of both performances. The magnitude of these components maintains similar amplitude, this method is robust to volume, noise, vibrato, articulation, and performer emotion.

The proposed model considers discrete probability distributions over the observations set. This entails a scalar quantization of the values of the components of the *eigen-vectors*. At first we used only one of the twenty components of each *eigen-vector* to form the observations sequence.

To quantize the data of the sequence, we adequate the *Gaussian mixture model* for that matter. This procedure consists of determining the weights, means and variances of the k gaussian densities that best fits the distribution of the data. We use the set of symbols $\Omega = \{1, 2, 3, ...\}$. When the *audio tracking* system gets an observation, it evaluates the observation over each gaussian component. The symbol assigned to the observation corresponds to the number of the gaussian component which emits the greatest probability. An example generated after applying this procedure to one of the data sets plotted in Fig. 3 using four gaussian components, is showed in Fig. 4.

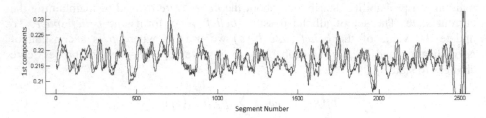

Fig. 3. Plot of the absolute magnitude of the first components

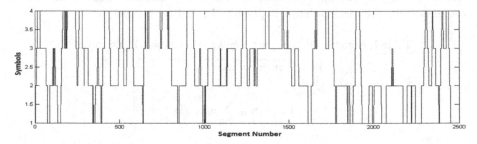

Fig. 4. Sequence of symbols generated from the *gaussian mixture model*

We propose an *ergodic* model, all the transitions are possible among states. The model is defined by a probability transition matrix among states P with elements p_{ij}, and an observation probability matrix Ψ with elements φ_{jk}. The initial estimate for Ψ can be obtained from the sequence of symbols. This estimate consists of determining the frequency of each symbol o_k by a histogram which determines the probability of symbol o_k in the sequence. The estimate assumes the same probability in all the states i (rows of the matrix) for observing symbol o_k, namely,

$$\Psi = \begin{bmatrix} \varphi_{11} \varphi_{12} & \cdots & \varphi_{1k} \\ \vdots & \ddots & \vdots \\ \varphi_{11} \varphi_{12} & \cdots & \varphi_{1k} \end{bmatrix}$$

which satisfies

$$\sum_{j=1}^{K} \varphi_{ij} = 1, \quad 1 \leq i \leq N$$

where K is the number of observed symbols. The transition matrix P can be initialized with random probabilities satisfying,

$$\sum_{j=1}^{N} p_{ij} = 1 \quad 1 \leq i \leq N$$

where N is the number of states. To find the optimal parameters of the model, $\lambda = (P, \Psi)$, we use the *Baum Welch* algorithm. For this, we need to introduce the probability vector of initial state, Π, which is simply initialized with probabilities of $1/N$, the model is trained so the probability of generating the observed sequence is maximized.

5   Preliminaries Results

5.1   Database

The database is composed by 10 songs, for each song we have two performances played sometimes by different musicians and even with different musical instruments. The genres used in these experiments are classical crossover, rock, and pop. All of the songs are WAV format, PCM signals coded to 16 bits and sampled to 44100Hz. The names of the songs are given below in Table 2.

5.2   Preparing the Songs

We take each couple of performances so that one of them is the target audio and the other one simulates the incoming audio stream. For extracting the observations sequence to train the model from the target audio, we split the audio signal, into overlapped segments, each one of them with length of 1s. The hop used between segments was 100ms. To each segment corresponds a 20×20 *entropy-chromagram*, the first component of the *eigen-vector* associated to DE was computed for all the *entropy-chromagrams*. To get the observations sequence from the rendition considered as the incoming audio stream, we followed the same procedure, but with a hop between segments of 1s.

5.3   Testing the Model

To assess the model we used sequences containing 4 symbols, i.e., $\Omega = \{1,2,3,4\}$, we use 4 symbols because that is the number of gaussians. The model is *ergodic* type with 4 states, i.e., $S = \{s_1, s_2, s_3, s_4\}$ (The number of states was obtained product of the experimentation). After training the model with the *Baum Welch* algorithm, we tested the model using the observations sequence from incoming audio stream. The goal was to obtain the decoding of the most probable sequence of states given the observations sequence and the model using both *Viterbi* and *belief path* algorithms. We use the *Viterbi* to obtain the real decoded sequence of states which the model should generate through the time while the rendition is being played live. If the path of the model through the *belief space* generated by the *belief state* $b_t(s)$ equals the sequence of states generated by the *Viterbi* algorithm, then, we can assert that the *belief path* algorithm is at least as good an estimator as Viterbi of the most probable sequence of states. In Fig. 5, we show an example of the sequences of states generated by both algorithms; the continuous line is the sequence generated by the *Viterbi* algorithm and the dashed line is the sequence generated by the *belief path* algorithm. Both sequences generate similar states sequences.

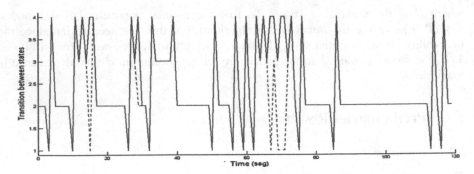

Fig. 5. Sequences of states generated by the *Viterbi* and *belief path* algorithms

Table 2. Results on estimate of states using *belief path* algorithm

Song	studio	Live	Length	Differe	%Diff
Yellow submarine (Beatles)	x		144	14	9.72
Dust in the wind (Sarah Brightman)	x	X	209	38	18.18
Mo Domine (by two different orchestras)	x		212	31	14.62
Hurts like heaven (Coldplay)	x	X	227	25	11.01
Puedes contar conmigo (La oreja de van gogh)	x	X	220	19	8.63
I am addicted (Madonna)	x	X	265	28	10.56
All by myself (Celine Dion)	x	X	288	8	2.7
Geografía (La oreja de van gogh)	x	X	184	16	8.69
You could be mine (Guns and Roses)	x	X	323	60	18.57
Yesterdays (Guns and Roses)	x	X	183	25	13.66

Table 2 shows the results product of comparing the sequences generated by both *Viterbi* and *belief path* algorithms. The first column shows the names of the songs; the second and third columns indicate if the experiment was carried out comparing performances recorded in studio, live or both; fourth column gives the average lengths of the songs; finally, fifth and sixth columns show the number differences and the difference in percent, respectively. The difference is always below 20%, which means the *belief path* algorithm performs well at making *audio-to-audio alignment* in real time.

6   Conclusions and Future Work

In this work we presented an efficient method to extract the most convenient feature to perform *audio-to-audio alignment* aligning performances recorded live and in studio. This feature consists of determining the *eigen-vector* associated to the *dominant eigen-value* which is extracted from *entropy-chromagrams*. This feature encompasses characteristics about the songs as volume, noise, vibrato, articulation and the performer emotion. On the other hand, a new methodology to implement *audio tracking* was introduced. This methodology is based on an estimate of parameters of a *partially observable Markov process*, which generates the most probable sequence of states in real time using a state estimator known as the *belief state*. The preliminary experiment consists of generating the most probable sequence of states from both *Viterbi* and *belief path* algorithms. We use *Baum Welch* algorithm to train the models which consist of 4 states and 4 observations for both HMM and POMP.

As it was described in the previous sections, we use discrete models, namely, we use symbols to refer the observations set, where these observations are the absolute magnitudes of the first components of a sequence the *eigen-vectors*. Besides, we consider *ergodic* models to train the model, so, we arrive to some comments about our results and proposals to future work. With respect to the percent of errors showed in Table 2, we are sure that involving more components will let down this percentage, in other words, we thing that increasing the dimensionality to the problem, the *belief path* algorithm will estimate the same states that the *Viterbi* algorithm. Therefore, these results motive us, since the system was able of estimating the mostly of states despite using a song recorded in studio and a live recorded song where different factors distorts the audio-signal. Also it is necessary to know if the alignment is carried out correctly, so, in the future we will consider *left-right* models where each state corresponds to a time interval. Finally, we will test models with different number of states and continuous models over the observations set.

References

[1] Orio, N., Lemouton, S., Schwarz, D.: Score following: state of the art and new developments. In: Proceedings of the Conference on New Interfaces for Musical Expression, Singapore, pp. 36–41 (2003)

[2] Dannenberg, R., Raphael, C.: Music score alignment and computer accompaniment. Communications of the ACM, Special Issue 49(8), 39–43 (2006)

[3] Suzuki, K., Ueda, Y., Raczynski, S.A., Ono, N., Sagayama, S.: Real-5time Audio to Score Alignment Using Locally-constrained Dynamic Time Warping of Chromagrams (2011)

[4] Montecchio, N., Cont, A.: A unified approach to real time audio-to-score and audio-to-audio alignment using sequential Montecarlo inference techniques. In: IEEE International Conference on Acoustics, Speech and Signal Processing (2011)

[5] Dixon, S.: Live tracking of musical performances using on-line time warping. In: 8th International Conference on Digital Audio Effects. Austrian Research Institute for Artificial Intelligence, Vienna (September 2005)

[6] Dixon, S., Widmer, G.: Match: A music alignment tool chest. In: 6th International Conference on Music Information Retrieval. Austrian Research Institute for Artificial Intelligence, Vienna (2005)

[7] Camarena-Ibarrola, A., Chávez, E.: Online music tracking with global alignment. International Journal of Matching Learning and Cybernetics 2(3), 147–156 (2011)

[8] Manzo-Martinez, A., Camarena-Ibarrola, J.A.: A robust characterization of audio signals using the level of information content per Chroma. In: IEEE International Symposium on Signal Processing and Information Technology (December 2011)

[9] Misra, H., Ikbal, S., Bourlard, H., Hermansky, H.: Spectral entropy based feature for robust asr. In: Proceedings of International Conference on Acoustics, Speech, and Signal Processing, pp. 193–196 (May 2004)

[10] Mohammad, A.: Entropy in signal processing. In: Traitement du Signal, pp. 87–116 (1994)

[11] Aucouturier, J., Defreville, B., Pachet, F.: The bag-of-frame approach to audio pattern recognition: A sufficient model for urban soundscapes but not for polyphonic music. Journal of Acoustical Society of America (2007)

[12] Poole, D.: Linear Algebra: A Modern Introduction. Cengage Learning (2011)

[13] Panju, M.: Iterative Methods for Computing Eigenvalues and Eigenvectors. In the Waterloo Mathematics Review, University of Waterloo, pp. 9–18

Statistical Features Based Noise Type Identification

Sohail Masood[2,3], Ismael Soto[4], Ayyaz Hussain[1], and M. Arfan Jaffar[2]

[1] Department of Computer Science, International Islamic University Islamabad, Pakistan
[2] Department of Computer Science, National University of Computer and Emerging Sciences, FAST-NU, Islamabad, Pakistan
[3] Departmento de Ingeneria Electrica de la Universidad de Chile, Santiago, Chile
[4] Departmento de Ingenieria Eléctrica de la Universidad de Santiago de Chile, Santiago, Chile
rsmbhatti@gmail.com, ismael.soto@usach.cl,
ayyaz.hussain@iiu.edu.pk, arfan.jaffar@nu.edu.pk

Abstract. In this paper, a new technique for automatically identifying the type of noise in digital images has been proposed. Our statistical features based noise Type identification scheme uses machine learning to distinguish different types of noises. Local features of 3x3 window are used to train the machine learning based classifier. Two types of noise (salt & peppers and random-valued) is catered for in this paper. Experiments show that the proposed technique gives promising results and can be enhanced to be a generic noise identification system for every type of noise.

Keywords: Noise Type Identification, Machine Learning, Digital Image Processing.

1 Introduction

Noise detection and removal from digital images is very primary task in most of digital image processing applications. Images corrupted with noise are first analyzed to find the type of noise and then specific noise detection and removal algorithm is applied for that type of noise. Different applications assume the type of expected noise depending upon their environment and apply algorithm for detection and removal of that noise type. With the increase in digital image processing applications for versatile and dynamic environment, the assumption of a specific type of noise is no more valid. Now a days, image processing applications are used in variety of way and in almost every discipline of life. So images can get corrupted with different types of noise in different times in a dynamic environment. There is a need of some mechanism to automatically identify the type of noise; so that one can apply specific algorithm for that type of noise.

Noise type identification is a very new topic of research and very little work has been done on it. In [1], Noise identification using Local Histograms method is proposed which consists of roughly segmenting and labeling the noisy image. The image of labels is then used for the selection of homogeneous regions.

In [2], a neural network based technique for identifying the type of noise present in a noisy image is proposed. The proposed method exhibits fast training process and

A. Gelbukh et al. (Eds.): MICAI 2014, Part II, LNAI 8857, pp. 231–241, 2014.
© Springer International Publishing Switzerland 2014

does not require any assumption in the given images such as homogeneous areas etc. Its accuracy gets down with the increase in noise density.

[3, 4, 5] implement statistical feature extraction for calculating the statistical properties and a simple pattern classification scheme is applied on the features to identify the noise type present in an image. This method first applies noise removal filters for all types of noises, subtracts the resulting image from original image to get noise and then tries to identify it.

In [14], Gonzalez and woods has given some methods for noise type identification, which are based on histogram analysis. These methods are based on global perspective and can be used to get an estimate about occurrence of a noise type in an image. These methods have some limitations or assumptions to work e.g. they require imaging system to be present or location information of noise is known or a single type of noise present in the image [14].

All the techniques available in literature simply inform about presence of a certain type of noise in an image but can't tell about the location of the noise. In this paper we have proposed a generic noise type identification method, which identifies noise type based of local window and thus can tell about the noise type in each corrupted pixel individually. Our technique not only works good for whole range of noise but also performs very well for mixed noise.

2   Major Contributions

In order to identify noise type, we have proposed a machine learning based approach which uses well-known statistical features to identify different types of noise. Main contributions of the proposed technique are:

- Novel approach for identification of noise type using statistical features and machine learning algorithm.
- Our method not only identifies the type of noise but also gives location of certain type of noise.
- Our technique identifies noise type on pixel by pixel bases, so it also has the capability to detect multiple types of noises present at different parts in a single image.
- Proposed technique identifies noise type with high accuracy without any prior knowledge about degradation process or original image.

Rest of the paper is organized as follows:

Section 3 explains the proposed technique. Section 4 discusses experimental results and discussions. Section 5 gives conclusion and future work.

3   Proposed Technique

The proposed technique uses well-known local statistical features of the images and utilizes Decision Tree algorithm (C4.5) [12] to solve the problem of noise type identification. Standard artificially generated training image [6, 7, and 13] is used to train machine learning (ML) algorithm and then tested over database of images. Ten well-known statistical features (which are discussed below) are used for the training of algorithm.

Figure 1 shows the proposed system architecture. Detailed procedure comprising of different steps is given below.

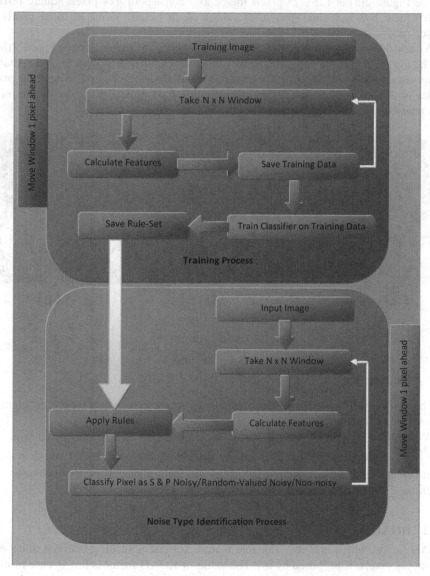

Fig. 1. Proposed System Architecture

3.1 Training Data Generation

Selection of a good training image is the most vital part of a trainable noise identification system. A synthetically created training image is used in [6, 7, and 13], which has more generalization capability. In Figure 2, we have shown the training and target images used by [6, 7, and 13].

The Figure 2(a) is 128x128 pixels image and consists of 4x4 pixels square boxes. Each square box has same gray level values of all pixels. Value of these pixels is chosen randomly between [0, 255].

We add 50% impulse noise to the first image to obtain the training image Figure 2(b).

The Figure 2(c) is the target image for our noise identification system, and contains white and black spots denoting the existence and absence of noise. Since the pixel values of the training image are chosen randomly, training a network for this training data provides more accurate results for all class of images.

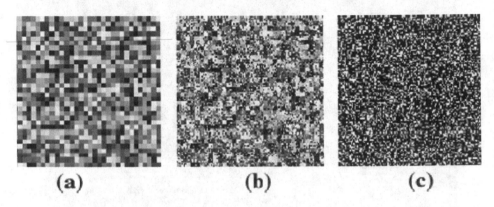

(a) **(b)** **(c)**

Fig. 2. Training Image [13]

3.2 Feature Set

We have used well-known statistical features in image processing for the problem of impulse noise detection.

We applied 10 well-known statistical functions on the N x N considered window. The N x N window is converted to a single dimensional 1x N^2 vector and then these functions are applied on it. Here is the detail and significance of each of the statistical function.

3.2.1 ROAD

ROAD factor, which is a very valuable feature for distinguishing between noisy and non-noisy pixels, is proposed by [8]. The value of ROAD factor is low in case of non-noisy pixels and high in case of noisy pixels. The ROAD factor is calculated using following steps:

First of all, absolute deleted difference is calculated among considered vector and the central pixel (for a 3x3 window, it consists of eight elements).

$$dn = |x - x\left(\frac{n}{2}\right)|$$

In the next step, this vector is sorted in increasing order. ROAD factor is the sum of the first four values of this sorted vector.

ROAD value is calculated for each pixel using its $N \times N$ window.

3.2.2 MAD

MAD (median of absolute deviations from the median) is a robust order statistics of the local variance [10] calculated according to the following equation:

$$MAD = median(abs(x - med))$$

Where x is the considered vector and med is the median of the considered vector.

MAD is a robust estimator and has the capability of accurately estimating distribution variance, even if the specified window has more than 50% corrupted samples.

3.2.3 Standard Deviation

Standard deviation of a vector is calculated as:

$$s = \left[\frac{1}{n-1}\sum_{i=1}^{n}(x_i - \bar{x})^2\right]^{\frac{1}{2}}$$

Where

$$\bar{x} = \frac{1}{n}\sum_{i=1}^{n}x_i$$

3.2.4 Variance

Variance is square of the standard deviation and is calculated as:

$$v = \frac{1}{n-1}\sum_{i=1}^{n}(x_i - \bar{x})^2$$

Where

$$\bar{x} = \frac{1}{n}\sum_{i=1}^{n}x_i$$

3.2.5 Median

Median is the value at middle index of a sorted vector and can be calculated as:

$$med = dx\left(\frac{n}{2}\right)$$

Where n is the size of the sorted difference vector dx, and dx is difference of the vector from central pixel.

3.2.6 Mean

Mean is calculated as:

$$\bar{x} = \frac{1}{n}\sum_{i=1}^{n} dx_i$$

Where dx is the difference of the vector from central pixel.

3.2.7 Min

Min returns the smallest value of the difference vector dx.

3.2.8 Max

Max returns the largest value of the difference vector dx.

3.2.9 Entropy

Entropy is a statistical measure of randomness and is calculated as:

$$entropy = -\sum_{k=1}^{m} p_k.* \log2(p_k)$$

Where p_k contains the histogram counts for k^{th} gray level and m is total number of gray levels in the image.

3.2.10 Rold

ROLD is proposed by [9] and is very good feature to detect random-valued impulse noise. It can be defined as:

$$ROLD_m(y_{i,j}) = \sum_{k=1}^{m} R_k(y_{i,j})$$

Where R_k is the kth smallest D_{st} for all $(s, t) \in \Omega_N^0$ and $D_{st}(y_{i,j})$ is defined as

$$D_{st}\left(y_{i,j}\right) = 1 + \frac{\max\left\{\log_2\left|y_{i+s,j+t} - y_{i,j}\right|, -5\right\}}{5} \qquad \forall(s,t) \in \Omega_N^0$$

3.3   Training of Classifiers

We take the training image and add 50% random-valued impulse noise. 3x3 window is taken from start of image and is moved through the image. Feature vector of each of the window is calculated and is used for training. The target value or class of the considered feature vector is 0, if central pixel of the window is noise-free and class is 1 for random-valued impulse noise.

Same training image is taken again and 50% salt & peppers noise is added to it. Same process is repeated except class is set to 2 for salt & peppers noise. Feature vectors and class of both types are merged to form the training data. So now we have feature vectors having salt & peppers noise, having random-valued noise, and having noise-free pixels.

This is a 3 class classification problem, which has been solved using machine learning based classifier.

After training, classifier generates a model or set of rules to be used in future for the process of noise detection. In the case of C4.5 [12], a set of rules are generated after the completion of training. These rules are in the form of IF-THEN-ELSE and can be directly used in real time. To detect noise type in a given image, same set of features of the current window (given in section 3.2) are calculated and are passed through to the rule set. The central pixel of the current window will be non-noisy if the output is 0, will have random-valued noise, if output is 1, and will have salt & peppers noise, if output is 2.

4   Experimental Results

We have performed comprehensive experiments to show the performance of the proposed technique. First of all we generated training data from training image (Fig. 3) as discussed in section 3. Classifier is trained on this training data. For testing purpose, we have used standard test images. Results have been reported on 4 standard images i.e. Baboon, Lena, Parrots, and Peppers. All these images have totally different texture pattern and dynamic range. So the results reported here are representative of wide range of image types.

Performance Measures used in the experiments are True Positive Rate, False Positive Rate, and Accuracy [11]. These measures are widely used in literature to gauge the performance of a classifier. Here is the description of these performance measures.

"The True Positive (TP) rate is the proportion of examples which were classified as class x, among all examples which truly have class x, i.e. how much part of the class was captured. In the confusion matrix, this is the diagonal element divided by the sum over the relevant row". [11].

"The False Positive (FP) rate is the proportion of examples which were classified as class x, but belong to a different class, among all examples which are not of class x. In the matrix, this is the column sum of class x minus the diagonal element, divided by the rows sums of all other classes". [11]

"Accuracy is defined as the total number of correctly classified instances for all classes divided by the total number of instances in the test set"[11].

Table 1 shows the overall accuracy of the classifier for whole range of noise density. We see that overall accuracy is above 96% for the whole range and for all test images.

Table 1. Noise Type Identification Accuracy

		Accuracy (%)			
		Baboon	**Lena**	**Parrots**	**Peppers**
	10%	97.628	96.643	97.128	96.517
	20%	96.772	96.551	96.681	96.555
	30%	97.043	97.118	97.121	96.969
	40%	97.166	97.392	97.254	96.994
Noise Density	50%	97.509	97.575	97.698	97.568
	60%	97.997	97.736	97.84	97.775
	70%	97.682	97.446	97.547	97.488
	80%	97.241	97.014	96.91	97.007
	90%	97.156	97.184	96.98	96.927

Table 2. TP and FP Rates for Baboon Image

		TP Rate (%)			FP Rate (%)		
		Non-Noisy	Random-Valued	Salt & Peppers	Non-Noisy	Random-Valued	Salt & Peppers
	10%	99.36	99.62	64.42	18.01	0.00	0.62
	20%	99.64	99.68	70.14	15.02	0.00	0.32
	30%	99.73	99.44	82.07	9.18	0.01	0.21
	40%	99.63	99.22	87.75	6.55	0.04	0.23
Noise Density	50%	99.43	98.74	92.50	4.40	0.13	0.25
	60%	98.53	98.61	96.69	2.36	0.57	0.27
	70%	96.64	98.42	97.86	1.86	1.29	0.27
	80%	90.98	98.66	98.96	1.19	2.77	0.24
	90%	77.69	99.20	99.48	0.66	3.99	0.09

Tables 2 and 3 show the TP and FP rates at different noise densities for the three classes i.e. Non-noisy, Random-valued noise, and salt & peppers noise. We see that TP rate for Noise-Free and random-valued class is high for whole range of noise density. But at 90% noise Noise-Free pixel detection performance is degraded. Similarly at low noise density, some salt & peppers noisy pixels are misclassified as Noise-Free pixels.TP and FP rates for random-valued class remain good and stable for whole range of noise density.

Table 3. TP and FP Rates for Lena Image

		TP Rate (%)			FP Rate (%)		
		Non-Noisy	Random-Valued	Salt & Peppers	Non-Noisy	Random-Valued	Salt & Peppers
	10%	98.28	99.821	63.831	17.672	0.0067	1.6145
	20%	99.00	99.545	74.002	13.405	0.0035	0.8925
	30%	99.51	99.684	83.504	8.4426	0.0037	0.4043
	40%	99.58	99.265	89.15	5.8754	0.0196	0.2967
Noise Density	50%	99.40	99.064	92.44	4.254	0.1594	0.2435
	60%	98.40	98.578	96.004	2.7054	0.6264	0.2877
	70%	96.06	98.217	97.874	1.9545	1.5206	0.3092
	80%	90.46	98.544	98.859	1.2989	3.0395	0.2038
	90%	78.75	99.10	99.474	0.7123	3.8295	0.1144

Table 4. TP and FP Rates for Parrots Image

		TP Rate (%)			FP Rate (%)		
		Non-Noisy	Random-Valued	Salt & Peppers	Non-Noisy	Random-Valued	Salt & Peppers
	10%	98.707	99.626	66.5	16.895	0.006634	1.2206
	20%	99.207	99.675	73.729	13.537	0.010461	0.7041
	30%	99.445	99.497	84.054	8.2116	0.007413	0.46396
	40%	99.48	99.46	88.494	6.0751	0.058937	0.33164
Noise Density	50%	99.262	98.886	93.328	3.8815	0.17188	0.32659
	60%	98.375	98.607	96.348	2.5223	0.56114	0.37258
	70%	96.101	98.605	97.729	1.8325	1.4729	0.32922
	80%	90.093	98.357	98.819	1.4127	2.9418	0.33067
	90%	76.228	99.25	99.356	0.6969	4.1857	0.16036

Table 5. TP and FP Rates for Peppers Image

		TP Rate (%)			FP Rate (%)		
		Non-Noisy	Random-Valued	Salt & Peppers	Non-Noisy	Random-Valued	Salt & Peppers
	10%	98.227	99.819	61.645	19.716	0.004428	1.682
	20%	99.134	99.652	73.682	13.72	0.014025	0.76268
	30%	99.421	99.327	83.107	8.725	0.014909	0.47151
	40%	99.425	99.169	87.489	6.6695	0.063171	0.37967
Noise Density	50%	99.326	98.892	92.593	4.2402	0.16836	0.28519
	60%	98.462	98.678	95.934	2.6941	0.60046	0.28822
	70%	96.39	98.46	97.469	2.0374	1.3339	0.33784
	80%	90.349	98.501	98.943	1.2793	2.9826	0.30724
	90%	78.084	98.833	99.332	0.91739	3.8877	0.19153

5   Conclusion

We proposed a novel method for identification of noise type in digital images. Experiments show promising results as we have achieved minimum accuracy of 96% for the whole range of noise density. Further experimentation is required to make this scheme more generic and reliable. For future work, here are some options to explore more.

- In this paper, we have taken 3x3 fixed window size. In future we can change window size to 5x5 or 7x7 etc.
- We have used C4.5 (Decision Tree) for classification purpose, which is not a specialized classifier for multi-class problems. We can use some evolutionary algorithm based classifier in future, which are known to perform better for multi-class problems.

Here we have considered only two types of noise. In future, we'll add more noise types to make it a generic noise identification system.

Acknowledgements. The authors acknowledge the financial support of the Higher Education Commission Pakistan and "Center for Multidisciplinary Research on Signal Processing" (CONICYT/ACT1120 Project) and the USACH/DICYT 061413SG Project.

References

1. Ghouse, M., Siddappa, M.: Adaptive Techniques based high Impulsive Noise Detection and Reduction of a Digital Image. Journal of Theoretical and Applied Information Technology 24(1) (2011)
2. Karibasappa, K.G., et al.: Neural Network Based Noise Identification in Digital Images. In: Proceedings of International Conference on Advances in Computer Engineering (2011)
3. Subashini, P., Bharathi, P.T.: Automatic Noise Identification in Images using Statistical Features. International Journal for Computer Science and Technology 2(3) (2011)
4. Raina, et al.: An approach for image noise identification using minimum distance classifier. International Journal of Scientific and Engineering Research 3(4) (2012)
5. Chen, Y., et al.: An automated technique for image noise identification using a simple pattern classification approach. In: Proceeding of Midwest Symposium on Circuits and Systems (2007)
6. Emin Yüksel, M., Besd_ok, E.: A simple neuro-fuzzy impulse detector for efficient blur reduction of impulse noise removal operators for digital images. IEEE Transaction on Fuzzy Systems 12(6) (2004)
7. Emin Yüksel, M.: A hybrid neuro-fuzzy filter for edge preserving restoration of images corrupted by impulse noise, IEEE Transaction on Image Processing 15 (4) (2006)
8. Garnett, R., Huegerich, T., Chui, C., He, W.: A universal noise removal algorithm with an impulse detector. IEEE Transaction on Image Processing 14(11) (2005)
9. Dong, Y., Chan, R.H., Xu, S.: A detection statistic for random-valued impulse noise. IEEE Transaction on Image Processing 16(4) (2007)
10. Huber, P.: Robust Statistics. Wiley, New York (1981)

11. Fawcett, T.: An introduction to ROC analysis. Pattern Recognition Letters 27(8), 861–874 (2006)
12. Quinlan, J.R.: C4.5: Programs for Machine Learning. Morgan Kaufmann Publishers, San Francisco (1993)
13. Kaliraj, G., Baskar, S.: An efficient approach for the removal of impulse noise from the corrupted image using neural network based impulse detector. Image and Vision Computing 28, 458–466 (2010)
14. Gonzalez, R.C., Woods, R.E.: Digital Image Processing. Addison-Wesley (1992)

Using Values of the Human Cochlea
in the Macro and Micro Mechanical Model
for Automatic Speech Recognition

José Luis Oropeza Rodríguez and Sergio Suárez Guerra

Computing Research Center, National Polytechnic Institute,
Juan de Dios Batiz s/n, P.O. 07038, Mexico
{joropeza,ssuarez}@cic.ipn.mx

Abstract. Recently the parametric representation using cochlea behavior has been used in different studies related with Automatic Speech Recognition (ASR). That is because this hearing organ in mammalians is the most important element used to make a transduction of the sound pressure that is received by the outer ear. This paper shows how the macro and micro mechanical model is used in ASR tasks. The values that Neely, Elliot and Ku founded in their works, related with the macro and micro mechanical model such as Neely were used to set the central frequencies of a bank filter to obtain parameters from the speech in a similar form as MFCC (Mel Frequency Cepstrum Coefficients) has been constructed.

An approach that considers a new form to distribute the bank filter in our parametric representation is proposed. Then this distribution of the bank filter to have a different representation of the speech in frequency domain compared with MFCC is applied. The response of these three values mentioned above into macro and micro mechanical model to create the central frequencies of the bank filter were used, then the Mel scale function substituted by a representation based in the cochlear response based on the Neely model. This model was used with a set of different parameters of the cochlea, used by Nelly, Elliot and Ku in their works, such as mass, damping and stiffness; among others. A performance of 98 to 100% was reached for a task that uses Spanish isolated digits pronounced by 5 different speakers. Corpus SUSAS with neutral sound records with some advantages in comparison with MFCC was applied.

Keywords: Speech recognition, cochlea, place theory and bank filter.

1   Introduction

For a long time Automatic Speech Recognition Systems (ASRs) have used parameters related with Cepstrum and Homomorphic Analysis of Speech [1], Linear Prediction Coefficient (LPC) [2], Mel Frequency Cepstrum Coefficients (MFCC) [3], and Perceptual Linear Prediction (PLP) [4], these last two being the most important. In each of these representations, the principal objective is to have a representation to compress speech data without irrelevant information not pertinent to the phonetic analysis of the data and to enhance aspects of the signal that contribute significantly to the detection of phonetic differences. MFCC and PLP coefficients employ Mel and Bark

A. Gelbukh et al. (Eds.): MICAI 2014, Part II, LNAI 8857, pp. 242–251, 2014.

scales respectively. These consider perceptual aspects to obtain a set of coefficients that represent the speech signal.

On the other hand, the most important organ in human hearing is the cochlea and various physiological models have been proposed [5] and [6]. Recently works related with the application of the cochlea behavior in ASR systems can be found, that is because in recent years the researchers have emphasized "human engineering", that is, to adopt the processing strategies of the human auditory perception. The application of such a human perceptual feature may improve ASR performance which has been established in literature [7][8][9][10][11][12]. In [12] an extraordinarily precise auditory model was used extracting the excitation dependent shapes of the delay trajectories and then a set of features were used without any other spectral information to carry out speech recognition task under different noise conditions on the TIMIT database. However, average recognition rates do not reach that of the MFCC features (except for very low noise SNRs), but the system behaves very stable under different noise conditions. In [11] they proposed a feature extraction method for ASR based on the differential processing strategy of the AVCN, PVCN and the DCN of the nucleus cochlear. The method utilized a zero-crossing with peak amplitudes (ZCPA) auditory model as synchrony detector to discriminate the low frequency formants. They used HMM recognition using isolated digits that showed better recognition rates in clean and non- stationary noise conditions than the existing auditory model. In [10] they employed a counterpart of the next physiological processing step in comparison with frequency decomposition and compression of amplitudes concepts. A simplified model of short-term adaptation was incorporated into MFCC feature extraction. They compared the proposal mentioned above with that structurally related to RASTA, CMS and Wiener filtering which performs well in combination with Wiener filtering. Compared with the structurally related RASTA, the adaptation model provides superior performance on AURORA 2, and, if Wiener filtering is used prior to both approaches, on AURORA 3 as well.

2   Characteristics and Generalities

The cochlea is a long, narrow, fluid-filled tunnel which spirals through the temporal bone. This tunnel is divided along its length by a cochlear partition into an upper compartment called scala vestibuli (SV) and lower compartment called scala timpani (ST). At the apex of the cochlea, SV and ST are connected to each other by the helicotrema [13]. A set of models to represent the operation of the cochlea has been proposed [14][15][16][17]; among others. In mammals, vibrations of the stapes set up a wave with a particular shape on the basilar membrane. The amplitude envelope of the wave is first increasing and then decreasing, and the position at the peak of the envelope is dependent on the frequency of the stimulus [18]. The amplitude of the envelope is a two-dimensional function of distance from the stapes and frequency of stimulation. The curve shown in Fig. 1 is a cross-section of the function for fixed frequency. If low frequencies excite the cochlea, the envelope is nearest to the apex, but if high frequencies excite it the envelope is nearest to the base.

This paper proposes an equation extracted from the fluid mechanical model to find a relationship between these frequencies and the place of the excitation into the cochlea. With that value a new distribution of the bank filter to extract parameters for ASR tasks is proposed.

In the micromechanical the anatomical structure of a radial cross-section (RCS) of the cochlear partition (CP) is illustrated in the following figure 2. In the model, the basilar membrane (BM) and tectorial membrane (TM) are each represented as a lumped mass with both stiffness and damping in their attachment to the surrounding bone. When the cochlea determines the frequency of the incoming signal from the place on the basilar membrane of maximum amplitude, the organ of Corti is excited, in conjunction with the movement of tectorial membrane; the inner and outer hair cells are excited obtaining an electrical pulse that travels by auditory nerve.

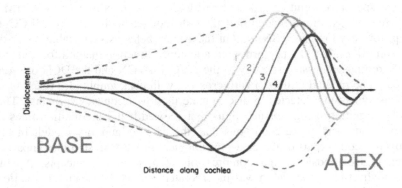

Fig. 1. Wave displacement inside cochlea

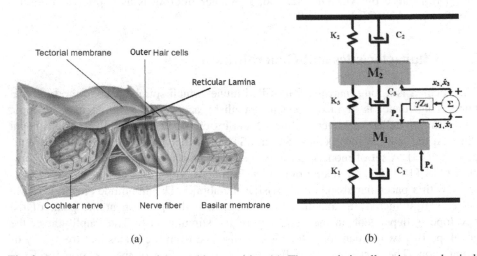

(a)   (b)

Fig. 2. Anatomical structure of the cochlear partition (a). The outer hair cells, micro mechanical representation (b).

Now the modeling cochlear will be divided in two ways of study. The first is the hydrodynamic movement that produced a movement on the basilar membrane and the second is the movement of the outer hair cells. This is named as the model of Macro and Micro Mechanical Cochlear [17]. The equations that describe the Macro Mechanical Cochlear are [17]:

$$\frac{d^2}{dx^2} P_d(x) = \frac{2\rho}{H} \ddot{\varepsilon}_p(x),$$ (1)

$$\frac{d}{dx} P_d(0) = 2\rho \ddot{\varepsilon}_s,$$ (2)

$$\frac{d}{dx} P_d(L) = 2\rho \ddot{\varepsilon}_h,$$ (3)

The equations (1), (2) and (3) were solved by finite difference, using central differences for (1), forward differences for the (2) and backward difference for (3), generating a tri-diagonal Matrix system[16] which we solved using the Thomas algorithm. It represents the Micro mechanical, because it uses the organ of Corti values.

$$
\begin{bmatrix}
\left(\frac{2\rho i \omega}{Z_m} - \frac{1}{\Delta}\right) & \frac{1}{\Delta} & \cdots & 0 & 0 & 0 & \cdots & 0 & 0 \\
\vdots & \ddots & \ddots & & \vdots & \vdots & \vdots & & \vdots \\
0 & & \ddots & & \vdots & \vdots & \vdots & & 0 \\
0 & 0 & \cdots & \frac{1}{\Delta^2} & -\left(\frac{2}{\Delta^2} + \frac{2\rho i \omega}{H Z_p(X_n)}\right) & \frac{1}{\Delta^2} & \cdots & 0 & 0 \\
0 & \vdots & \vdots & \vdots & \cdots & \cdots & & 0 \\
\vdots & \vdots & \vdots & \vdots & & \ddots & \ddots & 0 \\
0 & 0 & \cdots & 0 & 0 & \cdots & \frac{1}{\Delta} & -\left(\frac{1}{\Delta} - \frac{2\rho i \omega}{C_h}\right)
\end{bmatrix}
\begin{bmatrix}
P_d(X_1) \\
P_d(X_2) \\
\vdots \\
P_d(X_{n-1}) \\
P_d(X_n) \\
P_d(X_{n+1}) \\
\vdots \\
P_d(X_{N-1}) \\
P_d(X_N)
\end{bmatrix}
=
\begin{bmatrix}
\left(\frac{2\rho i \omega A_m}{Z_m G_m A_s}\right) P_e \\
0 \\
\vdots \\
0 \\
0 \\
0 \\
\vdots \\
0 \\
0
\end{bmatrix}
$$ (4)

The solution for P_d obtains the maximum amplitude on the basilar membrane shown in Figure 3. For these experiments the cochlear distance pattern is obtained manually. As can be seen, to solve equation 4 a set of variables related with the physiology of the cochlea is needed and some of these variables are described in table 1. These values are immersed into Z_p and Z_m; for example in [17].

Figures 3, and 4; show the behavior of the basilar membrane with the values shown in table 1. As is seen, before 300 Hz the behavior of the micro and macro mechanical model is not adequate, independently of the parameters used. This result is a consequence of the characteristics of the model proposed by [17]. Proposing our analysis from this frequency to 4.5 KHz was decided. Also, the response obtained has a behavior logarithmic. This is an important indication because the Mel function is related with a similar mathematical function.

Table 1. Values used in equation

Parameter	Neely & Kim 1986 (cgs)	Ku (human cochlea, 2008)IS	Elliot (2007)IS
$k_1(x)$	$1.1 * 10^9 e^{-4x}$	$1.65 * 10^8 e^{-2.79(x+0.00373)}$	$4.95 * 10^8 e^{-3.2(x+0.00375)}$
$c_1(x)$	$20 + 1500 e^{-2x}$	$0.9 + 999 e^{-1.53(x+0.00373)}$	$0.1 + 1970 e^{-1.79(x+0.00375)}$
$m_1(x)$	$3 * 10^{-3}$	$4.5 * 10^{-4}$	$1.35 * 10^{-3}$
$k_2(x)$	$7 * 10^6 e^{-4.4x}$	$1.05 * 10^6 e^{-3.07(x+0.00373)}$	$3.15 * 10^6 e^{-3.52(x+0.00375)}$
$c_2(x)$	$10 e^{-2.2x}$	$3 e^{-1.71(x+0.00373)}$	$11.3 e^{-1.76(x+0.00375)}$
$m_2(x)$	$0.5 * 10^{-3}$	$0.72 * 10^{-4} + 0.28710^{-2}x$	$2.3 * 10^{-4}$
$k_3(x)$	$1 * 10^7 e^{-4x}$	$1.5 * 10^6 e^{-2.79(x+0.00373)}$	$4.5 * 10^6 e^{-3.2(x+0.00375)}$
$c_3(x)$	$2 e^{-0.8x}$	$0.66 e^{-0.593(x+0.00373)}$	$2.25 e^{-0.64(x+0.00375)}$
$k_4(x)$	$6.15 * 10^8 e^{-4x}$	$9.23 * 10^7 e^{-2.79(x+0.00373)}$	$2.84 * 10^8 e^{-3.2(x+0.00375)}$
$c_4(x)$	$1040 e^{-2x}$	$330 e^{-1.44(x+0.00373)}$	$965 e^{-1.64(x+0.00375)}$
gamma	1	1	1
g	1	1	1
b	0.4	0.4	0.4
L	2.5	3.5	3.5
H	0.1	0.1	0.1
K_m	$2.1 * 10^5$	$2.63 * 10^7$	$2.63 * 10^7$
C_m	400	$2.8 * 10^3$	$2.8 * 10^3$
M_m	$45 * 10^3$	$2.96 * 10^{-3}$	$2.96 * 10^{-3}$
C_h	0.1	0.1	0.1
A_s	0.01	$3.2 * 10^{-1}$	$3.2 * 10^{-1}$
A_m	0.35 cm^2	0.429-0.55 cm^2	0.429-0.55 cm^2
Rho	0.35	1	1
N	250	500	500
Gm	0.5	0.5	0.5

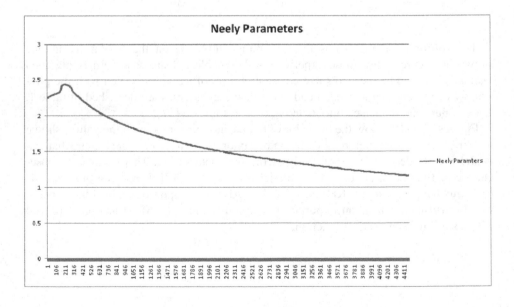

Fig. 3. Neely´s model using his parameters

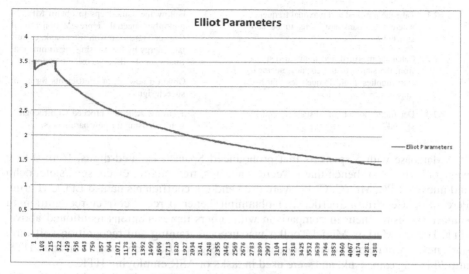

Fig. 4. Neely´s model using Elliot parameters

As mentioned above, the Neely model and later works have considered putting a number of these micro-mechanisms along the cochlea at the same distance between them. For that, this principle to establish the following relation between a minimal and maximal distance was used.

$$d(n) = dmax + \sum_{n=0}^{n=nint} n\frac{dmin - dmax}{nint + 1},$$

(5)

Where d_{min} and d_{max} are obtained from Figure 3 and 4, considering that $F_{min}=300$ Hz and $F_{max}=4.5$ KHz. This paper proposed a space equidistant between different points to analyze the cochlea. After that, for each distance one specifically frequency of excitation to the Basilar Membrane was obtained.

3   Experiments and Results

From the last analysis a computational model to obtain the distance where the maximum displacement of the basilar membrane occurs to a specific excitation frequency of the system was developed, which depends of the physical characteristics of the basilar membrane. The following procedure describes the computational model of the cochlea using this propose [20]. It is important to mention that the maximum response of the pressure curve used in [19] was obtained.

1. Obtain speech signal, realize preprocessing (It includes pre-emphasis, segmentation, windowing and feature extraction), for each sentence.

2. In the feature extraction, the same procedure as MFCC was used but the filter bank is constructed following the next steps.

2.4 Determine the frequency related with these distances, this represents the center of the filter bank.

2.5 Construct filter bank with frequency center obtained from the analysis of the Neely model using values in table 1.

2.1 Take the minimal and maximal frequency where filter bank are going to be constructed.

2.2 Calculate maximal and minimal distance from the stapes of the cochlea, nearer to start implies high frequencies, farthest implies low frequencies.

2.3 Determine a set of distances equally spaced

3. Follow the same steps to obtain MFCC, multiply spectral representation from Fourier Transform with filter bank, calculate energy by bands using logarithm, and finally, apply discrete cosine transform.

4. Obtain a new set of coefficients for each speech signal.

5. Train the ASR and proceed with recognition task using the new parameters.

A database with 5 speakers that pronounced Spanish isolated digits, from 0 to 9 was applied as workbench that is "cero, uno, dos, tres, cuatro, cinco, seis, siete, ocho and nueve". LPC, MFCC, CLPC were used and our coefficients named EPCC (Earing Perception Cepstrum Coefficients) obtaining better percent correct recognition in some tasks using them in comparison with others representations mentioned above. HTK Hidden Markov Model Toolkit was used as training and recognition software; our new parameters were added into HSigp.c file, contained inside HTK http://htk.eng.cam.ac.uk, and were used in tasks of ASR employing HTK.

This first experimental used a database that contains only digits in the Spanish language and the characteristics of the samples were frequency sample 11025, 8 bits per sample, PCM coding, mono-stereo. The evaluation of the experiment proposed involved 5 people (3 men and 2 women) with 300 speech sentences to recognize for each one (100 for training task and 200 for recognition task). 1500 speech sentences extracted from 5 speakers individually were taken, and the Automatic Speech Recognition trained using Hidden Markov Models with 6 states (4 states with information and 2 dummies to connection with another chain). Also, 3 Gaussian Mixture for each state in the Markov chain were employed. The parameters extracted from the speech signal were 39 (13 MFCC, 13 delta and 13 energy coefficients) when using MFCC or our proposal, and used to train the Hidden Markov Model. Table 1 contains results obtained in percentages when using LPC, CLPC, MFCC and our parametric representation to train as parameters. Table 2 shows results using Delta and Acceleration coefficients. It is important to mention that HTK give us results in two forms: by sentence and by words http://htk.eng.cam.ac.uk. We show both for reasons of consistency. Table 3 contains results obtained in percentage when using LPC, CLPC and MFCC, DELTA, ACCELERATION AND THIRD DIFFERENTIAL.

Table 2. LPC, CLPC and MFCC coefficients

SENTENCES				*WORDS*			
PARAMETERS/# STATES	*4*	*5*	*6*	PARAMETERS/# STATES	*4*	*5*	*6*
LPC	87.5	94	94	LPC	87.94	94.47	94.47
CLPC	90	97.5	98.5	CLPC	90.45	97.99	98.99
MFCC	97.5	97	99	MFCC	97.99	97.49	99.5
EPCC KU	98	99	99.5	EPCC KU	98.45	99.5	99.8
EPCC ELLIOT	98.5	98.5	99	EPCC ELLIOT	98.75	98.75	99.5
EPCC NEELY	98.7	99	99.5	EPCC NEELY	98.5	99.5	99.75

Table 3. LPC, CLPC, MFCC, DELTA AND ACCELERATION coefficient

SENTENCES				*WORDS*			
PARAMETERS/# STATES	*4*	*5*	*6*	PARAMETERS/# STATES	*4*	*5*	*6*
LPC	79	90.5	91.5	LPC	79.4	99.4	91.96
CLPC	93	99	99	CLPC	93.47	99.5	99.5
MFCC	99	99	99	MFCC	99.5	99.5	99.5
EPCC KU	100	100	100	EPCC KU	100	100	100
EPCC ELLIOT	100	100	100	EPCC ELLIOT	100	100	100
EPCC NEELY	100	100	100	EPCC NEELY	100	100	100

Table 4. LPC, CLPC, MFCC AND DELTA, ACCELERATION, DELTA, AND THIRD DIFFERENTIAL coefficients

SENTENCES				*WORDS*			
PARAMETERS/# STATES	*4*	*5*	*6*	PARAMETERS/# STATES	*4*	*5*	*6*
LPC	77	89.5	89	LPC	77.39	89.95	89.45
CLPC	89.5	99	99	CLPC	89.95	99.5	99.5
MFCC	98.5	99	99	MFCC	98.99	99.5	99.5
EPCC KU	100	100	100	EPCC KU	100	100	100
EPCC ELLIOT	100	100	100	EPCC ELLIOT	100	100	100
EPCC NEELY	100	100	100	EPCC NEELY	100	100	100

In the second experiment, a corpus elaborated by J. Hansen at the University of Colorado Boulder was used. He has constructed database SUSAS (Speech Under Simulated and Actual Stress) http://catalog.ldc.upenn.edu/LDC99S78.Only 9 speakers

Table 5. Results obtained using HTK, SUSAS Corpus and manual labeling

	MFCC		*EPCC Using Neely values*		*EPCC Using Ku values*		*EPCC Using Elliot values*	
	sen-tence	word	sen-tence	word	sen-tence	word	sen-tence	word
boston1	91.84	92.06	90.61	90.87	90.2	90.48	89.39	89.68
boston2	95.51	95.63	93.47	93.65	93.47	93.65	93.06	93.25
boston3	96.73	96.83	93.88	94.05	95.92	96.03	96.33	96.43
general1	96.73	96.83	92.24	92.46	93.88	94.05	93.88	94.05
general2	94.29	94.44	90.61	90.87	90.61	90.87	89.39	89.68
general3	93.47	93.65	88.16	88.49	93.47	93.65	93.06	93.25
nyc1	91.84	92.06	91.84	91.67	87.35	87.3	96.33	96.43
nyc2	91.02	91.27	91.84	92.06	86.53	86.9	93.88	94.05
nyc3	95.92	96.03	92.65	92.86	90.61	90.87	89.39	89.68

with ages ranging from 22 to 76 were used and we applied normal corpus not under Stress sentences contained into corpus. The words were "brake, change, degree, destination, east, eight, eighty, enter, fifty, fix, freeze, gain, go, hello, help, histogram, hot, mark, nav, no, oh, on, out, point, six, south, stand, steer, strafe, ten, thirty, three, white, wide, & zero". A total of 4410 files of speech were processed. Finally, Tables 4 and 5 show results when using our proposal (Earing Perceptual Cepstrum Coefficients –EPCC-) the best representations used in the state of the art and in the last experiment versus MFCC in SUSAS corpus.

4   Conclusions and Future Works

This paper describes new parameters for ASRs tasks. They employ the functionality of the cochlea, the most important hearing organ of humans and mammalians. At this moment, the parameters used for the MFCC analysis have been demonstrated to be the most important parameters and the most used for this task. For many years a great diversity of models that attempt describing the functionality of the ear have been proposed and are implicit that this phenomenon has been used for ASR based on phenomenological models. Another alternative was employed using a physiological model based in macro and micro mechanical proposed by Neely. This article demonstrated that the Neely cochlea model can be used to obtain speech signal parameters for Automatic Speech Recognition. In conclusion, the cochlea behavior can be used to obtain these parameters and the results are adequate.

Acknowledgment. We want to acknowledge The National Polytechnic Institute (IPN, Mexico), also Center for Computing Research and especially SIP project numbers 20141310 and 20141454 for their support.

References

1. Noll, A.M.: Shortime Spectrum and Cepstrum Techniques for Vocal Pitch Detection. Journal of Acoustical Society of America 36, 296–302 (1964)
2. John, M.: Linear Prediction: A Tutorial Review. Proceedings of the IEEE 63(4), 561–580 (1975)
3. Davis, S.B., Mermelstein, P.: Comparison of Parametric Representations for Monosyllabic Word Recognition in Continuously Spoken Sentence. IEEE Transactions on Acoustics, Speech and Signal Processing ASSP-28(4) (August 1980)
4. Hermansky: Perceptual Linear Predictive (PLP) analysis of speech. Journal of Acoustical Society of America, 1738–1752 (April 1990)
5. Dallos, P., Fay, R.R.: Mechanics of the cochlea: modeling effects. In: de Boer, S.E. (ed.) The Cochlea. Springer, USA (1996)
6. Luis, R., Ruggero, M.A.: Mechanics of the Mammalian Cochlea'. Physiological Reviews 81(3) (July 2001)
7. Kim, D.S., Lee, S.Y., Kill, R.M.: Auditory processing of speech signals for robust speech recognition in real word noisy environments. IEEE Trans. Speech Audio Processing 7(1), 55–69 (1999)

8. Geisler, C.D.: A model of the effect of outer hair cell motility on cochlear vibration. Hear. Res. 24, 125–131 (1996)
9. Geisler, C.D., Shan, X.: A model for cochlear vibration based on feedback from motile outer hair cells. In: Dallos, P., Geilser, C.D., Matthews, J.W., Ruggero, M.A., Steele, C.R. (eds.) The Mechanics and Biophysics of Hearing, pp. 86–95. Springer, New York (1990)
10. Holmberg, M., Gelbart, D., Hemmert, W.: Automatic speech recognition with an adaptation model motivated by auditory processing. IEEE Trans. Audio, Speech, Language Processing 14(1), 44–49 (2006)
11. Haque, S., Togneri, R.: A feature extraction method for automatic speech recognition based on the cochlear nucleus. In: 11th Annual Conference of the International Speech Communication Association, InterSpeech 2010, Makuhari, Chiba, Japan, September 26-30 (2010)
12. Harczos, T., Szepannek, G., Klefenz, F.: Towards Automatic Speech Recognition based on Cochlear Traveling Wave Delay Trajectories. In: Dau, T., Buchholz, J.M., Harte, J.M., Christiansen, T.U. (eds.) 1st International Symposium on Auditory and Audiological Research (ISAAR 2007), Auditory Signal Processing in Hearing-impaired Listeners (2007) ISBN: 87-990013-1-4. Print: Centertryk A/S
13. Keener, Sneyd, J.: Mathematical Physiology. Springer, USA (2008)
14. Elliot, S.J., Ku, E.M., Lineton, B.A.: A state space model for cochlear mechanics. Journal of Acoustical Society of America 122, 2759–2771 (2007)
15. Elliott, S.J., Lineton, B., Ni, G.: Fluid coupling in a discrete model of cochlear mechanics. Journal of Acoustical Society of America 130, 1441–1451 (2011)
16. Ku, E.M., Elliot, S.J., Lineton, B.A.: Statistics of instabilities in a state space model of the human cochlea. Journal of Acoustical Society of America 124, 1068–1079 (2008)
17. Neely, S.T.: A model for active elements in cochlear biomechanics. Journal of Acoustical Society of America 79, 1472–1480 (1986)
18. Békésy: Concerning the pleasures of observing, and the mechanics of the inner ear. Nobel Lecture (December 11, 1961)
19. Mario, J.H., Rodríguez, J.L.O., Guerra, S.S., Fernández, R.B.: Computational Model of the Cochlea using Resonance Analysis. Journal Revista Mexicana Ingeniería Biomédica 33(2), 77–86 (2012)
20. Mario, J.H.: Modelo mecánico acústico del oído interno en reconocimiento de voz, Ph. D. Thesis, Center for Computing Research-IPN (Junio 2013)

Identification of Vowel Sounds of the Choapan Variant of Zapotec Language

Gabriela Oliva-Juarez, Fabiola Martinez-Licona, Alma Martinez-Licona,
and John Goddard-Close

Universidad Autonoma Metropolitana, Electrical Engineering Depto., Mexico City, Mexico
{fmml,aaml,jgc}@xanum.uam.mx, gaby7884@gmail.com

Abstract. Many pre-hispanic languages in Mexico, including the Zapotec language, are faced with the real possibility of extinction in the near future. There are many reasons for this, such as the younger indigenous populations who prefer to speak Spanish instead and a dwindling number of older native speakers. This means that often there is a loss of information about the language's correct pronunciation. In particular, in the Choapan Zapotec variant there are six vowels, of which five are similar to those in Spanish; the sixth vowel is /ë/, and although it is similar to the /e/ vowel, some confusion arises due to the previously mentioned problems. In this paper, Dynamic Time Warping was applied in order to determine the phonetic sound from the two most important phonetic alphabets (IPA & SAMPA) for the /e/ vowels. Two databases of Choapan Zapotec were obtained and the vowel phonemes were segmented and their tonal characteristic prevailed for the symbol assignation in both alphabets. This paper aims to provide valuable information for modeling the sounds of this Zapotec variant, in order that it help conserve the language.

Keywords: Sound pattern recognition, Zapotec vowels, Prehispanic languages.

1   Introduction

Languages are by far the most representative way of communication for human beings. As a consequence of their dynamic and evolving behavior, some of them prevail and others disappear. The use and conservation of the essential characteristics of a particular language represent a critical issue towards providing a sense of identification among the communities that speak it. The extinction of a language, due to the disuse, is the result of several conditions such as the preference of the new generations to speak in modern languages, the disappearance of the native old speakers or the migration of groups of people to other places. Spanish and English are two examples of this phenomenon in relation with the Prehispanic and Native American languages. In Mexico languages like Wiyot, Mascouten, Pochuteco or Mangue have become extinct and many others are about to if there are no concerted efforts to keep them alive [1]; the Zapotec language is an example of a risk extinction language, since it is spoken by only 425,123 inhabitants [2].

A. Gelbukh et al. (Eds.): MICAI 2014, Part II, LNAI 8857, pp. 252–262, 2014.
© Springer International Publishing Switzerland 2014

A language can have variants within it, they are defined as variations around the standard language that identify groups of people, like families or neighbors, or even communities. Some of them may be so small that are hardly noticed, and the speakers can understand one another; some others are so huge that can prevent communication between speakers. The Zapotec language falls into the latter category. This language comes from the Southeast part of Mexico and it is spoken in the states of Oaxaca, Veracruz, partly in Chiapas and in a few places in Mexico City. In order to identify the language and its 57 variations the ISO639.3 standard assigned a three-letter code for each one [3], some representative examples are shown in Table 1.

The Zapotec is one of the languages of the Oto-Mangue linguistic family, which is the biggest and most diverse in Mexico. It also belongs to the linguistic group of Zapotecano that contains the macrolanguages chantino and zapoteca [1,4]. This linguistic family is well known to be tonal, that is, it is based on the tones of the voiced sounds making possible to distinguish words by focusing in the frequency shifts of the vocal folds. The fact that it contains so many variants means that the Zapotec language presents an interesting and challenging problem from a speech technologies point of view. Also, the fact that fewer people speak the language each year, represents an important problem for the preservation of the cultural heritage of these Prehispanic communities.

In this paper emphasis is on the vowel sounds of the Choapan variant of Zapotec. A database was collected by recording utterances of a list of words by a female native speaker of this variant. Vowel segmentation and recognition methods were used in order to identify the vowel sounds from a set of sounds found in the International Phonetic Association (IPA) and Speech Assessment Methods Phonetic Alphabet (SAMPA) phonetic alphabets [5,6]. The paper is organized as follows: section 2 describes the sounds of the Choapan variant of Zapotec, section 3 presents details of the development of the database as well as the selected pattern recognition method, section 4 reports the results of the sound identification, section 5 presents a discussion of the results and issues found during the recording process and the experimentation, and section 6 gives some conclusions and mentions further work that will be undertaken.

Table 1. ISO 639.3 coding for representative Zapotec variants

Zapotec variant	ISO639.3 Code
Mixtepec	zpm
Choapan	zpc
Istmo	zai
Mitla	zaw
Ocotlán	zac
Rincón	zar
Zoogocho	zpq

2   Sounds of the Variant of Zapotec from Choapan

The Zapotec variant of Choapan, also known as the San Juan Comaltepec Zapotec, is spoken in the municipality of Choapan, which is part of the state of Oaxaca and, according to the Summer Institute of Linguistics, also in the state of Veracruz. The recorded data was obtained from a speaker who lives in Arenal Santa Ana, a community of 1551 inhabitants located in Veracruz [7]; although differences have been reported between the Zapotec spoken in Choapan and Arenal Santa Ana, it should be noted that due to their geographically closeness, they are highly similar. It is important to notice that this particular variant is classified as a moribund language by the Expanded Graded Intergenerational Disruption Scale (EGIDS) [8]. According to EGIDS, this Zapotec variant has a very few number of fluent users, most of them are old people that are not able to restore the natural intergenerational transmission. The Choapan Zapotec alphabet consists of vowels and consonants [9], which are described in the following subsections.

2.1   Vowels in Choapan Zapotec

The number of vowels used in the alphabet of this variant of Zapotec is six, five of them are the same as in Spanish plus a sixth vowel, and they are spoken with three different kinds of pronunciation: simple, short and long, as shown in Table 2. The most important characteristic of the pronunciations is the vowel duration. Simple vowels have a duration that is between the short and the long vowels. The other two pronunciations use larynx modifications to produce an abrupt closure of the vocal cords in the case of the short vowels, and to produce a brief pause between the vowel sounds in the case of long vowels.

2.2   Consonants in Choapan Zapotec

In the Choapan Zapotec there are 23 consonants, most of them are similar to the Spanish sounds. The consonants are weak occlusive (b, d, g), strong occlusive (p, t, c, qu, k), weak affricative (dz, dy), strong affricative (tz, ch), weak fricatives (z, ž), strong fricatives (s, x, j), nasals (m, n), liquids (l, r) and semivowels (hu, y). The affricative sounds are not familiar sounds in Spanish, dz is the combination of the occlusive d plus the voiced z while dy sounds like a voiced ch; the consonant tz is produced by pronouncing the occlusive t and then a voiceless s. The weak fricative ž is not a Spanish sound, and is pronounced as a z but with a back position of the tongue; the rest of the phonemes are pronounced as in Spanish.

Table 2. Vowels of Choapan Zapotec

Pronunciations	A	E	Ë	I	O	U
Simple	a	e	ë	i	o	u
Short	a'	e'	ë'	i'	o'	u'
Long	a'a	e'e	ë'ë	i'i	o'o	u'u

3   Methods

The experimentation included the collection of a database, an automatic segmentation procedure and the identification of the vowel sounds by a method based on Dynamic Time Warping (DTW).

3.1   Data

A Mexican female from the community of Arenal Santa Ana, Veracruz was recorded uttering a list of chosen words. The list consisted of 188 words selected from the Swadesh list for Zapotec [10]. Swadesh, originally devised by the linguist Morris, contains the words that are present in almost all languages and form the basis for communication between humans. The selected words included nouns (numbers, colors, animals, parts of the body, etc.), pronouns and verbs. Each word was pronounced twice and the recording process took two sessions. The words were recorded on a desktop PC using Speech Filing System Version 4.8 [11], and a sampling frequency of 16 KHz. The speaker controlled the amplitude of the signals and the recording sessions were performed in a quite room. The speaker used headphones with an integrated microphone and repeated the word to be recorded if necessary; previously she checked the pronunciation of the words by asking the elder members of her family about the non-Spanish sounds. We also obtained a second dataset from a set of recordings texts read by a male speaker in Zapotec of the Choapan District [12]. The texts belong to the first five chapters of the Gospel of John from the Bible; since the verses are of different sizes only the segments that contained 16 words at most were considered.

3.2   Segmentation and Vowel Identification

The automatic segmentation was carried out using HTK [13]. We used the SAMPA phonetic symbol transcription for the determination of the Choapan Zapotec sounds. Since in this variant there are 18 vowel sounds, three realizations per the six vowels, we added a "s" to the short versions and a "l" to the long ones, so for vowel /o/ it would be "o" for o, "os" for o' and "ol" for o'o.

When dealing with a dying language is most likely to find sounds that can be confusable; the vowel realizations are not easy to differentiate because they share the same acoustic features, for example formants, and problems on the transcription may arise. We used DTW to identify those vowel sounds that presented this problem [14].

DTW is an algorithm for measuring similarity between two temporal sequences. It performs the comparison of the characteristics of the sequences using a measure of cost; this results in a cost matrix that contains the comparison results, then the trajectory with the minimum cost is selected meaning that this has the highest similarity between two sequences. In our case, the sequences to be compared were a prototype vowel that consisted in the defined sound for each realization of the phoneme and each one of the non-clear vowel realizations found during the segmentation. The prototypes were selected among those sounds that, according to the female speaker and the Choapan Zapotec grammar literature, were correctly pronounced.

We also used DTW to perform the identification of the sound for the "e" vowels, /e/ and /ë/. These sounds are so alike that it is very confusing to acoustically differentiate one another. In this case for the prototype sequence we used the sounds that were close to the /e/ Spanish vowel in the IPA Vowel Trapezoid (IPA_VT) [15].

The IPA_VT is a phonetic chart where all the vowels defined by the IPA alphabets are located according their realization. The "e" sounds correspond to vowels that can be front or central, meaning that the vowel is pronounced at the front of the oral cavity or at its center respectively, close-mid or open-mid. An open vowel is performed when the tongue is positioned as far as possible from the roof of the mouth, a close vowel when the tongue is positioned as close as possible from the roof of the mouth and a mid vowel when the tongue is positioned mid-way between an open and a close vowel. The close-mid and open-mid vowels are performed when the tongue is positioned just two-thirds of the way from the close to mid or to the open to mid vowels.

In order to obtain the prototype sequences we used the "e" sounds of the different languages that have an IPA alphabet and available sound realizations; those included English, German, Swedish, Portuguese, French, Italian and Polish. The sequence to be compared consisted on the set of realizations of the "e" vowels, /e/, /e'/, /e'e/, /ë/, /ë'/ and /ë'ë/, for the Veracruz Choapan Zapotec and the Choapan District Zapotec.

We used two different DTW approaches to run the experiments. The first one was the Matlab Ellis version that calculates a similarity matrix between specgram-like feature matrices using the cosine distance [16]. The other approach was implemented in Praat [17]; it calculates distances between the Mel Frecuency Cepstral Coefficients of the sequences and finds the optimum path through the distance matrix using the Viterbi-algorithm.

4   Results

The sounds transcribed were those that had duration of 60 milliseconds or more to guarantee a vowel phoneme. Thus the number of vowel utterances for the Veracruz Choapan Zapotec was 491 and for the Choapan District Zapotec was 5790. The distribution of the vowel phonemes and the vowel realizations are shown in Table 3. It is noticeable the low percentage of long vowel realizations in both datasets as well as the similar results for vowel /o/. It is also remarkable that more than half of the total of the sounds belong to simple realizations and that vowel /a/ has the highest number of examples of all. It finally draws attention to vowel /ë/ in the Veracruz dataset, the Swadesh word list, having more examples than the vowels /e/, /i/, /o/ and /u/.

In order to assess the DTW performance on our data, two preliminary tests were conducted with known data. When applied to the Veracruz Choapan Zapotec the method had a 76% of correct phoneme assignation while for the Choapan District Zapotec it had 81.67%. The Veracruz dataset had more undetermined vowel sounds because the speaker had doubts about the correct pronunciation. After applying DTW, the final number of vowel sounds for this Zapotec is shown in Table 4.

Table 3. Distribution of vowel phonemes (left) and vowel phoneme realizations (right) for the Veracruz Choapan Zapotec (Ver zpc) and the Choapan District Zapotec (zpc)

Vowel	Ver_zpc (%)	zpc (%)	Vowel Realization	Ver_ zpc (%)	zpc (%)
A	34.3	41.2	Simple	69.72	76.30
E	14.4	13.4	Short	23.64	18.76
Ë	19.5	3.7	Long	6.632	4.94
I	15.7	20.2			
O	5.0	5.4			
U	11.1	16.1			

Table 4. Number of Vowels extracted from the Veracruz Choapan Zapotec

Vowel realization	a	a'	a'a	e	e'	e'e	ë	ë'	ë'ë	i	i'	i'i	o	o'	o'o	u	u'	u'u
Known vowels	80	17	4	27	3	3	2	6	1	36	11	2	11	0	2	30	9	0
Unknown vowels	8	8	4	1	2	0	0	2	3	8	13	0	2	0	0	9	1	0

While performing DTW, emphasis was on vowels e and ë. The method was applied in order to determine the closest IPA and SAMPA sounds for these vowels. Table 5 shows the resulting symbols for the three realizations of the two vowels for the Choapan Zapotec of Veracruz using Matlab Ellis approach. In the case of the Choapan District Zapotec, all the vowel realizations had the IPA symbol " ɵ " and the SAMPA symbol " 8 " corresponding to the sound of the Swedish word *Buss* as shown in Table 6. In order to appreciate the acoustic characteristics of the found sounds we highlighted the IPA symbol ɵ on the IPA Vowel Trapezoid as shown in Figure 1; according to this, /ë/ and /e/ are central close-mid vowels.

Table 5. Phonetic symbols (IPA and SAMPA) assigned to vowels ë and e in all their realizations of the Choapan Zapotec of Veracruz, Matlab results

Vowel	Symbol		Word	Idiom	Gender
	IPA	SAMPA			
ë	ɵ	8	Buss[1]	Swedish	Feminine
ë'	ɵ	8	Buss	Swedish	Feminine
ë'ë	ɵ	8	Buss	Swedish	Feminine
e	ɔ	O	Ontem[2]	Portuguese	Feminine
e'	ɵ	8	Buss	Swedish	Feminine
e'e	ɵ	8	Buss	Swedish	Feminine

[1] Bus, [2] Yesterday

Table 6. Phonetic symbols (IPA and SAMPA) assigned to vowels ë and e in all their realizations of the Choapan District Zapotec, Matlab results

Vowel	Symbol		Word	Idiom	Gender
	IPA	SAMPA			
ë	ɵ	8	Buss	Swedish	Feminine
ë'	ɵ	8	Buss	Swedish	Feminine
ë'ë	ɵ	8	Buss	Swedish	Feminine
e	ɵ	8	Buss	Swedish	Feminine
e'	ɵ	8	Buss	Swedish	Feminine
e'e	ɵ	8	Buss	Swedish	Feminine

When the Praat DTW implementation was applied to the data, some differences were found compared to the Matlab results. Table 7 shows the resulting symbols for the three realizations of the two vowels for the Choapan Zapotec of Veracruz using

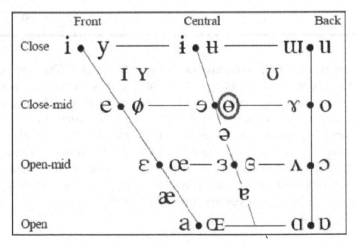

Fig. 1. IPA Vowel Trapezoid, the ë and e sounds symbol is highlighted, Matlab results

Praat. Table 8 shows the corresponding results for the Choapan District Zapotec. As it can be seen, the found IPA dominant sound in both Choapan Zapotec is ɛ. Figure 2 shows this symbol on the IPA Vowel Trapezoid; according to this, /ë/ and /e/ are mainly front open-mid vowels.

Table 7. Phonetic symbols (IPA and SAMPA) assigned to vowels ë and e in all their realizations of the Choapan Zapotec of Veracruz, Praat results

Vowel	Symbol		Word	Idiom	Gender
	IPA	SAMPA			
ë	ɛ	E	Gesetz[3]	German	Feminine
ë'	ɛ	E	Gesetz	German	Feminine
ë'ë	ɛ	E	Gesetz	German	Feminine
e	ɛ	E	Gesetz	German	Feminine
e'	ɛ	E	Gesetz	German	Feminine
e'e	ɐ	6	Besser[4]	German	Feminine

[3] Law, [4] Better

Table 8. Phonetic symbols (IPA and SAMPA) assigned to vowels ë and e in all their realizations of the Choapan District Zapotec, Praat results

Vowel	Symbol		Word	Idiom	Gender
	IPA	SAMPA			
ë	ɛ	E	Gesetz	German	Feminine
ë'	ə	@	Ce[5]	French	Masculine
ë'ë	ɛ	E	Gesetz	German	Feminine
e	ɛ	E	Gesetz	German	Feminine
e'	ɛ	E	Gesetz	German	Feminine
e'e	ə	@	Ce	French	Masculine

[5] This

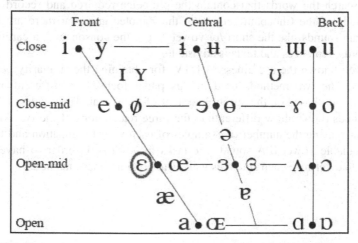

Fig. 2. IPA Vowel Trapezoid, the ë and e sounds symbol is highlighted, Praat results

5   Discussion

Zapotec is a language that has a number of variants that makes it complex to analyze. In the case of the Veracruz Choapan variant, the EGIDS moribund situation makes difficult the sound analysis due to the fact that it is not known some of the pronunciations. The DTW method allowed us to have certainty about the vowel phonemes; from the 18 vowel-realizations, short /o/ (o') and long /u/ (u'u) did not appear in the recorded database and there were a few examples of them in the Choapan District Zapotec records.

In this particular Zapotec variant the problem of pronunciation is evident. We had problems with the spelling of the recorded words because the speaker was not sure about the pronunciation of certain sounds. Although a consultation with a native speaker was made, we had to consult with some other Zapotec variants like Zogocho that has a 60% of intelligibility with the Choapan variant. Since this is a tonal language, the vowel sounds were clear to identify, but the imbalance of the number of examples for some of them does not allow having a complete analysis.

IPA trapezoid located the sounds /e/ and /ë/ as central vowels with the Matlab results. This means that their pronunciation is not similar to this of the Spanish vowel /e/ that is a front sound. In the other hand, the IPA trapezoid located the sounds /e/ and /ë/ as open vowels with the Praat results. This means that their pronunciation is wider than this of the Spanish vowel /e/ that is a mid-close sound. During the analysis of the /e/ and /ë/ vowels a mimic phenomenon could be observed: the speaker tended to pronounce the sound much like the Spanish, not allowing the differentiation of the simple, short and long pronunciations of both vowels.

The words selected for the recorded database of the Veracruz Choapan Zapotec belong to a generic list that was not phonetically balanced. Also the words contained in the Choapan District Zapotec are oriented toward the topic of the reading. This means that some of the phonemes have few examples, whilst others do not have any. The DTW results might improve with a larger number of examples for each phoneme; this leads to search the words that contain the phoneme required and record them. In a deeper study of the Choapam version of the Zapotec grammar there are few words that contain sounds like the short /o/ vowel (o') or the consonant ž, a careful analysis of the words, sentences and texts is advisable.

It is well known the usefulness of DTW for obtaining the similarity between two sequences. The two methods used in this paper focused on different approaches, though they are based on the spectral content of the signal. The results obtained with both methods didn't allow differentiate the three realizations of the two kinds of "e" vowels; increasing the number of examples of each vowel realization and the number of the available vowel IPA sounds are tasks to be done in order to have improved elements to determine each sound as well as to compare these methods.

6   Conclusions

A vowel analysis was carried out in two different databases of the Choapan Zapotec Variant. A Swadesh word list was recorded and some texts from the Bible were segmented to obtain a set of Zapotec phonemes. The problems that were encountered during the speech recording dealt with the confusion on the pronunciation of some words by the speaker and members of her community, which is a consequence of the language's high risk of disappearing. The impact it had on the /ë/ and /e/ vowel pronunciations lead to the determination of their sounds from a set of IPA and SAMPA alphabets by applying DTW in two different platforms. The assigned phonemes corresponded to those from tonal languages; more efforts on having a bigger, more reliable and balanced vowel database as well as experimenting with other pattern recognition methods are driven. The main objective is to obtain valuable information for modeling the sounds of this Zapotec variant that helps to conserve the language.

Acknowledgement. The first author would like to thank the Consejo Nacional de Ciencia y Tecnología (Conacyt), Mexico, for a grant given to her by them.

References

1. Catalogue of the National Indigenous Languages of Mexico, National Institute of Indigenous Languages INALI (2009), http://www.inali.gob.mx/clin-inali/
2. National populations statistics, National Institute of Statistics and Geography INEGI, http://www.inegi.org.mx
3. ISO639.3 standard, Summer Institute of Linguistics, http://www.sil.org
4. Ethnologue Languages of the World, http://www.ethnologue.com
5. International Phonetic Association Alphabet, http://www.langsci.ucl.ac.uk/ipa/ipachart.html
6. Speech Assessment Methods Phonetic Alphabet, http://www.phon.ucl.ac.uk/home/sampa/index.html
7. Social Development Secretary, Community information modules (2010), http://www.microrregiones.gob.mx/zap/datGenerales.aspx?entra=pdzp&ent=30&mun=130
8. Lewis, M.P., Simons, G.F.: Assessing Endangerment: Expanding Fishman's GIDS. Romanian Review of Linguistics 55(2), 103–120 (2010)
9. Lyman-Boulden, H.: Gramática Popular del Zapoteco de Comaltepec, Choapan, Oaxaca, 2a. Edición, Summer Institute of Linguistics (2010)
10. Swadesh lists for Oto-Manguean languages, http://en.wiktionary.org/wiki/Appendix:Swadesh_lists_for_Oto-Manguean_languages
11. Speech Filing System, University College London, http://www.phon.ucl.ac.uk/resource/sfs/
12. Choapan District Zapotec Bibble, http://www.scriptureearth.org/00e-Escrituras_Indice.php?sortby=country&name=all
13. Hidden Markov Model Toolkit, http://htk.eng.cam.ac.uk/
14. Rabiner, L., Juang, B.: Fundamentals of speech Recognition, p. 507. Prentice Hall (1993)

15. International Phonetic Association. Handbook of the International Phonetic Association: A guide to the use of the International Phonetic Alphabet. Cambridge University Press (1999)
16. Ellis, D.: Dynamic Time Warp (DTW) in Matlab (2003), http://www.ee.columbia.edu/~dpwe/resources/matlab/dtw/
17. Doing Phonetics by Computer, http://www.fon.hum.uva.nl/praat/

An Open-Domain Cause-Effect Relation Detection from Paired Nominals

Partha Pakray[1] and Alexander Gelbukh[2]

[1] Norwegian University of Science and Technology
Trondheim, Norway
parthapakray@gmail.com
www.parthapakray.com
[2] Centro de Investigación en Computación, Instituto Politécnico Nacional
Mexico City, Mexico
www.gelbukh.com

Abstract. We present a supervised method for detecting causal relations from text. Various kinds of dependency relations, WordNet features, Parts-of-Speech (POS) features along with several combinations of these features help to improve the performance of our system. In our experiments, we used SemEval-2010 Task #8 data sets. This system used 7954 instances for training and 2707 instances for testing from Task #8 datasets. The J48 algorithm was used to identify semantic causal relations in a pair of nominals. Evaluation result gives an overall F1 score of 85.8% of causal instances.

1 Introduction

Causality is the relation between two events, one of which being called CAUSE and the other one being called EFFECT, where EFFECT is a consequence of CAUSE. There are various forms of cause-effect expression such as in the form of intra-NP, inter-NP, and inter-sentence (Chang and Choi, 2004). Causality detection is one of the tasks in Question Answering domain. The natural language texts are generally complex and filled with ambiguity. The main challenging task is to detect the causality from natural language text. In this present task aims to develop the system for automatically recognizing cause-effect relations between pairs of nominal. In this paper we are trying to detect causal sentences.

Causal sentence can be either explicit or implicit, as it is shown in Figure 1. Explicit causal marker are "because", or "so", etc. These type of instances are relatively easy to recognize, using pattern that contain the marker (Khoo et al., 2000). There are no direct markers in implicit causal. An example of implicit causal is *"Nick ate double Cake. He was very hungry"*.

We develop a systems for automatically recognizing semantic relations for Cause-Effect between pairs of nominal. Nine relations such as Cause-Effect, Instrument-Agency, Product-Producer, Content-Container, Entity-Origin, Entity-Destination, Component-Whole, Member-Collection and Message-Topic are given for SemEval-

A. Gelbukh et al. (Eds.): MICAI 2014, Part II, LNAI 8857, pp. 263–271, 2014.

2010 Task #8 (Hendrix et al., 2010). For our experiments we used cause-effect relations as causals and remaining relations are non-causals.

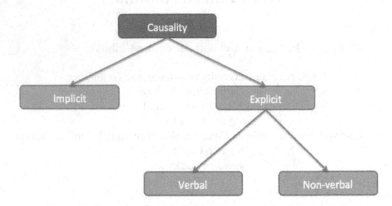

Fig. 1. Classification of causal relations

The paper is organized as follows. Related work is described in Section 2. Resource Processing and System Description is described in Sections 3 and 4, respectively. Features for Machine Learning are discussed in Section 5. Baseline system is described in Section 6. Evaluation Result is reported in Section 7. Finally, Section 8 concludes the paper.

2   Related Work

The system developed by Chang and Choi (2004) aims to extract causal relations that exist between two events expressed by noun phrases or sentences. They introduce the lexical pair probability and the cue phrase probability. These probabilities are learned from raw corpus in unsupervised manner. With these probabilities and the Naive Bayes classifier, they try to resolve the causal relation extraction problem. Their inter-NP causal relation extraction shows the precision of 81.29%.

Girju and Moldovon (2002) provide syntactic and semantic classification of cause-effect lexico-syntactic patterns for automatic detection and extraction of causation relationships in English texts. They also present a semi-automatic method of discovering generally applicable lexico-syntactic patterns that refer to the causation relation. The patterns are found automatically, but their validation is done semi-automatically. Their final purpose is to add a new module to their existing semantics, syntax and morphology. In this paper, a semi-automatic method and having the particular pattern <NP verb NP> was defined. The accuracy of this system was 65%.

Blanco et al. (2008) presented a supervised method for the detection and extraction of Causal Relations from open domain text. The system first identified the syntactic patterns that may encode causation, and then they used Machine Learning techniques to decide whether or not a pattern instance encodes causation. They focused on the most productive pattern, a verb phrase followed by a relator and a clause, and its reverse version, a relator followed by a clause and a verb phrase. As relators they considered the words as, after, because and since. They presented a set of lexical, syntactic and semantic features for the classification task. Their system is able to recognize sentences that contain causal relations with a precision of 98% and a recall of 84%.

The system developed by Pal et al. (2010) used Conditional Random Field (CRF) machine-learning framework, is adopted for classifying the pair of nominal. The system used WordNet, Name Entities, Direct dependency and transitive dependency features for machine learning. It achieved 75.60% of FScore for detecting Cause Effect relation.

The system developed by Sorgente et al (2013) proposed joins both rules and ML methods. In particular, their approach first identifies a set of plausible cause-e@ect pairs through a set of logical rules based on dependencies between words then it uses Bayesian inference to reduce the number of pairs produced by ambiguous patterns. This system achieved 63% for F-score.

Our system is similar to above-mentioned systems, but differs from them in that we introduced some more features like WordNet, Path distances, etc. Those features are described in Section 5.

3   Resource Preprocessing

For this experiment we used SemEval-2010 Task #8 (Hendrix et al., 2010) data sets. The annotated training corpus containing 8000 sentences was made available by the respective task organizers. The objective is to evaluate the effectiveness of the system in terms of identifying semantic relations between pair of nominal. In this corpus there is some noise, so among the 8000 sentences we used 7954 sentences as training corpus. The datasets is shown in Table 1.

Table 1. Dataset Description

SemEval 2010 Data Sets (Our System Used)		
	Total No of Instances	7954
Training Set	Total No of Causal Relation	995
	Total No of Non Causal Relation	6959
	Total No of Instances	2707
Test Set	Total No of Causal Relation	328
	Total No of Non Causal Relation	2379

An example for data sets is shown in Table 2.

Table 2. Example of SemEval-2010 Task #8

Sentence	Relation
"The **<e1>burst</e1>** has been caused by water hammer **<e2>pressure</e2>**."	Cause-Effect(e2,e1)
"He had chest pains and **<e1>headaches</e1>** from **<e2>mold</e2>** in the bedrooms."	Cause-Effect(e2,e1)
"Baker's yeast **<e1>enzymes</e1>** convert sugar (glucose, fructose) to **<e2>ethanol</e2>** and carbon dioxide."	Non-Causal

4   System Architecture

The system architecture is shown in Figure 2. In this system is defined three parts:
Pre-Processing, Feature Extraction and Machine Learning with decision phase.

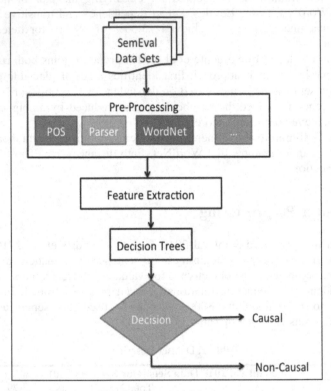

Fig. 2. System Architecture

Pre-Processing. Each of the training and test sentences is annotated by the paired
nominal tagged as <e1> and <e2>. The relation of the paired nominal and a comment
portion describing the detail of the input type follows the input sentence.

The sentences are filtered and passed through Stanford Dependency Parser
(Marneffe et al., 2006) to identify direct as well as transitive dependencies between
the nominal. The direct dependency is identified based on the simultaneous presence
of both nominal, <e1> as well as <e2> in the same dependency relation whereas the
transitive dependencies are verified if <e1> and <e2> are connected via one or more
intermediate dependency relations.

Different seed lists are prepared for different types of verbs. For example, the lists for
causal verbs were developed by processing the XML files of English VerbNet[1] (Kipper-
Schuler, 2005). The list of the causal verbs is prepared by collecting the member verbs
if their corresponding class contains the semantic type "CAUSE". The other verb lists

---

[1] http://verbs.colorado.edu/~mpalmer/projects/verbnet.html

for causals are prepared manually by reviewing the frequency of verbs in the training corpus. The WordNet[2] stemmer is used to identify the root forms of the verbs.

Feature Extraction is described in Section 6. There are various kinds of machine learning algorithm such as Support Vector Machines (SVM), Artificial Neural Networks (ANN), Decision Tree (DT) learning, etc. In this experiment we used decision tree algorithm for machine learning. A decision tree is a decision support tool that uses a tree-like graph or model of decisions and their possible consequences. C4.5[3] (or J48) is an algorithm used to generate a decision tree. Weka[4] is an open-source Java application produced by the University of Waikato in New Zealand. This software bundle features an interface through which many of the aforementioned algorithms can be utilized on preformatted data sets. From this Weka tool we used J48 algorithm.

5   Features for Machine Learning

Identification of appropriate features plays a crucial role in any machine-learning framework. The following features are identified heuristically by manually reviewing the corpus and based on the frequency of different verbs in different relations. Here is an example from SemEval-2 training data set:

"The <e1>burst</e1> has been caused by water hammer <e2>pressure</e2>."
In this experiment we generated 20 features for machine learning.

i.   Two nominals (e1 and e2) were used as Feature 1 and Feature 2.
ii.   System select the string and with its POS (after e1) as Feature 3 and Feature 4. For above example, Feature 3 is "has" and Feature 4 is "VBZ".
iii. System select the string and with its POS (before e2) as Feature 5 and Feature 6. For above example, Feature 5 is "hammer" and Feature 4 is "NN".
iv.   Surface Distance between e1 and e2 as Feature 6.
v.   Main Verb as Feature 7. After main verb string as Feature 8 and with that POS as Feature 9. Before main verb string as Feature 10 and with that POS as Feature 11.
vi.   We prepared a seed lists for different types of causals verbs. Then we check any causal verbs present or not with that list. If causals verb is present then we mark that token as a trigger as a Feature 12. For feature 13, we retrieved sense number from WordNet 2.1 of that trigger.
vii. We used WordNet distance between two nominal as feature 14. And also used the common parents of that two nominal as feature 15.
viii. For feature 16 and 17, we calculate the tree distance trigger to those arguments (Arg1 and Arg2).

---

[2] http://wordnet.princeton.edu/
[3] http://en.wikipedia.org/wiki/C4.5_algorithm
[4] http://www.cs.waikato.ac.nz/ml/weka/

ix. For feature 18, sentences are parsed through Stanford dependency parser. In this step we calculate distance between two arguments (e1 and e2). Parse tree of above example is shown in Figure 3. Here two arguments are "burst" and "pressure", and tree distance between them is 8.

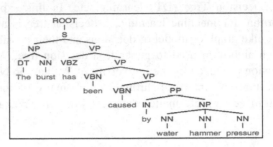

Fig. 3. Parse Tree

x. Check preposition before argument (e2) from parse tree. First we find the Noun Phrase (NP) of Noun Head and then check preposition before NP if there is any PP then select that preposition as Feature 19.

```
(ROOT
 (S
  (NP (DT The) (NN burst))
  (VP (VBZ has)                    ┈┈┈┈┈ CheckPPBeforeArg2
   (VP (VBN been)
    (VP (VBN caused)                       ∙∙∙∙∙∙∙∙∙∙∙∙∙∙∙∙∙∙∙ Arg2: Head of NP
     (PP (IN by) ◀┈┈┈┈
      (NP (NN water) (NN hammer) (NN pressure)))))))))
```

Fig. 4. Parse Tree

xi. Parse the sentence by Stanford Dependency Parser (in Figure 5) then Subject Arguments as Feature 20 and Feature 21. Object argument as Feature 22 and Feature 23.

```
det(burst-2, The-1)
nsubjpass(caused-5, burst-2)
aux(caused-5, has-3)
auxpass(caused-5, been-4)
root(ROOT-0, caused-5)
prep(caused-5, by-6)
nn(pressure-9, water-7)
nn(pressure-9, hammer-8)
pobj(by-6, pressure-9)
```

Fig. 5. Dependency Relation

6   Baseline Model

The baseline model is developed based on the similarity clues present in the phrasal pattern containing verbs and prepositions. Different rules are identified separately for the causals relations. A few WordNet features such as hypernym, meronym, distance and Common-Parents are added into the rule-based baseline model. Some of the relation specific rules are mentioned below.

The Cause-Effect relations are identified based on the causal verbs (cause, lead etc.). One of the main criteria for extracting these relations is to verify the presence of causal verbs in between the text segment of <e1> and <e2>. Different types of specific relaters (as, because etc.) are identified from the text segment as well. It is observed that such specific causal relaters help in distinguishing other relations from Cause-Effect.

The evaluation of the rule-based baseline system on gives an average F1- score of 55.02%. The rule base feature is not sufficient to detect causal relation between two nominal and the performance can be improved by adopting strategies for differentiating the nominal of a cause-effect pair.

7   Evaluation Result

Lexical, Syntactic and Semantic features were extracted from the text by using Stanford POS tagger, Stanford Parser, WordNet for machine learning representation. These representations were processed by filter *StringToWordVector*. This can be done through the WEKA GUI tools, the command line or through code using the API and there are a wide range of options to change the behavior of the filter, using vector normalization and converting all characters to lower case. We experiment with Decision Trees (J48 in WEKA).

Table 3. Training Set Result for Cross Validation

Data Sets	Cross Validations	Label	Precision	Recall	Fscore
Training Data	10 Folds	Causal	0.889	0.71	0.79
		Non-Causal	0.96	0.987	0.973
	5 Folds	Causal	0.891	0.70	0.786
		Non-Causal	0.95	0.95	0.95

An example of Receiver Operating Characteristic (ROC) curve is shown in Figure 5, obtained by applying a set of threshold to confidence output by a method. On the x-axis is plotted the proportion of false positive (how many times a method says the object class is present when it is not); on the y-axis is plotted the proportion of true positive (how many times a method says the object class is present when it is). The closer the curve follows the left-hand border and then the top borders of the ROC space, the more accurate the test.

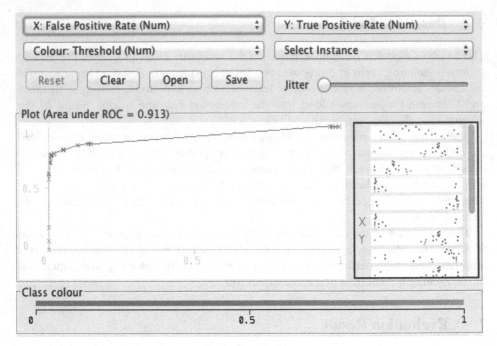

Fig. 6. ROC Curve

Table 4. Test Set Result

Data Set	Label	Precision	Recall	Fscore
Test	Causal	0.911	0.811	0.858
Set	Non-Causal	0.974	0.989	0.982

Table 5. Test Set Result

Test set	True Positive	False Negative	False Positive	True Negative
Causal	266	62	26	2353
Non-causal	2353	26	62	266

8   Conclusion

Sometimes it is very hard to differentiate between Causals and Non-causals relation by Machine Learning. For example, in the sentences "The <e1>blisters</e1> are caused by <e2>antibodies</e2> against desmogleins (Dsgs), which are glycoproteins present in the junctions between skin cells", the system detected this as Causal but it originally is Non-causal: the antibodies are actively involved in producing the blisters so it is not a causal relation. Another example: "Bacterial <e1>infections</e1> of the ear result in <e2>malodor</e2>, excessive exudation (drainage of pus-like material), and ulceration". The system detected this as Non-causal but originally it was Causal.

As to future work, our trigger list is small, so we need to increase our trigger list. Here "result" is a trigger, so it is not included in that trigger list.

References

1. Blanco, E., Castell, N., Moldovan, D.: Causal Relation Extraction. In: Proceedings of the Sixth International Conference on Language Resources and Evaluation (LREC), Marrakech, Morocco (2008)
2. Chang, D.-S., Choi, K.-S.: Causal relation extraction using cue phrase and lexical pair probabilities. In: Su, K.-Y., Tsujii, J., Lee, J.-H., Kwong, O.Y. (eds.) IJCNLP 2004. LNCS (LNAI), vol. 3248, pp. 61–70. Springer, Heidelberg (2005)
3. Hendrickx, I., Kim, S.N., Kozareva, Z., Nakov, P., Saghdha, D., Romano, L., Szpakowicz, S.: Semeval-2010 task 8: Multi-way classification of semantic relations between pairs of nominal
4. Sorgente, A., Vettigli, G., Mele, F.: Automatic Extraction of Cause-Effect Relations in Natural Language Text. DART@AI*IA 2013, pp. 37–48 (2013)
5. Girju, R., Moldovan, D.: Mining answers for causation questions. In: Symposium on Mining Answers from Texts and Knowledge Bases (2002)
6. Kipper-Schuler, K.: VerbNet. A broad coverage, comprehensive verb lexicon. Ph.D. thesis, University of Pennsylvania, Philadelphia, PA (2005)
7. Pal, S., Pakray, P., Das, D., Bandyopadhyay, S.: A Supervised Approach to Identify Semantic Relations from Paired Nominals. In: ACL-2010, SemEval 2010 Workshop, Uppsala, Sweden (2010)

An Alignment Comparator for Entity Resolution with Multi-valued Attributes

Pablo N. Mazzucchi-Augel and Héctor G. Ceballos

Tecnológico de Monterrey, Campus Monterrey, Mexico
{A00814519,ceballos}@itesm.mx

Abstract. Entity matching is a problem that concerns many data management processes. If we consider matching between entities represented by RDF individuals we might find attributes values lists with variable-length for some properties, which will lead us to the problem of comparing multi-valued attributes, e.g. comparing author names lists for determining publication matching. This matching technique would be more complex than comparing fixed-length records, but less complex than comparing XML documents. Instead of comparing a single string, representing the concatenation of these values, each value of one vector should be compared against all values of the other vector. We propose a set of heuristics to address the alignment and comparison process of multi-valued attributes and evaluate them in the context of bibliographic databases. Our first results show that it is possible to reduce the comparisons amount and provide an aggregated similarity metric that outperforms the average similarity of cross product comparisons.

Keywords: Entity Resolution, Author Matching, Multi-Valued Attributes, Bibliographic databases.

1 Introduction

Entity matching (also referred to as duplicate identification, record linkage, entity resolution or reference reconciliation) is a crucial task for data integration and data cleaning. It is the task of identifying entities (objects, data instances) referring to the same real world entity [10]. Nowadays, organizations maintain records referring to the same entity in distributed databases. Some attributes are redundant, but others complement the information. Problems arise when information must be put together in order to extract knowledge.

For instance, in the integration of bibliographic databases publications have multi-valued attributes like authors and keywords that traditionally have been represented as a single string with a concatenation of items, but in RDF these values can be found disaggregated. Similarity between multi-valued attributes must be summarized in a single value that could be pondered in the overall similarity score.

For Linked Data, data integration consists of adding links between equivalent entities (e.g. publications) by accessing the entity description in distributed repositories. Frameworks like Silk [17] provide facilities for this purpose, but treat similarity between multi-valued attributes as the average of the cross product comparisons. In this

A. Gelbukh et al. (Eds.): MICAI 2014, Part II, LNAI 8857, pp. 272–284, 2014.

paper, we propose a novel heuristic which increases the efficiency when comparing multi-valued attributes, as long as it reduces the amount of comparisons and improves the distinction between equivalent lists.

The paper is structured as follows: Section 2 present some of the string matching and aggregation techniques find in literature. Section 3 gives an overview of the proposed approach. In Section 4 we show results of the different heuristics proposed and discuss them in Section 5, in order to identify the most effective one to address this problematic.

2 Background

Next we describe some approaches proposed for approximate string matching (particularly on author names) and for aggregating individual comparisons.

2.1 String Matching Techniques

The entity resolution problem has been known for more than five decades, not just in the statistics area, but also in the database community as well as in the AI community. Entity resolution or duplicate detection relies on string comparison techniques, which deal with the typographical variation of string data. Multiple methods have been developed for this task, and each method works well for particular types of strings. It is not the objective of this paper to develop an exhaustive and detailed explanation of string matching techniques, but to mention which are the most useful and used the bibliographic database domain. For a comprehensive review refer to [1], [19], [6].

So, to deal with typographical errors, the most suitable approaches are the character-based similarity metrics. The *edit distance* calculate the minimum amount of edit operations (insert, delete or replace) of single characters needed to transform a string S_1 into S_2. The version of edit distance where each operation cost 1, is known as *Levenshtein* distance. If those strings are truncated or shortened, a better metric is the *Smith-Waterman* distance. Winkler modified the metric introduced by Jaro (a string comparison algorithm that was mainly used for the comparison of last and first names) to give higher weight to prefix matches since prefix matches are more important for surname matching [13]. It does not just find common characters, but focus also in their order.

Character-based similarity metrics work well for typographical errors. However, it is often the case that typographical conventions lead to rearrangement of words (e.g., "John Smith" versus "Smith, John"). In such cases, character-level metrics fail to capture the similarity of the entities. Token-based metrics try to compensate this problem. In this group, could be categorized the *Monge-Elkan* distance, the *cosine* or *tf.idf* similarities, the *Jaccard* similarity or the hybrid approach *Soft TF-IDF* that combines the token based with the string-based methods [6].

2.2 Aggregation

In this section we list the techniques found in the literature for generating an aggregated score, using the numerous comparisons performed. The linear sum assignment problem (LSAP) is one of the most famous problems in linear programming and in combinatorial optimization. Informally speaking, given an NxN cost matrix $C = (c_{ij})$ the objective is to match each row to a different column in such a way that the sum of the corresponding entries is minimized. In other words, to select N elements of C so that there is exactly one element in each row and one in each column, the sum of the corresponding costs should be the minimum [2]. Based on that approach, [18] introduced a linear sum assignment procedure to force 1-1 matching because he observed that greedy algorithms often made erroneous assignments. A greedy algorithm is one in which a record is always associated with the corresponding available record having the highest agreement weight. Subsequent records are only compared with available remaining records that have not been assigned. In [14] and [9] is used the Euclidean distance metric to combine distance similarity values, generated by the comparisons of multiples attributes of a tuple.

As the standard edit distance comparators did not work as well as the Jaro-Winkler formula in their experiments, [20] combined string distance's techniques (such as *Levenshtein* and *LCS*), averaging them, which seemed to produce better results. The objective was to use more information from the strings, and take advantage of each algorithm strength. The combined *root mean square (RMS)* has been also used by [8] to improve linkage accuracy over any single comparator.

In [3], a learning scheme is used to combine several of the distance functions detailed above. A binary SVM (support vector machine) classifier was trained, using as feature vector the numeric scores of those functions, and their confidence in the match task as the result of the comparison. It slightly outperforms the individual metrics. SVM do not generate an aggregated value like the other presented techniques, but combines partial results in order to improve the classification process.

3   The Matching Process

In this section we give an overview of the process that heuristics, presented in detail in Section 3.4, follow to increase the effectiveness in the alignment and comparison process of multi-valued attributes. Figure 1 illustrates the complete process, consisting of three stages: alignment, comparison and similarity aggregation.

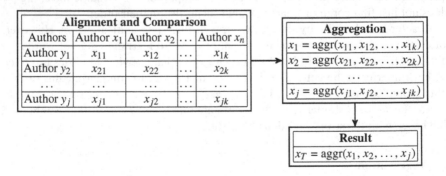

Fig. 1. Multi-valued attributes Alignment and Comparison Process

3.1   Alignment

The alignment phase consists on arranging elements of both lists for having a comparison matrix where the diagonal $\{(1,1),...,(N,N)\}$ denotes the right comparisons to make. In some cases, multi-valued attributes are already ordered hence this step might not be necessary, e.g. publication author lists.

According to the clustering and blocking methods used in the Google Refine project [7], Fingerprint [12] resulted the most useful and promising approach to align multiple attribute values in such a way that the comparison process performance is increased. Basically, Fingerprint splits a string in tokens and order them alphabetically.

For some heuristics we applied Fingerprint for sorting the item lists. In these cases, after executing FingerPrint over each element of the lists, each array was arranged in ascending order. The string obtained from FingerPrint was just used for ordering purpose. For comparison, the real name of authors was used.

3.2   Comparison Strategies

The proposed comparison strategies try to minimize the number of author name comparisons. The combination of comparison strategies determine which elements of the comparison matrix $\mathcal{M}$ are filled: the less author-name comparisons, the better. Consider the lists of authors $A_1[N]$ and $A_2[M]$, being $N \geq M$. The comparison strategies will determine which element of $A_1[i]$ ($0 < i < N$) and $A_2[j]$ ($0 < j < M$) will be compared. The result of the comparison (the individual similarity) is stored in $\mathcal{M}[i,j]$. The comparison strategies used were:

- **Full-Matrix**: compare all elements in $A_1[i]$ with all elements in $A_2[j]$.
- **Diagonal**: compare elements in $A_1[i]$ with elements in $A_2[j]$, only when i=j.
- **Row-Col-Deletion**: if $\mathcal{M}[i,j] \geq$ min-similarity, comparisons $\mathcal{M}[a,b]$ are skipped for $i < a < N$, $j < b < M$.
- **Row-Similarity-Threshold**: if $\mathcal{M}[i,j] \geq$ min-similarity, continue comparing in the next row of the matrix ($\mathcal{M}[i+1,j]$), i.e. $\mathcal{M}[i,b]$ is left empty for $j < b < M$.

We additionally defined a stop criterion for avoiding unnecessary comparisons:

- **Partial-Average-Threshold**: compare elements in $A_1[i]$ and $A_2[j]$ until reaching 80% of $\mathcal{M}$. If Max-Average (described in Section 3.3) is above min-similarity, continue with the comparison process; otherwise, stop.

Given the nature of the element comparison problem and based on the taxonomy described by [5] we used *Content-based* matching approaches to determine the similarity of two entities (author names in our case). We decided to combine two techniques that compare atomic values: one for character-to-character comparison (*Jaro Winkler*), and another for token-to-token comparison (*Longest Common Substring (LCS)*). For combining the results of both of them, we used the *root mean square (RMS)*, to improve the similarity grade over a single comparator [11,8]. Those author names which similarity score was above a defined threshold were considered similar.

3.3   Similarity Aggregation

Aggregation strategies try to determine the final similarity grade between the processed lists of authors. The strategies used are:

- **Average**: $\frac{\sum_{i=0}^{N}\sum_{j=0}^{M}\mathcal{M}[i,j]}{(N\times M)}$
- **Max-Average**: Max(Avg (x), Avg(y)), where $x = \sum_{i=0}^{N} Max(\mathcal{M}[i,*])$ and $y = \sum_{j=0}^{M} Max(\mathcal{M}[*,j])$.

In plain words Max-Average chooses between the maximum average of the sum of maximum values obtained from column or rows.

3.4   Evaluated Heuristics

We considered a heuristic as a selection of an alignment choice (original or Fingerprint), a combination of comparison strategies, and an aggregation style. A summary and a brief description of the self designed and evaluated heuristics (labeled $H_0, H_1, H_2, H_4, ..., H_7$), can be found in Table 1. Comparison strategies are decomposed in two criteria: one for choosing which elements to compare next, and another for determining when to stop comparing. The aim sought when designing the heuristics was to reduce the amount of comparisons needed to determine the similarity or not between two list of authors. It is expected that the comparison's strategies guide the heuristics to just compare the authors in the main diagonal, or to find the best possible match for one author, and then continue looking the next author's best matching candidate. If the lists do not match, for some heuristics will not be necessary to find the best matching candidate for each author. Just with a few comparisons would be enough to determine that has not sense continuing with the comparison process.

The heuristic H_0 which averages all possible author names comparisons, is the traditional process followed to establish a similarity grade between two lists of authors, so we select it as our baseline, in order to compare if the other heuristics generate any improvement in the process of establishing a similarity grade when comparing multivalued attributes.

Algorithm 1 shows an implementation of heuristic H_4, which implements the comparison's strategies Row-Col-Deletion and Row-Similarity-Threshold, and uses the Partial-Average-Threshold criterion to stop comparing if the temporary similarity is not good enough.

4   Experimental Results

In this Section we describe the datasets used in our experiments and the execution time for each heuristic. Finally, we present the results obtained in similarity classification and efficiency experiments.

Table 1. Evaluated Heuristics

Heuristic	Alignment	Comparisons			Aggregation
H_0 / H_1	Original Order	Full Matrix (NxM)			H_0 Average
		Who's Next		**Stop Criteria**	H_1 Max-Average
		if (j < M) then j=j+1 else j=0, i=i+1		i = N and j = M	
H_2	FingerPrint	1. Diagonal. 2. If sim < min-similarity then H_4.			Max-Average
		Who's Next		**Stop Criteria**	
		if (i<N) and (j<M) j=j+1, i=i+1		i = N and j = M	
H_4/ H_5	Original Order	Row-Col-Deletion + Partial-Average-Threshold			Max-Average
		Who's Next		**Stop Criteria**	
		if ($A_1 \wedge A_2$ are visible) then Row-Col-Deletion Row-Similarity-Threshold else if (j < M) then continue next column (j=j+1) else continue next row (i=i+1)		H_4 Partial-Average-Threshold or (i=N and j=M) H_5 i=N and j=M	
H_6/ H_7	H_6 Original Order H_7 FingerPrint	Row-Col-Deletion			Max-Average
		Who's Next		**Stop Criteria**	
		if ($A_1 \wedge A_2$ are visible) then H_6: Row-Col-Deletion H_7: Row-Col-Deletion, Row-Similarity-Threshold if (j < M) then continue next column (j=j+1) else continue next row (i=i+1)		H_6 i=N and j=M H_7 Partial-Average-Threshold or (i=N and j=M)	

Algorithm 1. Heuristic H_4 (Row-Col-Deletion + Row-Similarity-Threshold + Partial-Average-Threshold)

```
Input: alist_1 / alist_2
Result: Matrix M

1  for (i, i < alist_1.length , i++) {
2    if (alist_1[i] is available)
3      for(j, j < alist_2.length, j++) {
4        if (alist_2[j] is available)
5          M[i,j] = calculate_similarity(alist_1[i], alist_2[j])
6          if (M[i,j] >= threshold)
7            Turn off availability of alist_1[i], alist_2[j]
8            i = i+1 // Continue on next row
9          end-if
10       end-if
11       if (checkpoint)
12         if (Max-Average(M) < min-similarity)
13           Stop process
14     }
15   end-if
16 }
```

4.1 Datasets

We use two data-sets, one extracted from an internal repository and the other one from ISI Web of Knowledge. Both contain 548 records, the first one with information about papers published by our University researchers and the second one with the equivalent papers in the ISI Web database. From both datasets we used the publication ID and the author list (parsed for comparing individual author names).

Each author list of one file was compared against all the other author lists of the second file, performing a total of 300,304 comparisons. Of this total, 1,052 author-lists were equivalent (all the items in one list were in the other and vice versa). This is because the same group of authors could appear in multiple publications.

It is important to mention the difference between the author names comparison and the author lists comparison. The first one refers to the comparison performed between two authors, for example *Gutierrez-Vega, JC* against *Munoz-Rodriguez, D*, while the second one implies the aggregated similarity between two lists of authors, for example {*Gutierrez-Vega, JC; Chavez-Cerda, S; Rodriguez-Dagnino, RM*} versus {*Aleman-Llanes, E; Munoz-Rodriguez, D; Molina, C*}.

4.2 Running Time

To evaluate the computational cost of the algorithms, we measured the time each of them required to process the 300,304 author list comparisons. We used the average time of five trials for each heuristic. Previous to each trial, the warm-up stage last 1200 ms. A subset of the records were used multiple times during that period. The experiments had been run on an *Intel(R) Core(TM) i7 CPU Q 720 @ 1.60 GHz* machine, running a *64-bit Operating System (Windows 8 Pro)* with *4GB RAM*. The algorithms were implemented in Java. The average run time of each heuristic is shown in Table 2. It can be seen that heuristic H_4 run faster than H_0 and the rest of the evaluated heuristics.

Table 2. Total average processing time for 300,304 records

Heuristic ID	Run Time (in sec)	Heuristic ID	Run Time (in sec)
H_0	241	H_5	258
H_1	261	H_6	260
H_2	293	H_7	237
H_4	204		

4.3 Author Names Alignment

In the first place we evaluated if the proposed heuristics were capable of identifying one to one matches, and based on that determining how similar two author lists were. We used 0.82 as the minimum similarity threshold for our experiments. Author name comparisons with similarity above this threshold were considered as similar. Higher thresholds were tested, but resulted in a higher quantity of false-negatives. We also used the same threshold (0.82) to decide if two author's lists were similar or not.

We classified each pair of author lists in the following groups in order to assess the overall similarity in terms of one-to-one matches:

- **No match.** No pair of authors's names have a similarity above the threshold.
- **Some matches.** At least one pair of authors's names matched (this means that at least one pair of authors's names had a similarity value above or equal to the threshold), but not all of them.
- **All match.** All pairs of authors's names matched (both author lists have the same length ($N = M$) and N authors's name comparisons are above the min-similarity threshold).

In Figure 2 is shown the result of the classification. Note that in this experiment the baseline is not H_0. The baseline indicates how many authors actually shared the compared author-lists. It is convenient to mention the reason those heuristics which perform all possible comparisons, exceed the classified amount of authors-lists in the *Some matches* group. Cases like *Acevedo-Mascarúa, J.* and *Aceves, J* produce similarity values (0.84) above threshold (0.82), when in fact, those authors were not the same person. Then, when compared the following lists: {*Acevedo-Mascarúa, J.; Salguerio, M.*} and {*Arcos, D; Sierra, A; Nunez, A; Flores, G; Aceves, J; Arias-Montano, JA*}, the heuristics determined that one similarity existed, when actually was not the case as none of the authors were similar.

The small number of author list pairs classified in the *All match* group (in this case all the heuristics had a similar behavior) was due to a similar problem. We found for example the author lists {*Elías-Zúñiga, A.; Millard, B.*} and {*Zuniga, AE; Beatty, MF*} which are equivalent lists, but author name variants avoided to determine individual matches above the similarity threshold. Those are situations where it becomes difficult to identify that they refer to the same authors, even for a human expert. The heuristics classified this comparison into the *No match* group, when in fact it should be classified into the *All match* one. In spite of these particular situations, H_4 and H_7 were the heuristics which best classified the authors-lists into the groups *No matches* and *Some matches*.

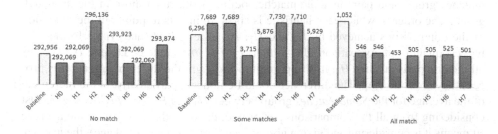

Fig. 2. Author Lists comparisons and average similarity percentage of each block

4.4 Author Lists Similarity

Next we evaluated if the similarity between author lists is better approximated by aggregating the individual author similarities chosen by each heuristic. Figure 3 shows the amount of author lists having an aggregated similarity above 0.82. As expected H_1 found out the biggest quantity of similar record pairs, but at cost of performing all versus all author name comparisons. The low amount of similarity found by H_0 is due to the aggregation strategy used, since it negatively impacts on the general average, allowing just a few authors-lists having an average similarity above the threshold.

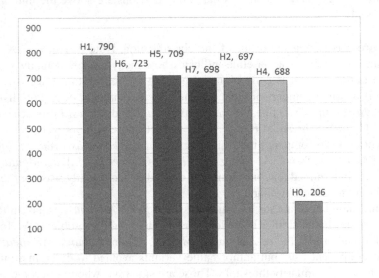

Fig. 3. Author Lists with aggregated similarity above threshold

Figure 4 shows both the amount of author name comparisons performed and the average aggregated similarity in each group for each heuristic. This time the groups are due to the classification made by a human being, so you would expect the average similarity of pairs of author lists in the all-match group to be higher than those in the some-matches group, and pairs in some-matches being greater than those in the no-match group. The order in which each heuristic is showed, intents to point out the reduction of the comparisons achieved by H_4 and H_7. As expected, H_0 and H_1 performed the biggest quantity of comparisons due to their *Full-Matrix* strategy. Despite H_1 executes all the comparisons, like H_0, it is important to highlight the different aggregation process they are following. The difference could be noticed, particularly, in the increment of the average for the *Some matches* group between H_0 and H_1. As *Max-Average* is just considering from all the comparisons performed, the ones that maximizes the average (it means it is considering and giving importance to author-names linkage), the average similarity grows up. The same occurs for the group *All match*. On the contrary this rise is not so evident in the average similarity of the group *No match* because there is not any author-name comparison value above the threshold (0.82) which impacts positively in the final result.

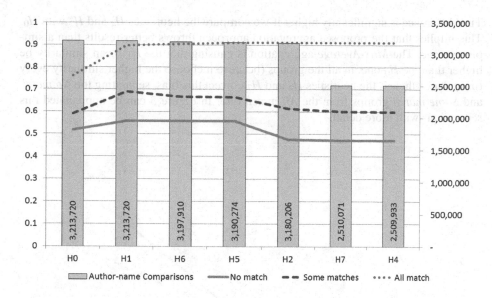

Fig. 4. Author Name comparisons with similarity average per group

This reduction in the amount of comparisons achieved by H_4 and H_7 could be noticed also in the reduction of the average similarity in the groups *some matches* and *no matches*. Since these heuristics, with the objective of increasing the performance, do not perform all the comparisons, it makes possible that even when a common author exists, it is not noticed as the comparison never takes place because of their logic. In this way, that similarity value (which is above the established threshold, 0.82) is prevented of impacting positively in the final average. This is more evident if heuristics H_4 and H_7 are compared with H_5 and H_6 respectively, as their only difference is that H_4 and H_7 make use of the *Partial-Average-Threshold* strategy, performing fewer comparisons as it evaluates if the Max-Average is above the threshold, once the 80% of the author-names have been compared. If it is not above the threshold, the comparison process finishes, as it is not expected that the remaining 20% of the authors impact on the final result, which is to determine if the authors-lists are similar or not.

5 Discussion

With the aim of comparing the results obtained by the heuristics, different statistical tests, available in the SPSS tool, were performed (ANOVA, Turkey HSD). The classification groups (*No match, Some matches, All matches*) as well as their respective similarity averages were used. We choose to evaluate the heuristics H_0, H_1, H_4 and H_7, because the first one makes use of the traditional approach, H_1 is an improvement of H_0, and H_4, H_7 obtained promising results during the experiments. Through those analyses could be observed, in the first place, that the highest difference between the medians was obtained by H_4 and H_7 in the *No match* and *All matches* groups (see Fig. 5).

This difference is significantly higher if we compare the heuristics H_4 and H_7 with H_0. This implies that the proposed aggregation approach throws better results than a simple average. The *Max-Average* aggregation is causing that the H_1 mean similarity be higher than the H_0 one, in all the groups (because it choose the higher similarity every time). Nevertheless the heuristics H_4 and H_7 correct this bias, separating the *No match* and *Some match* groups from the *All match* one. In Figure 5 can be appreciated this separations with more detail.

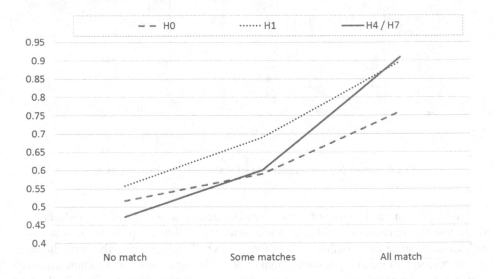

Fig. 5. Comparison of the rice of the similarity average between different groups

The reason of why H_4 and H_7 find a small amount of similar authors-lists pairs (Figure 3) is because of the previously mentioned difficult-to-resolve cases, just using the author name and surname attributes. Another justification could be that they perform less comparisons than the rest of the heuristics. It is important to mention that, Anyhow, the amount of similarity found by each heuristic does not differ much, except for H_0 and H_1, which perform much more comparisons.

Continuing with the authors-list comparisons analysis, in those cases where author lists are equivalent (all match), heuristics H_4 and H_7 reduce the number of comparisons due to the alignment and comparison process, managing to find, mostly, those similar authors. This is shown in Figure 4, in the (almost) constant line of the *All match* group. The fact of performing less comparisons also affect if those lists are quite similar (*Some match* group) or non similar at all (*No match* group). As the process could be stopped if at least 80% of the authors do not match, then the heuristics which perform more comparisons could increase the average similarity with the remaining 20%. But the final objective is not to link authors but to determine if two authors-lists are similar or not. Then, the heuristics H_4 and H_7, besides improving the difference between medians, reduce the number of comparisons.

Other problem which affects the heuristics H_0 and H_1 is when they process authors-lists which are very similar, but are not the same. In those situations, these heuristics would find higher amount of similarities than the ones that really exist. For example, consider the following lists: *Khan, M.A.;Maroof, S.A.; Khan, M.Y.* and *Uzair, M.;Khan, M.A.; Khan, M.Y.*. In this context H_0 and H_1 would found 4 similarities, when the maximum number of authors is 3. It is not the case for the heuristics which force the 1-1 matching, as H_4 and H_7. The difference with the approaches presented by [2] and [18], is that H_4 and H_7 do not need to perform all the comparisons to find the best alignment.

The FingerPrint approach has not made big contributions in these experiments because the lists were already ordered (in most cases). It would be of great help if we would have been comparing keywords or if those authors-lists were not ordered at all, as it happens with the Dublin Core [4] or SWRC [15] ontologies, where the authorship relation is not following any order.

6   Conclusions

In this paper we presented the first results of an approach to align, compare and aggregate the similarity of multi-valued attributes. It was compared against the traditional approaches, using different heuristics, and the results obtained were promising. It reduced in 22% the amount of comparisons performed, making the process more efficient. It also increased the classification quality, showing a considerable difference between the No match and All matches medians.

Despite these results seems promising we still need to improve the validation of its efficacy. We will divide the *Some matches* group in two smaller blocks: those that have a similarity value above 50% (for example) and those that are below that threshold. This would help to improve the quality assessment of the proposed heuristics. Besides, the use of public datasets (from DBLP or ACM), would help us to continue measuring the accuracy of the proposed heuristics.

Regarding those hard-to-determine similarities, we would add new different attributes (affiliation or common coauthors) to help the algorithms to determine if two authors represent the same entity or not. This would help the heuristics to increase the amount of similarities of the All matches group. Adding this approach to entity resolution frameworks like Silk [17] or OYSTER [16] would help us to verify if it is useful in the entity resolution process and if it improves the linkage between similar entities.

References

1. Bilenko, M., Mooney, R., Cohen, W., Ravikumar, P., Fienberg, S.: Adaptive name matching in information integration. IEEE Intelligent Systems 18(5), 16–23 (2003)
2. Burkard, R., Dell'Amico, M., Martello, S.: Assignment Problems. Siam, Philadelphia (2009)
3. Cohen, W.W., Fienberg, S.E.: A Comparison of String Distance Metrics for Name-Matching Tasks. In: Proceedings of the ACM Workshop on Data Cleaning, Record Linkage and Object Identification (2003)
4. DCMI: Dublin Core Ontology (2012), http://dublincore.org/documents/dces/
5. Dorneles, C.F., Gonçalves, R., Santos Mello, R.: Approximate data instance matching: a survey. Knowledge and Information Systems 27(1), 1–21 (2010)

6. Elmagarmid, A.K., Ipeirotis, P.G., Verykios, V.S.: Duplicate record detection: A survey. IEEE Transactions on Knowledge and Data Engineering 19(1), 1–16 (2007)
7. Google: Google Refine Project (2012), http://code.google.com/p/google-refine/
8. Grannis, S.J., Overhage, J.M., McDonald, C.: Real world performance of approximate string comparators for use in patient matching. Studies in Health Technology and Informatics 107(pt.1), 43–47 (2004)
9. Guha, S., Koudas, N., Marathe, A., Srivastava, D.: Merging the Results of Approximate Match Operations. In: Proceedings of The Thirtieth International Conference on Very Large Data Bases, pp. 636–647 (2004)
10. Köpcke, H., Rahm, E.: Frameworks for entity matching: A comparison. Data & Knowledge Engineering 69(2), 197–210 (2010)
11. Köpcke, H., Thor, A., Rahm, E.: Comparative evaluation of entity resolution approaches with FEVER. In: Proceedings of 35th Intl. Conference on Very Large Databases (VLDB) (2009)
12. Morris, T., Huynh, D.: FingerPrint Method (2010),
    https://github.com/OpenRefine/OpenRefine/wiki/Clustering-In-Depth
13. Porter, E.H., Winkler, W.E.: Approximate String Comparison and its Effect on an Advanced Record Linkage System. Tech. rep (1997)
14. Ravikumar, P., Cohen, W.W., Fienberg, S.E.: A secure protocol for computing string distance metrics. In: Proceedings of the Workshop on Privacy and Security Aspects of Data Mining at the Int. Conf. on Data Mining, pp. 40–46 (2004)
15. Sure, Y., Bloehdorn, S., Haase, P., Hartmann, J., Oberle, D.: The swrc ontology - semantic web for research communities. In: Bento, C., Cardoso, A., Dias, G. (eds.) EPIA 2005. LNCS (LNAI), vol. 3808, pp. 218–231. Springer, Heidelberg (2005)
16. Talburt, J.R.: Entity resolution and information quality. Elsevier (2011)
17. Volz, J., Bizer, C., Gaedke, M., Kobilarov, G.: Silk–a link discovery framework for the web of data. In: Proceedings of the 2nd Workshop on Linked Data on the Web (2009)
18. Winkler, W.E.: Advanced Methods For Record Linkage. Section on Survey Research Methods (American Statistical Association) (1994)
19. Winkler, W.E.: Overview of record linkage and current research directions. In: Proceedings of Bureau of the Census. Citeseer (2006)
20. Yancey, W.E.: Evaluating string comparator performance for record linkage. Statistical Research Division Research Report (2005)

Data Mining for Discovering Patterns in Migration

Anilu Franco-Arcega, Kristell D. Franco-Sánchez, Felix A. Castro-Espinoza, and Luis H. García-Islas

Universidad Autónoma del Estado de Hidalgo,
Área Académica de Computación y Electrónica,
Carr. Pachuca - Tulancingo km. 4.5, C.P.42084 Pachuca, Hidalgo, México
{afranco,luishg}@uaeh.edu.mx, kristell-daniella@hotmail.com,
fcastroe@gmail.com

Abstract. Nowadays, Data Mining has been successfully applied to several fields such as business administration, marketing and sales, diagnostics, manufacturing processes and astronomy. One of the areas where the use of Data Mining has not been well used is in the solution of social problems, where making effective decisions is essential to offering better social programs. In particular, this paper presents an analysis of Migration, which is an important social phenomenon that affects cultural, economic, ideological and demographic aspects of society, among others. This paper is based on an experiment with data processing and clustering analysis of demographic factors related to migration in the State of Hidalgo, Mexico. This study reveals the character and description of clusters obtained with data mining techniques. The knowledge from this characterization is potentially useful to government and social service agencies in the State of Hidalgo for the creation of specific social programs that might be device to mitigate the migration of the population.

Keywords: Data mining, clustering, migration.

1 Introduction

Currently, Data Mining has had a significant impact on the information industry, due to the wide availability of large datasets, which are stored in databases of different types. In order to make more informed decisions, institutions have responded to the urgent need to turn research and reformulate stored data into useful information and knowledge that can be used in a multitude of applications such as business management, production control, market analysis, engineering design, science exploration, etc. Accordingly, Data Mining tools and techniques greatly contribute to business strategies, knowledge bases, social and educational environments and scientific and medical research, to name just a few [20].

Data Mining techniques can help providing solutions of two significant types: prediction and description. The models generated by predictive methods estimate future and unknown values using known attributes or fields of a database

A. Gelbukh et al. (Eds.): MICAI 2014, Part II, LNAI 8857, pp. 285–295, 2014.

to make the prediction. Descriptive models, on the other hand, explore the properties of the processed data to identify patterns that explain or summarize the data, or to find relationships among the data [9],[21].

One of the areas where Data Mining has been applied is in the analysis of social problems. A social problem is the result of a process of collective definition that arises when a significant portion of the population considers some social situations as undesirable. These perceptions can also be transmitted to other social sectors. Consequently, a social problem is an aspect of society where a large number of people are involved [10]. If we are capable of analyzing the causes, consequences and factors of social problems, then we can characterize the behavior of the social problems and furthermore, identify new knowledge and relationships among different social problems such as poverty, marginalization, dealing trafficking, crime, etc. [25].

Data Mining has been successfully applied in several studies about social problems, such as identification of characteristics of a population [24], characterization of students [19],[1],[12], studies of residential segregation [2], academic performance[28],[11], unemployment [14], etc. Specifically, the social problem of human migration is a socio-spatial phenomenon [15], which occurs as a result of several changes in interdependent areas, social structures and spatial relations [8].

One of the most important social problem is migration, due to the fact that it can greatly influence the dynamics and magnitude of a given population. Migration is a social phenomenon that affects several important aspects, such as cultural, economics, ideology and demographics, to name just a few. Migration produces important changes in both the origin and destination places of migrants. This problematic behavior has motivated considerable analyses with the aim of identifying and thus, potentially, avoiding the negative effects of migration. Studying the phenomenon of migration in any country is very important, mainly because such studies can ultimately influence the dynamics of the population, it affects as well as the social, cultural and economic structures of a country or region. Such studies are essential to the formulation of development policies that impact the lives of people and societies which are seeking further growth, equity and quality of life [13]. The analysis of migration also allows the preparation of proposals supporting the implementation of programs that encourage investment by migrants in their own communities, and for the creation or improvement of proposals for mitigation and improvement by government agencies as well.

In Mexico, the state of Hidalgo is among the top ten sources of international migration; it is considered by the National Population Council as a state of high level contemporary emigration to the United States [5], according to the index of migration intensity of Mexican households, conducted in 2000 [27].

Typically, experts in the field of migration employ statistical techniques such as analyses of variance, paired t tests, Pearson correlation, Kruskal-Wallis tests, Spearman correlation, etc. [4] [3], [16], [17], [22] in order to understand the migration phenomenon. However, these techniques are not the most appropriate

when we want to obtain information about behavior patterns of different social groups. To overcome this restriction, the use of data mining techniques is
proposed in this paper.

This research work depicts and employs a model that describes the profiles
of migrants of Hidalgo State. This model is based on a large and significant
database, a Census of Population and Housing in the State of Hidalgo 2010
created by the Mexican National Institute for Geography and Statistics (INEGI:
Spanish acronym).

The paper is organized as follows. Section 2 presents the description of the
database of INEGI used for this study. Then, the results of applying Data Mining
tools on the outcome dataset are presented in Section 3. Finally, conclusions and
future recommended research are delineated.

2 Migrants' Demographic Data for the State of Hidalgo

We used the data about Population and Housing Census from INEGI collected in
2010, which contains, among other information, data from the individual homes
of the families that have migrant members. The attributes in the database from
INEGI provides information about the features of migrants's housing and the
conditions and the living quality of migrants' families.

2.1 Selection of the Data

In this phase, we integrated and collected the data from the international migrant's module from an expanded questionnaire from the Census mentioned
above. We linked the National Migrants Base with the National Housing Base
and we applied the necessary filters for obtaining the specific data from the
State of Hidalgo. We obtained registers where in the family had or haves had an
migrant to or from the United States.

2.2 Preprocessing and Transformation

In the preprocessing phase, the data was exported to a MySQL Server for a better
manipulation. We executed queries from SQL for obtaining only one table; after
that, we excluded the attributes without information (i.e. identifiers) and the
attributes with the same value for all the records. In the transformation phase
we edited the questions with answers of "Don't Know", with the same format
of the others answers, using the views of MySQL. Finally we got a dataset with
1567 records and 45 attributes, which are described in Table 1.

3 Migrant's Demographic Factor Analysis

We used the Open Source Software Weka version 3.7.9 for applying the clustering and evaluation algorithms for Data Mining. We applied four clustering

Table 1. Attributes' description from INEGI dataset

Attribute	Description
MUN	Township Code
MSEXO	Migrant's Gender
MEDAD	Migrant's Age
TAM_LOC	Size of locality
CLAVIVP	Kind of housing: independent, apartment, neighborhood, etc.
PAREDES	Wall's material: waste material, bamboo or palms, etc.
TECHOS	Roof's material: waste material, bamboo or palms, etc.
PISOS	Floor's material: earth, cement, tile, wood, etc.
COCINA	The housing has or hasn't a room for cooking
CUADORM	Number of rooms for sleeping (without hallways)
TOTCUART	Total rooms in the house (without hallways or bathrooms)
ELECTRI	The housing does or does not have electricity
DISAGU	Water availability: inside the house, outside the house, etc.
DOTAGUAD	Days/week with water: daily, twice a week, etc.
SERSAN	The housing does or does not have toilet
USOEXC	The housing does or does not share toilet with another house
CONAGU	Type of flushing the toilet: direct, with a bucket, etc.
DRENAJE	Drain connection: to public network, septic, etc.
COMBUST	The fuel commonly used for cooking: gas, wood, etc.
ELIBAS	Type of disposal of trash: car garbage collector, burning, etc.
TENVIV	Housing tenure: for rent, live in housing the owner, etc.
FADQUI	Acquisition of housing: bought, self-constructed, etc.
ESTUFAG	The housing does or does not have gas stove
ESTUFAL	The housing does or does not have wood stove
TINACO	The housing does or does not have tank
BOILER	The housing does or does not have heater
CISTERNA	The housing does or does not have cistern
REGADERA	The housing does or does not have shower
MEDLUZ	The housing does or does not have electric meter
RADIO	The housing does or does not have radio
TELEVI	The housing does or does not have television
REFRIG	The housing does or does not have refrigerator
LAVADORA	The housing does or does not have washing machine
AUTOPROP	Somebody in the housing does or does not have a car or truck
COMPU	The housing does or does not have computer
TELEFONO	The housing does or does not have telephone
CELULAR	Somebody in the housing does or does not have a cell phone
INTERNET	The housing does or does not have Internet
NUMPERS	Number of people in household
TIPOHOG	Type of household: basic or extended family, coresident, etc.
MNUMPERS	Number of international migrants
COMIO1VEZ	Some of the people in this house ate only once a day
NOCOMI1D	Some of the people in this house stopped eating all day
SINCOMER	Some of the people in this house ran out of food
INGTRHOG	Monthly income by work at home

algorithms to obtain different clusters' configurations of the data. First, we applied two algorithms where we do not have to specify the number of clusters to form, the EM algorithm [18] and the Self-Organizing Maps (SOM) [6]. When we applied the EM algorithm, we obtained five clusters; and with SOM four clusters were formed. According to these results, we decided to apply the Simple K -means [18] and the Make Density Based Clusterer (MDBC) [26] algorithms with three, four and five number of clusters, in order to compare the behavior of all the used algorithms and, furthermore, to obtain more consistent and appropiate clustering results.

In order to perform a successful and valid assessment for the clustering models obtained, we have applied a standard metric generally used in unsupervised learning, called cluster validity index (CVI). In specific, we used the Davies - Bouldin Index [23], which is one of the most commonly used in the literature, this metric is shown is Eq. 1.

$$DB(C) = \frac{1}{K} \sum_{C_k} \max_{C_l \in C \setminus C_k} \left\{ \frac{S(C_k) + S(C_l)}{d_G(\overline{C_k}, \overline{C_l})} \right\} \tag{1}$$

where

- K is the number of clusters,
- C_k represents the cluster k,
- $\overline{C_k}$ is the centroid of cluster k,
- d_G calculates the distance between two points, and
- $S(C_k) = 1/|C_k| \sum_{x_i \in C_k} d_G(x_i, \overline{C_k})$

This index applies the Euclidean distance to estimate the cohesion between the objects and its centroid, and the separation between centroids. However, since the Euclidean distance is traditionally used for numeric attributes and we have mixed attributes, we decided to use Gower's distance [7], which allows calculating the distance with heterogeneous attributes (numeric, boolean and categorical). This distance is shown in Eq. 2.

$$d_{G(ii')} = \sqrt{1 - S_{G(ii')}} \tag{2}$$

where,
$$S_{G(ii')} = \frac{\sum_{j=1}^{p} W_{ii'j} S_{ii'j}}{\sum_{j=1}^{p} W_{ii'j}}$$

The Davies - Bouldin Index was applied to the results of EM, SOM, Simple K-means and Make Density Based Clusterer algorithms, the two last with values of three, four and five groups. The results of this index for all the algorithms are shown in Table 2. The N/A value indicates that for the involved algorithm the Davies - Bouldin Index is not applicable due to the fact that, as have been stated before, in SOM and EM algorithms the number of clusters to obtain it is not compulsory.

According to the Davies - Bouldin Index, a lower value of this index means a better partition. Therefore, the best clustering model was obtained through the

Table 2. Davies - Bouldin Index for the different algorithms

Algorithm	3 groups	4 groups	5 groups
SOM	N/A	2.948	N/A
EM	N/A	N/A	4.358
Simple K-means	2.162	2.145	4.996
MDBC	2.137	2.228	5.064

Make Density Based Clusterer algorithm (MDBC) with three clusters obtaining a value of 2.137; however, the value obtained with Simple K-means (with four clusters) was also low, comparable with the other value, for this reason we perform a detailed analysis for these two results before to choose the clustering to characterize it.

For comparing both results, with three and four groups, we have checked the percentage of instances, that were colocated within the same group by the Simple K-means and the Make Density Based Clusterer (MDBC) algorithms. For the four clusters result, the 87.43% of the instances that the Simple K-means put into the groups stay in the same groups with the Make Density Based Clusterer algorithm (MDBC). With respect to the three-group result, we obtained 100% of the instances clustered in the same way, with both algorithms. With this findings, we have confirmed that the best result for this problem was obtained with the Make Density Based Clusterer algorithm (MDBC), forming three clusters.

3.1   Interpretation

Once we have obtained the best clustering model, we applied the InfoGainAttributeEval method from Weka with the purpose of finding the attributes with the highest information weight. This method evaluates the attributes' values with the information gain with respect to the cluster. It used the Ranker method that evaluates the attributes individually and listed them according to that evaluation. Table 3 shows the obtained value for this method by each attribute of the used dataset.

Figure 1 illustrates the behavior of the more representative attributes in this dataset. As we can notice, it is appreciated how the three clusters are formed.

We analyzed the results obtained by the selected algorithm at the end of section 3. In order to introduce this knowledge to social experts, a processable, comprehensible and interpretable characterization description has been produced. This clustering characterization is described as follows.

- **Cluster 0:** *Housing in exclusion and poverty.* This group is characterized by houses without basic services such as shower, water heater, water tank or washing machine; they do not have drain connections and they use a bucket of water to flush the toilet into a septic tank. They have piped water outside the house but inside the ground; the fuel that they use to cook is firewood, since they have wood stoves; the elimination of the garbage is done through burning. These houses are located mainly in the following

Table 3. Information Gain

Information Gain	Attribute	Information Gain	Attribute
0.44048	REGADERA	0.05912	TIPOHOG
0.43691	CONAGU	0.05428	TELEFONO
0.41677	BOILER	0.04776	TELEVI
0.35753	MUN	0.04599	INTERNET
0.30302	TINACO	0.04518	USOEXC
0.28859	COMBUST	0.04395	SERSAN
0.24461	DRENAJE	0.04252	PAREDES
0.24335	DISAGU	0.03981	MNUMPERS
0.17343	ELIBAS	0.03371	MEDLUZ
0.16468	ESTUFAL	0.03359	ELECTRI
0.15351	CELULAR	0.0306	FADQUI
0.15309	LAVADORA	0.02981	NUMPERS
0.12912	TAM_LOC	0.02742	CLAVIVP
0.12554	CUADORM	0.01783	CISTERNA
0.11418	TOTCUART	0.01662	MEDAD
0.11403	PISOS	0.01534	MSEXO
0.11338	INGTRHOG	0.01133	COCINA
0.10847	AUTOPROP	0.01059	RADIO
0.10592	ESTUFAG	0.01055	TENVIV
0.09471	REFRIG	0.00282	SINCOMER
0.09063	TECHOS	0.0022	NOCOMI1D
0.07984	COMPU	0.00212	COMIO1VEZ
0.06002	DOTAGUAD		

cities **Pisaflores, Tlahuiltepa, Omitlán de Juárez, Tepehuacán de Guerrero, Tenango de Doria, Chapulhuacán, La Misión, Tlanchinol, Eloxochitlán, Lolotla, Nicolás Flores. Pacula, Molango de Escamilla, Tecozautla, Juárez Hidalgo, Calnali, Cardonal y Tianguistengo.**

– Cluster 1: *Homes including over medium quantity of services and development.* This group is characterized by houses with services such as shower, water heater, water tank and washing machines; they have drain connection to the public network; they have piped water inside the house; the fuel that they use to cook is gas, from a gas cylinder or stationary tank; the garbage is collected by a garbage truck. These houses are located mainly in the following cities **Tulancingo de Bravo, Francisco I. Madero, Tasquillo, Zimapán, Pachuca de Soto, Acatlán, Mixquiahuala de Juárez, Atotonilco el Grande, Tezontepec de Aldama, Progreso de Obregón, San Agustín Metzquititlán, Santiago Tulantepec de Lugo Guerrero, Cuautepec de Hinojosa, Metepec, Tlanalapa, Tolcayuca e Ixmiquilpan.**

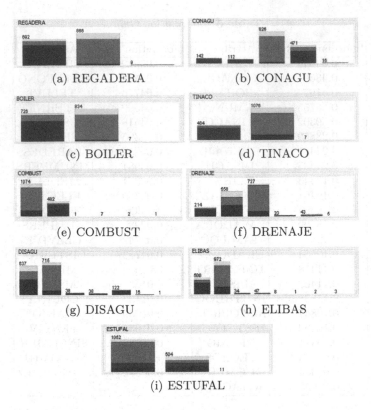

Fig. 1. More representative attributes for the demographic factor

– **Cluster2: *Housing in marginalization*.** This group is characterized by houses with services such as shower, water heater, water tank and washing machine; they have drain connection to a septic tank; they have piped water outside the house but inside the ground; the fuel that they use to cook is gas, from gas cylinder or stationary tank, but they also have wood or coal stove; the garbage is collected by a garbage truck. These houses are located mainly in the following cities **Huasca de Ocampo, Agua Blanca de Iturbide, Jacala de Ledezma, Alfajayucan, Chapantongo, Mineral del Chico, Huehuetla y Nopala de Villagrán.**

These characterizations can be used by experts or the government to develop social actions and decisions addressed to improve the quality of life of the migrants' families, and furthermore, reducing or attempting to mitigate the dinamics and forces that cause migration from in the State of Hidalgo.

In Figure 2 the location of the three characterized clusters obtained in this work is shown in the map of the State of Hidalgo. As we can see, cluster *housing in exclusion and poverty* dominates the north region of the state. Meanwhile, in the east and southeast regions of the state there are more migrants from cluster *homes including over medium quantity of services and development*. Finally, the majority of elements from cluster *housing in marginalization* are located in the southwest of Hidalgo. It is very important to note, that the clustering results described here, have been analyzed and validated by social experts in the migration phenomenon, and their opinion is that our results are consistent with their perception of the migration phenomenon in the state of Hidalgo.

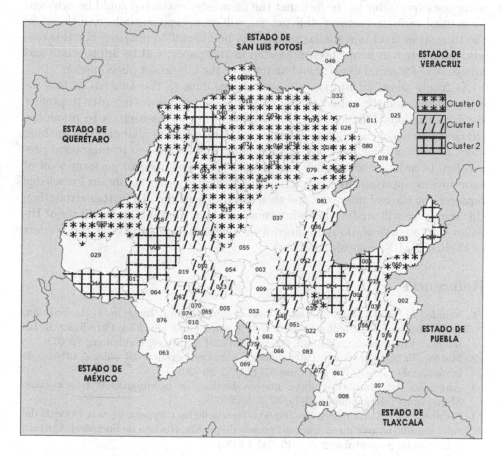

Fig. 2. Distribution of the discovered clusters in the State of Hidalgo

4   Conclusions and Future Remarks

This work presents a study that analyzes the data obtained from the Population and Housing Census made by INEGI and applied in 2010. We characterized these records into three groups, according to the application of several clustering algorithms. Moreover, we found the attributes (properties) that were more representative in differentiating those groups, and based on these attributes, we described the behavior of each of the groups. As have experimentally demonstrated in this paper, the social problem identification domain can be significantly informed through Data Mining techniques, due to the fact these results can be used by the administration of the State of Hidalgo for the creation of specific social programs addressed to providing assistance to the families abandoned through migration and to provide tenteative solutions to the problems of migration of the population.

In addition, the obtained results are very valuable for the migration phenomenon experts due to the fact that the knowledge extracted could be achieved by manual analysis; however, this process will grow exponentially, and therefore the time spent to obtain similar results will be difficult to manage. For this reason, automated, as it has been presented in this paper, will be appropriate and informative for social experts and analysts of the migration phenomenon.

As future work, we propose the use of new data to the analysis of this social problem, and the application of classification techniques in order to predict similar situations. Furthermore, the next step, in our research, is to refine the characterization of the identified groups with the ultimate goal of distinguishing more aspects of their behavior and applying this knowledge to migration prevention. In order to accomplish this ideas, we have planned to perform a set of experiments applying rules extraction algorithms in order to obtain knowledge representing the real migrants' and their families behavior. To further strengthen this study, we will analyze more information about migrants in the State of Hidalgo with additional, data obtained from the migration surveys at the borders of Mexico (EMIF: Spanish acronym).

References

1. Vellido, A., et al.: Data mining of virtual campus data. In: Jain, L.C., Tedman, R.A., Tedman, D.K. (eds.) Evolution of Teaching and Learning Paradigms in Intelligent Environment. SCI, vol. 62, pp. 223–254. Springer, Heidelberg (2007)
2. Mateos, P., Aguilar, A.M.: Diferenciación sociodemográfica del espacio urbano de la ciudad de méxico. Revista Eure 37(110), 5–30 (2011)
3. Anguiano, M.: Rumbo al norte: nuevos destinos de la emigración veracruzana. Migraciones Internacionales 3(1), 82–110 (2005)
4. Ramírez, A.G.B.: La migración como respuesta de los campesinos ante la crisis del café: Estudio en tres municipios del estado de puebla. Revista de Sociedad, Cultura y Desarrollo Sustentable 2(2), 319–341 (2006)
5. CONAPO. Índice de intensidad migratoria México Estados Unidos. Secretaria de Gobernación México (2000)
6. Banks, D., et al.: Classification, Clustering, and Data Mining Applications. In: Proceedings of the Meeting of the International Federation of Classification Societies (IFCS). Springer, Illinois (2004)
7. Chávez, D., et al.: Utilización del análisis de cluster con variables mixtas en la selección de genotipos de maíz (zea mays). Revista Investigación Operacional 30(3), 209–216 (2010)
8. Urry, J., Gregory, D.: Social Relations and Spatial Structures. Macmillan, Basingstoke (1985)
9. Dunham, M.H.: Data Mining. Introductory and Advanced Topics. Prentice Hall - Pearson Education (2003)
10. Ferrer, V., Bosch, E.: La violencia de género: De cuestión privada a problema social. Psychosocial Intervention 9(2), 7–19 (2000)

11. Castro, F., et al.: Applying data mining techniques to e-learning problems. In: Jain, L.C., Tedman, R.A., Tedman, D.K. (eds.) Evolution of Teaching and Learning Paradigms in Intelligent Environment. SCI, vol. 62, pp. 183–221. Springer, Heidelberg (2007)

12. Mugica, F., Castro, F., Nebot, A.: On the extraction of decision support rules from fuzzy predictive models. Applied Soft Computing 11, 3463–3475 (2011)

13. Franco, L.M.: Migración y Remesas en la ciudad de Ixmiquilpan. Fondo Editorial UAEH (2012)

14. Amaru-yawa, R., Colmenares, G.: Minería de Datos aplicada a los cambios en la estructura de la variable desempleo. Caso de estudio: El estado Mérida. Universidad de Los Andes. Mérida (2007)

15. Garrocho, C.: Distribución espacial de la población ZMCM 1950-1990 en Estudios Demográficos y urbanos. El Colegio de México (1995)

16. González, J.G.: Migración y remesas en el sur del estado de méxico. In: Papeles de Población, pp. 223–252 (2006)

17. Guillén, T.: Entre la convergencia y la exclusión. la deportación de mexicanos desde estados unidos de américa. In: Realidad, Datos y Espacio: Revista Internacional de Estadística y Geografía, pp. 164 – 179 (2012)

18. Frank, E., Witten, I.H.: Data Mining Practical Machine Learning Tools and Techniques. Morgan Kaufmann (2005)

19. Montoya, D.M., Díaz, I.B.: Una medida de similitud basada en las modas para la caracterización de una población estudiantil en edad extraescolar. Revista de Ingenierías Universidad de Medellín 4(7), 101–109 (2005)

20. Pei, J., Han, J., Kamber, M.: Data Mining: Concepts and Techniques. Morgan Kaufmann (2001)

21. Ferri, C., Hernández, J., Ramírez, M.: Introducción a la Minería de Datos. Prentice-Hall (2005)

22. Ávila, M.J., Jáuregui, J.A.: Estados unidos, lugar destino para los migrantes chiapanecos. In: Migraciones Internacionales, pp. 5–38 (2007)

23. Arbelaitz, O., et al.: et al. An extensive comparative study of cluster validity indices. Pattern Recognition 46, 243–256 (2013)

24. Gutiérrez, P., et al.: Identificación de patrones característicos de la población carcelaria mediante minería de datos. In: X Workshop de Investigadores en Ciencias de la Computación, pp. 461–465 (2008)

25. Tafolla, R., Aguilar, S., Benítez, J.L.: Problemas sociales, económicos y políticos de México. Editorial Universidad Nacional Autónoma de, México (2006)

26. Yadav, R., Godara, S.: Performance analysis of clustering algorithms for character. International Journal of Advanced Computer and Mathematical Sciences 4(1), 119–123 (2013)

27. Serrano, T.: Migración Internacional y Pobreza en el Estado de Hidalgo. Ediciones Universidad Autónoma del Estado de Hidalgo (2006)

28. Sabido, M., Maldonado, R.M.: Modelo clasificador para predecir el desempeño escolar terminal de un estudiante. In: International Institute of Informatics and Systemics. Décima Conferencia Iberoamericana en Sistemas, Cibernética e Informática, pp. 25–30 (2011)

Horizontal Partitioning of Multimedia Databases Using Hierarchical Agglomerative Clustering

Lisbeth Rodríguez-Mazahua, Giner Alor-Hernández,
Ma. Antonieta Abud-Figueroa, and S. Gustavo Peláez-Camarena

Division of Research and Postgraduate Studies
Instituto Tecnológico de Orizaba, Veracruz, México
lisbethr08@gmail.com, galor@itorizaba.edu.mx,
aabud@prodigy.net.mx, sgpelaez@yahoo.com.mx

Abstract. Horizontal partitioning is a database design technique widely used in relational databases in order to achieve query optimization. Recently, this technique has been applied in multimedia databases to improve query execution cost in these databases. Nevertheless, current algorithms are based on affinity between predicates to obtain an horizontal partitioning scheme (HPS). Affinity measures how a pair of predicates is accessed by the queries ("togetherness"). The main disadvantage of this measure is that it only involves two predicates, and hence does not show the "togetherness" of more than two predicates. In this paper we propose an horizontal partitioning method for multimedia databases which is based on a hierarchical agglomerative clustering algorithm. The main advantage of our method is that it does not use affinity to create the HPS. We present experimental results to clarify the soundness of the proposed method.

Keywords: Horizontal partitioning, Multimedia databases, Hierarchical clustering.

1 Introduction

Traditionally, partitioning techniques are used in the distributed system design to reduce accesses to irrelevant data. Three main partitioning techniques have been defined for relational and object-oriented databases: horizontal partitioning (HP), vertical partitioning (VP), and hybrid or mixed partitioning (MP) [20].

Currently, multimedia applications are highly available, such as audio/video on demand, digital libraries, electronic catalogues, among others. Rapid development of multimedia applications has created a huge volume of multimedia data and it is exponentially incremented from time to time. A multimedia database is crucial in these applications to provide an efficient data retrieval.

Distributed and parallel processing on database management systems (DBMS) may improve performance of applications which manipulate large volumes of data. This may be accomplished by removing irrelevant data accessed during the execution of the queries and by reducing the data exchange among sites or

A. Gelbukh et al. (Eds.): MICAI 2014, Part II, LNAI 8857, pp. 296–309, 2014.

nodes of a network, which are the two main goals on distributed database design [17]. Therefore, partitioning techniques have been used in multimedia databases to improve performance of applications.

In this paper, we address horizontal partitioning in distributed multimedia databases. Horizontal partitioning affects postively query performance, database manageability and availability. Horizontal partitioning divides a relation along its tuples. Thus each fragment has a subset of the tuples of the relation. There are two versions of horizontal partitioning: primary and derived. *Primary horizontal partitioning* of a relation is performed by using predicates that are defined on that relation. On the other hand, *derived horizontal fragmentation* is the partitioning of a relation that results from predicates being defined on another relation [17]. Our discussion about HP is mainly focused on the former.

Data partitioning requires the use of clustering techniques. A cluster is a data fragment. Currently, primary horizontal partitioning algorithms for multimedia databases are based on affinity, which measures the "togetherness" between a pair of predicates. The affinity of a pair of predicates is high if most of the queries executed against the database access that pair. The main disadvantage of affinity is that it does not show the "togetherness" when more than two predicates are involved. Hence this measure has no bearing on the affinity measured with respect to the entire cluster [3]. To solve this problem, in this paper a method for horizontal partitioning in multimedia databases is proposed. This method is based on hierarchical agglomerative clustering.

Hierarchical clustering algorithms produce a nested sequence of partitions of the data which can be depicted by using a tree structure that is popularly called as *dendrogram*. Hierarchical algorithms are either *divisive* or *agglomerative* [14]. The *agglomerative approach*, also called *bottom-up* approach, starts with each object forming a separate group. It successively merges the objects or groups that are close to one another, until all of the groups are merged into one (the topmost level of the hierarchy), or until a termination condition holds. The *divisive approach*, also called the *top-down* approach, starts with all of the objects in the same cluster. In each successive iteration, a cluster is split up into smaller clusters, until eventually each object is one cluster, or until a termination condition holds [10].

The basic hierarchical agglomerative clustering algorithm (HAC) is simple. It needs a measure of distance (or a similarity measure) between any two clusters. HAC begins by regarding each instance as a cluster in its own right; then it finds the two closest clusters, merges them, and keeps on doing until only one cluster is left [23].

This paper is structured as follows: In Section 2, the state of the art of horizontal partitioning in traditional and multimedia databases is presented. In Section 3, we describe the Multimedia Horizontal Partitioning Algorithm (MHPA), which is based on hierarchical clustering algorithm. In Section 4, we show the performance evaluation of the queries. Finally, Section 5 remarks the conclusion and future work.

2   State of the Art

In order to clarify the difference between the related work and our approach, we classify them into two classes described in the following subsections.

2.1   Horizontal Partitioning Methods for Traditional Databases

Several researches have worked on horizontal partitioning techniques in traditional databases, including [2], [21], [17], [15].

Ceri et al. [2] considered the database design problem consisting in the horizontal partitioning of an homogeneous file. They defined the concepts (simple predicate, minterm predicate, completeness and minimality of a set of predicates, among others) and the tools for the characterization of the access pattern of transactions. Also, a methodology for determining the access parameters was proposed.

Özsu and Valduriez [17] presented and iterative algorithm, called COM_MIN, to generate a complete and minimal set of predicates Pr' given a set of simple predicates Pr. They also proposed PHORIZONTAL, an algorithm for primary horizontal fragmentation. The input to PHORIZONTAL is a relation R that is subject to primary horizontal fragmentation, and Pr, which is the set of simple predicates that have been determined according to applications defined on relation R.

Shin and Irani [21] partitioned relations horizontally based on estimated user reference clusters (URCs). URCs were estimated from user queries but they were refined by using semantic knowledge of the relations.

Zhang and Orlowska [24] addressed two-phase horizontal partitioning of distributed databases. First, primary horizontal fragmentation was carried out on each relation based on the predicate affinity matrix and the bond energy algorithm. Second, the derived horizontal fragmentation was further performed by considering information related to the global relational database schema and its transactions.

Navathe et al. [15] proposed algorithms for generating candidate vertical and horizontal fragmentation schemes and a methodology for distributed database design by using these fragmentation schemes for relational databases. They applied in combination vertical and horizontal fragmentation schemes to form a grid. They used a technique similar to the graphical algorithm for vertical partitioning discussed in [16] to produce horizontal fragments.

Khalil et al. [11] developed a horizontal fragmentation algorithm and a replication protocol that increases the availability and reliability for a distributed database system. The proposed horizontal fragmentation algorithm is an extension of the vertical transaction-based algorithm [7].

Cheng et al. [6] explored the use of a genetic search-based clustering algorithm for data partitioning to achieve high database retrieval performance. They formulated the horizontal partitioning problem as a traveling salesman problem (TSP).

Khan and Hoque [12] presented a technique for horizontal fragmentation of the relations of a distributed database. This technique is capable of taking proper fragmentation decision at the initial stage by using knowledge gathered during requirement analysis phase whithout the help of empirical data about query execution.

Ezeife and Baker [8] proposed algorithms for horizontal fragmentation of four class object models: (1) simple attributes and methods, (2) complex atributes and simple methods, (3) attributes that support a class composition hierarchy using simple methods, and (4) complex attributes and complex methods. Ezeife and Barker [8] used the same algorithm defined by Özsu and Valduriez [17] with the same simple predicates. However, the number of minterms generated by this algorithm is exponential to the number of simple predicates.

Bellatreche et al. [1] presented algorithms for both primary and derived horizontal partitioning. Their primary algorithm is an extension of the algorithm proposed by [15].

2.2   Horizontal Partitioning Methods for Multimedia Databases

In the past few years, distributed multimedia applications and data have rapidly become available; as a result, data partitioning techniques have been adapted in a multimedia context to properly achieve high resource utilization and increased concurrency and parallelism [4].

Saad et al. [20] addressed primary horizontal fragmentation in distributed multimedia databases. They particularly focused on multimedia predicates implication required in traditional fragmentation algorithms such as [17], [15] [1]. Getahun et al. [9] considered semantic-based predicates implication required in traditional fragmentation algorithms in order to partition multimedia data efficiently. Chbeir and Laurent [4], [5] discussed a formal approach dedicated to multimedia query and predicate implication.

Table 1 introduces a comparative analysis that summarizes relevant contributions of related horizontal partitioning (HP) works.

According to Table 1, there are two problems in order to use current horizontal partitioning algorithms in multimedia databases: 1) most of the horizontal partitioning approaches for multimedia databases employ affinity to cluster predicates used in queries, and 2) Only, Chbeir and Laurent [4], [5] do not consider affinity, nevertheless its algorithm takes as input a set of frequently asked queries (FD) but they do not give any guideline to obtain FD and to evaluate the horizontal partitioning scheme generated by their algorithm. These deficiences can be improved by: 1) developing a horizontal partitioning algorithm for multimedia databases, which does not need affinity to create the fragments, and 2) by proposing a cost model to evaluate different horizontal partitioning schemes. In this paper, we propose a Multimedia Horizontal Partitioning Algorithm (MHPA) which tries to solve the aforementioned deficiences.

Table 1. Comparative of Some Horizontal Partitioning Algorithms

Authors	Horizontal Partitioning	Multimedia Data	Partitioning Strategy
Ceri et al. [2]	Yes	No	COM_MIN
Özsu and Valduriez [17]	Yes	No	COM_MIN
Shin and Irani [21]	Yes	No	URCs
Zhang and Orlowska [24]	Yes	No	Affinity
Navathe et al. [15]	Yes	No	Affinity
Khalil et al. [11]	Yes	No	Query Cost
Cheng et al. [6]	Yes	No	Affinity
Khan and Hoque [12]	Yes	No	Query Cost
Ezeife and Baker [8]	Yes	No	COM_MIN
Bellatreche et al. [1]	Yes	No	Affinity
Saad et al. [20]	Yes	Yes	Affinity
Getahun et al. [9]	Yes	Yes	Affinity
Chbeir and Laurent [4], [5]	Yes	Yes	Query Comparison
MHPA	Yes	Yes	Query Cost

3 Multimedia Horizontal Partitioning Algorithm (MHPA)

In order to clarify our approach we present the following scenario of a simple multimedia database used to manage equipment in a machinery sell company. The database consists of a table named EQUIPMENT (*id, name, image, graphic, audio, video*) where each tuple describes information about a specific equipment, including its image, graphic, audio, and video objects. Information of 10,000 equipments of four different types is stored: 2500 push mowers, 2500 string trimmers, 2500 chain saws, and 2500 water pumps. Let us also consider the following queries:

q_1:Find all images and graphics of chain saws
q_2:Find name, audio and video with id "WP01"
q_3:Find all graphic, audio and video
q_4:Find all image of water pumps

As in [4], we consider that data are stored in a table T defined over two kinds of attributes: atomic and multimedia attributes. Also, we assume a fixed attribute set $U = A \cup M$ where:

- $A = \{A_1, A_2, .., A_p\}$ and each A_i ($i = 1, 2, , p$) is an atomic attribute associate with a set of atomic values (such as strings, numbers, among others.) called the domain of A_i and denoted by $dom(A_i)$.
- $M = \{M_1, M_2, .., M_q\}$ and each M_j ($j = 1, 2, , q$) is a multimedia attribute, associated with a set of complex values (represented as sets of values or vectors) called multimedia features (such as, color, texture, shape, to mention but a few.). The domain of M_j is denoted by $dom(M_j)$.

Thus, given a table T defined over U, tuples t in T are denoted as $\langle a_1, a_2, .., a_p, m_1, m_2, ., m_q \rangle$ where a_i is in $dom(A_i)$ $(1 \leq i \leq p)$ and m_j is in $dom(M_j)$ $(1 \leq j \leq q)$. Every a_i (respectively m_j) is denoted by $t.A_i$ (respectively $t.M_j$).

3.1   Information Requirements of Horizontal Partitioning

Qualitative and quantitative information about queries is required in order to develop the horizontal partitioning process [17]. The fundamental qualitative information consists of predicates used in user queries. As in [4] the multimedia queries used in our approach are conjunctive projection-selection queries over T of the form $\pi_X \sigma_C(T)$ where X is a non empty subset of U and C is a conjunction of atomic select predicates, i.e., $C : P_1 \wedge \ldots \wedge P_m$ defined as follows.

DEFINITION 1: An atomic selection predicate P_j is an expression of the form $P_j = A_i \theta a$ where $A_i \in A$, $a \in dom(A)$ and $\theta = \{=, \leq, \geq, <, >, like\}$.

Two sets are required in terms of quantitative information about user queries:

1. **Predicate selectivity:** number of tuples of the relation that would be accessed by a user query specified according to a given predicate. If $Pr = \{P_1, P_2, ..., P_r\}$ is a set of predicates, sel_j is the selectivity of the predicate P_j.
2. **Access frequency:** frequency with which user query access data. If $Q = \{q_1, q_2, ..., q_s\}$ is a set of user queries, f_i indicates the access frequency of query q_i in a given period.

3.2   The Steps of the Multimedia Horizontal Partitioning Algorithm (MHPA)

Inputs: The table T to be horizontally partitioned, and a set of queries with their frequencies.

Step 1: Determine the set of predicates Pr used by queries defined on the table T. These predicates are defined on a subset of attributes $A'(A' \subseteq A)$. As in [1] we call each element of A' relevant predicate attribute. The third query does not have any predicate because the graphic, audio and video objects of all equipments are retrieved. Therefore this query is not relevant for horizontal partitioning. The predicates used by the queries q_1, q_2, q_4 of our running example are presented on Table 2.

Step 2: Build the predicate usage matrix (PUM) of table T. This matrix contains queries as rows and predicates as columns. In this matrix $PUM(q_i, P_j) = 1$ if a query q_i uses a predicate P_j; else it is 0. The PUM of our running example is shown in Table 3.

Table 2. Predicates used by queries

Q	Pr
q_1	$p_1 = name = $ "*CHAIN SAW*"
q_2	$p_2 = id = $ "*WP01*"
q_4	$p_3 = name = $"*WATER PUMP*"

Table 3. Predicate usage matrix

Q/Pr	P_1	P_2	P_3	f_i
q_1	1	0	0	15
q_2	0	1	0	10
q_4	0	0	1	20
sel_i	2500	1	2500	

Step 3: Construct a partition tree. MHPA is based on AGNES (AGglomerative NEsting), an agglomerative hierarchical clustering method. Initially AGNES places each object into a cluster of its own. The clusters are then merged step-by-step according to some criterion, e.g., minimum Euclidian distance between any two objects from different clusters. This is a single-linkage approach in that each cluster is represented by all of the objects in the cluster, and the similarity between two clusters is measured by the similarity of the closest pair of data points belonging to different clusters. The cluster merging process repeats until all of the objects are eventually merged to form one cluster [10]. MHPA first begins with single predicate fragments. And then, it forms a new fragment by selecting and merging two fragments of them. This process is repeated until a fragment composed of all predicates is made. This kind of bottom-up approach generates a dendrogram, which is called a partition tree (PT) [22]. Figure 1 shows the PT of the table EQUIPMENT obtained by MHPA.

When two fragments are merged the amount of relevant tuples accessed is decreased while the amount of irrelevant tuples accessed by the queries is increased. For example, if the predicates P_1, P_2 and P_3 are merged into a fragment, the query q_4 does not have to access 1 remote tuple, i. e., the tuple with the id "WP01" located in a different fragment. On the other hand, the query q_1 only accessed 2500 tuples, but it has to access 5000 tuples. Therefore the merged fragment will increase the amount of access to irrelevant tuples.

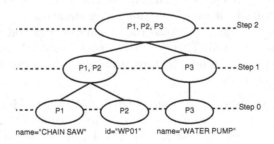

Fig. 1. Partition tree of the table EQUIPMENT obtained by MHPA

In order to optimize queries in distributed multimedia databases it is necessary to find the horizontal partitioning scheme that optimizes (minimizes) resource consumption. A good measure of resource consumption is the total cost that will be incurred in processing the query. Total cost is the sum of all times incurred in processing the query at various sites and in intersite communication. The total cost to be minimized includes I/O and communications costs. The I/O cost is the time necessary for disk access. This cost can be minimized by reducing the number of disk accesses needed for answer the query. The communication cost is the time needed for exchanging data between sites participating in the execution of the query [17].

In MHPA in each step during constructing a PT, two nodes (fragments) are selected which maximizes the merging profit defined below when they are merged into a node (fragment).

$$Merging\_Profit(MHPA) = DRT - IIT \tag{1}$$

where
DRT: the decreased amount of remote tuples accessed.
IIT: the increased amount of irrelevant tuples accessed.

DRT measures the minimization of communication costs, while IIT evaluates the reduction of I/O costs incurred in merging two fragments.

In each step during the construction process of a PT, MHPA produces an horizontal partitioning scheme hps_i merging two fragments which maximize the merging profit function defined in equation 1, so when the PT is finished we have a set of horizontal partitioning schemes $HPS = \{hps_1, hps_2, ..., hps_r\}$, every hps_i has a set of fragments $hps_i = \{fr_1, fr_2, ..., fr_s\}$.

To select two fragments of s fragments which can maximize the merging profit $\binom{s}{2} = (\frac{s(s-1)}{2})$ pairs should be examined. For example in Step 0 (ps_3) $s = r$ (where r is the number of predicates) because each predicate is located in a different fragment, so there are three fragments in Step 0 of Figure 1 and it is necessary to examine the merging profits of $(\frac{3(3-1)}{2}) = 3$ pairs and merge one pair with the maximum merging profit among them, which generates the hps_2 of Step 1 in Figure 1.

Table 4 shows MHPA Merging Profit Matrix (MPM) of the table EQUIPMENT in Step 0. In Algorithm 1, we show the process to get the MPM.

Algorithm 2 presents MHPA, it uses the PUM of the table T and generates the optimal horizontal partitioning scheme. Table 5 shows the horizontal partitioning schemes of the table EQUIPMENT obtained by using MHPA.

Table 4. Merging profits of table EQUIPMENT in Step 0

Pr	p_1	p_2	p_3
p_1		-25015	-87500
p_2			-25020
p_3			

Data: PUM of the table T (a set of predicates $Pr = \{P_1, P_2, ..., P_r\}$, the
selectivity sel_i of each predicate P_i, a set of queries $Q = \{q_1, q_2, ..., q_s\}$,
the frequency f_k of each query q_k

Result: MPM: Merging Profit Matrix

for each $P_i \in Pr \mid 1 \leq i \leq r-1$ **do**
    for each $P_j \in Pr \mid i+1 \leq j \leq r$ **do**
        $DRT = 0$;
        $IIT = 0$;
        $merging\_profit = 0$;
        for each $q_k \in Q \mid 1 \leq k \leq s$ **do**
            if $PUM(q_k, P_i) = 1$ & $PUM(q_k, P_j) = 1$ **then**
                $DRT = DRT + f_k * (sel_i + sel_j)$;
            else
                if $PUM(q_k, P_i) = 1$ **then**
                    $IIT = IIT + f_k * sel_j$;
                else
                    if $PUM(q_k, P_j) = 1$ **then**
                        $IIT = IIT + f_k * sel_i$;
                    end
                end
            end
        end
        $merging\_profit = DRT - IIT$;
        $MPM(P_i, P_j) = merging\_profit$;
    end
end

Algorithm 1: getMPM

Data: PUM

Result: optimal horizontal partitioning scheme (best_hps)

for each step $\in PT$ **do**
    getMPM(PUM, MPM) ;
    select two nodes with maximum merging profit ;
    merge the nodes ;
    compute the cost of each step;
    best_hps=step with minimum cost;
end

Algorithm 2: MHPA

Table 5. Resulting horizontal fragments of the table EQUIPMENT

PS	fr_1	fr_2	fr_3
hps_1	(P_1, P_2, P_3)		
hps_2	(P_1, P_2)	(P_3)	
hps_3	(P_1)	(P_2)	(P_3)

3.3 Cost Model

The cost of a hps_i is composed of two parts: irrelevant data access cost and transportation cost.

$$cost(hps_i) = ITAC(hps_i) + TC(hps_i) \tag{2}$$

ITAC measures the amount of data from both irrelevant tuples accessed during the queries. The transportation cost provides a measure for transporting between the nodes of the network.

The irrelevant tuple access cost is given by:

$$ITAC(hps_i) = \sum_{k=1}^{s} ITAC(fr_k). \tag{3}$$

In order to obtain the cost of a hps_i, it is necessary to use the PUM of a table T. The AUM has a set of atomic and multimedia attributes $U = A \cup M = \{A_1, A_2, ..., A_p, M_1, M_2, ..., M_q\}$, a set of queries $Q = \{q_1, q_2, q_m\}$, the frequency f_j of each query q_j, a set of predicates $Pr = \{P_1, P_2, ..., Pr\}$, the selectivity sel_t of each predicate P_t and a set of elements $PUM(q_j, P_t) = 1$ if query q_j uses the predicate P_t or $PUM(q_j, P_t) = 0$ otherwise. Also, it is needed a Fragment-Predicate Usage Matrix (FPUM). For instance, Table 6 shows the FPUM of the $hps_1 = \{fr_1, fr_2\}$. The FPUM shows the predicates used by each fragment fr_k and the cardinality $card_k$ of each fragment.

Table 6. FPUM

hps₁	P_1	P_2	P_3	$card_k$
fr_1	1	1	1	5000
fr_2	0	0	0	5000

The irrelevant tuple access cost of each horizontal fragment fr_k is given by:

$$ITAC(fr_k) = \sum_{q_j \in Q_k \wedge ITAC(q_j) \geq 0} ITAC(q_j) \tag{4}$$

$$ITAC(q_j) = \begin{cases} f_j(card_k - \sum_{P_t \in Pr_j} sel_t) & if\ n_p \geq 1 \\ 0 & otherwise \end{cases} \tag{5}$$

where Q_k is a set of queries which use at least one predicate and access at least one irrelevant predicate of the fragment fr_k. This is

$$Q_k = \{q_j | PUM(q_j, P_i) = 0 \wedge PUM(q_j, P_l) = 1 \wedge \{P_i, P_l\} \in fr_k\} \tag{6}$$

$$\{P_i, P_l\} \in fr_k \Rightarrow FPUM(fr_k, P_i) = 1 \wedge FPUM(fr_k, P_l) = 1 \tag{7}$$

Pr_j has the predicates used by a query q_j and located in the fragment fr_k, and n_p is the number of predicates in Pr_j.

$$Pr_j = \{P_t | PUM(q_j, P_t) = 1 \wedge FPUM(fr_k, P_t) = 1\} \tag{8}$$

We suppose that the network has nodes N_1, N_2, ..., N_s, the allocation of the fragments to the nodes gives rise to a mapping $\lambda : \{1, ..., p\} \rightarrow \{1, ..., p\}$ called location assignment [13]. The transportation cost of a hps_i is computed according to a given location assignment. The TC of hps_i is the sum of the costs of each query multiplied by its frequency squared, i. e.

$$TC(hps_i) = \sum_{j=1}^{m} TC(q_j)f_j^2 \tag{9}$$

The transportation cost of query q_j depends on the number of the relevant remote tuples and on the assigned locations, which decide the transportation cost factor between every pair of sites. It can be expressed by

$$TC(q_j) = \sum_{h} \sum_{h'} c_{\lambda(h)\lambda(h')} sel(h') \tag{10}$$

where h ranges over the nodes of the network for q_j, $sel(h')$ is the number of relevant remote tuples accessed by the query q_j, $\lambda(h)$ indicates the node in the network at which the query is stored, and c_{ij} is a transportation cost factor for data transportation from node N_i to node $N_j (i, j \in \{1, ..., p\})$ [13].

For instance, $TC(hps_1)$ of MHPA is calculated as follows. There are two fragments, so we suppose that there are two nodes N_1, N_2, and each fragment fr_i is located in each node N_i. We also assume that each query is located in the node where the fragment which contains the greater number of tuples that it uses is located and $c_{ij} = 1$. Figure 2 illustrates the local assignment of hps_1. Table 7 contains the costs of the horizontal partitioning schemes generated by MHPA. The optimal scheme is hps_3 with a cost of 3125400.

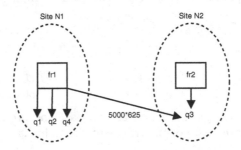

Fig. 2. Location assignment of hps_1

Table 7. Costs of the horizontal partitioning schemes

HPS	ITAC	TC	Cost
hps_1	137490	3125000	3262490
hps_2	25015	3125400	3150415
hps_3	0	3125400	3125400

4 Evaluation

We compared MHPA versus the affinity-based approach of most of the current horizontal partitioning methods for multimedia databases (Make-Partition). The benchmark used for the comparison was the database of a machinery sales company used in [18], [19], and described in Section 3. Some horizontal partitioning methods as [15], [11] have considered that the response time of a query is strongly affected by the amount of data accessed from secondary storage (disk). Hence, the objective functions of these methods are to minimize the number of disk accesses. The cost model proposed in this paper is used to compare the schemes obtained by MHPA, and the primary horizontal fragmentation algorithm Make-Partition of [15] since the cost to perform queries in distributed systems is dominated by the remote network communication as well as local disk accesses. Since Make-Partition is an affinity-based approach and the affinity between every pair of predicates is zero, then this algorithm does not partition the table EQUIPMENT. We present the comparison between the horizontal partitioning scheme of Make-Partition and MHPA in Table 8.

Table 8. Comparison of the Execution Cost of the Queries

query	Make-Partition			MHPA		
	ITAC	TC	Cost	ITAC	TC	Cost
q_1	112500	0	112500	0	0	**0**
q_2	99990	0	99990	0	0	**0**
q_3	0	0	**0**	0	3125000	3125000
q_4	150000	0	150000	0	400	**400**

As we can see in Table 8, the cost of queries q_1, q_2 and q_4 was lower when they were executed in the scheme obtained by MHPA. Only one query q_3 had a higher execution cost with MAHP, the reason of this is that q_3 require all the tuples of the database, since in the scheme of Make-Partition all the tuples are located in the same fragment, there is not transportation cost. Nevertheless, most of the queries in multimedia databases tend to only access subsets of the tuples.

5 Conclusion and Future Work

Horizontal partitioning techniques for multimedia databases has been recently proposed, nevertheless most of these techniques are based on affinity to cluster the predicates. In this paper, we have proposed a horizontal partitioning algorithm for multimedia databases based on hierarchical agglomerative clustering to avoid the problem of affinity. Also, we presented a cost model for the evaluation of horizontal partitioning schemes. The cost model measures the irrelevant tuple access cost and the transportation cost of queries in multimedia databases. We performed an evaluation of our algorithm and demonstrated that our algorithm outperforms Make-Partition in more cases. In the future we want to develop a hybrid partitioning algorithm for multimedia databases taking into account content-based (range, K-nearest neighbor) queries in the partitioning process.

Acknowledgments. The authors are very grateful to General Council of Superior Technological Education of Mexico (DGEST) for supporting this work. Also, this research paper was sponsored by the National Council of Science and Technology (CONACYT), as well as by the Public Education Secretary (SEP) through PROMEP.

References

1. Bellatreche, L., Karlapalem, K., Simonet, A.: Algorithms and support for horizontal class partitioning in object-oriented databases. Distrib. Parallel Databases 8(2), 155–179 (2000)
2. Ceri, S., Negri, M., Pelagatti, G.: Horizontal data partitioning in database design. In: Proceedings of the 1982 ACM SIGMOD International Conference on Management of Data, SIGMOD 1982, pp. 128–136. ACM, New York (1982)
3. Chakravarthy, S., Muthuraj, J., Varadarajan, R., Navathe, S.B.: An objective function for vertically partitioning relations in distributed databases and its analysis. Distrib. Parallel Databases 2(2), 183–207 (1994)
4. Chbeir, R., Laurent, D.: Towards a novel approach to multimedia data mixed fragmentation. In: Proceedings of the International Conference on Management of Emergent Digital EcoSystems, MEDES 2009, pp. 30:200–30:204. ACM, New York (2009)
5. Chbeir, R., Laurent, D.: Enhancing multimedia data fragmentation. Journal of Multimedia Processing and Technologies 1(2), 112–131 (2010)
6. Cheng, C.H., Lee, W.K., Wong, K.F.: A genetic algorithm-based clustering approach for database partitioning. IEEE Transactions on Systems, Man, and Cybernetics, Part C: Applications and Reviews 32(3), 215–230 (2002)
7. Chu, W.W., Ieong, I.T.: A transaction-based approach to vertical partitioning for relational database systems. IEEE Trans. Softw. Eng. 19(8), 804–812 (1993)
8. Ezeife, C.I., Barker, K.: A comprehensive approach to horizontal class fragmentation in a distributed object based system. Distrib. Parallel Databases 3(3), 247–272 (1995)
9. Getahun, F., Tekli, J., Atnafu, S., Chbeir, R.: The use of semantic-based predicates implication to improve horizontal multimedia database fragmentation. In: Workshop on Multimedia Information Retrieval on The Many Faces of Multimedia Semantics, MS 2007, pp. 29–38. ACM, New York (2007)
10. Han, J., Kamber, M., Pei, J.: Data Mining: Concepts and Techniques, 3rd edn. Morgan Kaufmann Publishers Inc., San Francisco (2011)

11. Khalil, N., Eid, D., Khair, M.: Availability and reliability issues in distributed databases using optimal horizontal fragmentation. In: Bench-Capon, T.J.M., Soda, G., Tjoa, A.M. (eds.) DEXA 1999. LNCS, vol. 1677, pp. 771–780. Springer, Heidelberg (1999)
12. Khan, S.I., Hoque, D.A.S.M.L.: A new technique for database fragmentation in distributed systems. International Journal of Computer Applications 5(9), 20–24 (2010)
13. Ma, H.: Distribution Design for Complex Value Databases. Ph.D. thesis, Massey University (2007)
14. Murty, M., Rashmin, B., Bhattacharyya, C.: Clustering based on genetic algorithms. In: Ghosh, A., Dehuri, S., Ghosh, S. (eds.) Multi-Objective Evolutionary Algorithms for Knowledge Discovery from Databases. SCI, vol. 98, pp. 137–159. Springer, Heidelberg (2008)
15. Navathe, S., Karlapalem, K., Ra, M.: A mixed fragmentation methodology for initial distributed database design. Journal of Computer and Software Engineering 3(4), 395–426 (1995)
16. Navathe, S.B., Ra, M.: Vertical partitioning for database design: A graphical algorithm. In: Proceedings of the 1989 ACM SIGMOD International Conference on Management of Data, SIGMOD 1989, pp. 440–450. ACM, New York (1989)
17. Özsu, M.T., Valduriez, P.: Principles of Distributed Database Systems, 3rd edn. Springer (2011)
18. Rodriguez, L., Li, X.: A vertical partitioning algorithm for distributed multimedia databases. In: Hameurlain, A., Liddle, S.W., Schewe, K.-D., Zhou, X. (eds.) DEXA 2011, Part II. LNCS, vol. 6861, pp. 544–558. Springer, Heidelberg (2011)
19. Rodríguez, L., Li, X., Cervantes, J., García-Lamont, F.: Dymond: An active system for dynamic vertical partitioning of multimedia databases. In: Proceedings of the 16th International Database Engineering & Applications Sysmposium, IDEAS 2012, pp. 71–80. ACM, New York (2012)
20. Saad, S., Tekli, J., Chbeir, R., Yétongnon, K.: Towards multimedia fragmentation. In: Manolopoulos, Y., Pokorný, J., Sellis, T.K. (eds.) ADBIS 2006. LNCS, vol. 4152, pp. 415–429. Springer, Heidelberg (2006)
21. Shin, D.G., Irani, K.B.: Fragmenting relations horizontally using a knowledge-based approach. IEEE Trans. Softw. Eng. 17(9), 872–883 (1991)
22. Son, J.H., Kim, M.H.: An adaptable vertical partitioning method in distributed systems. Journal of Systems and Software 73(3), 551–561 (2004)
23. Witten, I.H., Frank, E., Hall, M.A.: Data Mining: Practical Machine Learning Tools and Techniques, 3rd edn. Morgan Kaufmann Publishers Inc., San Francisco (2011)
24. Zhang, Y., Orlowska, M.E.: On fragmentation approaches for distributed database design. Information Sciences - Applications 1(3), 117–132 (1994)

Classification with Graph-Based Markov Chain

Ping He[*] and Xiaohua Xu[*]

Department of Computer Science, Yangzhou University, Yangzhou 225009, China
{angeletx,arterx}@gmail.com

Abstract. Markov chain is a popular graph-based model in data mining and machine learning areas. In this paper, we propose a novel intrinsic multi-class Markov chain classifier. It predicts the class label of arbitrary unseen data by setting the training data as the absorbing states of a Markov chain. It also incorporates kernel method for better generalization. Promising experiments on both artificial and real-world data sets demonstrate the effectiveness of our method.

Keywords: Graph model, Markov chain, Face recognition, Text classification.

1   Introduction

Data classification is a fundamental research area in the field of data mining. It refers to given a set of labeled data points, assigning labels to the unlabeled ones. According to the number of different pre-assigned labels, the problem can be further divided into two categories, binary classification and multi-classification. The former can only separate two classes, while the latter can handle multiple different classes. Various methods have been proposed to deal with classification in different ways. Among them, Support Vector Machine (SVM) [1] is one of the state-of-the-art sophisticated binary classification algorithms. It maximizes the margin of different classes to minimize the structural risk introduced by statistical theory. Two of the most commonly used SVMs are Linear-SVM and RBF-SVM, which adopt linear and Gaussian kernels to deal with linear and nonlinear separable data respectively. Different from SVM, KNN classifier [2] is one of the state-of-the-art lazy multi-class classifier, which assigns the unlabeled data with the label shared by most of its k neighbors.

In recent year, graph-based methods become more and more popular in machine learning and data mining areas. As a popular graph model, Markov chain [3] has been incorporated into different semi-supervised learning algorithms. Szummer and Jaakkola [4] first used Markov chain to estimate the posterior probability of each data in belonging to different classes by computing the probability of the labeled data reaching the unlabeled data. On the contrary, Zhu et. al. [5] estimate the posterior probability of the unlabeled data in belonging to different classes by computing its probability of reaching the labeled data in a Markov random walk. On the basis of that, Zhou et. al. [6] proposed a global and local consistency method that takes a

---

[*] Corresponding author.

A. Gelbukh et al. (Eds.): MICAI 2014, Part II, LNAI 8857, pp. 310–318, 2014.
© Springer International Publishing Switzerland 2014

balance between the spread label information in a Markov random walk and the initial label assignment. Wang et. al. [7] made further improvement by incorporating the Local Linear Embedding method [8] for weight estimation. However, in the development of classification algorithms, the application of graph-based Markov chain is not as popular as in semi-supervised learning. Hassan et al. [9] constructs a random walk model to represent how a particular word feature contributes to a given context. Islam et al. [10] introduce a new random walk term weighting method to improve text classification. Xu et al. [11] also proposed a random walk method for text classification with an out-of-sample extension. Bhagat et al. [12] gives a brief summarization about the label types, graph formulation, Markov chain based methods and their connections to iterative classification methods.

In this paper, we propose a multi-class Markov Chain Classifier model. It predicts the class labels of unseen data by setting the training data as the absorbing states of a Markov chain. To achieve better generalization, we also incorporate the kernel method into our model. Besides, the computational cost of our algorithm is provided as well. Comprehensive experiments are performed to evaluate the classification performance of our method. The promising experiments in comparison with the state-of-the-art SVM classifiers demonstrate that our method is effective.

The remainder of this paper is organized as follows. Section 2 provides some preliminaries and notations. Section 3 presents our algorithm in detail and analyzes the time complexity. Section 4 evaluates the algorithm with both artificial and real-world data sets. Section 5 concludes this paper.

2   Preliminaries

Given a training data set $\mathcal{D} = (\mathcal{X}, \mathcal{Y})$, where $\mathcal{X} = \{x_1, \cdots, x_n\}$ specifies the data set and $\mathcal{Y} = \{y_1, \cdots, y_n\}$ specifies the label set of $\mathcal{X}$, we map it onto an undirected and weighted graph $G=(V, E, W)$, where $V = \{v_1, \cdots, v_n\}$ is the vertex set, v_i corresponds to x_i, E is the edge set, and W is the weight set among V with its element w_{ij}=sim(v_i,v_j)=sim(x_i, x_j) indicating the pairwise similarity between two data points x_i and x_j.

Assume a Markov chain with the probability transition matrix $P=[P_{ij}]_{n \times n}$, the element of P, let us say p_{ij}, indicates the probability that one vertex v_i moves to another vertex v_j. Typically, P is computed in the following way,

$$P = D^{-1}W \tag{1}$$

where the diagonal matrix $D = \mathrm{diag}(W\mathbf{1}_n)$ and $\mathbf{1}_n$ is a n-dimensional vector with all entries equal to 1.

Let $Y = (y_{ij})_{n \times c}$ be a class indicating matrix, where c is the number of classes. The element of Y, let us say y_{ij}, indicates the degree of membership that vertex v_i belongs to class j. For the training data set whose class assignment is already known, $y_{ij} = 1$ if $y_i = c_j$ where c_j is the jth class label, and $y_{ij} = 0$ otherwise.

3   Markov Chain Classifier Models

We assume such a Markov chain: every class of data is an absorbing state, while every unseen (or test) data is a transitive state. A random walk starts when there is one or more transitive states added into the graph. At first, a particle is placed on each transitive state. It starts random walking with the transition probability P plus the new computed transition probability vector $p_v = (p(v_i, v))_{n \times 1}$, which indicates the transition probabilities from the test vertex v, corresponding to the test data x, to all the training data $v_i \in V$. The random walk ends when all the particles are absorbed. In another word, the random walk ends when the particles are absorbed by any training data.

To formulate the above Markov chain, we use y to denote the probability of the test vertex v in belonging to c different classes.

$$y = \sum_{v_i \in V} p(v_i, v) y_i = Y p_v \tag{2}$$

where

$$p_v \overset{def}{=} p(V, v) = \begin{bmatrix} p(v_1, v) \\ p(v_2, v) \\ \vdots \\ p(v_n, v) \end{bmatrix} \tag{3}$$

For each training vertex v_i in V, we have

$$p(V, v_i) = D^{-1} w_i = D^{-1} \begin{bmatrix} w_{1i} \\ w_{2i} \\ \vdots \\ w_{ni} \end{bmatrix} \tag{4}$$

Similarly, for the test vertex v absent in V, $p(V, v)$ is computed as follows.

$$p(V, v) = D^{-1} w(V, v) = D^{-1} \begin{bmatrix} w(v_1, v) \\ w(v_2, v) \\ \vdots \\ w(v_n, v) \end{bmatrix} \tag{5}$$

Therefore, the class indicating vector y has the following form,

$$\begin{aligned} y &= Y p(V, v) \\ &= Y D^{-1} w(V, v) \\ &= Y D^{-1} W W^+ w(V, v) \\ &= Y P W^+ w(V, v) \end{aligned} \tag{6}$$

where W^+ denotes the pseudo-reverse matrix of W, and $w(V, v)$ is a vector indicating the similarity between the test vertex v and the training vertices in V. We name this model **Markov Chain Classifier with 1-step transition** (MCC^1) because it absorbs the walking particles only in one step.

Next, we revise the above Markov chain a little by setting it absorbs the randomly walking particles after t steps. Obviously, it is a generalized form of MCC[1]. With the transition probability matrix P replaced with P^t, we get the new class indicating vector y under such model.

$$y = YP^t W^+ w(V, v) \tag{7}$$

We call it **Markov Chain Classifier with t**-step transition (MCC^t)

Note that a special case is that when $t = 0$, $P^t = I$, the resulting class indicating vector y is

$$y = YW^+ w(V, v) \tag{8}$$

We call this model **Markov Chain Classifier with 0**-step transition (MCC^0).

If we view the weight matrix W as a kernel, then we can incorporate the kernel matrix K into our model. By simply substitute the similarity metric $w(V, v)$ with the kernel function $k(X, x)$, we get.

$$w_{ij} \stackrel{def}{=} w(v_i, v_j) = k(x_i, x_j) \tag{9}$$

As a result, the weight matrix W in eq. (7) can accordingly be replaced by the kernel matrix K, leading to

$$F(x) = YP^t K^+ k(X, x) \tag{10}$$

If we define $\hat{F} = YP^t$ similar to eq. (2), then eq. (10) becomes

$$F(x) = \hat{F} K^+ k(X, x) \tag{11}$$

The class with the highest membership of x is assigned to it as its class label, i.e., $y(x) = \arg\max_i f_{ix}$, where $F(x) = [f_{1x}, f_{2x}, \ldots, f_{cx}]$.

However, K may be a singular matrix probably due to insufficient data or the existence of noise. To enhance the robustness of our classifier, we introduce a regularization parameter λ, leading to a **Regularized Markov Chain Classifier (RMCC)**.

$$F(x) = \hat{F}(K + \lambda I)^+ k(X, x) \tag{12}$$

To analyze the time complexity of our method, the computation of kernel matrix and pseudo-reverse matrix in the training stage is $O(mn^2)$ and $O(n^3)$ respectively. As to the out-of-sample stage, the computation of $\hat{F}K^+$ requires $O(cn^2)$. Nevertheless, if we consider the special case MCC^0, the computational cost of $\hat{F}K^+$ is reduced to $O(cn)$ because $\hat{F} = Y$.

4   Experiments

In this section, we evaluate the classification performance of our classifier RMCC, short for Regularized Markov Chain Classifier, in comparison with the state-of-the-art support vector machine classifier, on both artificial and real-world data sets.

We implement our algorithm in Matlab, and adopt the implementation of RBF-SVM and Linear-SVM in LibSVM [13], as well as the implementation of LDA by Cai et. al. [14]. We compute the weight between each pair of data using RBF function,

$$sim(v_i, v_j) = k(x_i, x_j) = e^{-\frac{\|x_i - x_j\|^2}{2\sigma^2}} \tag{13}$$

where σ is a scale parameter optimized over the interval $\{2^{-15}, 2^{-11}, ..., 2^{13}, 2^{15}\}$ using cross validation. The regularization parameter λ is fixed 0.0001 throughout the experiments.

In the following text, we first evaluate our algorithm on a nonlinear toy data set in comparison with RBF-SVM. Then we explore the impact of the number of transitions t on the classification performance of $RMCC^t$ on four UCI real-world data sets. Next, a face recognition data set is employed to compare our algorithm with the baseline and Linear Discriminate Analysis (LDA) method. Last, we test our algorithm along with SVM on text classification in the field of traditional Chinese medicine.

4.1   Toy Data Sets

Fig. 1 shows a non-linear artificial data set Yin-yang, where triangles and squares respectively represent two different classes of data, the solid symbols represent the training data, while the hollow symbols represent the test data. We test $RMCC^0$ and $RMCC^1$ on both the data sets, in comparison with the state-of-the-art RBF-SVM. Table 1 summarizes the comparison results. It can be seen that the test error ratios of both $RMCC^0$ and $RMCC^1$ produce lower error ratios than RBF-SVM.

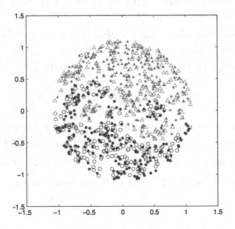

Fig. 1. Yin-yang dataset

Table 1. The comparison of error ratios (%) on Yin-yang data set

	RBF-SVM	$RMCC^0$	$RMCC^1$
Yin-yang	0.75	0.04	0.37

4.2   UCI Database

To explore the impact of the transition number t on the classification performance of our method, we set the maximum of t for $RMCC^t$ as 30, and compare our classifier with RBF-SVM and Linear-SVM on four real-world data sets from UCI database using 10-fold cross validation. Among them, there are two data sets that have been preprocessed: (1) The "name" attributes of PARKINSONS and YEAST data sets are removed. (2) The fifth and sixth attributes that contain only one value in YEAST are removed. Fig. 2 shows the learning curves of $RMCC^t$ with the increase of value t. Table 2 summarizes the averaged test error ratios as well as standard deviations of $RMCC^0$ and $RMCC^1$ in comparison with RBF-SVM and Linear-SVM.

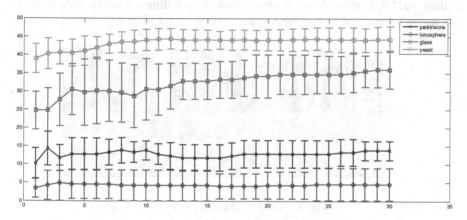

Fig. 2. The test error ratios and standard deviations of $RMCC^t$ on UCI data sets

Table 2. Comparison of error ratios (%) and standard deviations on UCI data sets

Data sets	Linear-SVM	RBF-SVM	$RMCC^0$	$RMCC^1$
parkinsons	15.39±5.51	11.71±4.61	**10.27±4.23**	14.38±4.66
ionosphere	13.97±6.25	4.83±3.00	**3.45±2.66**	4.31±3.98
glass	36.90±7.38	25.28±10.69	**24.73±5.15**	24.88±6.02
yeast	45.35±4.44	39.75±3.98	**38.99±3.96**	40.31±4.25

As we can see from Fig. 2, for each line that corresponds to a data set, the learning curves show comparatively stationary vibrations with the increase of t. Therefore, the stability is guaranteed. Combined with Table 2, it is quite interesting that, without the help of probability transition matrix, $RMCC^0$ model achieves impressive accomplishments instead of $RMCC^1$. Therefore, we conclude that Markov chain classifiers are well qualified for classification problem. The above experiments not only prove the effectiveness of our model but also indicate the best number of transitions t.

4.3   Face Recognition

In addition to the synthetic data and UCI data, we also select a face data, ORL illustrated in Fig. 3, for test. A random subset with p (=2,3,4,5,6,7,8) image per individual was taken with labels to form the training set, and the rest of the database was treated as the testing set. For each given p, we make 50 random splits to determine the training and test data. The averaged error ratios as well as standard deviation in comparison with baseline and LDA [14] are reported in Table 3. For the method LDA, both the training and testing images are mapped into low dimensional subspace where recognition was carried out by using nearest neighbor classifier (NN) and nearest centroid classifier (NC). For the baseline, the recognition is simply performed in the original 1024-dimensional image space without any dimensionality reduction. The data was pre-processed by normalizing each image vector to unit.

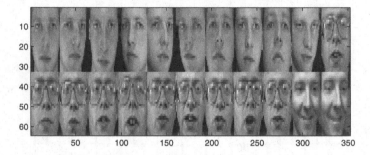

Fig. 3. Picture of 22 facial expressions

Table 3. Error ratios and standard deviations as a result of ORL data test

		2 Train	3 Train	4 Train	5 Train	6 Train	7 Train	8 Train
Baseline	NC	32.6±3.4	25.9±2.9	22.1±2.6	19.3±2.6	17.8±3.1	16.4±3.4	15.2±3.9
	NN	33.1±3.4	23.4±2.3	17.9±2.2	13.7±2.4	11.4±2.2	8.7±2.4	7.5±2.4
$RMCC^0$		**17.5±2.7**	**10.9±1.7**	**6.3±1.1**	**4.2±1.4**	**3.3±2.2**	**3.1±1.4**	**1.4±1.4**
$RMCC^1$		29.0±2.6	21.8±2.3	16.3±1.8	12.9±2.7	9.5±2.4	9.7±1.8	5.9±2.3
LDA	NC	22.3±3	13.9±2.4	10±1.8	7.3±1.4	6±2.1	5±1.9	3.8±2
PCARatio=1	NN	22.3±3	13.9±2.4	10±1.8	7.3±1.4	6±2.1	5±1.9	3.8±2
LDA	NC	28.4±3.7	15.9±2.2	10.3±2	6.9±1.5	5.6±2	4.6±2	3.6±1.8
Fisherface=1	NN	28.5±3.8	16±2.2	10.6±2	7.2±1.7	6±2.3	4.7±2.1	3.7±1.8

From table 4, we can see all the classifiers produce lower error ratios than baselines'. $RMCC^0$ again performs best of all with its error ratios drops more than 10% from 2 to 8 Train. Typically, the 5-Train partition is a rational division to determine the performance of a classifier. At that point, $RMCC^1$ produces the highest error ratios but shows the lowest rate of decline. This may because the transition matrix failed to provide more accurate transition probabilities. Thus, further work will address the improvement of the model in this aspect.

4.4   Text Classification

Text classification is another important branch of classification. In this experiment, we select articles from the field of Traditional Chinese Medicine (TCM). The data set is extracted from [15] and it contains 41 Tonics, 21 Exterior-Releasing Herbs and 46 Heat-Clearing Herbs, totally 108 tastes. For each Chinese herb, we record the description of its properties, flavors, meridian tropism and toxicity. For example, the description of Herba Menthae is "Bo He, property: pungent, cool; lung and liver meridians entered". To compute the weight matrix, we choose the method of Boolean weighting, $w_{ij} = 1$ if $TF_{ij} > 0$, otherwise $w_{ij} = 0$, where TF_{ij} is the term frequency, or the occurrence of term i in a description of herb j. The boolean matrix, whose rows denote the taste of herbs and columns denote the properties, are illustrated in Fig. 4. The cross validation method is adopted to test the error ratios and standard deviations of our models in comparison with RBF-SVM. The comparison result is summarized in Table 4.

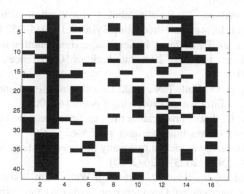

Fig. 4. The boolean weight matrix of Tonics

Table 4. The comparison of error ratios (%) on Tonics data set

	RBF-SVM	RMCC^0	RMCC^1
Tonics	18.98±1.33	**9.86±2.35**	39.13±0.1

5   Conclusion

A new graph-based classification algorithm is proposed and demonstrated. Built on the basis of stochastic theory, it incorporates Markov chain and kernel method to predict labels of unlabeled data. Compared with the state-of-the-art support vector machine classifier, our approach is an intrinsic multi-class classification algorithm, easy to understand and simple to implement. Experimental results demonstrate that our method is effective.

Acknowledgment. This research was supported in part by the Chinese National Natural Science Foundation under Grant nos. 61402395, 61003180, 61379066 and 61472343, Natural Science Foundation of Jiangsu Province under contracts BK20140492 and BK2010318, Natural Science Foundation of Education Department of Jiangsu Province under contracts 13KJB520026 and 09KJB20013, and the New Century Talent Project of Yangzhou University.

References

1. Vapnik, V.N.: The Nature of Statistical Learning Theory. Springer, New York (1995)
2. Cover, T.M., Hart, P.E.: Nearest Neighbor Pattern Classification. Knowledge Based Systems 8(6), 373–389 (1995)
3. Meyn, P., Tweedie, R.L.: Markov Chains and Stochastic Stability, 2nd edn. Cambridge University Press (2009)
4. Szummer, M., Jaakkola, T.: Patially labeled classification with markov random walk. Advances in Neural Information Processing Systems 14, 945–952 (2002)
5. Zhu, X., Ghahramani, Z., Lafferty, J.: Semi-supervised learning using Gaussian fields and harmonic functions. In: The 20th International Conference on Machine Learning, pp. 912–919 (2003)
6. Zhou, D., Bousquet, O., Lalf, T.N., et al.: Learning with local and global consistency. In: Advances in Neural Information Processing System 16 (2004)
7. Wang, F., Zhang, C.: Label propagation through linear neighborhoods. In: The 23th International Conference on Machine Learning, pp. 55–67 (2006)
8. Nonlinear dimensionality reduction by locally linear embedding. Sam Roweis & Lawrence Saul. Science 290(5500), 2323–2326 (2000)
9. Hassan, S., Mihalcea, R., Banea, C.: Random-Walk Term Weighting for Improved Text Classification. In: International Conference on Semantic Computing, pp. 242–249 (2007)
10. Rafiqul Islam, M., Rakibul, M.: An Effective Term Weighting Method Using Random Walk Model for Text Classification. In: Proceedings of 11th International Conference on Computer and Information Technology (ICCIT 2008), pp. 411–414 (2008)
11. Xu, Y., Yi, X., Zhang, C.: A Random Walks Method for Text Classification. In: Proceedings of SDM (2006)
12. Bhagat, S., Cormode, G., Muthukrishnan, S.: Node classification in social networks. Arxiv preprint arXiv:1101. 3291 (2011)
13. Chang, C.-C., Lin, C.-J.: LIBSVM: a library for support vector machines (2001), Software available at: http://www.csie.ntu.edu.tw/~cjlin/libsvm
14. Cai, D., He, X., Han, J.: Efficient kernel discriminant analysis via spectral regression, Technical Report 2888, Department of Computer Science, University of Illinois at Urbana-Champaign (August 2007)
15. Zhang, T.: Chinese Materia Medica. Higher Education Press (2008)

Solving Binary Cutting Stock with Matheuristics

Ivan Adrian Lopez Sanchez[1], Jaime Mora Vargas[1], Cipriano A. Santos[2],
and Miguel Gonzalez Mendoza[1]

[1] Instituto Tecnologico y de Estudios Superiores de Monterrey
{A01362066,jmora,mgonza}@itesm.mx
[2] Hewlett-Packard
cipriano.santos@hp.com

Abstract. Many Combinatorial Optimization (CO) problems are classifed as NP - complete problems. The process of solving CO problems
in an efficient manner is important since several industry, government
and scientific problems can be statedin this form. This work presents a
benchmark of three different methodologies to solve the Binary Cutting
Stock (BCS) problem; exact methodology by applying Column Generation (CG), a Genetic Algorithm (GA) and an hybrid between exact
methods and Genetic Algorithms in a Column Generation framework
which we denominate Matheuristic (MA). This benchmark analysis is
aimed to show Matheuristic solution quality is as good as the obtained
by the exact methodology. Details about implementation and computational performance are discussed.

1 Introduction

Many Combinatorial Optimization (CO) problems such as Vehicle Routing Problem (VRP), Traveling Salesman Person (TSP), Satisfiability Problem (SAT) and
Cutting Stock Problem (CS) are classifed as NP - complete problems. Solving
CO problems in an efficient manner could lead to a feasible practical implementation, in terms of computational requirements and costs. The Cutting Stock
(CS) problem is a well known combinatorial problem with application in the
paper industry allowing the minimization of the trim loss. In general a company
in the paper industry need to satisfy a demand of several products -or finals of
different widths. To achieve this objective companies define cutting patterns to
use in raw roll material and their usage level [16].

Previous research present a work in which they solve the Cutting Stock problem by applying Linear Programming [15], however the solution obtained is not
always integral and the need of using slack variables in order to remove fractional solutions arise. A special case of the Cutting Stock Problem is when the
demand of the products or finals is exactly one is called Binary Cutting Stock
(BCS) problem. Different to the Cutting Stock Problem that can be stated as a
Set Covering Problem (SCP), BCS can be stated as a Set Partitioning Problem
(SPP) which is a well known combinatorial problem classified as NP-Hard [9].

Since the wide field of applications of the SPP [2], [3], [11], [20], there have been
many solution methods like Genetic Algorithms (GA), [3], and greedy heuristics

A. Gelbukh et al. (Eds.): MICAI 2014, Part II, LNAI 8857, pp. 319–330, 2014.

[8]. Nevertheless, most of those research avenues are based on a explicit enumeration of all feasible subsets in order to choose the optimal or near optimal group of those subsets to minimize the cost.

Vance [20] presents a column generation approach with optimized set of branching rules which avoids explicit enumeration of all the feasible subsets from which this work is based, nonetheless implementation details are not explicit. Different from Vance work, in this work we will analyse the impact factor of including a column which reduced cost is not guarantee to be the most negative per iteration of the Column Generation process and by applying a metaheuristic to solve the problem.

Caprara, [5], study the most recent and relevant approaches (linear programming and heuristics) for the Set Covering Problem -which is a relaxed formulation of the SPP; by benchmarking with the Beasley's OR Library. As seen in [5], the exact methodologies uses branch and bond algorithm with linear programming and lagrangian relaxation, whereas the heuristics are based en neighberhood search, lagrangian relaxation and Genetic Algorithms, however any of the studied works use in a coupled fashion both methodologies.

In this work, the comparison of four different approaches are presented, an exact algorithm applying the branch and price algorithm desiged by [20], a classic heuristic denominated First Fit Decreasing [9], a Genetic Algorithm and a hybrid approach using the branch and price ideas from [20] and Genetic Algorithms.

1.1   The Set Partitioning Problem

Let J be a finite set of elements, where $J = j_1, j_2, j_3, ..., j_n$. Let P be a finite set, where $P = p_1, p_2, p_3, ..., p_M$. Let P_i be a subset of the finite set P with cost c_i, where $1 \leq i \leq M$. The SPP is about selecting m subsets p from a set of size M at a minimum cost C. Each subset m have an associated cost and covers one or more elements from a set J. This problem is constrained to cover each element from the set J exactly once. In the BCS problem each element j have a defined width w and restrict every subset -denominated as cutting pattern; m to a maximum lenght L, the solution of the BCS problem specify the minimum number of cutting patterns and its configuration satisfying all the constraints.

SPP Integer Programming formulation is as follows:

$$Min \sum_{i=1}^{M} c_i X_i \qquad (1)$$

s.t.

$$\sum_{i=i}^{M} X_i P_{i,j} = 1 \quad \forall j \in J \qquad (2)$$

$$X_i, P_{i,j} \in 0, 1 \qquad (3)$$

Where: $X_i = 1$ if the subset P_i is selected. $P_{i,j} = 1$ if the element j is part of the subset i.

Even though the previous formulation look straightforward, the size M of the set P grows exponentially as the number of elements n in the set J increases, leading to intractable solution times and memory usage. This matter create a disadvantage for both SCP and SPP IP traditional formulation -or any other solution approach which requires explicit enumeration; because of the need of the explicit enumeration of all the feasible subsets $P_{i,j}$. And if we consider complex rules and constraints to create those subsets, the explicit enumeration of those cant be achieved in a reasonable amount of time.

1.2   Column Generation

Dantzig-Wolfe decomposition (column generation) is an approach for solving large scale Linear Programming (LP) problems introduced by [10]. It consists in reformulating the original problem as a restricted master problem (RMP) and a sub-problem (SUB). While the restricted master problem handle few constraints and a huge number of variables the sub-problem tries to find a new variable for the restricted master problem that improves his current solution.

Given a linear problem with L columns:

$$Min\ z = c^T x \tag{4}$$

s.t.

$$Ax = b \tag{5}$$

$$lb \leq x \leq ub \tag{6}$$

Dantzig-Wolfe decomposition suggest to partition the $m \times n$ matrix A arbitrarily into an $m' \times n$ matrix A^1 and an $m'' \times n$ matrix A^2 generating the next two LP's:

With A having fewer rows but typically many more columns in L than A^1 with L' columns . This master problem may be solved even when A^1 and c'^T are not explicitly available, by applying a technique denominated delayed column generation we are able to find an entering column of A' and the corresponding component of c'^T in each iteration of the revised simplex method [7].

The column generation algorithm consists in execute sequentially the RMP followed by the SUB. At the end of the RMP the shadow prices of every restriction is sended as coefficients to the SUB, then the SUB find a promising column. For minimization problems if the promising column have a negative reduced cost $1 - reducedcost < 0$ then it enters to the RMP basis and we repeat the process until no other promising column with negative reduced cost is found Figure 3.

$$Min \; z_{RMP} = \sum_{k=1}^{L} \prime(c^T x_k)\alpha_k \tag{7}$$

s.t.

$$\sum_{k=1}^{L} \prime(A^1 x_k)\alpha_k = b^1 \tag{8}$$

$$\sum_{k=1}^{L} \prime \alpha_k = 1 \tag{9}$$

$$\alpha_k \geq 0 \forall k \tag{10}$$

Fig. 1. Restricted Master Problem (RMP)

$$Min \; z_{SUB} = (c^T - \pi^T A^1)\alpha_k \tag{11}$$

s.t.

$$A^2 x = b^2 \tag{12}$$

$$0 \leq x \leq ub \tag{13}$$

Fig. 2. Sub Problem (SUB)

Column Generation have been applied to solving the vehicle routing problem [17], branch and price algorithms[6] and timetabling problems [4].

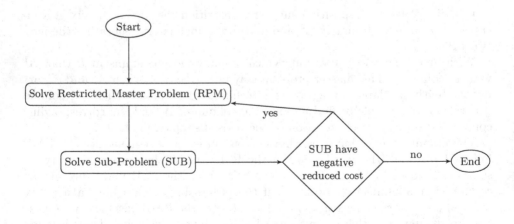

Fig. 3. Column generation algorithm

1.3   Genetic Algorithms

A Genetic Algorithm (GA) its a stochastic search methodology where the successor state is generated by combining two parent states rather than by modifying a single state [18]. Introduced by Holland a GA is an evolutionary algorithm based on natural selection theory [13].

GA's have been applied to solving many combinatorial optimization problems such as Traveling Salesman Problem (TSP), Vehicle Routing Problem (VRP), Set Covering Problem (SCP), scheduling problems and others [19] [12] [21], [1], [3].

A basic GA begin with a set of randomly generated individuals (states) called population, then each individual is evaluated by a fitness function (objective function), next, from that population we select (tipically) two parents and with certain probability (crossover rate) recombine those parents to generate two new individuals. Following with the evolutionary process with certain probability (mutation rate) we alter the individual genome string. This process is executed by a used defined number of iterations called generations. [18] [13].

At the end of the evoluionary process illustrated in Figure 4, the best individual represent the best solution found.

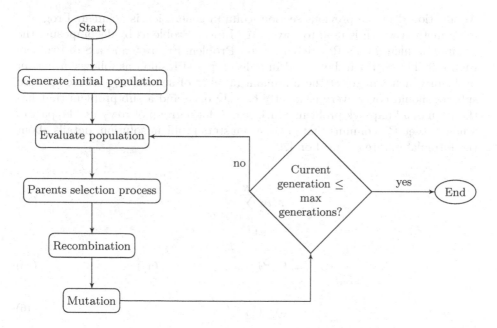

Fig. 4. Basic Genetic Algorithm flow

2   Implementation

As result of this research work four algorithms were implemented, a simple heuristic, a linear programming implementing branching rules, a genetic algorithm to solve the whole BCS -stated as an SPP;, and a genetic algorithm to be embedded in the column generation process. The outcomes from each algorithm and benchmarking are presented in the next section.

2.1 Heuristic

An heuristic $h(n)$ is a solution method supposed to estimate the cost of a solution designed from gained experience in the problem [18]. An intuitive process to solving the BCS problem is to build subsets by picking up elements that fits and don't violate any constraint. This heuristic is known as First Fit [14].

A better approximation algorithm is obtained by sorting the set of elements (finals) in a decreasing fashion such that $w(1) \geq w(2) \geq w(3) \geq ... \geq w(n)$ then selecting first the biggest elements and finding a small element that minimize the raw material waste an so on until no elements fits in the subset. It is proven that First Fit Decreasing algorithm guarantee solutions with no more 22 percent respect to the optimal solution [14].

2.2 Exact Mathematics with Column Generation

As mentioned in the previous section, column generation is a Linear Programming method which is used to solve large Linear Problems by decomposing the original problem into a Restricted Master Problem Figure 5 and a Sub-Problem Figure 6. The SPP can be stated in a decomposed fashion as follows: a master problem which will select the minimum number of subsets $P_{i,j}$, those selected subsets should cover every element j exactly once and a sub-problem that has the form of a knapsack problem which search for a group of rows j to be part of a new subset P_i (column) that enhance masters problem solution, details about the formulation are detailed on [20].

$$Min \ \sum_{i=1}^{K} c_i^T x_i \tag{14}$$

$$\text{s.t.}$$

$$\sum_{i=i}^{K} x_i P_{i,j} = 1 \quad \forall j \in J \qquad (\pi_j) \tag{15}$$

$$X_i, P_{i,j} \in 0,1 \tag{16}$$

Where:
K is the number of columns in the RMP base.
$x_i = 1$ if the subset P_i is selected.
$P_{i,j} = 1$ if the element j is part of the subset i.
π_j is the dual variable for row j.

Fig. 5. SPP restricted master problem

$$Max \sum_{j=1}^{m} \pi_j z_j \tag{17}$$

s.t.

$$\sum_{j=1}^{m} z_j w_j \leq L \tag{18}$$

$$z_j \in 0, 1 \tag{19}$$

Where:

$z_j = 1$ if the row j is selected to be part of the new subset P_i.

(y_j) is the dual variable for row j.

w_j a value for the row j.

L maximum value for a subset.

Fig. 6. SPP sub-problem

2.3 Metaheuristic

Genetics algorithms have been widely used to solve the SPP and SCP [21], [1], [3], however this implementations assume that an explicit enumeration of the feasible subsets is made and as we mention before, the number of feasible subsets grows exponentially and enumerating those could be a time consuming task if the number of rules and constraints is high.

Our approach applies the classic 0-1 genetic algorithm where the individual is a matrix $n \times n$. In this matrix each row represent a final and each column represent a subset. The size of the matrix is given by the upper bound of subsets to choose, in the worst case when all finals are the same width than the maximum lenght of a raw roll, the optimal solution will be to allocate one final per subset generating an identity matrix. Nonetheless this representation could generate infeasible solutions, in order to keep the spirit of evolutionary algorithms this work penalizes infeasible solutions.

Genetic Operators. The genetic operators implemented were designed specially for this problem. The main ideas were taken from the branching rules explained in [20] and the Column Generation Process.

Crossover operator takes two individuals from the population and with certain probability cp recombine column by column elements in such a way two new columns with minimum raw material waste are generated. In the other hand, mutation operator realizes a local search with probability mp is executed over each column of individuals by trying to maximize usage of the column and removing selected elements from other columns if exists.

2.4 Matheuristic

A Matheuristic is defined as the coupling of a Linear Problem and Computer Sciences methodologies to obtain the best parts of both sides. In this research work, the matheuristic is built by mixing a Linear Problem with a Genetic Algorithm in a Column Generation framework. Following the main idea of Column

Generation (CG), the RMP will be solved by a Linear Program and the entering columns are generated with a Genetic Algorithm. Since the task of the SUB is to find a new column that enhance the current solution, it isn't necessary to solve it to optimality. Even more, taking advantage of the genotype-phenotype map, we can add more than one column per CG iteration. In this case, the inserted columns will share similar phenotype but different genotype leafting the task of choosing the best of those to the RMP.

The Matheuristic were designed by using the framework built for the Column Generation experiments based on [20] and replacing the LP of the Knapsack Problem which tries to select the best subset of finals without violating capacity constraint that generates a negative reduced cost by a Genetic Algorithm that solve the same problem.

The implemented GA, uses the 0-1 genome codification where 1 means the final is part of the new column and 0 otherwise. Its objective function maximize the shadow costs of the selected elements creating a negative reduced cost implying enhance the current RMP solution. By looking for negative reduced costs the GA will be able to find different column configurations with equal or similar negative reduced cost.

Recombination operation is made by a sinple one point crossover meanwhile mutation process implies a local search which looks for feasible elements to add to the new column and selecting the most suitables.

3   Results

The different implementations were tested and benchmarked in 20 different scenarios. All 20 scenarios have a raw material lenght $L = 150$ and 100 finals with widths randomly generated $U(20, 100)$. Next we present graphs comparing the results obtained and performance.

All algorithms were tested in a computer with Intel i7 processor with 8 GB RAM. The implementatios were coded using Python, Gurobi and PyEvolve.

In Table 1 we summarize the results obtained in each methodology studied. Here we can notice that the exact methodology and math-heuristic methodologies solve the problem to optimallity were has the Genetic Algorithm obtain near optimal solutions. Also in the Table 1 the solution times and amount of explored nodes in the exact methodology and Matheuristics are benchmarked.

Figure 7 shows the solution obtained by each methodology studied, as noticed both exact methodology and matheuristic are solved to optimallity.

Figure 8 plot the required computational time for each methodology in every experiment. This result shows that the Metaheuristic is really fast but as showed earlier the solution found is not optimal. In the case of Matheuristics the performance is worst than Exact Methodology but obtains optimal solutions.

Figure 9 benchmark the amount of explored nodes by the exact Column Generation and Math-Heuristic. Just in four cases Matheuristic explored less nodes than Exact Methodology, however in average the number of explored nodes are very similar, Exact methodology explored 52.75 nodes in average whereas Matheuristic 53.85 nodes.

Table 1. Summary table

Experiment	Best integer solution			Explored nodes		Execution Time		
	Branch and Price	Math-Heuristic	Genetic Algorithm	Branch and Price	Math-Heuristic	Branch and Price	Math-Heuristic	Genetic algorithm
1	40	40	41	53	53	107.5710001	687.2379999	68.14199996
2	41	41	42	53	51	114.9919999	707.618	68.74699998
3	44	44	47	53	54	91.17799997	629.6259999	67.49799991
4	44	44	50	53	50	90.59800005	597.411	68.84800005
5	40	40	42	50	53	108.2819998	653.8200002	67.32999992
6	41	41	43	49	48	94.71199989	585.5580001	67.57800007
7	41	41	43	50	49	97.1869998	628.2869999	67.38000011
8	41	41	42	53	57	102.9190001	676.7639999	66.43000007
9	39	39	40	58	57	132.5509999	762.517	66.31200004
10	39	39	41	57	51	122.5980001	711.711	65.96899986
11	44	44	46	51	54	95.68499994	625.8990002	66.02699995
12	41	41	42	54	50	124.2410002	732.711	66.04400015
13	39	39	40	54	55	101.654	655.904	67.48699999
14	41	41	44	57	54	115.8800001	642.7149999	66.50300002
15	41	41	43	54	56	111.7089999	652.8309999	66.49799991
16	41	41	42	56	56	110.2189999	690.007	66.10400009
17	39	39	40	54	51	104.533	677.9679999	66.40599999
18	39	39	41	58	50	105.4170001	749.4619999	64.90100002
19	43	43	46	52	53	103.2319999	657.6660001	66.77600002
20	40	40	41	58	53	120.2690001	703.345	66.63999987

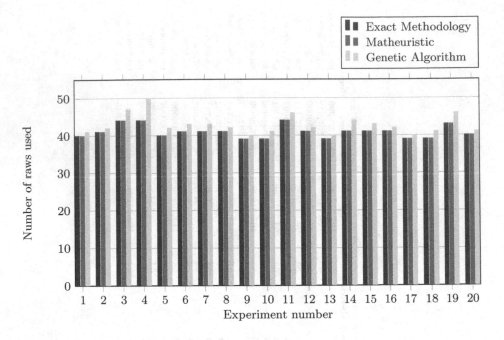

Fig. 7. Number of raws (solution) to use in each method

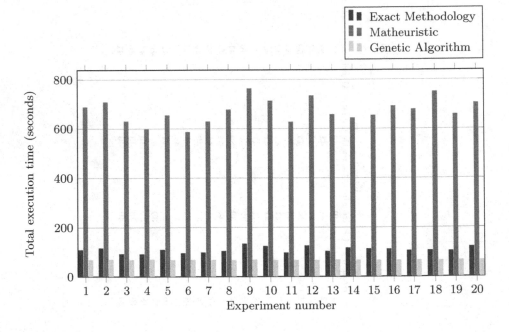

Fig. 8. Total solution time

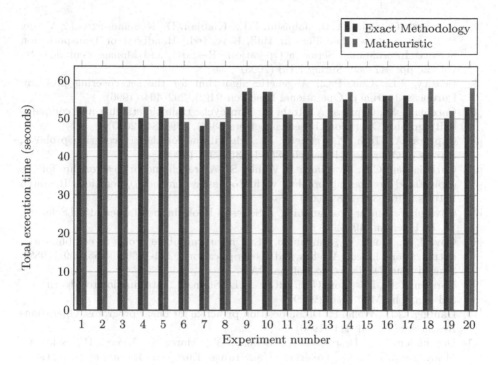

Fig. 9. Explored nodes

4   Conclusions and Future Work

Two conclusions were determined. First, at least for the proposed experiments, Matheuristics are as good as Exact Methodology, since both approaches find an optimal solution, then, if the subproblem is a non-linear program or contains fuzzy or subjective parameters, matheuristic will be easier to implement. Second, the number of explored nodes in the Branch and Price tree is affected by the quality of the entering column generated by the subproblem, in the case of matheuristics by designing better metaheuristics for the subproblem the number of explored nodes can be reduced.

As a future work, in order to improve solving time, the programming language is essencial, since Python is not a compiled language and performance from PyEvolve is not as good as a propertary implementation. In addition, obtained results leads to test Matheuristics to solving more complex problems such as Vehicle Routing Problem with Time Windows.

References

[1]   Aickelin, U., Dowsland, K.A.: An indirect genetic algorithm for a nurse-scheduling problem. Computers and Operations Research 31(5), 761–778 (2004)

[2] Barnhart, C., Cohn, A.M., Johnson, E.L., Klabjan, D., Nemhauser, G.L., Vance, P.H.: Airline crew scheduling. In: Hall, R.W. (ed.) Handbook of Transportation Science. International Series in Operations Research and Management Science, vol. 56, pp. 517–560. Springer US (2003)

[3] Beasley, J.E., Chu, P.C.: A genetic algorithm for the set covering problem. European Journal of Operational Research 94(2), 392–404 (1996)

[4] Cacchiani, V., Caprara, A., Toth, P.: Non-cyclic train timetabling and comparability graphs. Operations Research Letters 38(3), 179–184 (2010)

[5] Caprara, A., Toth, P., Fischetti, M.: Algorithms for the set covering problem. Annals of Operations Research 98(1-4), 353–371 (2000)

[6] Christiansen, C.H., Lysgaard, J., Wøhlk, S.: A branch-and-price algorithm for the capacitated arc routing problem with stochastic demands. Operations Research Letters 37(6), 392–398 (2009)

[7] Chvatal, V.: Linear Programming. A Series of Books in the Mathematical Sciences. W. H. Freeman (1983)

[8] Chvtal, V., Cook, W., Hartmann, M.: On cutting-plane proofs in combinatorial optimization. Linear Algebra and its Applications, 114-115(0), 455–499 (1989); Special Issue Dedicated to Hoffman, A.J.

[9] Cormen, T.H., Leiserson, C.E., Rivest, R.L., Stein, C.: Introduction to Algorithms, 3rd edn. The MIT Press (2009)

[10] Dantzig, G.B., Wolfe, P.: Decomposition principle for linear programs. Operations Research 8(1), 101–111 (1960)

[11] Desaulniers, G., Desrosiers, J., Dumas, Y., Marc, S., Rioux, B., Solomon, M.M., Soumis, F.: Crew pairing at air france. European Journal of Operational Research 97(2), 245–259 (1997)

[12] Drezner, Z.: Compounded genetic algorithms for the quadratic assignment problem. Operations Research Letters 33(5), 475–480 (2005)

[13] Eiben, A.E., Smith, J.E.: Introduction to Evolutionary Computing. Natural Computing Series. Springer (2003)

[14] Garey, R., Johnson, D.S.: Computers and Intractability: A Guide to the Theory of NP-Completeness. A Series of Books in the Mathematical Sciences. W.H. Freeman (1979)

[15] Gilmore, P.C., Gomory, R.E.: A Linear Programming Approach to the Cutting-Stock Problem. Operations Research 9(6), 849–859 (1961)

[16] Haessler, R.W., Sweeney, P.E.: Cutting stock problems and solution procedures. European Journal of Operational Research 54(2), 141–150 (1991)

[17] Jin, M., Liu, K., Eksioglu, B.: A column generation approach for the split delivery vehicle routing problem. Operations Research Letters 36(2), 265–270 (2008)

[18] Russell, S.J., Norvig, P.: Artificial intelligence: a modern approach. Prentice Hall series in artificial intelligence. Pearson Education/Prentice Hall (2010)

[19] Singh, G., Ernst, A.T.: Resource constraint scheduling with a fractional shared resource. Operations Research Letters 39(5), 363–368 (2011)

[20] Vance, P.H., Barnhart, C., Johnson, E.L., Nemhauser, G.L.: Solving binary cutting stock problems by column generation and branch-and-bound. Computational Optimization and Applications 3(2), 111–130 (1994)

[21] Zheng, Y.-L., Lei, D.-M.: Hybrid Niche Genetic Algorithm for Set Covering Problem. In: 2007 International Conference on Machine Learning and Cybernetics, pp. 1009–1013 (2007)

Nature-Inspired Optimization of Type-2 Fuzzy Systems

Oscar Castillo, Patricia Melin, and Fevrier Valdez

Tijuana Institute of Technology, Division of Graduate Studies Tijuana, Mexico
{ocastillo,pmelin,fevrier}@tectijuana.mx

Abstract. A review of the optimization methods used in the design of type-2 fuzzy systems, which are relatively novel models of imprecision, is presented in this paper. The main aim of the work is to study the basic reasons for optimizing type-2 fuzzy systems for solving problems different areas of application. Recently, nature-inspired methods have emerged as powerful optimization algorithms for solving complex problems. In the case of designing type-2 fuzzy systems for particular applications, the use of nature-inspired optimization methods have helped in the complex task of finding the appropriate parameter values and structure of the fuzzy systems. In this paper, we consider the application of genetic algorithms, particle swarm optimization and ant colony optimization as three different paradigms that help in the design of optimal type-2 fuzzy systems. A comparison of the different optimization methods for the case of designing type-2 fuzzy systems is also offered.

Keywords: Intelligent Control, Type-2 Fuzzy Logic, Interval Type-2 Fuzzy Logic.

1   Introduction

Uncertainty affects decision-making and arises in a number of different forms in real problems. The concept of information is related with the concept of uncertainty [17]. The most fundamental aspect of this relation is that the uncertainty involved in any problem-solving situation is a result of some information deficiency, which may be incomplete, imprecise, fragmentary, not fully reliable, vague, contradictory, or deficient in some other way. Uncertainty is an attribute of information [27]. The general framework of fuzzy reasoning allows handling much of this uncertainty and fuzzy systems that employ type-1 fuzzy sets represent uncertainty by numbers in the range [0, 1]. When something is uncertain, like a measurement, it is difficult to determine its exact value, and of course type-1 fuzzy sets make more sense than using crisp sets [14]. However, it is not reasonable to use an accurate membership function for something uncertain, so in this case what we need is higher order fuzzy sets, those which are able to handle these uncertainties, like the so called type-2 fuzzy sets [14]. So, the amount of uncertainty can be managed by using type-2 fuzzy logic because it offers better capabilities to handle linguistic uncertainties by modeling vagueness and unreliability of information [5] [26].

A. Gelbukh et al. (Eds.): MICAI 2014, Part II, LNAI 8857, pp. 331–344, 2014.

Recently, we have seen the use of type-2 fuzzy sets in Fuzzy Logic Systems (FLS) in different areas of application [1] [2] [6] [10] [12]. In this paper we deal with the application of interval type-2 fuzzy control to non-linear dynamic systems [3] [4] [5] [15] [19]. It is a well known fact, that in the control of real systems, the instrumentation elements (instrumentation amplifier, sensors, digital to analog, analog to digital converters, etc.) introduce some sort of unpredictable values in the information that has been collected [20] [21]. So, the controllers designed under idealized conditions tend to behave in an inappropriate manner [11] [22] [23].

2   Fuzzy Logic Systems

In this section, a brief overview of type-1 and type-2 fuzzy systems is presented. This overview is considered to be necessary to understand the basic concepts needed to develop the methods and algorithms presented later in the paper.

2.1   Type-1 Fuzzy Logic Systems

Soft computing techniques have become an important research topic, which can be applied in the design of intelligent controllers, which utilize the human experience in a more natural form than the conventional mathematical approach [16, 18]. A FLS, described completely in terms of type-1 fuzzy sets is called a type-1 fuzzy logic system (type-1 FLS). In this paper, the fuzzy controller has two input variables, which are the error e(t) and the error variation $\Delta e(t)$,

$$e(t) = r(t) - y(t) \tag{1}$$

$$\Delta e(t) = e(t) - e(t-1) \tag{2}$$

so the control system can be represented as in Figure 1.

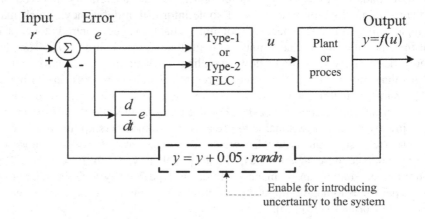

Fig. 1. System used for obtaining the experimental results

2.2   Type-2 Fuzzy Logic Systems

If for a type-1 membership function, as in Figure 2, we blur it to the left and to the right, as illustrated in Figure 3, then a type-2 membership function can be obtained. In this case, for a specific value x', the membership function (u'), takes on different values, which are not all weighted the same, so we can assign an amplitude distribution to all of those points.

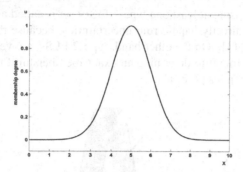

Fig. 2. Type-1 membership function

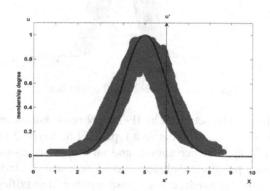

Fig. 3. Blurred type-1 membership function

A type-2 fuzzy set $\tilde{A}$, is characterized by the membership function [14, 17]:

$$\tilde{A} = \left\{ ((x,u), \mu_{\tilde{A}}(x,u)) \mid \forall x \in X, \forall u \in J_x \subseteq [0,1] \right\} \tag{3}$$

in which $0 \le \mu_{\tilde{A}}(x,u) \le 1$. Another expression for $\tilde{A}$ is,

$$\tilde{A} = \int_{x \in X} \int_{u \in J_x} \mu_{\tilde{A}}(x,u)/(x,u) \qquad J_x \subseteq [0,1] \tag{4}$$

Where $\int \int$ denotes the union over all admissible input variables x and u. For discrete universes of discourse $\int \dots$ is replaced by $\sum \dots$. In fact $J_x \subseteq [0,1]$ represents the primary membership of x, and $\mu_{\tilde{A}}(x,u)$ is a type-1 fuzzy set known as the secondary set. Hence, a type-2 membership grade can be any subset in [0,1], the primary membership, and corresponding to each primary membership, there is a secondary membership (which can also be in [0,1]) that defines the possibilities for the primary membership. Uncertainty is represented by a region, which is called the footprint of uncertainty (FOU). When $\mu_{\tilde{A}}(x,u) = 1, \forall u \in J_x \subseteq [0,1]$ we have an interval type-2 membership function, as shown in Figure 4. The uniform shading for the FOU represents the entire interval type-2 fuzzy set and it can be described in terms of an upper membership function $\overline{\mu}_{\tilde{A}}(x)$ and a lower membership function $\underline{\mu}_{\tilde{A}}(x)$.

A FLS described using at least one type-2 fuzzy set is called a type-2 FLS. Type-1 FLSs are unable to directly handle rule uncertainties, because they use type-1 fuzzy sets that are certain [14]. On the other hand, type-2 FLSs, are very useful in circumstances where it is difficult to determine an exact membership function, and there are measurement uncertainties [7, 8, 15].

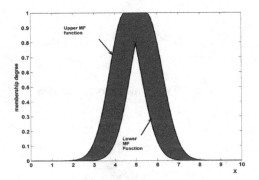

Fig. 4. Interval type-2 membership function

A type-2 FLS is also characterized by IF-THEN rules, but its antecedent or consequent sets are now of type-2. Similar to a type-1 FLS, a type-2 FLS includes a fuzzifier, a rule base, fuzzy inference engine, and an output processor, as we can see in Figure 5. The output processor includes type-reducer and defuzzifier; it generates a type-1 fuzzy set output (type-reducer) or a crisp number (defuzzifier).

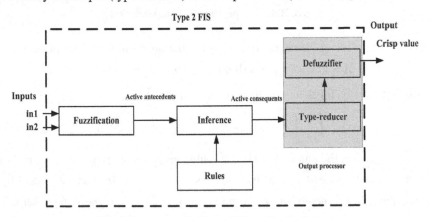

Fig. 5. Structure of a Type-2 Fuzzy Logic System

2.2.1. Fuzzifier

The fuzzifier maps a crisp point $x=(x1,...,xp)^T \in X_1 x X_2 x...x X_p \equiv X$ into a type-2 fuzzy set $\tilde{A}_x$ in X [17], interval type-2 fuzzy sets in this case. We will use type-2 singleton fuzzifier, in a singleton fuzzification, the input fuzzy set has only a single point on nonzero membership [14]. $\tilde{A}_x$ is a type-2 fuzzy singleton if $\mu_{\tilde{A}_x}(x) = 1/1$ for x=x' and $\mu_{\tilde{A}_x}(x) = 1/0$ for all other $x \neq x'$ [17].

2.2.2. Rules

The structure of rules in a type-1 FLS and a type-2 FLS is the same, but in the latter the antecedents and the consequents will be represented by type-2 fuzzy sets. So for a type-2 FLS with p inputs $x1 \in X1,...,xp \in Xp$ and one output $y \in Y$, Multiple Input Single Output (MISO), if we assume there are M rules, the lth rule in the type-2 FLS can be written as follows [14]:

$$R^l: \text{IF } x_1 \text{ is } \tilde{F}_1^l \text{ and } \cdots \text{and } x_p \text{ is } \tilde{F}_p^l \text{, THEN } y \text{ is } \tilde{G}^l \quad l=1,...,M \quad (5)$$

2.2.3. Inference

In the type-2 FLS, the inference engine combines rules and gives a mapping from input type-2 fuzzy sets to output type-2 fuzzy sets. It is necessary to compute the join ⊔, (unions) and the meet Π (intersections), as well as extended sup-star compositions (sup star compositions) of type-2 relations [14]. If $\tilde{F}^l{}_1 \times \cdots \times \tilde{F}^l{}_p = \tilde{A}^l$, equation (5) can be re-written as

$$R^l : \tilde{F}^l{}_1 \times \cdots \times \tilde{F}^l{}_p \to \tilde{G}^l = \tilde{A}^l \to \tilde{G}^l \quad l=1,...,M \quad (6)$$

R^l is described by the membership function $\mu_{R^l}(\mathbf{x}, y) = \mu_{R^l}(x_1,..., x_p, y)$, where

$$\mu_{R^l}(\mathbf{x}, y) = \mu_{\tilde{A}^l \to \tilde{G}^l}(\mathbf{x}, y) \quad (7)$$

can be written as [14]:

$$\mu_{R^l}(\mathbf{x}, y) = \mu_{\tilde{A}^l \to \tilde{G}^l}(\mathbf{x}, y) = \mu_{\tilde{F}_1^l}(x_1) \cap \cdots \cap \mu_{\tilde{F}_p^l}(x_p) \cap \mu_{\tilde{G}^l}(y)$$

$$= [\cap_{i=1}^{p} \mu_{\tilde{F}^l_i}(x_i)] \cap \mu_{\tilde{G}^l}(y) \quad (8)$$

In general, the p-dimensional input to Rl is given by the type-2 fuzzy set $\tilde{A}_x$ whose membership function is

$$\mu_{\tilde{A}_x}(\mathbf{x}) = \mu_{\tilde{x}_1}(x_1) \cap \cdots \cap \mu_{\tilde{x}_p}(x_p) = \cap_{i=1}^{p} \mu_{\tilde{x}_i}(x_i) \quad (9)$$

where $\tilde{X}_i (i = 1,..., p)$ are the labels of the fuzzy sets describing the inputs. Each rule Rl determines a type-2 fuzzy set $B^l = \tilde{A}_x \circ R^l$ such that [14]:

$$\mu_{B^l}(y) = \mu_{\tilde{A}_x \circ R^l} = \sqcup_{x \in X} [\mu_{\tilde{A}_x}(\mathbf{x}) \cap \mu_{R^l}(\mathbf{x}, y)] \quad y \in Y \ l=1,...,M \quad (10)$$

This equation is the input/output relation in Figure 5 between the type-2 fuzzy set that activates one rule in the inference engine and the type-2 fuzzy set at the output of that engine [14]. In the FLS we used interval type-2 fuzzy sets and meet under product t-norm, so the result of the input and antecedent operations, which are contained in the firing set $\Pi_{i=1}^{p}\mu_{F_{1i}}(x'_i \equiv F^l(x'))$, is an interval type-1 set [14],

$$F^l(\mathbf{x'}) = \left[\underline{f}^l(\mathbf{x'}), \overline{f}^l(\mathbf{x'})\right] \equiv \left[\underline{f}^l, \overline{f}^l\right] \qquad (11)$$

where

$$\underline{f}^l(\mathbf{x'}) = \mu_{\underline{F}_1^l}(x_1') * \cdots * \mu_{\underline{F}_p^l}(x_p') \qquad (12)$$

$$\overline{f}^l(\mathbf{x'}) = \mu_{\overline{F}_1^l}(x_1') * \cdots * \mu_{\overline{F}_p^l}(x_p') \qquad (13)$$

where * is the product operation.

2.2.4. Type Reducer
The type-reducer generates a type-1 fuzzy set output, which is then converted in a crisp output through the defuzzifier. This type-1 fuzzy set is also an interval set, for the case of our FLS we used center of sets (cos) type reduction, Ycos which is expressed as [14]:

$$Y_{\cos}(\mathbf{x}) = [y_l, y_r] = \int_{y^1 \in [y_l^1, y_r^1]} \cdots \int_{y^M \in [y_l^M, y_r^M]} \int_{f^1 \in [\underline{f}^1, \overline{f}^1]} \cdots \int_{f^M \in [\underline{f}^M, \overline{f}^M]} 1 / \frac{\sum_{i=1}^{M} f^i y^i}{\sum_{i=1}^{M} f^i} \qquad (14)$$

this interval set is determined by its two end points, yl and yr, which corresponds to the centroid of the type-2 interval consequent set $\tilde{G}^i$ [14],

$$C_{\tilde{G}^i} = \int_{\theta_1 \in J_{y1}} \cdots \int_{\theta_N \in J_{yN}} 1 / \frac{\sum_{i=1}^{N} y_i \theta_i}{\sum_{i=1}^{N} \theta_i} = [y_l^i, y_r^i] \qquad (15)$$

before the computation of Ycos (x), we must evaluate equation (15), and its two end points, y_l and y_r. If the values of f_i and y_i that are associated with y_l are denoted f_{li} and y_{li}, respectively, and the values of f_i and y_i that are associated with y_r are denoted f_{ri} and y_{ri}, respectively, from (14), we have [14]

$$y_l = \frac{\sum_{i=1}^{M} f_l^i y_l^i}{\sum_{i=1}^{M} f_l^i} \qquad (16)$$

$$y_r = \frac{\sum_{i=1}^{M} f_r^i y_r^i}{\sum_{i=1}^{M} f_r^i} \qquad (17)$$

2.2.5. Defuzzifier
From the type-reducer we obtain an interval set Ycos, to defuzzify it we use the average of y_l and y_r, so the defuzzified output of an interval singleton type-2 FLS is [14]

$$y(\mathbf{x}) = \frac{y_l + y_r}{2} \qquad (18)$$

3   Nature-Inspired Optimization Methods

In this section a brief overview of the basic concepts from some nature-inspired optimization methods needed for this work is presented.

3.1   Particle Swarm Optimization

Particle swarm optimization is a population based stochastic optimization technique developed by Eberhart and Kennedy in 1995, inspired by social behavior of bird flocking or fish schooling [1]. PSO shares many similarities with evolutionary computation techniques such as the GA [9].

The system is initialized with a population of random solutions and searches for optima by updating generations. However, unlike the GA, the PSO has no evolution operators such as crossover and mutation. In the PSO, the potential solutions, called particles, fly through the problem space by following the current optimum particles [16]. Each particle keeps track of its coordinates in the problem space, which are associated with the best solution (fitness) it has achieved so far (The fitness value is also stored). This value is called pbest. Another "best" value that is tracked by the particle swarm optimizer is the best value, obtained so far by any particle in the neighbors of the particle. This location is called lbest. When a particle takes all the population as its topological neighbors, the best value is a global best and is called gbest [19].

The particle swarm optimization concept consists of, at each time step, changing the velocity of (accelerating) each particle toward its pbest and lbest locations (local version of PSO). Acceleration is weighted by a random term, with separate random numbers being generated for acceleration toward pbest and lbest locations [1]. In the past several years, PSO has been successfully applied in many research and application areas. It is demonstrated that PSO gets better results in a faster, cheaper way when compared with other methods [19]. Another reason that PSO is attractive is that there are few parameters to adjust. One version, with slight variations, works well in a wide variety of applications. Particle swarm optimization has been considered for approaches that can be used across a wide range of applications, as well as for specific applications focused on a specific requirement.

The basic algorithm of PSO has the following nomenclature:

x_z^i	Particle position
v_z^i	Particle velocity
w_{ij}	Inertia weight
p_z^i	Best "remembered" individual particle position
p_z^g	Best "remembered" swarm position
c_1, c_2	Cognitive and Social parameters
r_1, r_2	Random numbers between 0 and 1

The equation to calculate the velocity is:

$$v_{z+1}^i = w_{ij} v_z^i + c_1 r_1 \left(p_z^i - x_z^i \right) + c_2 r_2 \left(p_z^g - x_z^i \right) \tag{19}$$

and the position of the individual particles is updated as follows:

$$x_{z+1}^i = x_z^i + v_{z+1}^i \tag{20}$$

The basic PSO algorithm is defined as follows:

1) Initialize

    a) Set constants z_{max}, c_1, c_2

    b) Randomly initialize particle position $x_0^i \in D$ *in* R^n *for* $i = 1, ..., p$

    c) Randomly initialize particle velocities $0 \le v_0^i \le v_0^{max}$ *for* $i = 1, ..., p$

    d) Set Z = 1

2) Optimize

    a) Evaluate function value f_k^i *using design space coordinates* x_k^i

    b) If $f_z^i \le f_{best}^i$ *then* $f_{best}^i = f_z^i, p_z^i = x_z^i.$

    c) If $f_z^i \le f_{best}^g$ *then* $f_{best}^g = f_z^i, p_z^g = x_z^i.$

    d) If stopping condition is satisfied then go to 3.

    e) Update all particle velocities v_z^i *for* $i = 1, ..., p$

    f) Update al particle positions x_z^i *for* $i = 1, ..., p$

    g) Increment z.

    h) Goto 2(a).

3) Terminate

3.2   Genetic Algorithms

Genetic Algorithms (GAs) are adaptive meta-heuristic search algorithms based on the evolutionary ideas of natural selection and genetic processes [8]. The basic principles of GAs were first proposed by John Holland in 1975, inspired by the mechanism of natural selection, where stronger individuals are likely the winners in a competing environment [9]. A GA assumes that the potential solution of any problem is an individual and can be represented by a set of parameters. These parameters are regarded as the genes of a chromosome and can be structured by a string of values in binary form. A positive value, generally known as a fitness value, is used to reflect the degree of "goodness" of the chromosome for the problem, which would be highly related with its objective value. The pseudocode of a GA is as follows:

1.   *Start with a randomly generated population of n chromosomes (candidate solutions to a problem).*

2.   *Calculate the fitness of each chromosome in the population.*

3. Repeat the following steps until n offspring have been created:
    a. Select a pair of parent chromosomes from the current population, the probability of selection being an increasing function of fitness. Selection is done with replacement, meaning that the same chromosome can be selected more than once to become a parent.
    b. With probability (crossover rate), perform crossover to the pair at a randomly chosen point to a form two offspring.
    c. Mutate the two offspring at each locus with probability (mutation rate), and place the resulting chromosomes in the new population.
4. Replace the current population with the new population.
5. Go to step 2.

The simple procedure just described above is the basis for most applications of GAs found in the literature [24] [25].

3.3   Ant Colony Optimization

Ant Colony Optimization (ACO) is a probabilistic meta-heuristic that can be used for solving problems that can be reduced to finding good paths along graphs. This method is inspired on the behavior presented by ants in finding paths from the nest or colony to the food source.

The S-ACO is an algorithmic implementation that adapts the behavior of real ants to solutions of minimum cost path problems on graphs [12]. A number of artificial ants build solutions for a certain optimization problem and exchange information about the quality of these solutions making allusion to the communication system of real ants [13].

Let us define the graph G = (V, E), where V is the set of nodes and E is the matrix of the links between nodes. G has $n_G = |V|$ nodes. Let us define L^K as the number of hops in the path built by the ant k from the origin node to the destiny node. Therefore, it is necessary to find:

$$Q = \{\, q_a,...,q_f \big| q_1 \in C \,\} \tag{21}$$

where Q is the set of nodes representing a continuous path with no obstacles; $q_a,...,q_f$ are former nodes of the path and C is the set of possible configurations of the free space. If xk(t) denotes a Q solution in time t, f(xk(t)) expresses the quality of the solution. The S-ACO algorithm is based on Equations (22), (23) and (24):

$$p_{ij}^k(t) = \begin{cases} \dfrac{\tau_{ij}^k}{\sum_{j \in N_{ij}^k} \tau_{ij}^\alpha(t)} & \text{if } j \in N_i^k \\ 0 & \text{if } j \notin N_i^k \end{cases} \tag{22}$$

$$\tau_{ij}(t) \leftarrow (1-\rho)\tau_{ij}(t) \tag{23}$$

$$\tau_{ij}(t+1) = \tau_{ij}(t) + \sum_{k=1}^{n_k} \tau_{ij}(t) \tag{24}$$

Equation (22) represents the probability for an ant k located on a node i selects the next node denoted by j, where, N_i^k is the set of feasible nodes (in a neighborhood) connected to node i with respect to ant k, τ_{ij} is the total pheromone concentration of link ij, and α is a positive constant used as a gain for the pheromone influence.

Equation (23) represents the evaporation pheromone update, where $\rho \in [0,1]$ is the evaporation rate value of the pheromone trail. The evaporation is added to the algorithm in order to force the exploration of the ants, and avoid premature convergence to sub-optimal solutions. For $\rho = 1$ the search becomes completely random.

Equation (24), represents the concentration pheromone update, where $\Delta\tau_{ij}^k$ is the amount of pheromone that an ant k deposits in a link ij in a time t.

The general steps of S-ACO are the following:

1. *Set a pheromone concentration τ_{ij} to each link (i,j).*
2. *Place a number k=1, 2,..., n_k in the nest.*
3. *Iteratively build a path to the food source (destiny node), using Equation (22) for every ant.*

    − *Remove cycles and compute each route weight $f\left(x^k(t)\right)$. A cycle could be generated when there are no feasible candidates nodes, that is, for any i and any k, $N_i^k = \varnothing$; then the predecessor of that node is included as a former node of the path.*

4. *Apply evaporation using Equation (23).*
5. *Update of the pheromone concentration using Equation (24)*
6. *Finally, finish the algorithm in any of the three different ways:*
    − *When a maximum number of epochs has been reached.*
    − *When it has found an acceptable solution, with $f(x_k(t)) < \varepsilon$.*
    − *When all ants follow the same path.*

3.4   General Remarks about Optimization of Type-2 Fuzzy Systems

The problem of designing type-2 fuzzy systems can be solved with any of the above mentioned optimization methods. The main issue in any of these methods is deciding on the representation of the type-2 fuzzy system in the corresponding optimization paradigm. For example, in the case of GAs, the type-2 fuzzy systems must be represented in the chromosomes. On the other hand, in PSO the fuzzy system is represented as a particle in the optimization process. In the ACO method, the fuzzy system can be represented as one of the paths that the ants can follow in a graph. Also, the evaluation of the fuzzy system performance must be represented as an objective function in any of the methods.

4   General Overview of the Area and Future Trend

In this section a general overview of the area of type-2 fuzzy system optimization is presented. Also, possible future trends that we can envision based on the review of this area are presented. It has been well-known for a long time that designing fuzzy systems is a difficult task, and this is especially true in the case of type-2 fuzzy systems [5]. The use of GAs, ACO and PSO in designing type-1 fuzzy systems has become a standard practice for automatically designing this sort of systems [1] [2] [13] [24]. This trend has also continued to the type-2 fuzzy systems area, which has been accounted for with the review of papers presented in the previous sections. In the case of designing type-2 fuzzy systems the problem is more complicated due to the higher number of parameters to consider, making it of upmost importance the use of bio-inspired optimization techniques for achieving the optimal designs of this sort of systems. In this section a summary of the total number of papers published in the area of type-2 fuzzy system optimization is presented, so that the increasing trend occurring in this area can be better appreciated. Also, the distribution of papers according to the used optimization technique is presented, so that a general idea of how these different techniques are contributing to the automatic design of optimal type-2 fuzzy systems is obtained.

Figure 6 shows the distribution of the published papers in optimizing type-2 fuzzy systems according to the different bio-inspired optimization techniques previously mentioned. From Figure 6 it can be noted that the use of GAs have been decreasing recently, on the other hand the use of PSO, ACO and other methods have been increasing. The reason for the increase in use of PSO and ACO may be due to recent works in which either PSO or ACO have been able to outperform GAs for different applications. Regarding the question of which method would be the most appropriate for optimizing type-2 fuzzy systems, there is no easy answer. At the moment, what we can be sure of is that the techniques mentioned in this paper and probably newer ones that may appear in the future, would certainly be tested in the optimization of type-2 fuzzy systems because the problem of designing automatically these types of systems is complex enough to require their use.

There are other nature-inspired techniques that at the moment have not been applied to the optimization of type-2 fuzzy systems that may be worth mentioning. For example, membrane computing, cuckoo search, firefly algorithm, harmony computing, electromagnetism based computing, and other similar approaches have not been applied (to the moment) in the optimization of type-2 fuzzy systems. It is expected that these approaches and similar ones could be applied in the near future in the area of type-2 fuzzy system optimization. Of course, as new nature-inspired optimization methods are being proposed at any time in this fruitful area of research, it is expected that newer optimization techniques would also be tried in the near future in the automatic design of optimal type-2 fuzzy systems.

No. Publications

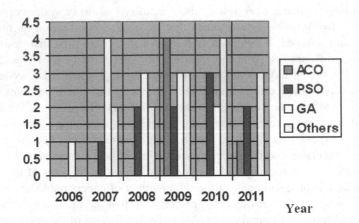

Fig. 6. Distribution of publications per area and year

5   Conclusions

In the previous sections we have presented a representative account of the different optimization methods that have been applied in the optimal design of type-2 fuzzy systems. To the moment, genetic algorithms have been used more frequently to optimize type-2 fuzzy systems. However, more recently PSO and ACO have attracted more attention and have also been applied with some degree of success to the problem of optimal design of type-2 fuzzy systems. There have been also other optimization methods applied to the optimization of type-2 fuzzy systems, like artificial immune systems and the chemical optimization paradigm. At this time, it would be very difficult to declare one of these optimization techniques as the best for optimizing type-2 fuzzy systems, as different techniques have had success for different applications of type-2 fuzzy logic. In any case, the need for nature-inspired optimization methods is justified due to the complexity of designing type-2 fuzzy systems.

References

[1] Bingül, Z., Karahan, O.: A Fuzzy Logic Controller tuned with PSO for 2 DOF robot trajectory control. Expert Systems with Applications 38(1), 1017–1031 (2011)
[2] Cao, J., Li, P., Liu, H., Brown, D.: Adaptive fuzzy controller for vehicle active suspensions with particle swarm optimization. In: Proceedings of SPIE-The International Society of Optical Engineering, vol. 7129 (2008)
[3] Castillo, O., Huesca, G., Valdez, F.: Evolutionary computing for topology op-timization of type-2 fuzzy controllers. STUDFUZZ, vol. 208, pp. 163–178. Springer, Heidelberg (2008)

[4] Castillo, O., Aguilar, L.T., Cazarez-Castro, N.R., Cardenas, S.: Systematic de-sign of a stable type-2 fuzzy logic controller. Applied Soft Computing Journal 8, 1274–1279 (2008)

[5] Castillo, O., Melin, P., Alanis, A., Montiel, O., Sepulveda, R.: Optimization of interval type-2 fuzzy logic controllers using evolutionary algorithms. Journal of Soft Computing 15(6), 1145–1160 (2011)

[6] Castro, J.R., Castillo, O., Melin, P.: An Interval Type-2 Fuzzy Logic Toolbox for Control Applications. In: Proceedings of FUZZ-IEEE 2007, London, pp. 1–6 (2007)

[7] Castro, J.R., Castillo, O., Martinez, L.G.: Interval type-2 fuzzy logic toolbox. Engineering Letters 15(1), 14 (2007)

[8] Cordon, O., Gomide, F., Herrera, F., Hoffmann, F., Magdalena, L.: Ten years of genetic fuzzy systems: current framework and new trends. Fuzzy Sets and Systems 141, 5–31 (2004)

[9] Cordon, O., Herrera, F., Villar, P.: Analysis and guidelines to obtain a good uni-form fuzzy partition granularity for fuzzy rule-based systems using simulated annealing. International Journal of Approximate Reasoning 25, 187–215 (2000)

[10] Dereli, T., Baykasoglu, A., Altun, K., Durmusoglu, A., Turksen, I.B.: Industrial applications of type-2 fuzzy sets and systems: A concise review. Computers in Industry 62, 125–137 (2011)

[11] Hagras, H.: Hierarchical type-2 fuzzy logic control architecture for autono-mous mobile robots. IEEE Transactions on Fuzzy Systems 12, 524–539 (2004)

[12] Juang, C.-F., Hsu, C.-H.: Reinforcement ant optimized fuzzy controller for mobile-robot wall-following control. IEEE Transactions on Industrial Electronics 56(10), 3931–3940 (2009)

[13] Juang, C.-F., Hsu, C.-H.: Reinforcement interval type-2 fuzzy controller de-sign by online rule generation and Q-value-aided ant colony optimization. IEEE Transactions on Systems, Man, and Cybernetics, Part B Cybernetics 39(6), 1528–1542 (2009)

[14] Karnik, N.N., Mendel, J.M.: An Introduction to Type-2 Fuzzy Logic Systems, Technical Report, University of Southern California (1998)

[15] Martinez, R., Castillo, O., Aguilar, L.T.: Optimization of interval type-2 fuzzy logic controllers for a perturbed autonomous wheeled mobile robot using genetic algorithms. Information Sciences 179(13), 2158–2174 (2009)

[16] Martinez, R., Rodriguez, A., Castillo, O., Aguilar, L.T.: Type-2 fuzzy logic controllers optimization using genetic algorithms and particle swarm optimization. In: Proceedings of the IEEE International Conference on Granular Computing, GrC 2010, pp. 724–727 (2010)

[17] Mendel, J.M.: Uncertainty, fuzzy logic, and signal processing. Signal Processing Journal 80, 913–933 (2000)

[18] Mohammadi, S.M.A., Gharaveisi, A.A., Mashinchi, M.: An evolutionary tuning technique for type-2 fuzzy logic controller in a non-linear system under uncertainty. In: Proceedings of the 18th Iranian Conference on Electrical Engineering, ICEE 2010, pp. 610–616 (2010)

[19] Oh, S.-K., Jang, H.-J., Pedrycz, W.: A comparative experimental study of type-1/type-2 fuzzy cascade controller based on genetic algorithms and particle swarm optimization. Expert Systems with Applications 38(9), 11217–11229 (2011)

[20] Sepulveda, R., Castillo, O., Melin, P., Rodriguez-Diaz, A., Montiel, O.: Experimental study of intelligent controllers under uncertainty using type-1 and type-2 fuzzy logic. Information Sciences 177(10), 2023–2048 (2007)

[21] Sepúlveda, R., Montiel, O., Lizárraga, G., Castillo, O.: Modeling and simulation of the defuzzification stage of a type-2 fuzzy controller using the xilinx system generator and simulink. In: Castillo, O., Pedrycz, W., Kacprzyk, J. (eds.) Evolutionary Design of Intelligent Systems in Modeling, Simulation and Control. SCI, vol. 257, pp. 309–325. Springer, Heidelberg (2009)

[22] Sepulveda, R., Montiel, O., Castillo, O., Melin, P.: Modelling and Simulation of the defuzzification Stage of a Type-2 Fuzzy Controller Using VHDL Code. Control and Intelligent Systems 39(1) (2011)

[23] Sepulveda, R., Montiel, O., Castillo, O., Melin, P.: Embedding a high speed interval type-2 fuzzy controller for a real plant into an FPGA. Appl. Soft Comput. 12(3), 988–998 (2012)

[24] Wagner, C., Hagras, H.: A genetic algorithm based architecture for evolving type-2 fuzzy logic controllers for real world autonomous mobile robots. In: Proceedings of the IEEE Conference on Fuzzy Systems, London (2007)

[25] Wu, D., Tan, W.-W.: Genetic learning and performance evaluation of interval type-2 fuzzy logic controllers. Engineering Applications of Artificial Intelligence 19(8), 829–841 (2006)

[26] Yager, R.R.: Fuzzy subsets of type II in decisions. J. Cybernetics 10, 137–159 (1980)

[27] Zadeh, L.A.: The concept of a linguistic variable and its application to approximate reasoning. Information Sciences 8, 43–80 (1975)

Hierarchical Genetic Algorithms for Fuzzy Inference System Optimization Applied to Response Integration for Pattern Recognition

Daniela Sánchez, Patricia Melin, and Oscar Castillo

Tijuana Institute of Technology, Tijuana, BC 22379, Mexico
danielasanchez.itt@hotmail.com,
{pmelin,ocastillo}@tectijuana.mx

Abstract. In this paper, a new method for fuzzy inference system optimization is proposed. The optimization consists in find the optimal parameters of fuzzy inference system used to combine the responses of modular neural networks using a hierarchical genetic algorithm. The optimized parameters are: type of fuzzy logic (type-1 and interval type-2), type of system (Mamdani or Sugeno), type of membership functions, number of membership functions in each variable (inputs and output), their parameters and the consequents of the fuzzy rules. Four benchmark databases are used to test the proposed method where, each database is a different biometric measure (face, iris, ear and voice) and each database is learned by a modular neural network. The main objective of the fuzzy inference system is to combine the different responses of the modular neural network and achieve final good results even when one (o more) biometric measure has individually a bad result. The results obtained in a previous work are used to compare with the results obtained in this paper.

Keywords: Modular Neural Networks, Type-1 Fuzzy Logic, Interval Type-2 Fuzzy Logic, Hierarchical Genetic Algorithms, Pattern Recognition, Human Recognition, Biometric Measures.

1 Introduction

The biometric systems have emerged because the security is nowadays something needed. There are four categories of biometric systems. The first one is for the control of the access to data. The second is for the control of access to areas. The third one to perform the identification against an existing credential. The fourth one to identify individuals whose identities need to be established using perhaps a biometric measure [1][10][17].

These systems use various physiological characteristics of the human, such as face [15][23], fingerprint [8], iris [21][24] , ear [3][20], voice [16] among others. The hybrid intelligent systems integrate different competent intelligent techniques to perform the human recognition using biometric measures [14][29], some of these techniques are neural networks, fuzzy logic and genetic algorithms. Using these

A. Gelbukh et al. (Eds.): MICAI 2014, Part II, LNAI 8857, pp. 345–356, 2014.

techniques good results have been achieved [8][16][23] where using one o more biometric measure the human recognition is performed, for this reason, in this paper these techniques are used. The biometric measures in this work are face, iris, ear and voice, using a modular neural network for each biometric measure their responses are combined using a fuzzy integrator. The parameters of this fuzzy integrator is optimized using a hierarchical genetic algorithm.

This paper is organized as follows: the basic concepts used in this research work are presented in Section 2. Section 3 contains the description of the proposed method. Section 4 presents experimental and comparison results and in Section 5, the conclusions of this work are presented.

2   Basic Concepts

In this section, a brief overview of the basic concepts used in this research work are presented.

2.1   Modular Neural Network

Artificial Neural networks (ANNs) have the remarkable ability to derive meaning from complicated or imprecise data. A trained neural network can be thought of as an "expert" in the category of information it has been given to analyze [12]. A neural network is said to be modular if the computation performed by the network can be decomposed into two or more modules that operate on distinct inputs without communicating with each other [2]. Each of the neural networks is built and trained for a specific task. The final decision is based on the results of the individual networks, called agents or experts. The results of the different applications involving Modular Neural Networks (MNNs) lead to the general evidence that the use of modular neural networks implies a significant learning improvement comparatively to a single NN and especially to the backpropagation NNs [14].

2.2   Fuzzy Logic

Fuzzy logic is a useful tool for modeling complex systems and deriving useful fuzzy relations or rules [18]. However, it is often difficult for human experts to define the fuzzy sets and fuzzy rules used by these systems [26]. The basic structure of a fuzzy inference system consists of three conceptual components: a rule base, which contains a selection of fuzzy rules, a database (or dictionary) which defines the membership functions used in the rules, and a reasoning mechanism that performs the inference procedure [11][28].

The concept of a type-2 fuzzy set, was introduced by Zadeh (1975) as an extension of the concept of an ordinary fuzzy set (henceforth called a "type-1 fuzzy set"). A type-2 fuzzy set is characterized by a fuzzy membership function, i.e., the membership grade for each element of this set is a fuzzy set in [0,1], unlike a type-1 set where the membership grade is a crisp number in [0,1]. Fuzzy logic is a useful tool for modeling complex systems and deriving useful fuzzy relations or rules However, it is often difficult for human experts to define the fuzzy sets and fuzzy rules used by these systems, for that reason different techniques to perform the optimization are used to set the fuzzy system architecture [4][18].

2.3   Hierarchical Genetic Algorithms

Genetic Algorithms (GAs) are nondeterministic methods that work by maintaining a constant-sized population of candidate solutions known as individuals (chromosomes). GAs have proven to be a useful method for optimizing the membership functions of the fuzzy sets used by these fuzzy systems [9][13]. A Hierarchical genetic algorithm (HGA) is a type of genetic algorithm. Its structure is more flexible than the conventional GA. The basic idea under hierarchical genetic algorithm is that for some complex systems, which cannot be easily represented, this type of GA can be a better choice. The complicated chromosomes may provide a good new way to solve the problem [22][25][27].

3   General Architecture of the Proposed Method

The proposed method combines the responses of modular neural networks (MNNs) using the fuzzy logic as response integrators. The main idea of the proposed method is to minimized the error of recognition when the responses of the different modular neural networks are combined. In this work, each modular neural network represents a different biometric measure and each MNNs is represented as an input in the fuzzy integrator. In this work four biometric measure are used. An example of the fuzzy inference system used is shown in Fig. 1. This fuzzy integrator has 4 inputs and 1 output, 4 inputs because 4 biometric measure are used, and the final results is given by the output.

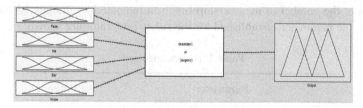

Fig. 1. Example of the fuzzy inference system

3.1   Description of the Hierarchical Genetic Algorithm for the Optimization

The optimization of some parameters of the fuzzy integrator is performed. These parameters are type of fuzzy logic (type-1 and interval type-2 fuzzy logic), type of system (Mamdani or Sugeno), type of membership functions (Trapezoidal or gBell), number of membership functions in each variable (inputs and output), their parameters and the consequents of the fuzzy rules. The chromosome of the proposed hierarchical genetic algorithm is shown in Fig. 2.

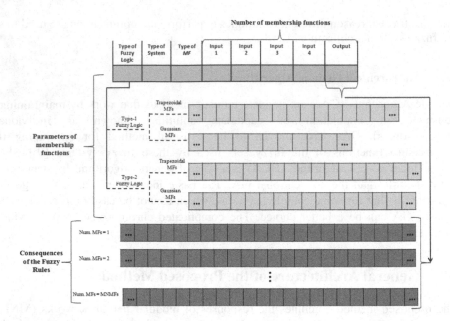

Fig. 2. The chromosome of the proposed hierarchical genetic algorithm

To perform the consequents optimization, depending of the maximum number of membership function (MNMFs) used in each variable (this number is freely established before the evolution) all the possible rules are generated. When an individual of the HGA is going to be evaluated, depending of the number of membership functions indicated by the genes for the inputs, the possible rules for this combination are taken with their respective consequents. The consequents are taken depending of the number of membership function indicated by the gen for the output. In Table 1, the parameters established for the fuzzy integrator are shown.

Table 1. Parameters used

Parameter	Value
Maximum number of MFs in each variable	5
Number of inputs	4
Number of outputs	1
Maximum number of possible rules	625

The genetic parameters used to test the proposed hierarchical genetic algorithm are shown in Table 2.

Table 2. Genetic parameters of the hierarchical genetic algorithm

Genetic Operator	Value
Population size	10
Maximum number of generations	100
Selection	Roulette wheel
Selection Rate	0.85
Crossover	Single Point
Crossover Rate	0.9
Mutation	bga
Mutation Rate	0.01

3.2   Databases

In this section, the databases used in this work are presented. The human recognition is performed to 77 persons, for this reason only the first 77 persons of each database are used.

3.2.1. Face Database

The database of human iris from the Institute of Automation of the Chinese Academy of Sciences was used [6]. Each person has 5 images. The image dimensions are 640 x 480, BMP format. Fig. 3 shows examples of the human iris images.

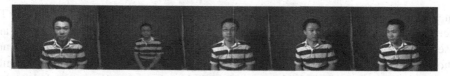

Fig. 3. Examples of the face images from CASIA database

3.2.2. Iris Database

The database of human iris from the Institute of Automation of the Chinese Academy of Sciences was used [7]. Each person has 14 images (7 for each eye). The image dimensions are 320 x 280, JPEG format. Fig. 4 shows examples of the human iris images.

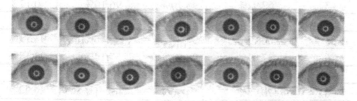

Fig. 4. Examples of the human iris images from CASIA database

3.2.3. Ear Database

The database of the University of Science and Technology of Beijing was used [5]. Each person has 4 images, the image dimensions are 300 x 400 pixels, the format is BMP. Fig. 5 shows examples of the human ear images.

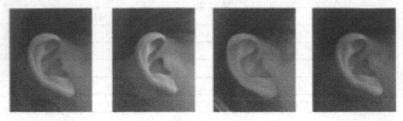

Fig. 5. Examples of Ear Recognition Laboratory from the University of Science & Technology Beijing (USTB)

3.2.4. Voice Database

In the case of voice, the database was made from students of Tijuana Institute of Technology. Each person has 10 voice samples, WAV format. The word that they said in Spanish was "ACCESAR". To preprocess the voice the Mel Frequency Cepstral Coefficients were used.

4   Experimental Results

In this section, the results obtained using the proposed method are presented. To perform the experimental results the modular neural networks presented in [19] are used. Ten non-optimized results of modular neural networks for each biometric are shown in Table 3. The architectures of these modular neural networks are randomly established, i.e. their number of neurons in 2 hidden layers, goal error and learning algorithm are randomly fixed.

Table 3. The best results for each biometric measure

Training	Face	Iris	Ear	Voice
1	87.01%	79.10%	94.81%	87.79%
2	85.71%	81.82%	77.92%	91.77%
3	52.92%	96.10%	96.10%	90.17%
4	45.78%	82.58%	79.22%	91.88%
5	60.17%	94.37%	97.40%	91.23%
6	37.01%	90.91%	57.14%	93.18%
7	47.19%	63.20%	81.82%	90.04%
8	70.78%	84.96%	90.91%	89.94%
9	68.83%	92.73%	82.47%	92.86%
10	68.83%	98.27%	67.53%	86.36%

The different trainings presented above were combined and 5 cases were considered to be presented and test the proposed method. As you noticed, each database contains different persons, the criteria to consider that the face, iris, ear, voice are for one person is for example that the first face, the first iris, the first ear and the first voice are of the first person, and so on. The same cases were used in [19], these cases are shown in Table 4. It can be observed that the biometric measures do not have perfect results, for this reason the proposed method must provide a good result even when one (o more) biometric measure has individually a bad result.

Table 4. The best results for each biometric measure

Case	Face	Iris	Ear	Voice
1	FT4	IT5	ET5	VT2
	45.78%	98.27%	82.47%	91.88%
2	FT1	IT4	ET2	VT1
	87.01%	63.20%	77.92%	91.77%
3	FT2	IT2	ET4	VT5
	85.71%	96.10%	97.40%	93.18%
4	FT6	IT7	ET6	VT10
	37.01%	63.20%	57.14%	86.36%
5	FT4	IT7	ET9	VT4
	45.78%	63.20%	82.47%	91.88%

For each case previously established, 30 evolutions were performed. In this case, the maximum number of membership functions for each variable was equal to 5, but this number can be modified. The total number of possible rules was 625, but as above was described, depending on the number of membership functions in each input variables is the number of rules used. In Table 5, the obtained results are shown (bests and average) when the HGA considered better Type-1 Fuzzy Logic than Type-2 Fuzzy Logic, and in Table 6 when the HGA considered better Type-2 Fuzzy Logic than Type-1 Fuzzy Logic.

Table 5. Type-1 Fuzzy Logic Results

Case	Num. of Evolutions	Best	Average
1	5	99.78%	99.35%
		0.0022	0.0065
2	15	95.13%	93.20%
		0.0487	0.0680
3	11	98.44%	96.89%
		0.0156	0.0311
4	3	89.72%	88.46%
		0.1028	0.1154
5	10	94.70%	94.03%
		0.0530	0.0597

Table 6. Type-2 Fuzzy Logic Results

Case	Num. of Evolutions	Best	Average
1	25	100%	99.51%
		0	0.0049
2	15	95.89%	93.51%
		0.0411	0.0649
3	19	98.70%	97.72%
		0.0130	0.0228
4	27	91.02%	88.69%
		0.0898	0.1131
5	20	97.19%	95.62%
		0.0281	0.0438

In Fig. 6, the best fuzzy integrator for the case #1 with 225 rules and Mamdani type is shown.

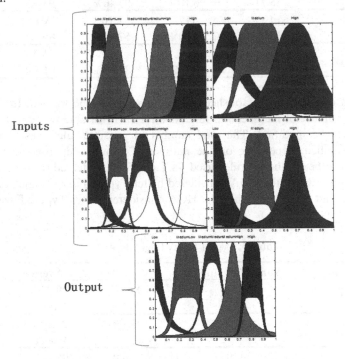

Fig. 6. Best fuzzy integrator for the case #1

In Fig. 7, the best fuzzy integrator for the case #2 with 120 rules and Sugeno type is shown. This fuzzy integrator has 4 constants values in the output.

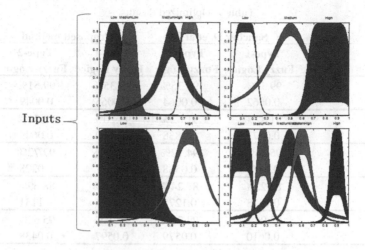

Fig. 7. Best fuzzy integrator for the case #2

In Fig. 8, the best fuzzy integrator for the case #5 with 64 rules and Sugeno type is shown. This fuzzy integrator has 3 constants values in the output.

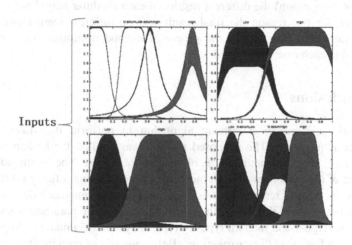

Fig. 8. Best fuzzy integrator for the case #5

4.1 Comparison Results

In [19] also a optimization is proposed, but the number of membership function or constant values in the output was always fixed (5 membership functions). To observe what happen when this part is optimized, the averages obtained in [19] when the optimization is performed and in this work are shown in Table 7.

Table 7. Optimized Results

Case	Sanchez D. et al [4]		Proposed method	
	Type-1 Fuzzy Logic	Type-2 Fuzzy Logic	Type-1 Fuzzy Logic	Type-2 Fuzzy Logic
1	99.38%	99.35%	99.35%	99.51%
	0.0062	0.0064	0.0065	0.0049
2	91.22%	91.62%	93.20%	93.51%
	0.0877	0.0838	0.0680	0.0649
3	95.44%	94.12%	96.89%	97.72%
	0.0455	0.0588	0.0311	0.0228
4	85.22%	87.24%	88.46%	88.69%
	0.1478	0.1275	0.1154	0.1131
5	93.90%	94.21%	94.03%	95.62%
	0.0610	0.0579	0.0597	0.0438

It can be observed that almost in all the cases, the proposed method in this work is better than when the number of membership function or the constant values for the output is fixed as in [19] using type-1 or type-2 fuzzy logic. The proposed method provides better results because, depending of the application and for example in this case (human recognition) the different results of each modular neural network can be different and, for this reason the final result will be different even using the same fuzzy integrator. For this reason, the proposed method optimizes fuzzy integrators appropriated to each case established.

5   Conclusions

In this work, a hierarchical genetic algorithm to perform the fuzzy integrator optimization is proposed. The proposed method was applied for human recognition based on face, iris, ear and voice biometric measures. The main idea is the combination of the responses of each biometric measure using a fuzzy integrator, and to minimize the error of recognition. As have a good fuzzy integrator depends on their parameters, in this work the idea is the optimization of some parameters such as type of fuzzy logic (type-1 and interval type-2), type of system (Mamdani or Sugeno), type of membership functions (Trapezoidal or gBell), number of membership functions in each variable (inputs and output), their parameters and the consequents of the fuzzy rules. A comparison with a previous work where the number of membership functions or the constant values for the output is fixed was presented, and we can observed that better results are obtained when also the optimization of this parameter is optimized. As future work the combination of different type of membership function in the same variable will be implemented and the minimization of the number of rules.

References

1. Abiyev, R., Altunkaya, K.: Personal Iris Recognition Using Neural Network, Near East University, Department of Computer Engineering, Lefkosa, North Cyprus (April 2008)
2. Azamm, F.: Biologically Inspired Modular Neural Networks. PhD thesis, Virginia Polytechnic Institute and State University, Blacksburg, Virginia (May 2000)
3. Carreira, M.: Aplicación de las redes neuronales de compresión a la extracción de características para el reconocimiento a partir de imágenes de la oreja. Universidad Politécnica de Madrid, España (September 1995)
4. Castillo, O., Melin, P.: Type-2 Fuzzy Logic Theory and Applications, pp. 29–43. Springer, Berlin (2008)
5. Database Ear Recognition Laboratory from the University of Science & Technology Beijing (USTB). Found on the Web page, http://www.ustb.edu.cn/resb/en/index.htm (accessed September 21, 2009)
   Database of Face. Institute of Automation of Chinese Academy of Sciences (CASIA). Found on the Web page, http://biometrics.idealtest.org/dbDetailForUser.do?id=9 (accessed November 11, 2012)
6. Database of Human Iris. Institute of Automation of Chinese Academy of Sciences (CASIA). Found on the Web page, http://www.cbsr.ia.ac.cn/english/IrisDatabase.asp (accessed September 21, 2009)
7. Hidalgo, D., Castillo, O., Melin, P.: Optimization with genetic algorithms of modular neural networks using interval type-2 fuzzy logic for response integration: The case of multimodal biometry. In: International Joint Conference on Neural Networks (IJCNN), pp. 738–745 (2008)
8. Huang, J., Wechsler, H.: Eye Location Using Genetic Algorithm. Department of Computer Science, George Mason University, Washington, DC (1999)
9. Jain, A.K., Li, S.Z.: Encyclopedia of Biometrics. Springer (2009)
10. Jang, J., Sun, C., Mizutani, E.: Neuro-Fuzzy and Soft Computing. Prentice Hall, New Jersey (1997)
11. Khan, A., Bandopadhyaya, T., Sharma, S.: Classification of Stocks Using Self Organizing Map. International Journal of Soft Computing Applications 4, 19–24 (2009)
12. Man, K.F., Tang, K.S., Kwong, S.: Genetic Algorithms: Concepts and Designs. Springer (1999)
13. Melin, P., Castillo, O.: Hybrid Intelligent Systems for Pattern Recognition Using Soft Computing: An Evolutionary Approach for Neural Networks and Fuzzy Systems, 1st edn., pp. 119–122. Springer (2005)
14. Melin, P., Mendoza, O., Castillo, O.: Face Recognition With an Improved Interval Type-2 Fuzzy Logic Sugeno Integral and Modular Neural Networks. IEEE Transactions on Systems, Man, and Cybernetics, Part A 41(5), 1001–1012 (2011)
15. Melin, P., Urias, J., Solano, D., Soto, M., Lopez, M., Castillo, O.: Voice Recognition with Neural Networks, Type-2 Fuzzy Logic and Genetic Algorithms. Tijuana Institute of Technology, Tijuana México, Agosto (2006)
16. Moreno, B., Sanchez, A., Velez, J.: F., On the Use of Outer Ear Images for Personal Identification in Security Applications. In: IEEE 33rd Annual International Carnahan Conference on Security Technology, pp. 469–476 (1999)
17. Okamura, M., Kikuchi, H., Yager, R., Nakanishi, S.: Character diagnosis of fuzzy systems by genetic algorithm and fuzzy inference. In: Proceedings of the Vietnam-Japan Bilateral Symposium on Fuzzy Systems and Applications, Halong Bay, Vietnam, pp. 468–473 (1998)

18. Sanchez, D., Melin, P., Castillo, O.: Optimization of type-1 and type-2 fuzzy systems applied to pattern recognition. In: The 4th World Conference on Soft Computing, pp. 203–207 (2014)
19. Sánchez, R.: El Iris Ocular como parámetro para la Identificación Biométrica. Universidad Politécnica de Madrid, España (September 2000)
20. Sarhan, A.: Iris Recognition Using Discrete Cosine Transform and Artificial Neural Networks. Department of Computer Engineering, University of Jordan, Amman-11195, Jordan (2009)
21. Tang, K.S., Man, K.F., Kwong, S., Liu, Z.F.: Minimal Fuzzy Memberships and Rule Using Hierarchical Genetic Algorithms. IEEE Trans. Ind. Electron. 45(1), 162–169 (1998)
22. Vázquez, J.C., López, M., Melin, P.: Real Time Face Identification Using a Neural Network Approach. In: Melin, P., Kacprzyk, J., Pedrycz, W. (eds.) Soft Computing for Recognition Based on Biometrics. SCI, vol. 312, pp. 155–169. Springer, Heidelberg (2010)
23. Verma, B., Blumenstein, M.: Pattern Recognition Technologies and Applications, pp. 90–91. Information Science Reference, Hershey (2008)
24. Wang, C., Soh, Y.C., Wang, H., Wang, H.: A Hierarchical Genetic Algorithm for Path Planning in a Static Environment with Obstacles. In: Canadian Conference on Electrical and Computer Engineering, IEEE CCECE 2002, vol. 3, pp. 1652–1657 (2002)
25. Wang, W., Bridges, S.: Genetic Algorithm Optimization of Membership Functions for Mining Fuzzy Association Rules. Department of Computer Science Mississippi State University (March 2, 2000)
26. Worapradya, K., Pratishthananda, S.: Fuzzy supervisory PI controller using hierarchical genetic algorithms. In: 5th Asian Control Conference, vol. 3, pp. 1523–1528 (2004)
27. Zadeh, L.A.: Fuzzy Sets. Journal of Information and Control 8, 338–353 (1965)
28. Zhang, Z., Zhang, C.: An Agent-Based Hybrid Intelligent System for Financial Investment Planning. In: Ishizuka, M., Sattar, A. (eds.) PRICAI 2002. LNCS (LNAI), vol. 2417, p. 355. Springer, Heidelberg (2002)

Low-Cost Fuzzy-Based Obstacle Avoidance Method for Autonomous Agents

Luis Carlos Gonzalez-Sua, Ivan Gonzalez, Leonardo Garrido, and Rogelio Soto

Tecnológico de Monterrey
Monterrey, NL, Mexico 64849
{lc.gonzalezsua,ni.gonzalez.phd.mty,
leonardo.garrido,rsoto}@itesm.mx
http://www.itesm.mx

Abstract. In this article, there lies an implementation of a novel fuzzy-based methodology that will reduce the amount of operations per iteration, reducing the computational cost of traditional fuzzy systems. This was achieved by implementing adaptive control theories like gain scheduling. Also, the method was implemented with a self-tuning technique using Genetic Algorithms (GA) that increases the method's efficiency, improving the following metrics: amount of collisions and time spent to finish the task. Two experiments were implemented to test the previously mentioned metrics; the first experiment will test the agent with several intersecting dynamic obstacles, in a long path. The second experiment will deal with two aggressive agents that will attempt to collide with the test agent. For comparison purposes, the Potential Fields' Method (PFM) was implemented and tested under the same metrics and experiments. The obtained results show for experiment 1 an improvement on the average collisions by 25.03% less compared to the PFM statistics and only and increase of 1.43% of the average time spent. And for experiment 2, there was an improvement of 93.46% of less average collisions compared to PFM and a reduction of 10.27% of average time spent. The contribution of this work is to implement a faster and less processing expensive method than traditional fuzzy ones.

Keywords: Fuzzy logic, Self-tuning, Autonomous agents, Obstacle avoidance, Potential fields.

1 Introduction

Obstacle avoidance and navigation are closely together, however it is not the same thing, because navigation requires to create a path with several waypoints from a point A to a point B, but in the middle of the way they will meet some other points according to the terrain and some obstacles [4]. However, this article will focus on the obstacle avoidance part due to its importance to a safe navigation [7]. There has been plenty of research for obstacle avoidance [14], nonetheless, fuzzy has demonstrated to be quite a good choice [16], it has demonstrated to be a worthy option [11], and has demonstrated that in can be a

A. Gelbukh et al. (Eds.): MICAI 2014, Part II, LNAI 8857, pp. 357–369, 2014.

feasible option for obstacle avoidance [8]. Notwithstanding, there is the need for comparison, and potential fields has proven to be a worthy adversary [10]. The use of fuzzy for obstacle avoidance purposes gives a more human approach [9], but it has shown some drawbacks [2], highlighting the high number of required calculations and the necessity for an optimal tuning [15]. Withal the difficulties, fuzzy still can be use as a practical obstacle avoidance method [5]. In this article, the authors proposed two practical solutions to the previously mentioned drawbacks of fuzzy. To resolve the high number of calculations requirements, they establish a novel methodology based on the gain-scheduling theory and obtain a method that can maintain the fuzzy original structure, and also, can process several inputs without having an exponential increase in the number of calculation per iteration. The other drawback, as mentioned before, was the tuning issue. Implementing standard simple tuning algorithms [6] was not a viable solution due to the high level of uncertainties of the model, however, heuristic methods offers an alternative. Previous research has demonstrated that using genetic algorithms (GA) could be a feasible way to find a viable solution [13], [1].

Some recent work has demonstrated that by implementing GA with another optimization method like particle swarm optimization (PSO), can obtain better results [12], and that some other biology inspired methods like ant colony optimization (ACO) can also improve the performance [3]. Although, those methods requires a higher order magnitude (like 10 or 100 times bigger than implemented) and communication among the searching agents, but they excel in parallel simulations. Therefore, the singular case treated in this article was not able to take advantage of this features and GA was the best available option.

The following sections explains the proposed method and the implementation of GA to obtain an applicable option with an acceptable performance.

2   Methods

This section contains all the implemented methods and a brief explanation, commencing with the potential fields method, the fuzzy staged method and the optimisation by genetic algorithms.

2.1   Potential Fields Method (PFM)

The PFM has proven to be a feasible method for obstacle avoidance purposes, due to the effectiveness and relatively easy implementation, this method is by far one of the most used methods [17]. The easy implementation of the PFM is due to the simplicity of the algorithm, it calculates a resulting vector based on the distance and direction to goal and obstacles, the magnitude of the vector is given by a particular formula, for this article, an inverse equation was implemented as the equation (1) shows.

$$f(x) = \frac{a}{dist - b} + c \qquad (1)$$

Where a, b and c are constants that modify the behaviour of the graph and *dist* is the distance between the agent and the goal/obstacle.The implemented PFM uses the following values for the goal: $a = -20$, $b = -0.9$ and $c = -0.5$, and for the obstacles $a = 12.5$, $b = -0.8$ and $c = -1.5$. The figure 1 shows the graphs for the behaviour towards the goal and the obstacles.

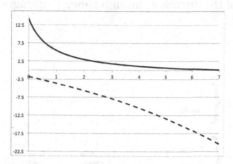

Fig. 1. Graphs for potential fields equations. The solid line shows the behaviour for obstacles and dashed line shows the behaviour for goal.

It can be noticed, that the obstacles will generate a higher repel force the closer it gets, and the goal generates a higher attraction the far it gets. this was considered to make the agent to go straight to the goal the far it gets and react if gets close to any obstacle. This configuration was selected to make the agent faster and less reactive, because if the agent's reaction to obstacles is too sensitive, the agent will spend most of the time changing directions and not moving. Also, if the reaction is too loose, the collisions will be more common.

2.2   Proposed Fuzzy Staged Method (FSM)

The Fuzzy Staged Method, proposes a new alternative to traditional fuzzy systems when the computational costs are important. This method split the current set of rules in several stages according to the relations between the inputs. In this article, the authors implemented this method to an obstacle avoidance algorithm, that requires six input variables to control three outputs, that will manipulate an agent through a field avoiding any type of obstacles without getting too far from the destination. If a traditional fuzzy method were implemented, the total amount of evaluated rules per iteration will be as high as 810 $(2*3*3*3*5*3)$ rules per iteration, because a fuzzy system to have a proper function needs that for every combination of inputs a rule will be evaluated. Therefore, instead of evaluating so many rules, the FSM will reduce the total number of rules per iteration to only 30 $(2*3+3*3+3*5)$ without breaking the condition that for each combination of inputs there must be a rule.

To implement FSM, first, it is necessary to analyse the relationships among the variables to group them in stages. In this case, the relation between the variables was palpable among pairs, for the first stage, the stamina and the effort both are variables directly related to the agent's motion model that determines how fast it moves. Then, for the second stage, the distance to the target and the relative speed are linked by a a derivate, because the relative speed is the change of the distance through time. And the same happens int the third stage with the direction to obstacle and angular speed of the obstacle, because the angular speed is the change of the direction through time. The stages where implemented as shown on figure 2.

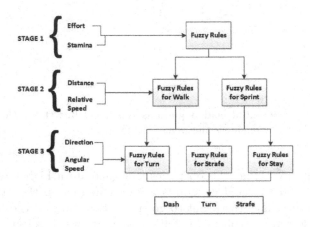

Fig. 2. Block Diagram for Fuzzy Staged Method

The rules implemented in each stage will be explained in the following subsections, is worth to notice that all the outputs go at the bottom of the block diagram, however, the power output can be separated from the rest to simplify the implementation (less rules to be written and most of them will be repetitive).

Stage 1. As mentioned before, the stamina and the effort defines the rules for the first stage, it also controls directly the power output, because the effect of the other stages is minimum and negligible, thus it can be isolated from the rest of the rules, therefore instead of writing six sets of rules for the third stage, there was only needed to write three sets of rules. However, the total amount of written rules does not affect the number of evaluated rules per iteration, it only simplifies the implementation process.

The table 1 shows the implemented rules for this stage. Notice that for every combination of inputs, there is a rule to be evaluated, getting only six rules at this stage.

Stage 2. The stage 2 was composed by distance and relative speed inputs, that as mentioned before, they are strongly related. The total amount of rules to be

Table 1. Rules for Stage 1

	Effort	
Stamina	Tired	Fresh
Critical	Walk	Walk
Normal	Sprint	Walk
High	Sprint	Sprint

Table 2. Rules for Stage 2

	Distance		
Rel. Speed	V. Close	Close	Far
Away	Stay	Stay	Stay
Slow	Dodge	Turn	Stay
Fast	Dodge	Turn	Stay

evaluated for this stage is nine. Compared to the first stage, the outputs could not be separated from the rest, because the turn angle and the strafe angle are mutually exclusive, because if the agent strafes and turns in the same cycle, will result in a very inefficient move.

The output from this stage does not controls directly any output, but they selects. as stage 1, the set of rules that will apply to the next stage. For the current one, the rules are shown on table 2.

Stage 3. This is the final stage, from now on, the output from here will affect directly the direction where to the agent will displace. The variables are direction and angular speed. These two variables were left last, because the direction by itself do not give an accurate localisation of the obstacle, it means that it will only describe where is the obstacle but not far, and it is necessary to know how far the obstacle is, because if the obstacle is too far away, there is no need for course corrections. However, if the agent is too close, it is necessary to determine if the obstacle will have a chance get in the agent's path or if only will be close but not in the middle of the way, that is why three set of rules was defined from the previous stage.

In this last stage, the three set of rules decide if whether do nothing about the obstacle (Refer to table 3 Stay), make a slight correction (Refer to table 4 Turn) or make a strong course correction (Refer to table 5 Strafe). Despite that the strong correction will be mostly efficient to avoid obstacles, it has a trade off, because the higher the strafing angle, the less effective will be the dash.

2.3   Optimization by Genetic Algorithm

To improve the FSM efficiency, a genetic algorithm was implemented to find a combination of membership functions. The enforced GA searches for the best

Table 3. Rules for Stage 3 - Stay

	Angular Speed		
Direction	To Left	Static	To Right
Far Left	Straight/Face	Straight/Face	Straight/Face
Left	Straight/Face	Straight/Face	Straight/Face
Center	Straight/Face	Straight/Face	Straight/Face
Right	Straight/Face	Straight/Face	Straight/Face
Far Right	Straight/Face	Straight/Face	Straight/Face

Table 4. Rules for Stage 3 - Turn

	Angular Speed		
Direction	To Left	Static	To Right
Far Left	Straight/Face	Straight/Face	Straight/Face
Left	Straight/Face	Right/Face	Hard Right/Face
Center	Right/Face	Right or Left*/Face	Left/Face
Right	Hard Left/Face	Left/Face	Straight/Face
Far Right	Straight/Face	Straight/Face	Straight/Face

possible combination by obtaining the maximum possible value of the equation (2).

$$eval = 2000 + (800 - t) - 100 * coll \tag{2}$$

Where *eval* stands for the evaluation value, t is the time spent for the current individual and *coll* is the times that the agent collides with an obstacle. The value of 2000 was selected to set an acceptable evaluation value of the individual (i.e. individuals with 2000 evaluation was considered as decent). The value of 800 was taken as the minimum time to be beaten, so if the time that the agent spent to complete the test was higher, it will take it as a punishment. The 100 coefficient that multiplies the collisions, was set to define a higher punishment for each collision, this was designed to make the GA to find a viable combination to reduce the collisions to a minimum.

The GA was conceived with a 0.8 cross probability and 0.2 mutating probability. Also, the individual chromosome has 92 segments of 32 bits each, which defines the different values of the membership functions, therefore, more than one segment was required to define a single membership function. The initial population was of 30 individuals, and left searching for 56 generations. The best individual was taken and enforced, the values were fine tuned to get a more centred approach (remove the unbalance in the MFs), resulting in the values shown in the figures 3, 4, 5, 6 and 7.

The resulting individual was tested at the same conditions and experiments of the PFM. The following section will explain in detail the experiments and the results from both methods.

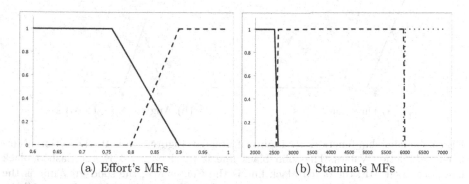

(a) Effort's MFs (b) Stamina's MFs

Fig. 3. Membership functions for inputs of Stage 1. Figure 3(a) is the Effort Membership Function Values. The solid line is the Tired MF and the dashed line is the Fresh MF. Range (-1, 1). Figure 3(b) is the Stamina Membership Function Values. The solid line is the Critical MF, the dashed line is the Normal MF and the doted line is High MF. Range (0, 8000).

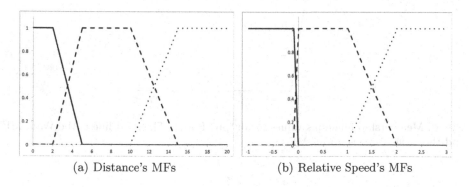

(a) Distance's MFs (b) Relative Speed's MFs

Fig. 4. Membership functions for inputs of Stage 2. Figure 4(a) is the Distance Membership Function Values. The solid line is the Very Close MF, the dashed line is the Close MF and the doted line is Far MF. Range (0, 150). Figure 4(b) is the Relative Speed Membership Function Values. The solid line is the Away MF, the dashed line is the Slow MF and the doted line is Fast MF. Range (-4, 4).

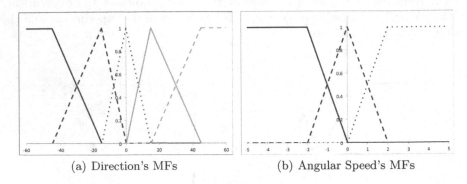

(a) Direction's MFs   (b) Angular Speed's MFs

Fig. 5. Membership functions for inputs of Stage 3. Figure 5(a) is the Direction Membership Function Values. The solid black line is the Far Left MF, the dashed black line is the Left MF, the doted black line is the Center MF, the solid grey line is the Right MF and the dashed grey line is Far Right MF. Range (-90, 90). Figure 5(b) is the Angular Speed Membership Function Values. The solid line is the To Left MF, the dashed line is the Static MF and the doted line is To Right MF. Range (-180, 180).

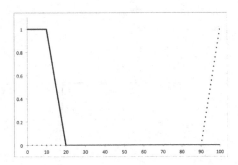

Fig. 6. Membership functions values for output Power. The solid line is the Walk MF and the dashed line is Sprint MF.

Table 5. Rules for Stage 3 - Strafe

	Angular Speed		
Direction	**To Left**	**Static**	**To Right**
Far Left	Straight/Face	Straight/Face	Straight/Face
Left	Straight/Face	Straight/Dodge Right	Straight/Avert Right
Center	Straight/Dodge Right	Straight/Dodge Left or Right*	Straight/Dodge Left
Right	Straight/Avert Left	Straight/Dodge Left	Straight/Face
Far Right	Straight/Face	Straight/Face	Straight/Face

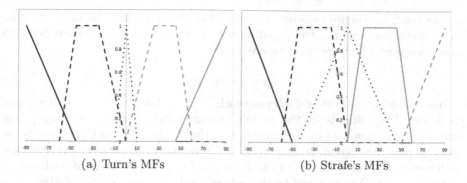

(a) Turn's MFs   (b) Strafe's MFs

Fig. 7. Membership functions for outputs Turn and Strafe. Figure 7(a) is the Turn Membership Function Values. The solid black line is the Hard Left MF, the dashed black line is the Left MF, the doted black line is the Straight MF, the solid grey line is the Right MF and the dashed grey line is Hard Right MF. Range (-90, 90). Figure 7(b) is the Strafe Membership Function Values. The solid black line is the Dodge Left MF, the dashed black line is the Avert Left MF, the doted black line is the Face MF, the solid grey line is the Avert Right MF and the dashed grey line is Dodge Right MF. Range (-90, 90).

3   Experiments and Results

In order to test the proposed method two types of experiments were implemented in the Robocup 2D simulator server. The first experiment was designed to analyse the behaviour of the agent in long runs, with some static and dynamic obstacles. The second experiment was conceived in a more aggressive approach to watch the ability of the agent to react facing incoming obstacles. The following subsections will explain in detail how the experiments were created and implemented.

3.1   Experiment 1

The experiment number 1 is an hexagonal path with six obstacles and six waypoints, the first three obstacles that the agent encounters are three dynamic ones that maintains a constant speed with small differences among them in order to collide with the agent if the agent tries a straight line path at maximum speed. The other three agents are static in a straight line pattern, hence if the agent tries to go straight from one waypoint to the next one, it will collide with each obstacle. The figure 8 shows the current global coordinates on the server from the left side. This experiment was designed to test the agent's ability to maintain maximum speed through a better stamina management, because the server simulates fatigue by giving the agent a value of a maximum stamina of 8000, and if the level drops below 2500, the effort value decreases and the agent cannot reach maximum velocity, meaning that the agent will use more stamina but obtains less impulse, the equation (3) shows the current relation between consumed power and the effective dash power.

$$edp = e * dpr * p \tag{3}$$

Where edp is the effective dash power which is the final value that will impulse the agent. The e stands for the agent's current effort value, dpr is dash power rate, which is a constant of the agent, and p that is the value of the energy to be spent to move the agent. It is clear that the relationship between the effective dash power and the power is lineal, however, because the value of dash power rate is constant, the effort will be the only variable that affects the effective dash power, thus if this value is less than 1, the effective dash power will be less than supplied power, translating in an inefficient use of stamina and less speed.

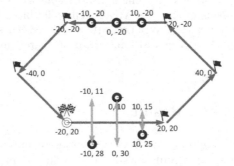

Fig. 8. Layout for Experiment 1. Dark grey lines show the agent's path and light grey shows the obstacle's path. Flag conventions: checkered flags - start/end, solid flags - waypoints.

Table 6. Results for experiment 1

Simulations	7000			
	Time Spent Avg.	Std. Dev.	Collisions Avg.	Std. Dev.
FSM	850.25	38.49	0.71	1.15
PFM	838.20	24.23	0.95	1.72

A total of 7000 experiments were made, for each of the methods (FSM and PFM), the results are shown in the table 6. It worth to notice that the PFM's statistics shows a very good performance regarding to the collisions average, however, the FSM demonstrates that it was able to even improve the amount of collision compared to its counterpart reducing it by a 25.03%. However, the time spent does not show an improvement, the FSM have an average 1.43% higher that the PFM in the time spent metrics, maybe, due to the evaluation function that gives the collisions more punishment than the reward given to time savings.

3.2   Experiment 2

The second experiment was designed to test the method's ability to avoid incoming obstacles. It consists of two aggressive agents located along a straight path from the test agent's start position to the goal zone. The aggressive agents will focus on the test agent and will attempt to ram it at maximum speed, until the test agent reaches the goal zone or the aggressive agents loss sight of the test agent. Figure 9 shows the initial coordinates of the agents, the initial positions and the goal position.

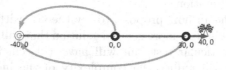

Fig. 9. Layout for Experiment 2. Dark grey arrows shows the agent's path and light grey indicates that the obstacles will go to the current agent's position. The checkered flags signals the goal

To evaluate both methods in this test, a total of 12000 experiments were made for each of the methods. Table 7 shows the obtained statistics for both methods. It is noticeable that the FSM excels the PFM in this tests, a reduction of 93.46% in the collisions average stablishes that the FSM is better to avoid dynamic obstacles such as the aggressive agents, specially because they do not move in a predictable path like the obstacles from experiment 1, because they change their path according to the current location of the test agent. Also, due to the fact that the test agents has less collisions, the average time spent is also improved by 10.27%, indicating that the FSM can be faster than the PFM.

Table 7. Results for experiment 2

Simulations	12000			
	Time Spent Avg.	Std. Dev.	Collisions Avg.	Std. Dev.
FSM	102.78	6.71	0.18	0.57
PFM	114.55	12.97	2.71	2.40

4   Conclusions and Future Work

The obtained results shows that the FSM can successfully avoid obstacles even better than the PFM, however, the tuning of the inputs and outputs is crucial to the method's efficiency. GA offers a viable option for tuning purposes, although, the evaluation function's focus is critical to decide whether the agent is aimed to spent less time to complete the test or if the agent focus on reducing the collisions to a minimum. In this work, as mentioned before, the target was to reduce the amount of collisions, rather than the time spent, but the GA provides a solution that reduces the collisions' average and maintains an average value close to the time spent of the PFM. Is also worth to be mentioned, that the more generations that are allowed to run the GA, the better solution it will obtain, but again it strongly relies on the evaluation function. As the main contribution of this work, the total amount of operations per iteration, was significantly reduced. For this particular case, a traditional fuzzy method will need 810 rules to work properly. This method only uses 30 rules per iteration, a reduction of almost 96% of the rule evaluations per iteration.

As future work, the authors propose, to try the GA with different evaluation functions in order to obtain a more general solution that will not only have a good performance on a particular test, but will have a decent behaviour on almost every scenario, and will reduce the complexity of the individual to converge faster into an optimal solution. Also, as a part of a wider program, the authors will implement the method on mobile robots, provided by the Tecnológico de Monterrey. The implementation of those tests, will have some limitations (i.e. limited space, limited amount of bots, battery limitations etc.) and may will take longer than the experiments with the simulated agents.

Acknowledgments. This works was possible thanks to the support of the CONACYT and the Tec de Monterrey through the Autonomous agents and e-Robots research chairs. Also the authors will like to extend a special thanks to Carlos Hernandez, Cesar Osimani, David Chapa and Jazzmin Novelo for their collaboration during this work. Also a special thanks to Claudia Valenzuela for her support and patience. Last but not least, the authors appreciate the never-ending work of Nova, Athos, Wolf and the rest of the SC lab crew.

References

1. Benbouabdallah, K., Qi-dan, Z.: Genetic fuzzy logic control technique for a mobile robot tracking a moving target. International Journal of Computer Science Issues 10(1), 607–613 (2013)
2. Castillo, O., Melin, P.: A review on the design and optimization of interval type-2 fuzzy controllers. Applied Soft Computing 12(4), 1267 (2012)
3. Castillo, O., Melin, P.: A review on interval type-2 fuzzy logic applications in intelligent control. Information Sciences 279, 615–631 (2014)
4. Cepeda, J.S., Chaimowicz, L., Soto, R., Gordillo, J.L., Alanís-Reyes, E.A., Carrillo-Arce, L.C.: A behavior-based strategy for single and multi-robot autonomous exploration. Sensors 12(9), 12772–12797 (2012)
5. Chiu, C.-S., Lian, K.-Y., Liu, P.: Fuzzy gain scheduling for parallel parking a car-like robot. IEEE Transactions on Control Systems Technology 13(6), 1084–1092 (2005)
6. Cortes-Rios, J.C., Gomez-Ramirez, E., Ortiz-De-La-Vega, H.A., Castillo, O., Melin, P.: Optimal design of interval type 2 fuzzy controllers based on a simple tuning algorithm. Applied Soft Computing 23, 270–285 (2014)

7. Fox, D., Burgard, W., Thrun, S., Cremers, A.B.: A hybrid collision avoidance method for mobile robots. In: Proceedings of the 1998 IEEE International Conference on Robotics and Automation, vol. 2, pp. 1238–1243 (1998)
8. Gonzalez-Sua, L.C., Barron, O., Soto, R., Garrido, L., Gonzalez, I., Gordillo, J.L., Garza, A.: Design and implementation of a fuzzy-based gain scheduling obstacle avoidance algorithm. In: 2013 12th Mexican International Conference on Artificial Intelligence (MICAI), pp. 45–49. IEEE (2013)
9. Hwang, C.-L., Chang, L.-J.: Internet-based smart-space navigation of a car-like wheeled robot using fuzzy-neural adaptive control. IEEE Transactions on Fuzzy Systems 16(5), 1271–1284 (2008)
10. Lee, J., Nam, Y., Hong, S., Cho, W.: New potential functions with random force algorithms using potential field method. Journal of Intelligent & Robotic Systems 66(3), 303–319 (2012)
11. Lee, T.-L., Wu, C.-J.: Fuzzy motion planning of mobile robots in unknown environments. Journal of Intelligent and Robotic Systems 37(2), 177–191 (2003)
12. Martínez-Soto, R., Castillo, O., Aguilar, L.T.: Type-1 and type-2 fuzzy logic controller design using a hybrid pso-ga optimization method. Information Sciences (2014)
13. Martínez-Soto, R., Castillo, O., Castro, J.R.: Genetic algorithm optimization for type-2 non-singleton fuzzy logic controllers. In: Castillo, O., Melin, P., Pedrycz, W., Kacprzyk, J. (eds.) Recent Advances on Hybrid Approaches for Designing Intelligent Systems. SCI, vol. 547, pp. 3–18. Springer, Heidelberg (2014)
14. Masehian, E., Sedighizadeh, D.: Classic and heuristic approaches in robot motion planning–a chronological review. In: Proc. World Academy of Science, Engineering and Technology. Citeseer (2007)
15. Meléndez, A., Castillo, O., Valdez, F., Soria, J., Garcia, M.: Optimal design of the fuzzy navigation system for a mobile robot using evolutionary algorithms. Int. J. Adv. Robotic. Sy. 10(139) (2013)
16. Pradhan, S.K., Parhi, D.R., Panda, A.K.: Fuzzy logic techniques for navigation of several mobile robots. Applied Soft Computing 9(1), 290–304 (2009)
17. Pradhan, S.K., Parhi, D.R., Panda, A.K., Behera, R.K.: Potential field method to navigate several mobile robots. Applied Intelligence 25(3), 321–333 (2006)

Fuzzy Controller for a Pneumatic Positioning Nonlinear System

Omar Rodríguez-Zalapa[1,2], Antonio Hernández-Zavala[1],
and Jorge Adalberto Huerta-Ruelas[1]

[1] Centro de Investigación en Ciencia Aplicada y Tecnología Avanzada CICATA- IPN,
Querétaro, México
{anhernandezz,jhuertar}@ipn.mx
[2] Universidad Tecnológica de Querétaro UTEQ, Querétaro, México
omar.rodriguez.2013@ieee.org

Abstract. The design of controllers for nonlinear uncertain dynamical systems is one of the most important challenging tasks in control engineering. In this paper, we propose a fuzzy system for controlling a nonlinear uncertain plant. We show that alternative techniques of fuzzy control can improve or complement conventional techniques in these kind of plants.

The case of use is a real pneumatic positioning system with no mechanically coupling with the final effector, and with nonlinearities and uncertainties. We used a webcam as a feedback sensor with an image processing algorithm.

Conventional control techniques for linear systems such as proportional-derivative (PD), proportional-integral (PI), and proportional-integral-derivative (PID), can be applied to control the pneumatic levitation system. However, its response is uncertain for the case of vertical position setpoint variations (due to different indices of turbulence along the tube) and in object characteristics (weight, shape, roughness and size). To overcome that problem, we designed a set of fuzzy control rules considering response of the system under conventional controllers and considering the non-linear dynamics of the plant. The optimal parameters of the conventional controllers were estimated through ITAE performance index. We show the performance of a PD, PI, PID and a fuzzy controller under the same operating conditions with a fixed set point. The results obtained for the proposed fuzzy control system, demonstrates good performance in rising time, settling time, reduced overshoot and greater flexibility than conventional (PD, PI and PID) controllers.

Keywords: Control of non-linear uncertain systems, fuzzy controller, PID controller, performance index, rule base.

1 Introduction

Non-linear systems are the most common in the real world, and are usually difficult to describe mathematically. There are no general methods available to address a wide variety of non-linear systems. As a first approximation analysis, it has been practical to design the controller based on a linear model of the system discriminating

A. Gelbukh et al. (Eds.): MICAI 2014, Part II, LNAI 8857, pp. 370–381, 2014.
© Springer International Publishing Switzerland 2014

nonlinearities. The designed controller is then applied to the nonlinear system (real system) for evaluation and potential redesign by analyzing its performance results and comparing these values with those resulting from computer simulation. The linear approximation of a nonlinear system is acceptable if the operating value of the plant is set to an equilibrium point, and if the range of input values around that point is small [1].

Despite much research and a large amount of various solutions proposed, most industrial control systems are based on conventional classic controllers such as PID. Different sources estimate that application rate for PID controllers at industrial level is between 90 % and 99% compared to others. A reason is a clear relationship between the response of the system and the parameters of the PID. Plant operators have a systematic knowledge about the influence of these parameters and their specific response. Over the past decades there have been development of many PID tuning techniques. In most classical industrial controllers, special procedures to automate its parameter settings are integrated (tuning and self-tuning) [2]. However, when the process becomes too complex to be described by an analytical model, it is unlikely to be controlled by conventional approaches. In this case, a classical control methodology can simplify the model of the plant, but does not provide good performance. Human control is vulnerable and highly dependent on the experience and qualifications of the operator. As a result, many PID controllers are poorly tuned in practice [2].

Therefore, an alternative way to address the problem in such cases is to use an artificial intelligence technique such as fuzzy control. The development and implementation of controllers using fuzzy logic has been increasing day by day. As mentioned by Takatsu [3], models of predictive control, fuzzy control and neural network controllers, have promoted in its applications a large expectation, and have even better prospects for the future than other 15 control techniques reported in this survey.

However, if there is no knowledge of the behavior of the system and its features, the design of a fuzzy controller becomes complex as you need to set different parameters for the input and output variables of the system. Control rules are based on the experience of the system operator, but what kind and how many rules and membership functions are necessary [4]. This is an optimization problem, and to obtain an optimal set of fuzzy membership functions and control rules is not straightforward. It requires time, experience and skills of the designer. In principle there is no general rule or method for the fuzzy inference system setup [5], [6], [7]. Several methods, techniques and algorithms have been developed to solve optimization problems that were inspired by processes, observed from nature and they were named Nature Inspired Algorithms (NIA) [8], [9].

Levitation systems have different applications like contactless transport of materials and parts, and product position such as silicon wafers, glass sheets, solar cells, or food, and are required to avoid shocks, friction, contamination, magnetism, and statics [10]. Additional advantages generate low heat and are almost maintenance free.

Our system to probe control algorithms was an air levitation system with nonlinearities as function of vertical position of the sphere within the tube. Since there is no linear relationship between the air flow rate and the vertical distance of the sphere with respect to the base of the tube (height h), as reported by Escano [11], the physical variables involved and the assumptions made to obtain an approximate mathematical model, also apply in our work plant. Mosquera [12], published a paper on the design, modeling, and position control of a pneumatic levitation system using a PID controller. They propose an approximate mathematical model considering that the levitating sphere was confined in a variable diameter pipe, smooth walls and laminar air flow. In both papers, nonlinear differential equations of second order are obtained in the approximation of the mathematical model of the pneumatic levitation system by discriminating other effects and variables. As the rate of air flow is modified by the fan, it implies that the dynamics of the motor-fan should also be considered and modeled.

In real control systems, uncertainties are unavoidable, and can be classified into two categories: disturbance signals and dynamic perturbations. Disturbances include input and output disturbance (such as a gust on an aircraft), sensor noise and actuator noise, etc. Perturbations represent the discrepancy between the mathematical model and the actual dynamics of the system in operation [13]. In our case the dynamic of the pneumatic levitation system has many variables involved with non-linear interrelationships between them, such as height of the centroid of the sphere to the base, its mass and acceleration, air flow speed, drag effect, rotational and lateral movements, sphere roughness, sphericity, pipe diameter, roughness of tube walls, air pressure distribution around the sphere, level of turbulence, etc. Therefore, it is complicated to obtain an accurate dynamic model of the vertical motion of the sphere along the pipe. Also, as the rate of air flow is modified by the speed of the fan, this implies that its dynamics should be also considered and modeled.

We analyzed at first a linear approach to prove the performance of conventional classics controllers and then, considering that modelling errors may adversely affect the stability and performance of a control system, we proposed a fuzzy controller and compared its performance with the others.

2   Control System Architecture

The location of each component of the system is shown in Fig. 1: A) A webcam is used to capture *RGB* images that are sent to a computer for its processing and to obtain an approximate measure of the sphere height, based in [14], b) a fan motor at the base of the column has the function to generate air flow, and its speed is modified via PWM (Pulse Width Modulation) from a control board based on microcontroller, c) A clear acrylic pipe that contains the air flow and provides its movement trajectory from the bottom to the top of the pipe with the sphere contained in it, finally d) a computer which has two major tasks, 1) it processes and analyze each image captured to obtain a measure of the distance of the centroid of sphere to a fixed point on the acrylic base, and 2) it provides the control action based on the error magnitude to obtain the value of PWM required.

The acrylic column is separated by 1425 mm from the center of the camera. The dimensions of the cylindrical column are 1395 mm in height with an outer diameter of

76.2 mm and a wall thickness of 3 mm. The half of the column was covered in the back with a black vinyl film, leaving the open side towards the focal axis of the camera. Base dimensions are 299x248x295 mm, made of acrylic material as the column. Expanded polystyrene sphere has a diameter of 60 mm, it is freely movable along the vertical direction. The PWM speed control of the fan motor is located inside the base at the bottom. The air flow injected lifts the ball inside the column and leaves through the top.

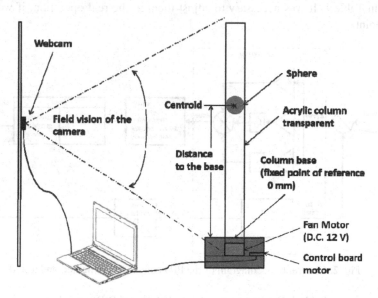

Fig. 1. Main components of pneumatic levitation system with a feedback control

A proposed algorithm coded in C++ measures the distance from the centroid of a segmented object in a color image with respect to a fixed reference point. The average time for this process is 0.08 s and percentage error in a static point of the sphere was less than 1.64% with respect to a laser instrument [14]. The algorithm processes each image to find the location of the sphere within the column, obtaining the distance from its centroid to the origin position in millimeter. This magnitude is fed to the control system to compare its value with the desired position (setpoint). The error magnitude is calculated, to determine corresponding value of Pulse Width Modulation (PWM) to modify the fan motor speed.

3   Controller Design

The general block diagram of the PID controller implemented is shown in Fig. 2. In every triangle is represented each of parameters: K_p, K_i, and K_d as the proportional, integral and derivative constants respectively, there is represented the PID action although the same model was used to obtain the response of the PD and PI controller in an independent way, omitting the other control action in each case. The dashed line shown the operations that the computer made, the modules of processing images and the controller actions.

Using as a first approach a set of operating points to obtain an approximated linear model of the system. Applying the ITAE (integral of time multiplied by the absolute value of error) criteria for tuning the PID parameters [15], [16] through the Toolbox Identification System of MatLab™ [17]. The final PD, PI and PID parameters are shown in Table I. It was necessary to adjust them in the real operation, if we change the setpoint.

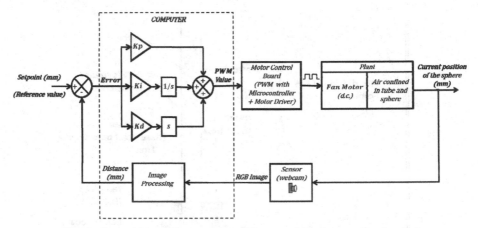

Fig. 2. General block diagram of the PID control implemented and tested

Table 1. Parameters used on the PD, PI and PID controllers

Controller	K_p	K_i	K_d
PD	4	----	0.075
PI	4	200	----
PID	2	50	0.075

The equations on time domain for each conventional controller [18] that were implemented and discretized to create an algorithm are,

For PD controller:

$$y(t) = K_p e(t) + K_p T_d \frac{de(t)}{dt} \tag{1}$$

For PI controller:

$$y(t) = K_p e(t) + \frac{K_p}{T_i} \int_o^t e(t) dt \tag{2}$$

For PID controller:

$$y(t) = K_p \left[e(t) + \frac{1}{T_i} \int_o^t e(t) dt + T_d \frac{de(t)}{dt} \right] \tag{3}$$

Where $y(t)$ is the output of the system (current position of the sphere), $e(t)$ is the error between the setpoint and the current output value, K_p is the proportional gain, T_i is the integral time and T_d is the derivative time. They are also named proportional, integral and derivative gains if they are written as K_p, $K_i = \frac{K_p}{T_i}$, $K_d = K_p T_d$.

Due to a lack of an accurate model of the plant, it is mandatory to adjust parameters of conventional controllers every time that we change setpoint, we propose a controller using fuzzy logic. The general block diagram of the fuzzy controller is shown in Fig. 3. The block named Fuzzy Controller was developed using the Fuzzy Toolbox of MatLab[TM] [19].; Once that Fuzzy Inference System was tuned and tested, we created a script code to call it from the main program in C++.

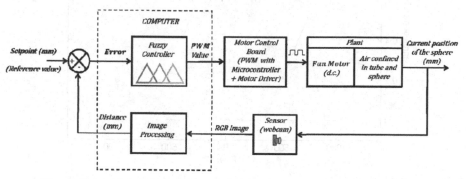

Fig. 3. General block diagram of the Fuzzy Controller implemented and tested

We use the general block diagram of a Fuzzy Inference System (FIS) based on Mamdani fuzzy model [20] and it is represented in Fig. 4,

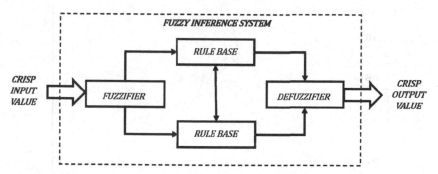

Fig. 4. General block diagram of the Fuzzy Inference System based on Mamdani model [20]

Proposed membership functions used for the Fuzzier to change the input crisp error magnitude to a fuzzy value are shown in Fig. 5. The input universe of the Error (Crisp Input Value) was defined in the interval of -1400 mm to 1400 mm and we defined 5 membership functions: Big Negative (BN), Medium Negative (MN), Zero, Medium Positive (MP) and Big Positive (BP). The output universe (Crisp Output Value: PWM) was defined in the interval of 90 to 130 of an enabled interval from 0 to 255, because there are a dead zone where the object cannot move and a maximum value reached in the upper limit of the tube. Three membership functions were defined for the PWM output: Slow, Medium and Fast, shown in Fig. 6. Output behavior versus the input is illustrated in Fig. 7.

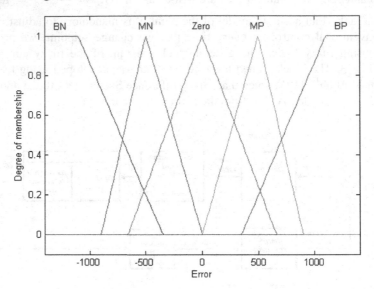

Fig. 5. Membership functions defined for the input Error

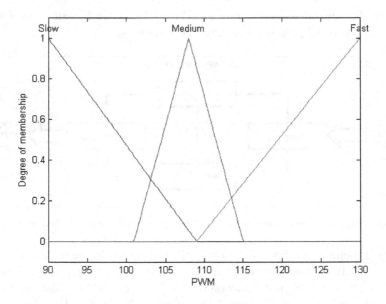

Fig. 6. Membership functions of PWM output

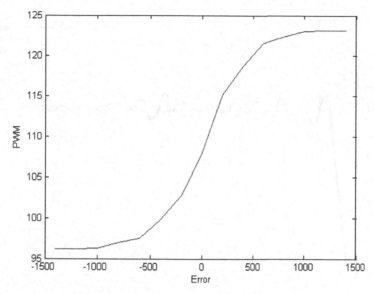

Fig. 7. Output function graph of Fuzzy Controller

The rules defined for these Fuzzy Controller were:
1. If (Error is Big Negative: BN) then (PWM is Slow)
2. If (Error is Medium Negative: MN) then (PWM is Slow)
3. If (Error is Zero) then (PWM is Medium)
4. If (Error is Medium Positive: MP) then (PWM is Fast)
5. If (Error is Big Positive) then (PWM is Fast)

4   Results

The responses of every controller implemented and tested are shown in Fig. 8 and 9. The results of the 3 experiments are represented in every graph (A, B, C) that were tested under the same operating conditions, with the same parameters and a setpoint of 800 mm. The resultant points were generated with no uniform sampled data with an average period of time of 0.16 s in a total time of 50 s.

Oscillations around the setpoint depend on the accumulative error due to different sources like air turbulence, noise of sensor (webcam), and no uniform delay times (processing images, controller actions, decision making, etc.). Averaging response of the three experiments in each type of controller, we can analyze its performance.

Considering the underdamped response in the time, we selected three parameters (or indexes) to measure and compare controller´s performance: Percent over shoot (%OS), Rise time (Tr) and Settling time (Ts). In Table 2 averaged values are shown calculated of these parameters. The fuzzy controller had a minimun value in settling time (Ts), to   maintain the error minor or equal to 2%. The PI controller had a minimum value in settling time (Ts), to maintain the error minor or equal to 5%. The PD and PI controllers did not reach an error minor or equal to 2% in the total sampled time (50 s) of the experiments. The fuzzy controller also had minimum values of percent over shoot (%OS) and rise time (Tr).

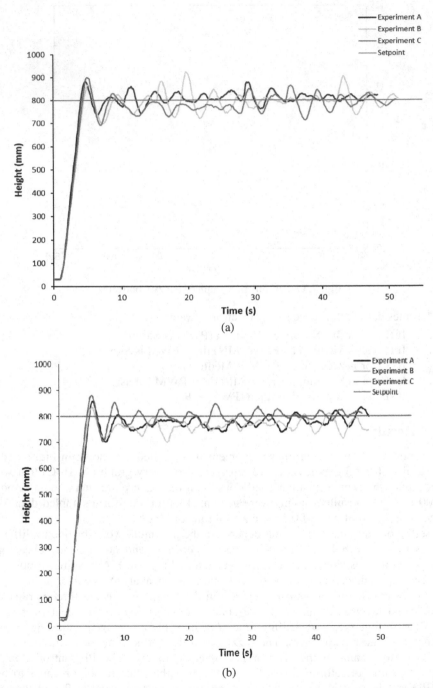

Fig. 8. Responses of (a) PD controller and (b) PI controller, for three independent experiments (A, B, C) with a setpoint of 800 mm

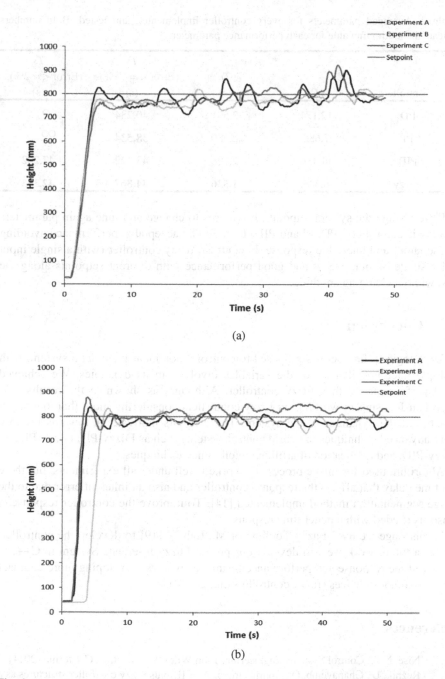

(a)

(b)

Fig. 9. Responses of (a) PID controller and (b) Fuzzy controller, for three independent experiments (A, B, C) with a setpoint of 800 mm

Table 2. Averaged parameters for every controller implemented and tested. Bold numbers indicate the minimum value for each performance parameter.

Controller	%OS	Tr (s)	Ts (Error <= 5%) (s)	Ts (Error <= 2%) (s)
PD	12,174	2,581	40,234	∞
PI	7,680	2,680	**38,534**	∞
PID	11,130	2,796	43,322	47,202
Fuzzy	**6,325**	**1,536**	44,867	**42,333**

If we change the system setpoint , it requires to change and tune again parameters for classic controllers (PD, PI and PID) to obtain an acceptable performance avoiding an oscillatory and unestable response. In contrast, fuzzy controller (with a single input and a single output: SISO) had good performance with diferent setpoints along the tube without changing anything.

5   Conclusion

A fuzzy logic technique was proposed to control a nonlinear pneumatic system, with multiple interdependencies of the variables involved in its dynamics. We achieved good performance with a fuzzy controller. Although, as shown in the results it is important focusing in working on fuzzy controllers considering more than one input variable of the dynamics of the system. These results motivate us towards propose more advanced techniques in hybrid control systems such as Fuzzy-PD, Fuzzy-PI, and Fuzzy-PID, and application of artificial intelligence techniques.

Algorithm used for image processing worked well under all experiments, but there is a time delay that affects the response controller and also an inherent error due to the image segmentation method implemented [14]. To improve the controller response, a sensor is needed with a better time response.

In this stage we used Fuzzy Toolbox of MatLab [TM] [19] to develop the controller, but, as a future work we will develop our proper Fuzzy Inference System in C++, to improve time response and performance results, as well as, developing more compact and autonomous devices (fuzzy controllers embedded).

References

1.   Nise, N.S.: Control Systems Engineering. John Wiley & Sons, Inc., California (2011)
2.   Reznik, L., Ghanayemb, O., Bourmistrovc, A.: PID plus fuzzy controller structures as a design base for industrial applications. Engineering Applications of Artificial Intelligence 13(4), 419–430 (2000)

3. Takatsu, H., Itoh, T.: Future Needs for Control Theory in Industry-Report of the Control Technology Survey in Japanese Industry. IEEE Transactions on Control Systems Technology 7(3), 298–305 (1999)

4. Barua, A., Mudunuri, L.S., Kosheleva, O.: Why Trapezoidal and Triangular Membership Functions Work So Well: Towards a Theoretical Explanation. Journal of Uncertain Systems 8(3), 164–168 (2014)

5. Castillo, O., Huesca, G., Valdez, F.: Evolutionary Computing for Topology Optimization of Fuzzy Systems in Intelligent Control. In: Applied Soft Computing Technologies: The Challenge of Complexity, vol. 34, pp. 633–647. Springer (2006)

6. Olivas, E.L., Castillo, O., Valdez, F., Soria, J.: Ant Colony Optimization for Membership Function Design for a Water Tank Fuzzy Logic Controller. In: IEEE Workshop on Hybrid Intelligent Models and Applications, HIMA (2013)

7. Fierro, R., Castillo, O., Valdez, F., Cervantes, L.: Design of optimal membership functions for fuzzy controllers of the water tank and inverted pendulum with PSO variants. In: IFSA World Congress and NAFIPS Annual Meeting (IFSA/NAFIPS) 2013 Joint, pp. 1068–1073. IEEE (2013)

8. Parul Agarwal, S.M.: Nature-Inspired Algorithms: State-of-Art, Problems and Prospects. International Journal of Computer Applications 100(14), 14–21 (2014)

9. Valdez, F., Melin, P., Castillo, O.: A survey on nature-inspired optimization algorithms with fuzzy logic for dynamic parameter adaptation. Expert Systems with Applications 41(14), 6459–6466 (2014)

10. Delettre, A., Laurent, G.J., Fort-Piat, L.: A New Contactless Conveyor System for Handling Clean and Delicate Products Using Induced Air Flows. In: 2010 IEEE/RSJ International Conference on Robots and Systems (IROS), pp. 2351–2356. Taipei, Taiwan (2010)

11. Escano, J.M., Ortega, M.G., Rubio, F.R.: Position control of a pneumatic levitation system. In: 10th IEEE Conference on Emerging Technologies and Factory Automation, ETFA 2005, Catania (2005)

12. Leyton, V.H.M., Bacca, G., Meneses, O.Q., Fernández, J.A.D.: Control de posición de un sistema de levitación. Revista Universitaria en Telecomunicaciones Informática y Control 1(2), 9–17 (2012)

13. Gu, D.-W., Petkov, P.H., Konstantinov, M.M.: Robust Control Design with MATLAB. Springer, London (2005)

14. Zalapa, O.R., Zavala, A.H., Ruelas, J.A.H.: Sistema de medición de distancia mediante imágenes para determinar la posición de una esfera utilizando el sensor Kinect XBOX. Polibits (49), 59–67 (2014)

15. Martins, F.G.: Tuning PID controllers using the ITAE criterion. International Journal of Engineering Education 21(5), 867–873 (2005)

16. Awouda, A.E.A., Mamat, R.B.: New PID Tuning Rule Using ITAE Criteria. International Journal of Engineering (IJE) 3(6), 597–608 (2010)

17. Ljung, L.: System Identification Toolbox for Use with {MATLAB} (2007)

18. Golnaraghi, F., Kuo, B.C.: Automatic control systems. Wiley Publishing (2009)

19. MathWorks, I., Wang, W.C.: Fuzzy Logic Toolbox: for Use with MATLAB: User's Guide, MathWorks, Incorporated (1998)

20. Mamdani, E.H.: Application of fuzzy algorithms for control of simple dynamic plant. In: Proceedings of the Institution of Electrical Engineers, vol. 121(12), pp. 1585–1588 (1974)

Yager–Rybalov Triple Π Operator as a Means of Reducing the Number of Generated Clusters in Unsupervised Anuran Vocalization Recognition

Carol Bedoya[1], Julio Waissman-Villanova[2], and Claudia Victoria Isaza-Narvaez[1]

[1] SISTEMIC, Departamento de Ingeniería Electrónica, Facultad de Ingeniería, Universidad de Antioquia UdeA, Calle 70 No. 52-21, Medellín, Colombia
{carol.bedoya,victoria.isaza}@udea.edu.co
[2] Departamento de Matemáticas, Universidad de Sonora, Blvd. Encinas y Rosales C.P. 8300, Hermosillo, Sonora, México
juliowaissman@mat.uson.mx

Abstract. The Learning Algorithm for Multivariate Data Analysis (LAMDA) is an unsupervised fuzzy-based classification methodology. The operating principle of LAMDA is based on finding the datum-cluster relationship obtained by means of the Global Adequacy Degrees (GADs) of the Marginal Adequacy Degrees (MADs) of all the data attributes. In comparison with other unsupervised clustering algorithms, LAMDA does not require the number of classes as input parameter; however, in some applications, the quantity of obtained clusters does not correspond with the number of desired classes. Typically, this issue is overcome by merging interrelated clusters within the same class; nevertheless, in some applications the number of generated clusters related to the same class reaches a non-desired and impractical number. In LAMDA, the number of generated clusters is controlled by using a linear mixed connective with an exigency index α. This connective is an unnatural aggregation operator of the MADs, which adds an additional parameter to set up. In this paper, a full reinforcement operator (Yager–Rybalov Triple Π) is used as aggregation operator for merging the information contained in the MADs. This approach significantly reduces the number of generated classes and suppresses the LAMDA dependence of the parameter α. The proposed approach was tested in a case study related to unsupervised anuran vocalization recognition. A database of advertisement calls of six anuran (frog) species for testing this proposal was selected. All 102 vocalizations were correctly identified (100% of accuracy) and solely the desired classes were generated by the algorithm (establishing a cluster-class bijection).

Keywords: Fuzzy clustering, Fuzzy connective, Bioacoustics, Anuran, Aggregation operator, Bipolar scale.

1 Introduction

Classification techniques with unsupervised learning regularly need the number of clusters as input parameter (e.g., K-means, Fuzzy C-means, Gustafson-Kessel), even

A. Gelbukh et al. (Eds.): MICAI 2014, Part II, LNAI 8857, pp. 382–391, 2014.
© Springer International Publishing Switzerland 2014

when it is unknown. In some specific algorithms (e.g., LAMDA) it is not necessary; however, the fact of not constraining the number of generated clusters in datasets with high levels intra-class uncertainty, could result in large amounts of clusters related to the same class. In the Learning Algorithm for Multivariate Data Analysis LAMDA [1], a cluster-class bijection (one-to-one correspondence) is typically desired; nevertheless, this cannot be constantly achieved. In general, when the dataset is noisy and there exist high levels of intra-class uncertainty, the number of desired classes is significantly less than the number of generated clusters.

In this document a case study related to unsupervised frog vocalization recognition was selected to illustrate the problem. The automated recognition of animal vocalizations has become an interesting tool in the noninvasive extraction of ecological information. When the studied species possess mimetic or cryptic attributes, the personnel costs, the habitat invasiveness, and the time consuming could be considerably reduced without any loss of information implementing an automated acoustic recognition system.

Acoustic recognition systems consist of three main stages: pre-processing, where recordings are noise-reduced and segmented in order to obtain separated vocalizations; feature extraction, where acoustic features are extracted from the waveforms with the purpose of increasing the dissimilarity among classes (i.e., species); and classification, where each vocalization is assigned to an specific cluster according to a similarity measure. Acoustic recognition systems (and every pattern recognition system) could be categorized in accordance with the learning approach used in their classification stage: supervised and unsupervised. In the supervised approach, each datum (in this case each vocalization) is labeled by an expert in order to bias the algorithm parameters according to the training data [2]. On the other hand, in the unsupervised approach, the classification algorithm infers by itself the feature space division and classifies each datum based on it (i.e. labeled data are not necessary) [2].

The unsupervised learning is useful, in comparison with the supervised learning, when the labeling of datasets is expensive or exhausting, when patterns change over time, or when the content of the data is unknown and a categorization of the data is needed. Nonetheless, unsupervised learning is significantly more difficult to achieve [3]. In bioacoustics (the study of animal sound generation), supervised techniques have been widely used during the last decade with acceptable results [4]. Nowadays the implementation of unsupervised techniques in automated animal vocalization recognition is an open issue in bioacoustics [5]; worldwide contributions in this field are limited. Unsupervised approaches are especially useful in cases with no *a priori* knowledge of all the existent species in a specific area, when the obtained information is particularly large and could not be labeled, or when language structures need to be found.

In this paper, a modification to the LAMDA methodology is proposed in order to notably reduce the large amounts of clusters produced by minimal data variations. The proposed modification consists on replacing the actual linearly compensated hybrid connective (min-max) [6], used as aggregation operator for obtaining the membership degrees, with the Yager-Rybalov Triple Π operator (3Π) [7]. The modified methodology was applied to a case study related to animal vocalization recognition (specifically anuran vocalizations). 100% of accuracy results and a one-to-one correspondence between the generated clusters and the desired classes (anuran species) were obtained. Anurans (commonly known as frogs and toads) is the name given to the members of the Anura order [8]. Anurans, and the rest of the members of the Amphibia class in general, are highly sensitive to the variations of the habitat conditions, which makes the monitoring of the fluctuations of their populations a valuable estimator of the environmental quality.

This paper is presented as follows: in Section 2, the clustering algorithm and the modifications made to the classification technique are explained, in Section 3 the bioacoustical analysis of the anuran vocalizations is presented, in Section 4 the results are analyzed and discussed, and finally, in Section 5 conclusions and future work are exposed.

2   LAMDA Clustering Methodology

2.1   Clustering Algorithm

The Learning Algorithm for multivariate data analysis (LAMDA) [1] is a Fuzzy-based clustering algorithm that does not require the number of clusters as input parameter. It is not a distance-based method, which allows it to perform a similitude analysis among data in order to establish a relationship between each object with its respective cluster [9]. Furthermore, LAMDA estimates the membership degree of a datum to a cluster in a non-iterative process (i.e., results are obtained solely with one data reading). Due to the previously mentioned features, LAMDA stand out over other fuzzy classification algorithms (e.g., Fuzzy C-means and Gustafson-Kessel) [10]. LAMDA clustering usefulness has been showed in several applications; however, when the dataset is noisy (e.g., recordings of animal vocalizations), the number of generated clusters by LAMDA is considerably larger than the number of desired classes.

LAMDA is based on the use of adequacy degrees to establish similarities among data with the purpose of generating clusters. Let $\hat{m} \in [0,1]^n$ be the vector of input features, where $\hat{m}_j$ is the membership of the input to the jth descriptor, then the input in LAMDA is a vector of membership degrees of simple concepts or features. The contribution of each feature to a global concept is called the marginal adequacy degree (MAD). The MAD M_{lj} of each jth descriptor (feature) $\hat{m}_j$ to the cluster l is estimated by:

$$M_{lj} = \rho_{lj}{}^{\hat{m}_j}(1 - \rho_{lj})^{1-\hat{m}_j} \qquad (1)$$

where $\hat{m} \in \mathbb{R}^n$ is a vector that contains all normalized features, $\hat{m}_j$ is the datum belonging to the jth descriptor in $\hat{m}$, $\rho \in \mathbb{R}^{h \times n}$ is a matrix with the mean values for each j-th descriptor in each lth cluster respectively, ρ_{lj} is the element belonging to the l cluster and to the jth descriptor in the matrix ρ, h is the number of clusters, and n is the number of features. The value of ρ_{lj} represents the adequacy degree in which the feature $\hat{m}_j$ is presented in the lth cluster. If the value of ρ_{lj} is close to 1, then $\hat{m}_j$ has to be close to 1 to model correctly the cluster. On the other hand, a value of ρ_{lj} close to 0 implies that the value of $\hat{m}_j$ has to be close to 0 (a high degree of confidence related to de absence of the feature in the object) in order to model correctly the cluster. Note that if $\rho_{lj} = 0.5$ then $\forall\, \hat{m}_j \in [0,1]$, $M_{l,j} = 0.5$. It means that the adequacy of this feature will be the same independently of its value (i.e. this feature is considered as non-informative).

Fuzzy aggregation operators are used to establish the adequacy of each object to each cluster [6]. In LAMDA these operators are used to estimate the global adequacy degrees (GADs) $g \in \mathbb{R}^h$ [10] of an object in a cluster. The process consists on synthesize Marginal adequacy degrees (MADs) $M \in \mathbb{R}^{h \times n}$, coming from different sources, using a linearly compensated hybrid connective [6]:

$$g_l\left(M_{l,1}, ..., M_{l,n}\right) = \alpha\, C\left(M_{l,1}, ..., M_{l,n}\right) + (1 - \alpha)\bar{C}\left(M_{l,1}, ..., M_{l,n}\right) \tag{2}$$

where g_l is the GAD associated to the cluster l in g, C is a Triangular norm (T-norm), $\bar{C}$ represents the dual connective of C (also known as Triangular conorm, T-conorm, or S-norm) [11], and $0< \alpha <1$ is an exigency index (parameter to adjust the influence of the T-norm and T-conorm in the fuzzy aggregation). Usually, minimum and maximum are used as T-norm and T-conorm respectively [12]. This is made with the purpose of obtaining the GAD of an object to a class. Nonetheless, in some applications the T-norm and T-conorm (min-max in this case) could be changed according to the database requirements (e.g., nilpotent minimum - nilpotent maximum, product-probabilistic sum, Łukasiewicz-Bounded sum, etc.).

A "Non-Information" class could be defined as the class where all features are non-informative and thus, independently of the object:

$$g_0 = \alpha\, C(0.5, ..., 0.5) + (1 - \alpha)\bar{C}(0.5, ..., 0.5), \; \forall\, \hat{m} \tag{3}$$

Regarding the operation of LAMDA, the algorithm is initialized with only one pre-defined cluster, commonly known as the Non-Information class (NIC), cluster 0 in this case, with $\rho_{0j} = 0.5 \,\forall\, j = 1, ..., n$. The first object is classified in the NIC because it is considered unrecognized; then, a new cluster ($l = 1$) is created using Eq. (4), and the mean values $\rho_{lj}[k]$ of the first step $k = 1$ are initialized with the NIC parameters ($\rho_{lj}[k - 1] = 0.5 \,\forall\, j = 1, ..., n$) and $n_l[k - 1] = 1$. Subsequently, a new object is entered at updated step k, and the GADs are calculated with the values ($\hat{m}_j[k]$) of the new object. If the object is assigned to the NIC (i.e., maximum GAD corresponds to the NIC cluster), a new cluster is created and initialized with the NIC parameters modified by the data values as additional information. Otherwise, the mean values of the previously created cluster ($\rho_{lj}[k - 1] \,\forall\, j = 1, ..., n$) are updated with the values of that object in order to contain the new entry value (in this case $n_l[k - 1]$ is the number of objects previously classified in this cluster).

$$\rho_{lj}[k] = \rho_{lj}[k - 1] + \left[\frac{\hat{m}_j[k] - \rho_{lj}[k-1]}{n_l[k-1]+1}\right] \tag{4}$$

Where $\rho_{lj}[k]$ is the updated mean value for the j-th descriptor in the l-th cluster respectively, $\rho_{lj}[k-1]$ is the preceding ρ_{lj} value (the same used for calculating MADs in Eq. 1), and $n_l[k-1]$ is the number of objects previously classified in the cluster l.

This process continues until all objects are analyzed. If the generated clusters do not correspond with the number of desired classes, the similar clusters could be merged within the same class according to an expert opinion or a similarity measure. In LAMDA, the use of the min-max aggregation operator together with a high exigency level tends to generate large amounts of clusters. In some cases, this can be surpassed reducing the exigency index, but this generally produces misclassified data. Nowadays, there exist some methods proposed for automatically merging the generated clusters [13]; however, always is preferable a parameterless algorithm producing a practical number of generated clusters.

2.2   Full Reinforced LAMDA Clustering Algorithm

The inherent necessity of using the α index in the linearly compensated hybrid connective implies that, in some cases, the values of the MADs could contradict each other (being cancelled out by the aggregation operation). This produces as consequences, a deviation regarding the expected outcome and a misclassification regarding the desired class. The cause of this issue could be that MADs and GADs do not share similar properties. In order to overcome the presented issue, a different aggregation operator is proposed for the GAD calculation.

The MAD for the lth cluster from the jth feature $M_{l,j}$, is independently computed from other clusters and features. This means that the MAD is in fact a fuzzy membership function, whose inputs are also values of fuzzy memberships. These fuzzy sets have some particular properties: First, if $\rho > 0.5$, then the maximal value of $M_{l,j}$ is reached with $\hat{m}_j = 1$. Respectively, if $\rho < 0.5$, then the maximal value of $M_{l,j}$ is reached with $\hat{m}_j = 0$. The MADs are fuzzy membership functions in a bipolar scale; they represent a degree from a total distrust (0) to a total trust (1), including a non-informative degree value (0.5). This suggests that the use of an aggregation operator well adapted to bipolar scales could be used more naturally in the calculation of the GADs. Particularly, if $M_{l,j} = 0.5$, the MAD is equivalent to the degree of a non-informative feature; hence, it is desirable that the GAD is not going to be affected by this feature. Additionally, in order to keep the homogeneity of the fuzzy system, is expected that $g_0 = 0.5$, which is the fixed point of the bipolar scale.

The Yager-Rybalov Triple Π operator [7] is a full reinforcement operator that can be viewed as a generalization of a symmetric sum [14]. The GAD computed by the Triple Π operator becomes:

$$g_l\left(M_{l,1}, \ldots, M_{l,n}\right) = \frac{\prod_{j=1}^{n} M_{lj}}{\prod_{j=1}^{n} M_{lj} + \prod_{j=1}^{n} 1 - M_{lj}} \tag{5}$$

The main properties of the Triple Π operator in the GAD calculation are: **(i)** $g_l\left(M_{l,1}, \ldots, M_{l,n}\right)$ is commutative. **(ii)** $g_l(0.5, \ldots, 0.5) = 0.5$ represents the NIC as a midpoint in a bipolar scale. (iii) $g_l(M_{l,1}, ..., M_{l,n}, 0.5) = g_l(M_{l,1}, ..., M_{l,n})$ is not affected by a non-informative feature. (iv) $g_l(M_{l,1}, ..., M_{l,n}) \geq \max(M_{l,1}, ..., M_{l,n})$ if $M_{l,j} \geq 0.5 \ \forall j = 1, ..., n$. This is known as positive reinforcement; it means that all the marginal adequacies are evident for this cluster and the global adequacy is higher than each mad individually analyzed. (v) $g_l(M_{l,1}, ..., M_{l,n}) \leq \min(M_{l,1}, ..., M_{l,n})$ if $M_{l,i} \leq 0.5 \ \forall i = 1, ..., n$. This is known as negative reinforcement; it means the opposite of positive reinforcement: marginal adequacies are against the cluster l and the global adequacy is lower than each mad individually analyzed.

3   Case Study: Unsupervised Anuran Vocalization Recognition

3.1   Materials

A dataset by the Smithsonian Tropical Research Institute (STRI) [15] constituted by 103 calls of six anuran species was used. The advertisement calls were recorded at Monumento Nacional Barro Colorado, Panama (9°09'N, 79°51'W) but only those species located in Colombia (Chocó department) with a significant number of calls were selected [12]: *Rhinella margaritifer* (RM), *Diasporus diastema* (DD), *Hypsiboas boans* (HB), *Leptodactylus fuscus* (LF), *Leptodactylus savagei* (LS), and *Scinax ruber* (SR).

3.2   Methods

The identification of the animal vocalizations (in this case anuran calls) was performed using the three previously-mentioned stages in Section 1. The methodology consists of: a digital filter, for noise reduction; an energy-based thresholding, for segmentation; Mel Frequency Cepstral Coefficients (MFCCs), as acoustic features; and a modified LAMDA, for clustering. The goal is to identify anuran vocalizations of the same species using unsupervised learning.

Preprocessing
Initially, the signals were oversampled to attain a sampling rate of 44100 Hz. Then an IIR Butterworth band-pass filter [16] centered on the average species frequencies ± the maximal variation among individuals of the same species was applied: RM - 1626 Hz, DD – 3046 Hz, HB – 506 Hz, LF – 2240 Hz, LP – 400 Hz, SR – 835 Hz, DA – 1576 Hz, and DT – 2939 Hz. Finally, each advertisement call existent in the recordings was segmented using a thresholding algorithm [17] over the energy of the signals; the root mean square value (RMS) was selected as threshold.

Feature Extraction
12 Mel Frequency Cepstral Coefficients (MFCCs) [18] were used as acoustic features – parameters of the call that maximize the variability among anuran species (inter-class) and minimize the variability within anuran species (intra-class) –. The MFCCs redistribute the frequencies across the spectrum in order to benefit specific bands before the

feature extraction. They evidence several advantages over the typically used time-frequency features, e.g., small variation over time, high accuracy, and recognition regardless of the call type [19]. The MFCCs were calculated over each previously-segmented vocalization; then, each feature was averaged, obtaining a vector $\bar{m} \in \mathbb{R}^n$ per vocalization. Finally, $\bar{m}$ was rescaled – range [0,1] – (Eq. 6) and used as input for the classification stage.

$$\hat{m}_j = \frac{\bar{m}_j - \bar{m}_{min}}{\bar{m}_{max} - \bar{m}_{min}} \tag{6}$$

where $\bar{m}_{min}$ and $\bar{m}_{max}$ are the minimum and maximum values of $\bar{m}$ respectively, $\hat{m} \in \mathbb{R}^n$ is the vector $\bar{m}$ normalized, $\hat{m}_j$ is the datum belonging to the j-th MFCC in $\hat{m}$, and $n = 12$ is the number of features (12 descriptors).

Classification
After extracting the acoustic features, the clustering algorithm was applied using the procedure of section 2.1 with the section 2.2 modification. The clustering was used to identify each profile of anuran specie (six total species).

4   Results and Discussion

Table 1 shows the classification results of the LAMDA methodology before and after the proposed modification. The number of generated clusters was significantly higher when the min-max operator was used (39 clusters for 6 anuran species). These clusters were obtained after testing the algorithm with different α values; $\alpha = 0.9$ was selected because with this value there were not misclassified data. In contrast, when the Yager-Rybalov Triple Π operator was used, only the desired clusters were generated, i.e., six clusters corresponding to six classes (anuran species). The 3Π operator allowed LAMDA to establish a cluster-class bijection, by means of solely generating the desired clusters (see Figure 1). If the min-max operator is used, the set of clusters corresponding to a similar class should be merged at the end of the classification procedure (see figure 2).

100% of accuracy was achieved with both aggregation operators. Although the number of generated clusters by min-max was significantly higher than the number generated by 3Π, none of them could be associated with two or more classes; therefore, results after merging are the same for both operators. However, it is important to clarify that the used database is constituted by only 102 data. In this case, 102 data generated 38 clusters (a very large amount); with a larger and noisier database the algorithm could yield amounts of clusters that could make the manual merging process prohibitive. Additionally, the 3Π operator avoids the use of the α parameter, which turns LAMDA in a parameterless methodology.

Table 1. Clustering results of the LAMDA methodology using min-max and 3Π as aggregation operators. Each vocalization was correctly classified using both operators; however, min-max (α = 0.9) generated extra quantities of clusters related to the same class (species).

Class	Species	Acronym	vocalizations	Number of Clusters 3Π	Number of Clusters Min-Max	Accuracy
1	*Rhinella margaritifer*	RM	13	1	7	100 %
2	*Diasporus diastema*	DD	10	1	1	100 %
3	*Hypsiboas boans*	HB	31	1	8	100 %
4	*Leptodactylus fuscus*	LF	14	1	7	100 %
5	*Leptodactylus savagei*	LP	18	1	2	100 %
6	*Scinax ruber*	SR	16	1	13	100 %

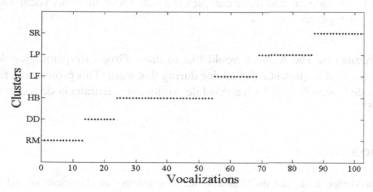

Fig. 1. Clustering results of the LAMDA methodology using the Yager-Rybalov Triple Π operator as fuzzy connective. Only six clusters were generated by the algorithm. Each clusters is related to solely one class (anuran specie), establishing a one-to-one relationship between clusters and classes.

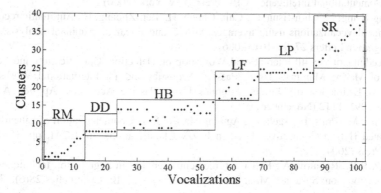

Fig. 2. Clustering results with the min-max duple in the linearly compensated hybrid connective (aggregation operator of Eq. 3). 38 clusters related to 6 classes were generated.

5   Conclusions and Future Work

In this research, the use of the Yager-Rybalov Triple Π operator as fuzzy connective in the LAMDA methodology was proposed. This aggregation operator allowed the algorithm to significantly reduce the number of generated clusters in comparison with the min-max connective. The 3Π suppressed the existing dependence of the methodology with this α index (the only parameter to set up) and transformed LAMDA in a parameterless algorithm.

Regarding the results, six anuran species were correctly identified (100% of accuracy) using unsupervised learning with both aggregation operators; however, was the 3Π operator the only connective that could establish a one-to-one relationship between clusters and classes. Future work will consist on apply this classification technique to a larger, noisier, and more complex dataset, which involves vocalizations of different animal species.

Acknowledgments. The Authors would like to thank Grupo Herpetológico de Antioquia for its valuable guidance and advice during this work. This project was financed by "Fondo de Sostenibilidad Universidad de Antioquia – Estrategia de sostenibilidad 2014-2015".

References

1. Aguilar-Martin, J., López de Mantarás, R.: The process of classification and learning the meaning of linguistic descriptors or concepts. Approximate Reasoning in Decision Analysis, 165–175 (1982)
2. Duda, R.O., Hart, P.E., Stork, D.G.: Pattern Classification. John Wiley & Sons, New York (2001); J. Classif. 24(2) (September 2007)
3. Tzanakou, E.M.: Supervised and Unsupervised Pattern Recognition: Feature Extraction and Computational Intelligence. CRC Press, New York (2000)
4. Chang-Hsing, L., Chih-Hsun, C., Chin-Chuan, H., Ren-Zhuang, H.: Automatic recognition of animal vocalizations using averaged MFCC and linear discriminant analysis. Pattern Recognition Letters 27, 93–101 (2006)
5. Proceedings of the 4th International Workshop on Detection, Classification and Localization of Marine Mammals Using Passive Acoustics and 1st International Workshop on Density Estimation of Marine Mammals Using Passive Acoustics. Applied Acoustics 71(11), 991–1112 (November 2010)
6. Sánchez, M., Prats, F., Agell, N., Aguilar-Martin, J.: A Characterization of Linearly Compensated Hybrid Connectives Used in Fuzzy Classifications. In: ECAI, pp. 1081–1082. IOS Press (2004)
7. Yager, R.R., Rybalov, A.: Full reinforcement operators in aggregation techniques. IEEE Transactions on Systems, Man, and Cybernetics, Part B: Cybernetics 28(6), 757–769 (1998)
8. McCallum, M.L.: Amphibian Decline or Extinction? Current Declines Dwarf Background Extinction Rate. Journal of Herpetology 41, 483–491 (2007)
9. Bedoya, C., Uribe, C., Isaza, C.: Unsupervised Feature Selection Based on Fuzzy Clustering for Fault Detection of the Tennessee Eastman Process. In: Proceedings of the 13th

Ibero-American Conference on Artificial Intelligence (IBERAMIA), Cartagena de Indias, Colombia, pp. 350–360 (2012)

10. Botía, J.F., Isaza, C., Kempowsky, T., Le Lann, M.V., Aguilar-Martín, J.: Automaton based on fuzzy clustering methods for monitoring industrial processes. Engineering Applications of Artificial Intelligence 26(4), 1211–1220 (2013)

11. Piera-Carrete, N., Desroches, P., Aguilar-Martin, J.: Variation Points in Pattern Recognition. Pattern Recognition Letters 11, 519–524 (1990)

12. Bedoya, C., Isaza, C., Daza, J.M., López, J.D.: Automatic Recognition of Anuran Species Based on Syllable Identification. Ecological Informatics 24, 200–209 (2014)

13. Isaza, C.: Diagnostic par Techniques d'apprentissage Floues: Conception d'une Methode de Validation et d'optimisation des Partitions. PhD thesis, Laboratoire d'Analyse et d'Architecture des Syst'emes du CNRS (October 2007)

14. Emilion, R., Regis, S., Doncescu, A.: A General Version of the Triple Pi Operator. International Journal of Iintelligent Systems, 1–18 (2013)

15. Ibañez, R., Stanley, A., Ryan, M., Jaramillo, C.: Vocalizaciones de ranas y sapos del Monumento Natural Barro Colorado. Parque Nacional Soberanía y áreas adyacentes. Sony MusicEntertaiment (Central America) S.A. (1999)

16. Selesnick, I.W., Burrus, C.S.: Generalized Digital Butterworth Filter Design. In: Proceedings of the IEEE Int. Conf. Acoust., Speech, Signal Processing, vol. 3 (May 1996)

17. Zhao, X., O'Shaughnessy, D.: A new hybrid approach for automatic speech signal segmentation using silence signal detection, energy convex hull, and spectral variation. In: Canadian Conference on Electrical and Computer Engineering, CCECE 2008, pp. 4–7 (May 2008)

18. Mermelstein, P.: Distance measures for speech recognition, psychological and instrumental. Pattern Recognition and Artificial Intelligence, 374–388 (1976)

19. Fox, E.: A new perspective on acoustic individual recognition in animals with limited call sharing or changing repertoires. Animal Behaviour 75, 1187–1194 (2008)

AI-Based Design of a Parallel Robot Used as a Laser Tracker System: Intelligent vs. Nonlinear Classical Controllers

Ricardo Zavala-Yoé[1], Ricardo A. Ramírez-Mendoza[1],
and Daniel Chaparro-Altamirano[2]

[1] Instituto Tecnológico de Monterrey
Puente 222. Ejidos de Huipulco. 14380. Mexico City
[2] Computer Science Dept.,Columbia University, New York, NY, USA

Abstract. Classical ways for coordinate measuring devices are manual theodolites, photogrammetry-based systems, total stations and a recently-introduced device referred to as laser tracker systems. Basically, a laser tracker system is a more accurate and reliable 3D measurement tool that allows to increase and maintain accuracy as time goes by. Laser tracker systems deals with industry-based measuring problems which can be alignment, reverse engineering, tool building, part inspection, installation, and manufacturing and assembly integration. A very interesting case of the latter is robot-tracking calibration in an welding line. In a welding line, robots are controlled in order to keep a prescribed trajectory to accomplish its welding task properly. Nevertheless, in spite of a good control algorithm design, as time goes by, deviations appear and some maintenance has to be done on the robotic unit. So, robot calibration can be done with a laser tracker. Although laser tracker systems are made by very well established and serious companies, their laser products may be very expensive for small or medium size industries. Our contribution is to offer a parallel robot-based laser tracker system model whose implementation would result cheaper than sophisticated laser devices and takes advantage of the parallel robot bondages as high payload. As a first step, simulations of the controlled systems are done here. This parallel robot-based laser tracker is designed to help in the calibration process which consists in repeating some specified trajectory for the serial (welding) robot. The laser tracker system tracks the welding robot trajectory in a day-by-day period of time (for instance) in order to identify the moment when a deviation of the reference trajectory happens. Hence, corrections can be done avoiding greater problems in the welding line. In order to design the parallel robot-based tracker system, a kinematic analysis and a dynamical modeling have to be done in order to design a set of controllers which will be assessed. All of it assisted by AI (artificial intelligence) algorithms. The laser tracker kinematic analysis was done assisted by ANN (artificial neural networks) and by GA (genetic algorithms). This fact allowed to compute numerically/graphically the laser tracker workspace in order to warrant the right accessibility of the corresponding 3D (three dimensional) space. A dynamical model which represents the parallel robot-based laser tracker system was also

A. Gelbukh et al. (Eds.): MICAI 2014, Part II, LNAI 8857, pp. 392–409, 2014.

obtained. This model was used by our set of controllers. The controller design is split into two groups: One considers AI-based algorithms and the second one, classical design-based controllers. A comparison between the two groups is done and advantages/disadvantages are shown in terms of performance in the presence of a persistent perturbation which models ground vibrations in the factory the welding robots are. Such vibrations are endlessly present because they are produced by other assembling machines which disturb the welding process. So, in spite of this perturbation our parallel robot-based laser tracker system showed to behave well with Intelligent Control keeping good tracking of a sinusoidal welding calibration trajectory in the serial robot. In this work it is assumed that a laser device is mounted in the parallel robot with inertial dynamical effect on the parallel robot. Analytical developments are provided as well as numerical/graphical solutions done in MATLAB/SIMULINK to deal with this complex dynamical system. An integral viewpoint with ANN, GA, and Fuzzy Logic was used in this study.

1   Introduction

The laser tracker was conceived as a portable coordinate measuring device that can measure very large or not regular bodies. However, its application is not only restricted to static measuring but also to moving machines as robotic arms. For instance, consider a robot tracking calibration in a welding line. In a such manufacturing process, robots are controlled in order to keep a prescribed trajectory to accomplish its task properly. Nevertheless, in spite of a good control algorithm design, as time goes by, deviations appear and the robot has to be adjusted. This paper proposes a laser tracker system based on a 3SPS-1S parallel manipulator. So, the laser tracker unit will be mounted on the end effector (the moving platform) of a parallel robot (see figure 1 and section 1.2). Note that in this paper an interaction between a serial manipulator and a parallel robot is being modeled, controlled and simulated assisted by AI algorithms. A serial robot consists of a fixed based mechanically connected to a lower limb which is linked by joints to upper limbs. The last one moves an end effector. In contrast, a parallel robot has both extremes of its limbs attached to a fixed platform and to a moving platform, which is the end effector in this case (see figure 2 and [16], [5], [20]).

1.1   Laser Tracker Systems

As mentioned, until recently, coordinate measuring devices were coordinate-measuring machines, manual theodolites,collimators, photogrammetry-based systems, and total stations. However, a modern system which surpasses those ones is the laser tracker. A laser tracker measures the three dimensional position of a moving target with an accuracy of a few microns over a range of tens of meters. Basically, a laser tracker system combines a laser interferometer to measure relative distance and optical encoders to measure azimuth and elevation of a

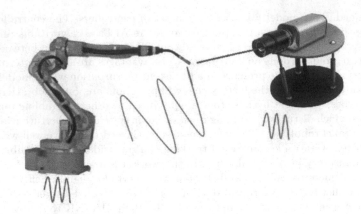

Fig. 1. Interaction between two different kinds of robots via AI and classical control in the presence of disturbances

beam-steering mirror. This mirror directs a laser beam in a wide range of directions. In order to accomplish its tracking task, a laser tracker uses a reflexion device referred to as SMR (sphere mounted retro reflector). This SMR consists of a corner cube reflector made carefully so the apex of the mirrors coincides with the center of curvature of a precision tooling ball. These balls works as interface between the optical measurement from the tracker and the moving system, the robot arm which needs to be adjusted described in this paper. A SMR is placed at the far end of the welding robot end effector. Once that this robot starts moving following a sinusoid signal reference (simulating a welding process) the laser tracker (mounted in the parallel robot) tracks the robot arm trajectory directing its laser beam to the SMR positioned at the welding arm (see figure 1 and [2], [11]).

1.2   The Parallel Robot 3SPS-1S

Parallel manipulators have received a lot of attention from researchers over the past couple of decades, due to the advantages they present over their serial counterparts, such as more accuracy, higher load capacity/robot mass ratio and more rigidity.

Researchers have taken an interest in parallel robots with less than six degrees of freedom (DOF), because in some applications there is no need to be able to move and rotate the end effector in every direction, and using less than six DOF manipulators decreases the costs. Three DOF spherical manipulators, also known as parallel wrists, can be used as an alternative to the wrists with three revolute joints for applications where there is need to orient something. Parallel robots takes their names from their links structure. So, 3SPS-1S means that there are three identical limbs which have spherical (S) joints at the extremes and a prismatic (P) joint in the middle (3SPS) plus one passive (non actuated) link in the middle (of the platforms) whose extrems are also spherical (S) joints, i.e., 3SPS-1S. The base platform is static and the end effector is the (upper) moving platform [16], [8], [9].

A particular case of the 3SPS-1S manipulator proposed by Cui and Zhang [6] is shown in Figure 2. It has three identical legs, made of two bodies, linked by an actuated prismatic joint. The legs are attached to the platform and the base by spherical joints. It is assumed that the platform and the base are circular, with radii r_p and r_b respectively, and that the spherical joints of the legs are located along these circumferences. There is also a central passive leg that connects the center of the base to the center of the platform using a spherical joint. See figure 2. There are two coordinate systems. The general coordinate system xyz is located at the center of the base (point O), and the coordinate system of the platform uvw with origin on point P is located at the center of the spherical joint of the central leg. The orientation of the platform is given in terms of the Euler angles which are three angles introduced by Euler to describe the orientation of a rigid body [14], [16]. The central constraining leg of the mechanism increases the stiffness of the system and forces the manipulator to have three pure rotation degrees of freedom. In order to design the control algorithm for the parallel robot, the kinematics and dynamics of this robot has to be obtained. The former will help to determine the manipulator's work space, the latter will provide a model to design the control algorithms. The workspace indicates the zone of the 3D space the robot can move in. The work space computation is aboard below. Later, the kinematics problems are also deduced. Both are taken from [3].

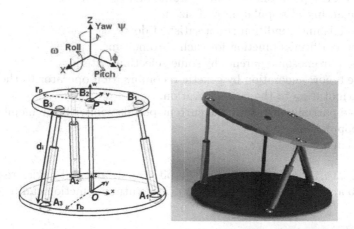

Fig. 2. Model of the 3SPS-1S parallel wrist and corresponding Euler angles for the end effector (moving platform)

2   Computing the Workspace of the Parallel Robot-Based Laser Tracker with Genetic Algorithms

Some times complex analytical problems needs powerful numerical methods as genetic algorithms [10], [12], [1]. As a result of such analytical complexity of the equations which describe the workspace manipulator, a numerical method has been developed in [3] to compute and plot such workspace. That numerical method is based in *five* algorithms which look for the right points in the 3D space while the following conditions are checked: rightness of limbs length, avoiding collision among limbs, and restriction in the Euler angles. The resulting workspace is shown in figure 3, left panel. This region defines a smaller zone in the 3D space than the one provided by the Genetic Algorithm optimization described next. It is known that the 3SPS-1S parallel wrist is characterized by its lack of a big workspace; therefore, optimizing the parameters of the robot in order to maximize the workspace is very important. Nevertheless it is also important for the manipulator to have its parameters r_b, r_p and h as close as possible to a set of desired parameters, mainly because many times there are size limitations in the location where the manipulator is to be placed. Such numerical optimization for the workspace computation was done by means of a genetic algorithm (described partially in [3]). This method tries to maximize the workspace and at the same time, keep the robot parameters as close as possible to a set of desired parameters. The algorithm is given here:

Algorithm 1. Computation of manipulator's workspace

1. Fix size of population, n=3 and parameters, r_b, r_p, h.
2. Create an initial population p of size n.
3. While finishing condition is not satisfied do:
4. Compute a fitness function for each chromosome.
5. Choose chromosome parents by some selection criterion.
6. Create a new generation by genetic recombination operator to the parents.
7. Apply mutation to the new generation.
8. Replace partially or totally the current population with the members of the new population.
9. End While.

Let $\Delta\omega, \Delta\phi, \Delta\psi$, be the range of the pitch, yaw and roll angles respectively, and hd, rb and rp the desired parameters. The fitness function can be expressed as

$$fitness = a\Delta\phi + b\Delta\psi + c\Delta\omega - d|h - h_d| - e|r_b - r_{bd}| - f|r_p - r_{pd}|$$

Where a, b, c, d, e, and f are weights given to each parameter and "d" stands for desired. The value of such weights depends on the importance of each of them for a specific application. Starting with the following set of desired parameters $h_d = 20, r_b = 15, r_p = 15$ with corresponding weights,a=2, b=2, c=0.05, d=10,

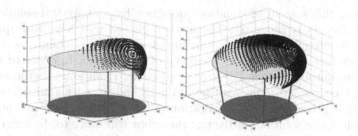

Fig. 3. Left: Workspace computed with conventional algorithms (no GA). Right: Optimized workspace determined via GA.

e=5, f=5 a numerical/graphical solution was found for the optimized workspace. See figure 3, right hand side panel.

Linked with determination of the workspace is the computation of singularities which were calculated numerically in [3]. by an algorithm which checks the Jacobian matrix of the manipulator. Singularities appear at $\omega \in \mathbb{R}, \phi = \psi = 0$, where $\mathbb{R}$ is the set of all real numbers.

3   Inverse Kinematics

In order to move the laser tracker, the end effector of the parallel robot has to be moved to a desired position. So, given the Euler angles ω, ϕ, ψ, the length of the limbs d_i has to be calculated (see figure 2). This problem is referred to as *inverse kinematics*. It is well known that solving the inverse kinematics problem is easy for parallel robots. Nevertheless it is the other way around for serial robots. The 3SPS-1S inverse kinematics problem was also solved in [3] and is given by the following expression:

$$d_i = \sqrt{(b_{xi} - a_{xi})^2 + (b_{yi} - a_{yi})^2 + (b_{zi} + h)^2} \tag{1}$$

Where $\mathbf{a}_i = [a_{xi}, a_{yi}, 0]^T$ be the vector from origin O to point $\mathbf{A}_i$ in the xyz system, $^B b_i$ the vector from origin P to point $\mathbf{B}_i$ in the rotating system uvw, $\mathbf{p} = [0, 0, h]^T$ the vector between points O and P. See figure 2. Rotation matrices are not included here but they are well explained in [4], [16].

4   Solving Direct Kinematics with ANN

The direct or forward kinematics problem is to deduce the orientation of the moving platform (ω, ϕ, ψ) when the limbs length $d_i, i = 1, 2, 3$ are known (see equation 1 and figure 2). This means that a system defined by equations 1 and 2 has to be solved:

$$\begin{bmatrix} b_{xi} \\ b_{yi} \\ b_{zi} \end{bmatrix} = {}^A R_B \begin{bmatrix} b_{xi} \\ b_{yi} \\ b_{zi} \end{bmatrix}, {}^A R_B = \begin{bmatrix} c_\phi c_\psi & -c_\phi s_\psi & s_\phi \\ c_\omega s_\psi + c_\psi s_\omega s_\phi & c_\omega c_\psi - s_\omega s_\phi s_\psi & -c_\phi s_\omega \\ s_\omega s_\psi - c_\omega c_\psi s_\phi & c_\psi s_\omega + c_\omega s_\phi s_\psi & c_\omega c_\phi \end{bmatrix} \tag{2}$$

Obviously this system of equations does not have analytical solution and a numerical method is necessary. The method chosen was Newton-Raphson but this algorithm requires to provide an initial value close enough to the actual solution but such solution is the unknown of the system. In order to find such approximate initial value an ANN was proposed. Traditional methods to solve the direct kinematics problem in the 3SPS-1S end up with multiple solutions, meaning that given an initial orientation of the platform it is not possible to know which of the solutions is the one the robot will move to. In order to allow only one solution, an ANN-based method was proposed in [3] to calculate the direct kinematics but based in the current position of the platform. So, this ANN consists of six inputs, three outputs, and two hidden layers. One of them with eight neurons and the other with two. See figure 4. The inputs of the ANN are the length of the three limbs and the octant of point B_i. The outputs are the three angles used to construct a rotation matrix $^A R_B$ (see equation 2 and [3]). The ANN is trained with a back propagation scheme. A data set of 1000 samples was obtained by varying the Euler angles (one at a time) with a resolution of 1 degree and determining d_1, d_2, d_3 was done by means of inverse kinematics (see equation 1).

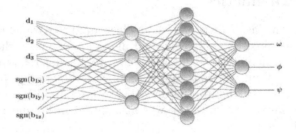

Fig. 4. ANN used to determine the 3SPS-1S forward kinematics

For any given length of the limbs and initial position of the platform, it is possible to find an approximate solution to the direct kinematics using the trained ANN. Once the approximate solution is found, equation 1 can be written three times (one for each limb) and the system of three nonlinear equations can be solved using the Newton-Raphson's method. A validation set consisting of 100 positions was used to check the method. The result error between the two trajectories was negligible. The direct kinematics numerical/graphical computation is shown in figure 5.

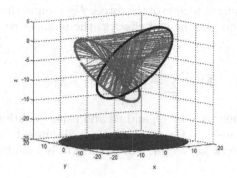

Fig. 5. Direct or forward kinematics determined by an ANN

5 Dynamics

In kinematics there exists two issues: direct and inverse problems (see section 4 and 3). Linked with this, there are also two issues in dynamics, direct and inverse problems. Direct (or forward) dynamics means that given the forces or torques in the actuators which move a robot, determine the trajectory (and its time derivatives) of the end effector. Inverse dynamics means that given the trajectory of the end effector (moving platform), compute the necessary forces/torques required to get such trajectory [16], [9]. In [4] the direct and inverse dynamics models were obtained. Specially for this kind of parallel robot, getting the direct dynamics model is more suitable because its input model is a set of torques or a set of forces. The computation of a control law will provide the right forces/torques, so in order to simulate the behavior of the system, the forward dynamics of the manipulator is needed [4]. In order to simplify the notation, for any vector e with x, y and z components, a matrix e^* will be defined as follows (recall that $\times$ means vector cross product):

$$e \times a = e^*a, \quad with \quad e^* = \begin{bmatrix} 0 & -z & y \\ z & 0 & -x \\ -y & x & 0 \end{bmatrix} \tag{3}$$

where a is an arbitrary 3×1 vector.

In order to simplify the model, it is considered that each leg is just one body that changes its length. Let J_i be the inertia moment of the leg around its x and y axis, τ_i be the force produced by the actuator on point $\mathbf{B}_i$ along the unit vector $\mathbf{s}_i$, and $\mathbf{f}_N$ a force perpendicular to $\mathbf{s}_i$, where $\mathbf{s}_i$ is the unit vector going from point $\mathbf{A}_i$ to point $\mathbf{B}_i$, due to the inertia. We have:

$$\mathbf{f}_i = \tau_i \mathbf{s}_i + \mathbf{f}_{Ni} \tag{4}$$

Let $\mathbf{M}_N$ be the resultant torque of the forces f_{Ni} around the center of the platform. If $\mathbf{M}$ is the torque on the end effector, the moment equilibrium equation may be written as:

$$\mathbf{M} = \sum_{i=1}^{3} \tau_i \left(\mathbf{PB}_i \times \mathbf{s}_i \right) + \mathbf{M}_N \tag{5}$$

Following the method used by [9] and [4] and using equations (4) and (5), the forward or direct dynamics of the manipulator is obtained below where $\ddot{\mathbf{x}}_p$ is the moving platform acceleration vector. Notice that (6) is a nonlinear vector-matrix differential equation:

$$\ddot{\mathbf{x}}_p = (\mathbf{T}_1 - \mathbf{V}_1)^{-1} \left(J^T \tau - \mathbf{T}_2 + \mathbf{V}_2 \right) \tag{6}$$

where

$$T_1 = I_p$$

$$T_2 = \boldsymbol{\omega}_p \times (I_p \boldsymbol{\omega}_p)$$

$$U_{1i} = -\mathbf{b}_i^*$$

$$U_{2i} = \boldsymbol{\omega}_p \times (\boldsymbol{\omega}_p \times \mathbf{b}_i)$$

$$\mathbf{V}_1 = \sum_{i=1}^{3} \frac{J_i}{d_i^2} \mathbf{b}_i^* \mathbf{s}_i^{*2} \mathbf{U}_{1i}$$

$$\mathbf{V}_2 = \sum_{i=1}^{3} \frac{J_i}{d_i^2} \mathbf{b}_i^* \mathbf{s}_i^{*2} \mathbf{U}_{2i}$$

and I_p is the inertia matrix of the platform, ω_p the angular velocity of the platform, $\mathbf{b}_i$ the vector going from point P to point B_i, and d_i the length of the ith leg, $i = 1, 2, 3$, [4], [15], [9]. The inertial effect caused by the laser unit mass was considered by increasing the moving platform mass, altering global inertial effects in equation 6. So, the parallel robot plus the laser beam unit, i.e., the laser tracker system considered here is represented by equation 6. The latter will be the plant controlled by AI algorithms and by classical control schemes according to the next section.

6   Modelling the Interaction between the Two Robots in Industrial Environment

Recall that it is assumed that the parallel robot-based laser tracker system is used to asses a serial robot tracking performance. As it was explained in the Abstract, the serial manipulator suffers deviations from its reference signal as time goes by. Time to check up. Naturally, the serial arm works in industrial environment, which implies that its tracking control algorithm can deal with disturbances (vibrations) produced in the factory, i.e., welding line. This fact implies that the parallel robot also has to deal with these disturbances in order to warrant a good deviation test for the serial manipulator. In order to accomplish this goal, two classical controllers were evaluated: a linear one, a PID (proportional, derivative, integral) controller and a nonlinear one, a SMC (sliding mode controller). Later, two fuzzy logic controllers were tested: a fuzzy proportional-derivative (F-PD) controller and a fuzzy sliding mode controller (F-SMC), which is actually a fuzzy sliding mode proportional controller. See sections 7 and 8. The persistent perturbation $p(t)$ which models the vibration of other machines and which affects our laser tracker performance is defined as $p(t) = 0.1sin(2\pi(5)t)$. The reason about why to consider 0.1 as amplitude and 5 Hz as frequency will be given next. It is assumed that the serial arm moves according to a reference signal given by $r(t) = 0.5sin(2\pi(0.5)t)$. Although the serial robot is an industrial arm with six degrees of freedom, for the purposes of tracking calibration it will move as a three degrees of freedom robot. The base will rotate from left to right and, by keeping fixed three joints, the equivalent upper structure will be a two degrees of freedom serial robot (see figure 1). The latter structure will develop an up-down sinusoid motion for its end effector. This equivalent two degrees of freedom serial robot is a well known nonlinear dynamical system [13] which was modeled, controlled (by a F-SMC) and simulated in [18]. As this serial arm exhibited a very good performance with the above mentioned controller [18], for the current experiment its output position was recorded in Simulink. This signal was used as the reference signal for the parallel robot, modeling in this way that the laser beam mounted on the parallel robot is linked to the SMR on the serial robot end effector. As a consequence, the parallel robot (laser tracker) will have to move considering $\omega = 0.01$, ϕ is the signal recorded in Simlink from the serial manipulator and which has to approximate $\phi = 0.5sin(2\pi(0.5)t)$, and $\psi = t$. The latter provide a side to side swiping in order to track the y-axis motions of the serial arm and ϕ tracks the sinusoid signal done by the serial robot. Finally, $\omega = 0.01$ keeps a fixed $\omega \neq 0$ away from its singularity. On the other hand, the disturbance amplitude is considered as one fifth of the parallel robot's reference signals ϕ and the frequency is ten times higher, 5 Hz.

7   Classical Controllers: PID and SMC

As it was mentioned before, two classical (crisp) controllers are tested here in terms of performance. Later, they will be compared with their AI-based counterparts. The general control loop used in this work is shown in figure 6 where the controller will be generic and will be either classical or intelligent. It is remarkable that the blocks are very complex and details are omitted. Note for instance that the Euler angles have to be transformed to actuator variables by means of the inverse kinematics blocks (see expression 1). Although equations are mathematically enough to describe a dynamical system, the gap between models and numerical implementation is huge. See also section 8.3. It is remarkable that in figure 6 each block contains many sub blocks and MATLAB scripts (not provided here). They contain the equations described through all the paper.

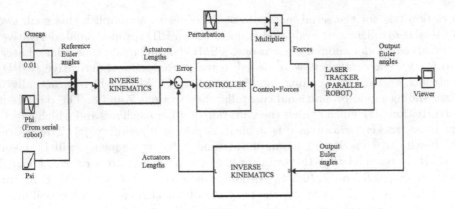

Fig. 6. Generic closed loop for all the control schemes

7.1 Proportional Derivative Integral Controller (PID)

A PID controller was implemented in the model environment described above. Recall that a PID-control law is defined by

$$u = K_P \tilde{x} + K_D \dot{\tilde{x}} + \int \tilde{x} dt \tag{7}$$

Where u is the control law, $\tilde{x} = x_d - x$ is the error of the closed loop system, x_d is a desired variable (reference, see figure 7), and x is an actual variable to be compared with the reference. The resulting positions of the perturbed laser tracker are given in figure 8. It is clear that the PID can not deal neither with disturbances nor with the parallel robot dynamics.

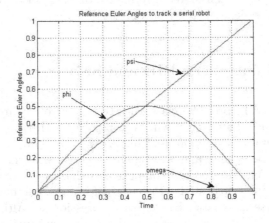

Fig. 7. Euler angles references for the parallel robot to track the serial manipulator

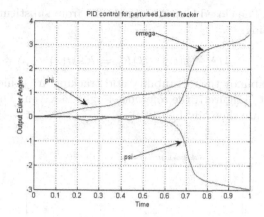

Fig. 8. PID control of the laser tracker parallel robot disturbed

7.2 Nonlinear Control: Sliding Mode Controller (SMC)

It was mentioned that equation 6 is referred to as direct or forward dynamics. In this section, it is more convenient to consider its dual, i.e., the inverse dynamics. The inverse dynamics model is more suitable to design nonlinear controllers as the SMC. Renaming $M_p = T_1 - V_1$, $K_p = T_2 - V_2$, $u = J^T \tau$ where "p" stands for platform, equation 6 can be written as equation 8:

$$M_p \ddot{\mathbf{x}}_p + K_p = u \tag{8}$$

It is well known that a sliding mode regime allows asymptotic stability and asymptotic tracking via Lyapunov theory [13]. Such regime is accomplished by a suitable controller designed in terms of the sliding variable s which allows the state variables of the dynamical model to converge to an invariant set referred to as sliding hyperplane. The sliding variable s and its corresponding time derivative are given by the following equations [13]:

$$s = \dot{\tilde{x}} + \lambda \tilde{x}, \, \tilde{x} = x_d - x, \lambda > 0 \tag{9}$$

$$\dot{s} = \ddot{\tilde{x}} + \lambda \dot{\tilde{x}} \tag{10}$$

Where x_d is the desired variable (reference to follow) and x is the interest variable, a state variable or a generalized coordinate. In the sense of [13] the control law which can deal with the above mentioned disturbance in sliding mode regime was designed as follows:

$$u = (M_p \ddot{x}_{pd} + p(t)K_p + M_p \Lambda \dot{\tilde{x}}_p) - K sat(s), \Lambda = \lambda I, K = kI, k > 0 \tag{11}$$

Where $sat(s)$ stands for saturation function of s and I is the identity matrix. The last summand in the latter equation is a compensation term which achieves the sliding regime. The closed loop system results from substituting equation 11 in equation 8 yielding:

$$M\dot{s} + (p(t)I - I)K_p = K sat(s) \qquad (12)$$

By means of Lyapunov theory stability and tracking are achieved [13],[18]. In figure 9 a zoom out of figure 7, the reference angles, is given. The corresponding perturbed outputs are shown in figure 10.

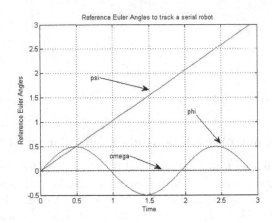

Fig. 9. Reference angles for the laser tracker parallel robot

Notice that the SMC in figure 10 takes three seconds of transient time to control the angles of the laser tracker. The steady state comes after the third second of simulation (not shown to increase detail). So, this performance is relatively good (via irregular transient time). It is noteworthy mention that although SMC is very robust and -in general- provide good close loop performance, its computation may take long time and frequently ends up with numerical stiff problems as a consequence of the highly nonlinear closed loop, i.e., plant plus controller. The SMC parameters used were $\lambda = 0.33$ and $k = 1$.

8   Artificial Intelligence-Based Controllers

Next, the AI version of the latter PID and SMC controllers are assessed here. It is well known that AI-based controllers have good performance in difficult situations as partially known models of a plant, complex (nonlinear) systems, etc, [7].

8.1   Fuzzy Proportional-Derivative Controller (F-PD)

Given the reference inputs shown in figure 9 the performance achieved by this controller can be examined by observing the laser tracker outputs in picture 12.

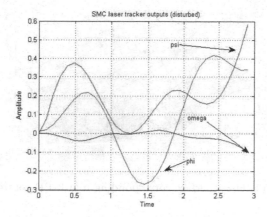

Fig. 10. Disturbed laser tracker outputs with SMC

It can be seen that the tracking goal is reasonably well achieved after a transient period of five seconds. It is noteworthy mention that the fuzzy algorithm is rather simple (a Mamdani -based one [7], [17]) but it could deal reasonably well with the disturbance in order to have a good performance. The decision table is given below where, as usual, symbols mean N=Negative, ZE=Zero, P=Positive, B=Big, M=Medium, S=Small.

Table 1. Fuzzy Rules for the F-PD

$\tilde{x}\|\dot{\tilde{x}}$	NB	N	ZE	P	PB
NB	NB	NB	NB	N	ZE
N	PB	PB	N	ZE	P
Z	NB	N	ZE	P	PB
P	N	Z	P	PB	PB

Notice that the irregular surface (static nonlinearity) helps to deal well with the disturbance and keeps a good closed loop performance. The transient time is about three seconds and the slope of the ramp signal is maintained from second four. The F-PID succeeded because its input/output characteristic approximates statically a sliding mode regime [18], [7]. Of course the classical PID controller can not compete with this F-PD controller (compare figures 8 and 12).

8.2   Fuzzy Sliding Mode Controller (F-SMC)

The idea behind this controller is to become fuzzy the sliding variable s via a fuzzy decision vector. The sliding mode regime requires for s to stay in the plane (or hyperplane) defined by equation 9. A control law u will be in charge of

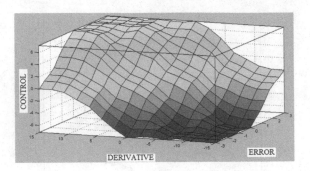

Fig. 11. Fuzzy surface corresponding to a F-PD control

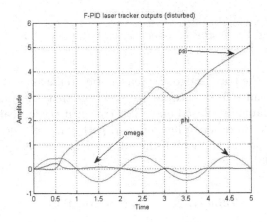

Fig. 12. Disturbed outputs in the laser tracker system controlled by a F-PID

that. Such control law will be designed quite close to the one given by equation 11, but an extra term w will be added. This w will give a fuzzy component in the controller. As there are three Euler angles to control, there must exist three identical sets of fuzzy rules, respectively. These fuzzy rules have to provide the control to reach the sliding plane.

1. if s is NB then u is PB
2. if s is NM then u is PM
3. if s is NS then u is PS
4. if s is ZE then u is ZE
5. if s is PS then u is NS
6. if s is PM then u is NM
7. if s is PB then u is NB

Membership functions were chosen triangular in the middle and trapezoids at the extremes. Fuzzy controllers of this type define *nonlinearities as well but static.* More precisely, fuzzy rules surfaces are *nonlinear static (memory-less) bounded sector nonlinearities* [18], [7]. The input-output surface (actually a curve) for the set of rules shown above is a distorted straight line (not shown). That is why this fuzzy control is only proportional. Now it is necessary to define the sliding control law as it was done in equation 11. Adding an extra compensation term w to equation 11 yields equation 13:

$$u = (M_p \ddot{x}_{pd} + p(t)K_p + M_p \Lambda \dot{\tilde{x}}_p) - K sat(s) + w, \Lambda = \lambda I, K = kI, k > 0 \quad (13)$$

Again, by Lyapunov theory a positive definite function was chosen in such a way that its derivative can be negative definite in order to warrant stability and tracking (see section 7.2 and [13], [18]).

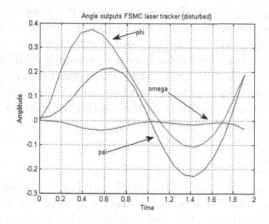

Fig. 13. Outputs from laser tracker system controlled by a FSMC

In this case the performance obtained is poor with respect to the reference signal. Compare figures 9, 10 and 13. The reason is that the fuzzy decision rules have one input and one output and this construction is not enough to deal with this problem. Lyapunov theory indicates that the control law given by equation 13 will work properly as long as the variable w provides enough energy. This is not the case for this system. Note that the set of rules of the F-SMC defines only a *proportional sliding mode controller*. Nevertheless a F-SMC did achieved a good performance for a simpler nonlinear dynamics, the robot described in [18].

8.3   Numerical Considerations for Both Sets of Controllers

Consider the crisp PID and SMC controllers. The former defines a linear structure which uses the error signal $\tilde{x}$ as an input. It is a very simple controller which can not go further. The latter, the SMC is a nonlinear controller which uses the sliding variable s and its derivative $\dot{s}$ as inputs. The general success of a SMC is that the states variables converges to an attractive (invariant) set.

However, as the control law is discontinuous (switching variable) as a result of the saturation (or signum) functions [13], the entire closed loop may produces numerical stiffness. In addition, as known, plants as serial or parallel robots are highly nonlinear with coupled equations which worsen the discretization process from the continuous domain. The simulations presented in this work were done in MATLAB/Simulink and a multiplicity of another numerical problems were present as tolerances, integration method, step size, algebraic loops, data dependency violations (as a result of the sorting order and asynchronous tasks associated with the subsystems), etc. On the other hand, in the case of the fuzzy controllers, the F-PID was designed in terms of a set of rules which defines a *proportional derivative fuzzy controller* which showed a relatively good performance. Note in this case that the fuzzy control output w is a function of $\tilde{x}, \dot{\tilde{x}}$, i.e., $w = f(\tilde{x}, \dot{\tilde{x}})$ and that makes w richer to compute a control signal. Nevertheless, when a F-SMC was implemented, as a result of a the poverty of the rules (in spite of being computed with respect to the sliding variable s) and because of the complexity of the plant model (the parallel robot) the general performance was poor. In contrast, compare for instance a successful F-SMC implementation to control a serial robot in [18]. Nevertheless, that serial robot model was simpler than the parallel robot representation studied here. In general, parallel robots have more complicated dynamics than their serial counterparts as a result of existence of closed kinematic chains [19], [13].

9   Conclusions

An integral viewpoint with ANN, GA, and Fuzzy Logic was used in this study. In this work, a parallel robot-based laser tracker system was designed step-by-step analytically, from kinematics and workspace to the dynamic model and controllers. In particular cases, analytical solutions could not be found and conventional (not AI-based) numerical algorithms had to be created. However, even these numerical solutions were not precise enough and AI had to be applied (recall the case of the computation of the workspace and direct kinematics of the laser tracker, where ANN and GA were needed). Although it was possible to mathematically obtain a dynamical model, its numerical implementation was difficult to do as a result of the implicit nonlinear and cross products expressions. It is famous that parallel robots are very difficult to deal with, either modeling them or simulating them. In addition to the laser tracker model proposed, an interacting environment with another robot and industry perturbations was mathematically designed to mimic a calibration process of the welding serial robot. All the later creates a complex system to deal with. That is why classical controllers and AI (fuzzy based) controllers were assessed. For this application, the F-PID controller achieved better performance (specially during the transient period). In addition, its complexity is much more lower than the SMC and the F-SMC. All of these can be improved by some auto adjusting extra mechanism but definitely, it has to be helped by other crisp nonlinear controllers. It has to be remarked that the gap between mathematical models and numerical simulations always has to be taken into account.

References

1. Bai, S., Hansen, M.R.: Evaluation of Workspace of a Spherical Robotic Wrist. In: 2007 IEEE/ASME International Conference on Advanced Intelligent Mechatronics, pp. 1–6. IEEE (2007)
2. Burge, J., Peng, S., Zobrist, T.: Use of a commercial laser tracker for optical alignment. In: Proc. of SPIE, pp. 1–12. Optical System Alignment and Tolerancing (2007)
3. Chaparro-Altamirano, D., Zavala-Yoé, R., Ramírez-Mendoza, R.: Kinematic and Workspace Analysis of a Parallel Robot used in Security Applications. In: Proc. IEEE International Conference on Mechatronics, Electronics and Automotive Engineering, Cuernavaca, Morelos, Mexico. IEEE (2007)
4. Chaparro-Altamirano, D., Zavala-Yoé, R., Ramírez-Mendoza, R.: Dynamics and Control of a 3SPS-1S Parallel Robot Used in Security Applications. In: 21st International Symposium on Mathematical Theory of Networks and Systems, MTNS, Groningen, The Netherlands (2014)
5. Craig, J.J.: Introduction to Robotics: Mechanics and Control. Prentice Hall (2004)
6. Cui, G., Zhang, Y.: Kinetostatic Modeling and Analysis of a New 3-DOF Parallel Manipulator. In: 2009 International Conference on Computational Intelligence and Software Engineering, pp. 1–4. IEEE (December 2009)
7. Driankov, D., Hellendorn, H., Reinfrank, M.: An Introduction to Fuzzy Control. Springer (1996)
8. Gan, D., Dias, J., Seneviratne, L.: Design and Analytical Kinematics of a Robot Wrist Based on a Parallel Mechanism. In: World Automation Congress, pp. 1–6 (2012)
9. Merlet, J.P.: Parallel Robots. Solid Mechanics and its Applications. Springer (2006)
10. Mitchell, M.: An Introduction to Genetic Algorithms. The MIT Press, Cambridge (1996)
11. Prenninger, J.P., Filz, K.M., Incze, M., Gander, H.: Use of a commercial laser tracker for optical alignment. Measurment 4, 255–264 (1995); Optical System Alignment and Tolerancing
12. Shang, Y., Li, G.J.: New crossover operators in genetic algorithms. In: Proceedings of the T hird International Conference on Tools for Artificial Intelligence, pp. 150–153 (1991)
13. Slotine, J., Li, W.: Applied Nonlinear Control. Pearson Education (1991)
14. Tsai, L.-W.: Kinematics of A Three-Dof Platform with Three Extensible Limbs. In: Recent Advances in Robot Kinematics, ch. 8, pp. 401–410. Springer (1996)
15. Tsai, L.W.: Solving The Inverse Dynamics of Parallel Manipulators by The Principle of Virtual Work. In: ASME Design Eng. Tech. Conf., pp. 451–457 (1998)
16. Tsai, L.W.: Robot Analysis: The Mechanics of Serial and Parallel Manipulators. John Wiley & Sons, Inc. (1999)
17. Zadeh, L.A.: Fuzzy sets. Information and Control, 338–353 (1965)
18. Zavala-Yoé, R.: Fuzzy Control of Second Order Vectorial Systems: L2 Stability. In: Proc. of European Control Conference, Brussels, Belgium (1997)
19. Zavala-Yoé, R.: Modelling and Control of Dynamical Systems: Numerical Implementation in a Behavioral Framework. SCI, vol. 124. Springer, Heidelberg (2008)
20. Zlatanov, D., Bonev, I., Gosselin, C.: Constraint Singularities as C-Space Singularities. In: 8th International Symposium on Advances in Robot Kinematics, Caldes de Malavella, Spain (2002)

Simple Direct Propositional Encoding
of Cooperative Path Finding Simplified Yet More[*]

Pavel Surynek

Charles University Prague, Faculty of Mathematics and Physics
Malostranské náměstí 25, 118 00 Praha 1, Czech Republic
pavel.surynek@mff.cuni.cz

Abstract. This paper addresses makespan optimal solving of cooperative path-finding problem (CPF) by translating it to propositional satisfiability (SAT). The task in CPF is to relocate a set of agents to given goal locations so that they do not collide with each other. Recent findings indicate that a simple direct encoding outperforms the more elaborate encodings based on binary encodings of multi-value state variables. The direct encoding is further improved by a hierarchical build-up that uses auxiliary variables to reduce its size in this work. The conducted experimental evaluation shown that the simple design of the encoding together with new improvements which reduced its size significantly are key enablers for faster solving of the encoded CPFs than with existing encodings. It has been also shown that the SAT based methods dominates over A* based methods in environments with high occupancy by agents.

Keywords: Cooperative path-finding (CPF), propositional satisfiability (SAT), SAT encodings, A*.

1 Introduction, Motivation, and Related Works

The problem of *cooperative path-finding* (CPF) [13, 18, 20, 24] represents an abstraction for variety of problems where the task is to relocate some physical agents, robots, or other objects so that they do not collide with each other. Each agent is given its initial position in a certain environment and its task is to reach a given goal position. It is assumed that all the agents are the same (same size and velocity) and are controlled centrally.

The major difficulty in CPF comes from possible interactions among relocated agents, which is imposed by the requirement that they must not collide with each other. The more agents appear in the instance the more complex interaction arises and consequently the instance is harder to solve.

There are many **motivations** for introducing CPF. Classical multi-robot relocation problems where agents are represented by actual mobile robots can be viewed as CPF. Planning movements of units in real-time strategy games is another application [24]. Even data relocation in a network can be regarded a CPF (agent is represented by a data packet and spatial occupancy turns into storage occupancy).

---

[*]This work is supported by the Czech Science Foundation (contract no. GAP103/10/1287).

A. Gelbukh et al. (Eds.): MICAI 2014, Part II, LNAI 8857, pp. 410–425, 2014.
© Springer International Publishing Switzerland 2014

The indifference between agents in terms of their properties allows abstraction where the environment is modeled as an undirected graph and agents as items placed in vertices of this graph [20, 24]. At most one agent is placed in each vertex. The time is discrete and the move is possible only into a currently unoccupied vertex while no other agent is allowed to enter the same target vertex.

Contemporary approaches to solving CPF include polynomial time sub-optimal algorithms [13, 25] as well as methods that generate optimal solutions in certain sense [21, 22]. This work focuses on generating *makespan optimal* solutions to CPF where the makespan is the maximum of arrive times over all the agents. **Related** makespan optimal methods for CPF currently include methods employing translation of CPF to *propositional satisfiability* (SAT) [22, 23], methods based on *conflict resolution* between paths for individual agents [19], and classical *A* based methods* equipped with powerful heuristics [21]. The first mentioned approach excels in relatively small environments with high density of agents while latter two approaches are better in large environments with few agents.

This work tries to contribute to SAT-based methods. It is inspired by our recent (unpublished) findings that quite complex and elaborate propositional encodings called INVERSE and ALL-DIFFERENT proposed in [22] and [23] can be easily outperformed by an encoding of a straightforward design. The direct encoding design is further simplified here by introducing auxiliary variables. The introduces simplifications reduced the size of the encoding significantly which in turn enabled faster solving of CPFs encoded using the proposed encoding. It is also shown how the SAT-based solving stands in comparison with A* based methods.

The **organization** of the paper is as follows. The CPF problem is introduced formally first. Then a theoretical study of sizes of CPF encodings is provided. A novel propositional encoding of CPF is described thereafter and its theoretical properties are summarized. Experimental evaluation in which existing encodings and the A* based method are compared with the novel encoding constitute the last part.

2   Cooperative Path Planning Formally

An arbitrary **undirected graph** can be used to model the environment where agents are moving. Let $G = (V, E)$ be such a graph where $V = \{v_1, v_2, ..., v_n\}$ is a finite set of vertices and $E \subseteq \binom{V}{2}$ is a set of edges. The placement of agents in the environment is modeled by assigning them vertices of the graph. Let $A = \{a_1, a_2, ..., a_\mu\}$ be a finite set of *agents*. Then, an arrangement of agents in vertices of graph G will be fully described by a *location* function $\alpha: A \longrightarrow V$; the interpretation is that an agent $a \in A$ is located in a vertex $\alpha(a)$. At most **one agent** can be located in each vertex; that is α is uniquely invertible. A generalized inverse of α denoted as $\alpha^{-1}: V \longrightarrow A \cup \{\bot\}$ will provide us an agent located in a given vertex or $\bot$ if the vertex is empty.

Definition 1 (COOPERATIVE PATH FINDING). An instance of *cooperative path-finding* problem is a quadruple $\Sigma = [G = (V, E), A, \alpha_0, \alpha^+]$ where location functions α_0 and α^+ define the initial and the goal arrangement of a set of agents A in G respectively. $\square$

The dynamicity of the model supposes a discrete time divided into time steps. An arrangement α_i at the i-th time step can be transformed by a transition action which instantaneously moves agents in the non-colliding way to form a new arrangement α_{i+1}. The resulting arrangement α_{i+1} must satisfy the following *validity conditions*:

(i) $\forall a \in A$ either $\alpha_i(a) = \alpha_{i+1}(a)$ or $\{\alpha_i(a), \alpha_{i+1}(a)\} \in E$ holds   (1)
        (agents move along edges or not move at all),

(ii) $\forall a \in A \ \alpha_i(a) \neq \alpha_{i+1}(a) \Rightarrow \alpha_i^{-1}(\alpha_{i+1}(a)) = \bot$ (2)
        (agents move to vacant vertices only), and

(iii) $\forall a, b \in A \ a \neq b \Rightarrow \alpha_{i+1}(a) \neq \alpha_{i+1}(b)$ (3)
        (no two agents enter the same target/unique invertibility of resulting arrangement).

The task in cooperative path finding is to transform α_0 using above valid transitions to α_+. An illustration of CPF and its solution is depicted in Figure 1.

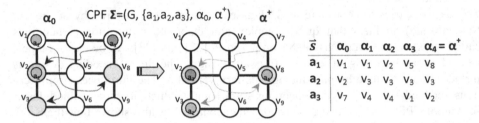

Fig. 1. Cooperative *path-finding (CPF)* on a *4-connected grid.* The task is to relocate three agents a_1, a_2, and a_3 to their goal vertices so that they do not collide with each other. A solution $\vec{s}$ of makespan 4 is shown.

Definition 2 (SOLUTION, MAKESPAN). A *solution* of a *makespan* m to a cooperative path finding instance $\Sigma = [G, A, \alpha_0, \alpha^+]$ is a sequence of arrangements $\vec{s} = [\alpha_0, \alpha_1, \alpha_2, ..., \alpha_m]$ where $\alpha_m = \alpha^+$ and α_{i+1} is a result of valid transformation of α_i for every $= 1, 2, ..., m - 1$.   □

If it is a question whether there exists a solution of Σ of the makespan at most a given bound η we are speaking about a *bounded CPF (bCPF)*. It is known that bCPF is NP-complete and finding makespan optimal solution to CPF is NP-hard [15].

3   Theoretical Analysis of SAT Encodings of CPF

The goal is to build a propositional formula $F(\Sigma, \eta)$ for a given bCPF Σ and a makespan bound η so that $F(\Sigma, \eta)$ has a model (is satisfiable) if and only if Σ has a solution of makespan η. A sequence of arrangements of agents $\alpha_0, \alpha_1, \alpha_2, ..., \alpha_\eta$ over the graph forming the solution should be readable from the model of $F(\Sigma, \eta)$. The idea of *time expansion graph* [1, 12] is adopted to construct such formula.

If it is known how many propositional variables are needed to express sequence of consecutive arrangements of agents over the graph, then it can seen how far from these bounds the suggested encoding is. Following propositions summarize estimations of the number of necessary propositional variables considering various approaches to express the arrangements. The presented estimations assume that almost every arrangement is possible at any time step.

Also, encodings need to be considered as sparse representations. Otherwise it would be possible to count the total number of distinct sequences of arrangements and take binary logarithm of this number as the estimation. Such an encoding is however impractical as it is hard to decode.

Proposition 1 (LOCATION-ESTIMATION). *Let η be a makespan bound. Then $\eta \cdot \mu \cdot \lceil \log_2 n \rceil$ propositional variables are sufficient to express consecutive arrangements of agents up to the time step η.* ∎

Proof. A technique of expressing a multi-value state variable using vectors of propositional variables that encode individual values as binary numbers will be used. There are n possible states of an agent at every time – the agent can appear in any vertex of the input graph. To represent an n-state variable, $\lceil \log_2 n \rceil$ bits (propositional variables) are needed. Hence, we have $\eta \cdot \mu \cdot \lceil \log_2 n \rceil$ propositional variables in total to represent locations of all the agents (there are μ agents) at every time step. ∎

Proposition 2 (INVERSE- ESTIMATION). *Consecutive arrangements of agents up to the time step η can be expressed by $\lceil \frac{\eta}{2} \rceil \cdot n \cdot \lceil \log_2 \mu \rceil + \eta \cdot n$ propositional variables.* ∎

Proof. Instead of expressing where each agent is located, the content of vertices will be recorded. The crucial observation is that at most $\lceil \eta/2 \rceil$ changes of agents can occur in a single vertex (an agent must leave the vertex after which another agent can enter the vertex – the change consumes 2 time-steps). Information what agent entered the vertex is again multi-value state variable with μ states. Hence, $\lceil \log_2 \mu \rceil$ bits are needed to record it. Altogether, $\lceil \eta/2 \rceil \cdot n \cdot \lceil \log_2 \mu \rceil$ bits are needed to record possible changes for all the agents. Additional η bits per vertex indicate time-steps at which the change in the vertex occurred. ∎

The INVERSE encoding [22] partially use the idea presented in the proof. However, the content of vertices is recorded for all the time-steps (not only for half of them as here). An interesting way to represent arrangements of agents at all the time-steps is to record changes between consecutive arrangements while only the initial arrangement is recorded completely.

Proposition 3 (NEIGHBORHOOD-ESTIMATION). *Let $\delta = max_{v \in V} \, deg(v)$ and let the initial arrangement α_0 be expressible using $a \in \mathbb{N}$ propositional variables, then consecutive arrangements of agents up to the time step η can be expressed by $a + \eta \cdot \mu \cdot \lceil \log_2 (\delta + 1) \rceil$ propositional variables.* ∎

Proof. The idea is to record what move has been taken by each agent. Assume that neighbors of each vertex in G have a fixed order, then the move of an agent can be encoded as an order number of the neighbor into which it moved. Assuming that the degree (the number of edges incident with the given vertex) of all the vertices in G is at most δ, the move of an agent can be recorded by $\lceil \log_2 (\delta + 1) \rceil$ bits (an extra state is needed to represent the no move action). Altogether, $\eta \cdot \mu \cdot \lceil \log_2 (\delta + 1) \rceil$ bits are sufficient to record moves of all the agents at all the time steps. ∎

The estimation gives good results in sparse graphs since each vertex has few neighbors in such a case. This property is partially used in the INVERSE encoding again. However, the estimation may degenerate up to the location-based estimation if the graph is highly connected.

Note that up to now two of three options of how to regard the 3-dimensional space of vertices, agents, and time-steps have been discussed. It remains to show an estimation in which we ask at what time-steps a given agent appears in given vertex. As a single agent may enter a vertex multiple times, the simple scheme in which multi-value state variable representing the third dimension is indexed by remaining two dimensions can no longer be used. Little of the structural properties of the CPF problem can be used in the estimation.

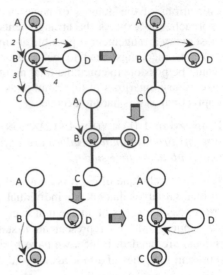

Fig. 2. Illustration *of the **minimum number** of time steps before returning to the same vertex.* The next visit to the vertex can be separated by at least 4 time steps.

Proposition 4 (TIME-BASED ESTIMATION). *Consecutive arrangements of agents in an optimal solution up to the time step η can be expressed by $\left\lceil\frac{\eta}{4}\right\rceil \cdot n \cdot \mu \cdot \lceil \log_2 \eta \rceil$ propositional variables.* ∎

Proof. The most important observation is that at least 4 time steps are allowed to elapse before an agent returns into a given vertex in a makespan optimal solution. Step 1 is for leaving the vertex, steps 2, 3 are for entering and leaving by the other agent, and step 4 is for returning to the vertex – the situation is illustrated in Figure 2. If the agent returns earlier, then the movement can be eliminated from the solution without compromising its optimality or correctness. Hence, a single agent can visit the given vertex at most $\lceil \eta/4 \rceil$ times. Expressing the time step, at which the visit occurs, needs $\lceil \log_2 \eta \rceil$ bits. All these information are recorded for every vertex and every agent, which in total gives $\lceil \eta/4 \rceil \cdot n \cdot \mu \cdot \lceil \log_2 \eta \rceil$ bits. ∎

Other measures and characteristics than the size of the encoding are difficult to be captured as the dependence of behavior of SAT solvers on the structure of the formula is too complex.

4   A Simplification of Simple SAT Encoding

Let us recall a so called DIRECT encoding of bCPF $\Sigma = [G = (V, E), A, \alpha_0, \alpha_+]$ with makespan bound η where $V = \{v_1, v_2, ..., v_n\}$ and $A = \{a_1, a_2, ..., a_\mu\}$ with $n, \mu \in \mathbb{N}$. The DIRECT encoding is part of our unpublished work. As discussed in the previous section, arrangements of agents over the graphs at all the time steps from 1 to μ will be represented. The encoding will use a propositional variable for each vertex, agent, and a time step which will be assigned $TRUE$, if and only if the given agent appears in a given vertex at given time step.

Unlike representations of arrangements using binary encoding of multi-value state variable, this encoding has a propositional variable for every state. Although more propositional variables are needed to encode arrangements, we expect that the benefit of better Boolean constraint propagation outweighs the larger size of the encoding. The suggested encoding will be called DIRECT and is formally introduced in the following definition.

Definition 3 (DIRECT ENCODING). A DIRECT encoding of a given bCPF $\Sigma = [G = (V, E), A, \alpha_0, \alpha_+]$ with makespan bound η consists of propositional variables $\mathcal{X}^i_{j,k}$ for every $i = 0, 1, ..., \eta$, $j = 0, 1, ..., n$, $k = 0, 1, ..., \mu$. The interpretation is that $\mathcal{X}^i_{j,k}$ is assigned $TRUE$ if and only if a_k appears in v_j at time step i. The following constraints modeling validity conditions on consecutive arrangements are introduced:

(a) $\bigwedge^n_{j,l=1, j<l} \neg \mathcal{X}^i_{j,k} \vee \neg \mathcal{X}^i_{l,k}$ for every $i \in \{0, 1, ..., \eta\}$,   (4)
   $\bigvee^n_{j=1} \mathcal{X}^i_{j,k}$ and $k \in \{1, 2, ..., \mu\}$
   (an agent is placed in exactly one vertex at each time step)

(b) $\bigwedge^\mu_{k,h=1, k<h} \neg \mathcal{X}^i_{j,k} \vee \neg \mathcal{X}^i_{j,h}$ for every $i \in \{0, 1, ..., \eta\}$,   (5)
   and $j \in \{1, 2, ..., n\}$
   (at most one agent is placed in each vertex at each time step)

(c) $\mathcal{X}^i_{j,k} \Rightarrow \mathcal{X}^{i+1}_{j,k} \vee \bigvee_{l:\{v_j,v_l\}\in E} \mathcal{X}^{i+1}_{l,k}$ for every $i \in \{0, 1, ..., \eta - 1\}$,   (6)
   $\mathcal{X}^{i+1}_{j,k} \Rightarrow \mathcal{X}^i_{j,k} \vee \bigvee_{l:\{v_j,v_l\}\in E} \mathcal{X}^i_{l,k}$ $j \in \{1, 2, ..., n\}$, and $k \in \{1, 2, ..., \mu\}$
   (an agent relocates to some of its neighbors or makes no move)

(d) $\mathcal{X}^i_{j,k} \wedge \mathcal{X}^{i+1}_{l,k} \Rightarrow \bigwedge^\mu_{h=1} \neg \mathcal{X}^i_{l,h} \wedge \bigwedge^\mu_{h=1} \neg \mathcal{X}^{i+1}_{l,h}$ (7)
   for every $i \in \{0, 1, ..., \eta - 1\}$, $j, l \in \{1, 2, ..., n\}$ such that $\{v_j, v_l\} \in E$
   and $k \in \{1, 2, ..., \mu\}$
   (target vertex of a move must be vacant and the source vertex will be vacant after the move is performed). □

Observe that all the constraints are now written as *clauses* (disjunctions of *literals*, where literal is a variable or its negation) or can be easily rewritten as clauses. Thus, a *conjunctive normal form* (*CNF*) [5] can be easily obtained from Definition 3. The resulting formula modeling existence of solution of given bCPF Σ with makespan bound η in the CNF form will be denoted as $F_{DIR}(\Sigma, \eta)$.

The DIRECT encoding has a significant drawback, which is its size. Particularly (d) constraints produce too many clauses – (d) constraints stand for $2 \cdot \eta \cdot |E| \cdot |A|$ ternary clauses. Using auxiliary variables, this number can be reduced to $2 \cdot \eta \cdot |E|$.

The DIRECT encoding can be improved in another way as well. Constraints (a) can be eliminated without compromising equisatisfiability of bCPF Σ with η and $F_{DIR}(\Sigma, \eta)$. Omitting (a) constraints may cause that a single agent appears multiple times in the graph. Nevertheless, populating a single only makes it harder to find a solution thus does not matter if occurs. The same can be done with the second implication in (c) constraints. Again, it does not compromise equisatisfiability if it is omitted. The absence of constraints may cause appearance of an agent from nothing at a certain time step. Nevertheless, the first implication propagates all the agents towards the last time steps. Hence, extra-appeared agents just only make it harder to find a solution. Note that omitted constraints are not entailed by the rest at the logical level. The equisatisfiability after omitting mentioned constraints need to be seen at the abstract level of the solution existence in bCPF. The resulting encoding will be called SIMPLIFIED and is formally introduced in the following definition.

Definition 4 (SIMPLIFIED ENCODING). A SIMPLIFIED encoding of a given bCPF $\Sigma = [G = (V, E), A, \alpha_0, \alpha_+]$ with makespan bound η consists of propositional variables $\mathcal{X}_{j,k}^i$ and $\mathcal{E}_j^i$ (auxiliary for macros) for every $i = 0,1,\dots,\eta$, $j = 0,1,\dots,n$, $k = 0,1,\dots,\mu$. The interpretation is that $\mathcal{X}_{j,k}^i$ is assigned *TRUE* if and only if a_k appears in v_j at time step i and $\mathcal{E}_j^i$ is *TRUE* if and only if v_j is vacant at time step i. The following constraints modeling validity conditions on consecutive arrangements are introduced:

(A) $\bigwedge_{k,h=1,k<h}^{\mu} \neg \mathcal{X}_{j,k}^i \vee \neg \mathcal{X}_{j,h}^i$ for every $i \in \{0,1,\dots,\eta\}$,   (8)

                             and $j \in \{1,2,\dots,n\}$

  (at most one agent is placed in each vertex at each time step)

(B) $\mathcal{X}_{j,k}^i \Rightarrow \mathcal{X}_{j,k}^{i+1} \vee \bigvee_{l:\{v_j,v_l\}\in E} \mathcal{X}_{l,k}^{i+1}$ for every $i \in \{0,1,\dots,\eta-1\}$,   (9)

                             $j \in \{1,2,\dots,n\}$, and $k \in \{1,2,\dots,\mu\}$

  (an agent relocates to some of its neighbors or makes no move)

(C) $\mathcal{X}_{j,k}^i \wedge \mathcal{X}_{l,k}^{i+1} \Rightarrow \mathcal{E}_l^i \wedge \mathcal{E}_j^{i+1}$ (10)

    for every $i \in \{0,1,\dots,\eta-1\}$, $j,l \in \{1,2,\dots,n\}$ such that $\{v_j, v_l\} \in E$

    and $k \in \{1,2,\dots,\mu\}$

    (target vertex of a move must be vacant and the source vertex will be vacant after the move is performed)

(D) $\mathcal{E}_j^i \Rightarrow \bigwedge_{h=1}^{\mu} \neg \mathcal{X}_{j,h}^i$ (11)

    for every $i \in \{0,1,\dots,\eta\}$, $j \in \{1,2,\dots,n\}$

  (empty vertex macro connected through auxiliary variable). □

Again, all the constraints of the SIMPLIFIED encoding can be written as clauses. Let the resulting formula for bCPF Σ with makespan bound η be denoted $F_{SIM}(\Sigma, \eta)$.

Properties of the DIRECT and SIMPLIFIED Encodings

Let us summarize basic properties of the proposed SIMPLIFIED encoding. The fact that the encoding does what is what designed for is summarized in the following proposition. Further, a discussion is devoted to the size of the encoding.

Proposition 5 (ENCODING SOUNDNESS). *Let* $\Sigma = [G, A, \alpha_0, \alpha_+]$ *be a bCPF and* η *a makespan bound, then* $F_{DIR}(\Sigma, \eta)$ *as well as* $F_{SIM}(\Sigma, \eta)$ *is satisfiable if and only if* Σ *has a solution of makespan* η. *Moreover, the solution of* Σ *can be reconstructed from the model of* $F_{DIR}(\Sigma, \eta)$ *or from* $F_{SIM}(\Sigma, \eta)$. ∎

Sketch of Proof. First, note that the second part of the proposition is important to be stated as it is possible to establish equisatisfiability between a propositional formula and Σ even for trivial cases of the formula from which a solution of Σ cannot be reconstructed.

If there is a solution $\vec{s}$ of Σ with makespan bound η then a model of $F_{DIR}(\Sigma, \eta)$ and $F_{SIM}(\Sigma, \eta)$ can be constructed from $\vec{s}$. Arrangements of agents at individual time-steps within $\vec{s}$ can be directly used to set up variables $\mathcal{X}^i_{j,k}$. Values of auxiliary variables $\mathcal{E}^i_j$ are implied by constraints (C). Validity constraints (i), (ii), and (iii), that the solution $\vec{s}$ has to satisfy, ensure satisfaction of constraints of $F_{DIR}(\Sigma, \eta)$ and $F_{SIM}(\Sigma, \eta)$.

Conversely, if we have a model of $F_{DIR}(\Sigma, \eta)$ or $F_{SIM}(\Sigma, \eta)$ then a sequence of arrangements of agents at individual time-steps can be read out from variables $\mathcal{X}^i_{j,k}$. Constraints of $F_{DIR}(\Sigma, \eta)$ or $F_{SIM}(\Sigma, \eta)$ ensure that valuation of variables $\mathcal{X}^i_{j,k}$ correspond to valid arrangements. Moreover, constraints within the encodings also ensure that movement validity constraints are preserved as well. ∎

Proposition 6 (ENCODING SIZE). *Let $\Sigma = [G = (V, E), A, \alpha_0, \alpha_+]$, where with a bound η be an instance of bCPF. The DIRECT encoding $F_{DIR}(\Sigma, \eta)$ requires*

$$(\eta + 1) \cdot |A| \cdot |V| \qquad (12)$$

$$(\eta + 1) \cdot \left(\binom{|V|}{2} \cdot (|A| + 1) + \binom{|A|}{2} \cdot |V| \right) + \eta \cdot |A| \cdot (|V| + 2 \cdot |E|)$$

propositional variables and clauses respectively.

The SIMPLIFIED encoding $F_{SIM}(\Sigma, \eta)$ requires

$$(\eta + 1) \cdot (|A| + 1) \cdot |V| \qquad (13)$$

$$(\eta + 1) \cdot \left(|V| \cdot |A| + \binom{|A|}{2} \cdot |V| \right) + \eta \cdot |A| \cdot (|V| + 2 \cdot |E|)$$

propositional variables and clauses respectively. ∎

Proof. Let us investigate the DIRECT encoding first. The number of propositional variables can immediately seen from the scope of indexes. The number of clauses appearing in (4), (5), and (6) can be calculated as a product of the size of index scopes. Clauses in (7) will develop into $2 \cdot |A|$ ternary clauses. An analogical calculation can be done for the SIMPLIFIED encoding. ∎

Note that most of clauses in the DIRECT encoding are binary or ternary which supports good performance of Boolean constraint propagation (unit propagation [5]). The same holds for the SIMPLIFIED encoding.

Asymptotically, the number of variables is $\mathcal{O}(\eta \cdot |V| \cdot |A|)$ and the number of clauses is $\mathcal{O}(\eta \cdot |V|^2 \cdot |A|)$ in the DIRECT encoding. If this is compared with the INVERSE encoding [22] where the number of variables is reported to be $\mathcal{O}(\eta \cdot |V|^2 \cdot \log_2|A|)$ and the number of clauses $\mathcal{O}(\eta \cdot |V|^2 \cdot \log_2|A|)$ and with the ALL-DIFFERENT encoding [23] where the number of variables is $\mathcal{O}(\eta \cdot \log_2|V| \cdot |A|^2)$ and the number of clauses is $\mathcal{O}(\eta \cdot \log_2|V| \cdot |V|^2)$, then the size of the DIRECT encoding is larger approximately by the factor of $\mathcal{O}\left(\frac{|A|}{\log_2|A|}\right)$ or $\mathcal{O}\left(\frac{|V|}{\log_2|V|}\right)$ respectively (note that

$|A|$ is dominated by $|V|$). However, the size of clauses is much smaller in case of DIRECT encoding.

The asymptotic number of variables is $O(\eta \cdot |V| \cdot |A|)$ and the number of clauses is $O(\eta \cdot |A| \cdot \max\{|V| \cdot |A|, |E|\})$ in the SIMPLIFIED encoding. Although factor $\max\{|V| \cdot |A|, |E|\}$ in the number of clauses may be up to $|V|^2$, it is smaller in typical CPF instances. Hence in theory, $F_{SIM}(\Sigma, \eta)$ will be smaller than $F_{DIR}(\Sigma, \eta)$ typically.

5   SAT-Based Optimal CPF Solving

The suggested SIMPLIFIED encoding is intended for makespan optimal CPF solving. As it is possible to solve bCPF with given makespan bound η by translating it to SAT, an optimal makespan and corresponding solution can be obtained using multiple queries to a SAT solver with encoded bCPF. Various strategies exist for getting the optimal makespan. The simplest one and very efficient one at the same time is to try sequentially makespan bounds $\eta = 1, 2, \ldots$ until η equal to the optimal makespan is encountered. This strategy will be further referred as *sequential increasing*. The sequential increasing is also used in domain independent planners such as SAT-PLAN [12], SASE [11] and others. Pseudo-code of the strategy is listed as Algorithm 1.

The focus here is on SAT encoding while querying strategies are out of scope of the paper; though let us mention that in depth study of querying strategies is given in [17]. There is a great potential in querying strategies as they can bring speedup of planning process in orders of magnitude, especially when combined with parallel processing.

Algorithm 1. SAT based optimal CPF solving.
  input: a CPF instance Σ
  output: a pair consisting of the optimal makespan
                  and corresponding optimal solution

---

function *Find-Optimal-Solution-Sequentially* $(\Sigma = (G, A, \alpha_0, \alpha^+))$: **pair**
  1:          $\eta \leftarrow 1$
  2:          **loop**
  3:              $F(\Sigma, \eta) \leftarrow$ *Encode-CPF-as-SAT* (Σ, η)
  4:              **if** *Solve-SAT* $(F(\Sigma, \eta))$ **then**
  5:                  $s \leftarrow$ *Extract-Solution-from-Valuation*$(F(\Sigma, \eta))$
  6:                  **return** (η, s)
  7:              $\eta \leftarrow \eta + 1$
  8:          **return** $(\infty, \emptyset)$

Any complete SAT solver [5] may be used as the external module of the suggested optimal CPF solving algorithm. Notice however that a CPF solver following the framework of Algorithm 1 is *incomplete*. If the given CPF instance Σ has no solution then the algorithm runs infinitely. The treatment of incompleteness is easy. The solvability of Σ can be checked by some of sub-optimal polynomial time solving algorithms such as that suggested in [13] or by PUSH-AND-ROTATE [25] (which corrects the previous algorithm [14]) before optimal SAT solving is started. The speed of the solving process is not compromised by solving the instance sub-optimally first since the runtime of solving encoded bCPFs by a SAT solver significantly dominates in the overall runtime.

6   Experimental Evaluation

The proposed SIMPLIFIED encoding has been competitively evaluated with respect to other existing two propositional encodings of bCPF called INVERSE [22] and ALL-DIFFERENT [23] and with respect to the unpublished DIRECT encoding. Various static characteristics of encodings such as its size and runtime behavior, when the encoding is built-in to the SAT-based optimal CPF solving, were compared. The SAT-based solving with all the encodings has been compared with another state-of-the-art method developed around A* algorithm called OD+ID [21]. The comparison with OD+ID interestingly extends results shown in [22, 23] where SAT-based CPF solving was compared with domain independent SAT-based planners SASE [11] and SATPLAN [12] only.

The experimental setup employs random CPF instances over 4-connected grids with randomly placed obstacles. This is a standard benchmark for evaluating CPF solving methods suggested in [20]. Although it is not very general, it provides easy comparison with results in existing literature. Initial locations and goals of agents were distributed randomly over the grid. Grids of sizes 6×6, 8×8, and 12×12 were used in experiments; 10% were occupied by obstacles. All CPF the instances in the evaluation were solvable.

All the encodings were further augmented with *reachability heuristic* as proposed in [23]. That is, locations that are unreachable from the initial position or from the goal in the given number of time steps are forbidden and associated constraints (clauses) are omitted. This heuristic significantly reduces the size of all the encodings and speeds up the solving process.

Glucose version 3.0 [1] SAT solver has been used in the experimental evaluation. According to the 2013 SAT Competition [3] Glucose is one of few top SAT solvers in terms of performance in solving hard combinatorial problems. As CPF can be regarded as a combinatorial problem, this choice of SAT solver is justified.

Let us also briefly summarize properties of all the encodings and A* based method used in competitive comparison. The IVERSE encoding is build around the *inverse location function* α^{-1}, which is used to represent arrangements of agents. The primary motivation is to keep the encoding as small as possible, hence it uses multi-value state variables encoded by bit vectors, which eliminates additional constraints. However, no attention is paid to Boolean constraint propagation. Relatively long clauses appear in the encoding.

The ALL-DIFFERENT encoding on the other hand uses standard *location function* α to represent arrangements of agents. Again, locations are modeled as bit-vectors. The main idea is to express the requirement that each agent must occupy a unique location by the *all-different* relation over bit vectors [4]. Note that no propagator based on network flows, as it is known in constraint programming [16], is used here. Boolean constraint propagation is considered at the level of the all-different relation, which is designed in that sense [4]. However, the encoding of the all-different relation grows as quadratically which makes the encoding complicated for higher number of agents.

OD+ID is a search method. It is always trying to separate agents into groups for which shortest paths to their goals can be found independently on other agents.

The best case occurs if each agent is in its own group. That is, the cooperative solution consists of shortest paths between initial positions and goals of agents. The worst case is on the other hand if all the agents are considered as a single group. If agents become too interdependent in the densely occupied environment, the performance of the method considerably degrades.

All the source codes used to conduct experiments are posted on website to allow full reproducibility of presented results: http://ktiml.mff.cuni.cz/~surynek/research/micai2014.

Static Evaluation of Encodings

There are several static characteristics of propositional formulae in CNF that are correlated with performance of their solving by most SAT solvers. Obviously, the size of the formula in terms of the *number of variables* and the *number of clauses* determines the time needed to find a solution significantly. Typically the larger the formula is the longer runtime of its solving should be expected though the solving runtime is also affected by other factors (easily solvable large formula is possible).

How the formula is *constrained* determines the difficulty of its solving as well. It is known that in random 3-SAT case (clauses has exactly three literals) the most difficult formulae have the *ratio of the number of clauses to the number of variables* around 4.24 [5] which is called a *phase transition*. Formulae that are over-constrained (tend to be unsatisfiable) or under-constrained (tend to be satisfiable), that is, have the clause to variable ratio far from the phase transition can be solved easily in most cases. Hence, encodings producing such formulae are preferred. Another important characteristic is the *length of clauses* while short clauses are preferred. This is implied by the *Boolean constraint propagation* represented by the *unit propagation* [5], which always assigns *TRUE* to the last unassigned literal in a clause during search. Short clauses promote frequent use of unit propagation, which significantly speeds up the process of solving the formula [6].

Note that preferences in the mentioned characteristics are sometimes contradictory. We want the formula to be small, hence the number of clauses should be small, but over-constraining by many clauses is desirable at the same time. Therefore, discussed preferences should not be considered literally – also because the considered behavior of SAT solvers appears in most cases but does not appear absolutely. They are rather a simple guidance that was kept in mind when an encoding is designed.

Static characteristics of the SIMPLIFIED encoding are compared with other three propositional encodings – INVERSE, ALL-DIFFERENT, and DIRECT – in Table 1. A 4-connected grid of size 8×8 various numbers of agents is shown. The winner according to discussed preferences in each characteristic is shown in bold (results over 6×6 and 12×12 indicate same conclusions and thus are omitted for space limitations).

It can be observed that the smallest encoding in terms of the number of variables and clauses is the INVERSE one while the biggest one is the DIRECT encoding with ALL-DIFFERENT and SIMPLIFIED encodings standing in the middle. This aspect seems to be disadvantageous for the proposed DIRECT encoding. However in terms of the clause to variable ratio and the size of clauses, the DIRECT encoding seems to be the best followed by the SIMPLIFIED one as they have highest number of shortest clauses.

Whether these static advantages prevail over disadvantages of encodings, must be evaluated in runtime experiments.

Table 1. Static *characteristics* of encodings over 8×8 grid. INVERSE, ALL-DIFFERENT, DIRECT, SIMPLIFIED and encodings – all with compiled distance heuristics [23] – are compared. bCPF instances are generated over the 4-connected grid of size 8×8 with 10% of cells occupied by obstacles. Makespan bound η is always 16. The number of variables and clauses, the ratio of the number of clauses and the number of variables, and the average clause length are listed for different sizes of the of agents A. The DIRECT encoding is biggest in terms of the length of formula but has smallest clauses in average and is most constrained out of all the encodings, which suggests good behavior in Boolean constraint propagation (unit propagation) and pushes the formula far from the *phase transition*. The SIMPLIFIED encoding inherited a promising clause to variable ratio and short clauses from the DIRECT encoding.

Grid 8×8			INVERSE		ALL-DIFFERENT		DIRECT		SIMPLIFIED	
|Agents|										
1	#Variables	*Ratio*	8 358.7	*3.748*	1 489.3	*5.325*	814.4	*28.539*	1 628.8	*2.078*
	#Clauses	*Length*	31 327.9	*2.616*	7 930.4	*3.057*	23 241.9	*2.149*	3 384.6	*2.550*
4			10 019.5	*5.532*	7 834.5	*4.440*	3 257.6	*35.589*	4 072.0	*4.420*
			55 437.0	*2.641*	34 781.9	*3.103*	115 934.3	*2.272*	17 997.8	*2.374*
16			11 680.3	*7.820*	67 088.3	*3.231*	13 030.4	*64.506*	13 844.8	*10.853*
			91 344.5	*3.127*	216 745.4	*3.147*	840 540.6	*2.505*	150 259.2	*2.180*
32			12 510.7	*9.765*	230 753.0	*2.802*	26 060.8	*105.084*	26 875.2	*19.002*
			122 170.3	*3.733*	646 616.2	*3.168*	2 738 584.7	*2.621*	510 672.1	*2.111*

Runtime Evaluation of Encodings

The speed of SAT-based optimal CPF solving with the three discussed encodings has been evaluated. Again, 4-connected grids of various sizes were used in experiments. The *runtime*[1] needed for finding an optimal solution has been measured for the number of agents ranging from 1 up to the number for which at least one method solves all the instances (the increasing number of agents makes the CPF instance more difficult). The timeout of 256 seconds has been used. For each number of agents, 10 random instances of bCPF have been generated and solved. All the testing instances were solvable. The average runtime and makespan is reported.

Evaluation of SAT-based CPF solving would be incomplete if it is not compared with other state-of-the-art solving methods. Therefore A*-based method OD+ID [15] is included into competitive comparison.

Runtime results are shown in Figure 3. Also average optimal makespans are shown for the sake of completeness. Results for the 8×8 grid indicate that SAT-based solving with the SIMPLIFIED encoding is the best option if the occupancy of the graph with agents is non-trivial, that is > 10%. Almost identical results can be observed in case of 6×6 and 12×12 grids.

The DIRECT encodings follows the SIMPLIFIED one in term of solving speed. It outperforms remaining two encodings INVERSE and ALL-DIFFERENT if the occupancy of the graph with agents exceeds approximately 30%. The closest competitor to

---

[1] All the runtime measurements were done on an experimental server with the 4-core CPU Xeon 2.0GHz and 12GB RAM under Linux kernel 3.5.0-48.

presented encodings seems to the ALL-DIFFERENT encoding which is a better option for less occupied graphs.

In very sparsely occupied graphs, OD+ID method is the best as lot of independence among agents can be found. However, OD+ID degrades dramatically if there is higher concentration of agents in the graph since agents become more interdependent and independence heuristics no longer work.

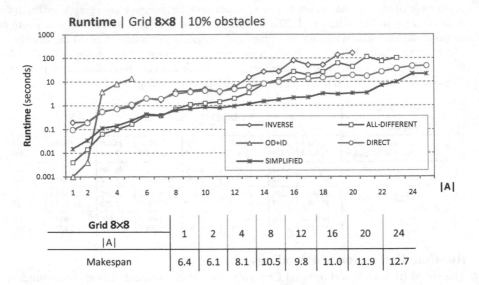

Grid 8×8 |A|	1	2	4	8	12	16	20	24
Makespan	6.4	6.1	8.1	10.5	9.8	11.0	11.9	12.7

Fig. 3. Runtime *of SAT-based CPF solving – grid 8×8*. Glucose 3.0 is used as an external solver in SAT-based solving. For each number of agents, 10 random instances were solved and the average runtime is reported. The SIMPLIFIED encoding can be solved the fastest for the occupancy with agents greater than 10%. The SIMPLIFIED and the DIRECT encoding are the only encodings for which all the instances have been solved in a given timeout of 256 seconds. Note that the DIRECT encoding becomes faster than the IVERSE and ALL-DIFFERENT encodings when the occupancy exceeds 30%. The average optimal makespan for selected numbers of agents is shown in the table in the bottom (again it is the average makespan out of makespans of 10 instances). Note that OD+ID is fastest for sparsely populated graphs but its increases runtime quickly with higher number of agents.

The INVERSE encoding was always the worst option out of all the tested methods. We consider that the reason for its weak performance is that relatively long clauses appear in it. On the other hand, short clauses of the DIRECT encoding and their abundance promoting unit propagation are the main reasons for the good performance of this encoding. We observed that solving of formulae of the DIRECT encoding by the SAT solver is relatively fast while large portion of the time is consumed by generating the formula (the formula is generated into file, which is subsequently read by the SAT solver). Hence, there is still room to increase the speed of SAT-based solving if the solving process is better engineered.

7   Discussion, Conclusions, and Future Works

A new propositional encoding of the makespan bounded cooperative path-finding problem (bCPF) has been proposed. The idea of the work was to simplify further our unpublished encoding whose design was very simple with no elaborate technique behind. The next goal was to check how simple encodings stands with respect to existing relatively elaborate encodings for the problem. The new encoding has been called SIMPLIFIED as it simplifies our previous encoding called DIRECT.

The SIMPLIFIED encoding has been used within the SAT-based framework for solving CPF (unbounded version) optimally. The comparison of SIMPLIFIED and DIRECT encodings with existing two encodings INVERSE [22] and ALL-DIFFERENT [23] as well as with A* search based method OD+ID [21] on random CPF instances over 4-connected grids has been done and showed surprising results. The DIRECT encoding despite its relatively naive design performed better than the ALL-DIFFERENT encoding on instances with occupancy by agents > 30% and almost always better than the INVERSE encoding. The SIMPLIFIED encoding was even better and it prevailed over all the other encodings in case with occupancy higher than approximately 10%.

Generally, the SAT-based approach turned out to be better whatever encoding has been used than the A* based OD+ID whenever occupancy with agents has been higher than trivial. This can be explained by the fact that OD+ID's heuristic cannot detect independence among agents in cases with high occupancy. Note also that this method can be regarded as all-in-one while in the SAT-based approach the SAT solver itself is an external module. It is quite unrealistic to implement equivalent number of propagation, learning, and heuristic techniques in the all-in-one solution as they are in SAT solvers. Through an encoding of the problem in the SAT formalism, we can access all these elaborate techniques almost for free. We hope that lessons learned from the design of encodings for CPF can be applied in other areas as well.

It would be interesting to study models of CPF also in other formalisms than SAT. The promising candidate seems to be *constraint satisfaction problem* (CSP) [7] where *global constraints* can be used. *Integer programming* (IP) model are also worth studying. Recently an attempt to model the problem in the *answer set programming* (ASP) formalism has been made [9]. Also, it seems that existing encodings are still far from theoretically smallest possible sizes. Hence, we see an opportunity in further reductions of the size of SAT encodings.

Another interesting question is if finding *makespan sub-optimal* solution can be modeled as SAT. It is known that sub-optimal methods such as [13, 25] generate solutions that have excessively long makespans. Their shortening is a difficult process as shown in [22]. The optional way may be to propose a SAT encoding that prefers sub-optimal solution of short makespans.

We are also investigating the possibility of *automated generation* of encodings. Our first examination of the problem of finding an encoding automatically indicates that it belongs to Σ_1^P class. Hence, the encoding can be theoretically found by a QBF solver. The open question is if this process is practically feasible.

References

1. Ahuja, R.K., Magnanti, T.L., Orlin, J.B.: Network flows: theory, algorithms, and applications. Prentice-Hall (1993)
2. Audemard, G., Simon, L.: The Glucose SAT Solver (2013), http://labri.fr/perso/lsimon/glucose/ (accessed in June 2014)
3. Balint, A., Belov, A., Heule, M., Järvisalo, M.: SAT 2013 competition (2013), http://satcompetition.org/ (accessed in June 2014)
4. Biere, A., Brummayer, R.: Consistency Checking of All Different Constraints over Bit-Vectors within a SAT Solver. In: Proceedings of Formal Methods in Computer-Aided Design (FMCAD 2008), pp. 1–4. IEEE Press (2008)
5. Biere, A., Heule, M., van Maaren, H., Walsh, T.: Handbook of Satisfiability. IOS Press (2009)
6. Bjork, M. Successful SAT Encoding Techniques. Journal on Satisfiability, Boolean Modeling and Computation, Addendum (2009)
7. Dechter, R.: Constraint Processing. Morgan Kaufmann Publishers (2003)
8. Eén, N., Sörensson, N.: An Extensible SAT-solver. In: Giunchiglia, E., Tacchella, A. (eds.) SAT 2003. LNCS, vol. 2919, pp. 502–518. Springer, Heidelberg (2004)
9. Erdem, E., Kisa, D.G., Oztok, U., Schüller, P.: Experimental Evaluation of Multi-Agent Pathfinding Problems using Answer Set Programming. In: Proceedings of the 20th International Workshop on Knowledge Representation and Automated Reasoning (RCRA 2013), AI*IA (2013)
10. Gent, I.P., Walsh, T., The, S.A.T.: Phase Transition. In: Proceedings of the 11th European Conference on Artificial Intelligence (ECAI 1994), pp. 105–109. John Wiley and Sons (1994)
11. Huang, R., Chen, Y., Zhang, W.: A Novel Transition Based Encoding Scheme for Planning as Satisfiability. In: Proceedings of AAAI 2010. AAAI Press (2010)
12. Kautz, H., Selman, B.: Unifying SAT-based and Graph-based Planning. In: Proceedings of the 16th International Joint Conference on Artificial Intelligence (IJCAI 1999), pp. 318–325. Morgan Kaufmann (1999)
13. Kornhauser, D., Miller, G.L., Spirakis, P.G.: Coordinating Pebble Motion on Graphs, the Diameter of Permutation Groups, and Applications. In: Proceedings of the 25th Annual Symposium on Foundations of Computer Science (FOCS 1984), pp. 241–250. IEEE Press (1984)
14. Luna, R., Berkis, K.E.: Push-and-Swap: Fast Cooperative Path-Finding with Completeness Guarantees. In: Proceedings of the 22nd International Joint Conference on Artificial Intelligence (IJCAI 2011), pp. 294–300. IJCAI/AAAI Press (2011)
15. Ratner, D., Warmuth, M.K.: Finding a Shortest Solution for the N × N Extension of the 15-PUZZLE Is Intractable. In: Proceedings of AAAI 1986, pp. 168–172. Morgan Kaufmann (1986)
16. Régin, J.-C.: A Filtering Algorithm for Constraints of Difference in CSPs. In: Proceedings of the 12th National Conference on Artificial In-telligence (AAAI 1994), pp. 362–367. AAAI Press (1994)
17. Rintanen, J., Heljanko, K., Niemelä, I.: Planning as satisfiability: parallel plans and algorithms for plan search. Artificial Intelligence 170(12-13), 1031–1080 (2006)
18. Ryan, M.R.K.: Exploiting Subgraph Structure in Multi-Robot Path Planning. Journal of Artificial Intelligence Research (JAIR) 31, 497–542 (2008)
19. Sharon, G., Stern, R., Goldenberg, M., Felner, A.: The increasing cost tree search for optimal multi-agent pathfinding. Artificial Intelligence 195, 470–495 (2013)

20. Silver, D.: Cooperative Pathfinding. In: Proceedings of the 1st Artificial Intelligence and Interactive Digital Entertainment Conference (AIIDE 2005), pp. 117–122. AAAI Press (2005)
21. Standley, T.S., Korf, R.E.: Complete Algorithms for Cooperative Pathfinding Problems. In: Proceedings of the 22nd International Joint Conference on Artificial Intelligence (IJ-CAI 2011), pp. 668–673. IJCAI/AAAI Press (2011)
22. Surynek, P.: Towards Optimal Cooperative Path Planning in Hard Setups through Satisfiability Solving. In: Anthony, P., Ishizuka, M., Lukose, D. (eds.) PRICAI 2012. LNCS, vol. 7458, pp. 564–576. Springer, Heidelberg (2012)
23. Surynek, P.: On Propositional Encodings of Cooperative Path-Finding. In: Proceedings of the 24th International Conference on Tools with Artificial Intelligence (ICTAI 2012), pp. 524–531. IEEE Press (2012)
24. Wang, K.C., Botea, A.: MAPP: a Scalable Multi-Agent Path Planning Algorithm with Tractability and Completeness Guarantees. In: JAIR, vol. 42, pp. 55–90. AAAI Press (2011)
25. de Wilde, B., ter Mors, A., Witteveen, C.: Push and rotate: cooperative multi-agent path planning. In: Proceedings of International Conference on Autonomous Agents and Multi-Agent Systems (AAMAS 2013), pp. 87–94. IFAAMAS (2013)

Pendulum Position Based Fuzzy Regulator of the Furuta Pendulum – A Stable Closed-Loop System Design Approach

Nohe Ramon Cazarez-Castro[1], Luis T. Aguilar[2], Selene L. Cardenas-Maciel[3], and Carlos A. Goribar-Jimenez[3]

[1]Instituto Tecnologico de Tijuana, Division de Estudios de Posgrado e Investigacion
[2]Instituto Politecnico Nacional, Centro de Investigacion y Desarrollo de Tecnologia Digital
[3]Instituto Tecnologico de Tijuana, Departamento de Ingenieria Electrica y Electronica
{nohe,lilettecardenas}@ieee.org, laguilarb@ipn.mx,
cgoribar@tectijuana.edu.mx

Abstract. This paper reports the design of a Mamdani type fuzzy controller to solve the regulation problem of a Furuta pendulum. The fuzzy rule-base is designed following the fuzzy Lyapunov synthesis, allowing to guarantee stability of the closed-loop system equilibrium point, minimizing heuristics in the fuzzy controller design stage. An important result of this paper is that the dynamic model of the Furuta pendulum it is not necessary in the design process and only angular position of the pendulum is available for measurements.

1 Introduction

The solution of the regulation problem for an inverted pendulum is a classical problem in control engineering due to its applications on robotics as in the balancing stage in a biped robot. Different control techniques have been used to solve this problem as variable structure control [1,2], control based on dynamic surface [3,4], energy based control [5], optimal control [6], and saturation techniques [7]. A disadvantage of the above mentioned techniques is that identification of the parameters of the plant is needed.

Some computational intelligence techniques have been used as control strategy to solve the regulation problem. In [8], bioinspired methods are used to optimize gains of a proportional-derivative-integral (PID) controller to solve the regulation problem for an inverted pendulum. In [9], a type-2 fuzzy inference system is proposed to control an inverted pendulum. In [10] is presented a genetic-fuzzy type-2 hybridization to solve the regulation problem for a non-minimum phase servomechanism with nonlinear backlash. The above mentioned computational intelligence methods solve the problem on hand, but each one of the approaches require of the mathematical model of the plant. This work differs from the previous references in the fact the fuzzy controller design approach does not require

A. Gelbukh et al. (Eds.): MICAI 2014, Part II, LNAI 8857, pp. 426–435, 2014.
© Springer International Publishing Switzerland 2014

of the mathematical model of the plant, and only the angular position of the pendulum is available for measurements.

In this paper a fuzzy system is proposed to solve the stabilization problem for a Furuta pendulum [11].

Typically a heuristics based methodology is used to design the rule-base for a fuzzy inference system, which have been widely criticized by the traditional control community due that stability can not be demostrated following this design approach. On this paper the design of a Mamdani [12] type fuzzy controller to stabilize the Furuta pendulum on its open loop unstable equilibrium point is reported. The design is based on the Lyapunov stability theory [13] to guarantee stability of the closed-loop system.

The rest of the paper is organized as follows. The dynamic model for the Furuta pendulum and the problem statement are given in Section 2. In Section 3 the controller design based on Lyapunov theory is presented. Results to the control problem are shown in Section 4. Finally, conclusions can be found in Section 5.

2   Dynamic Model for the Furuta Pendulum

The purpose of this Section is to provide the dynamic model of the Furuta pendulum in order to test the forthcoming synthesized fuzzy controller.

The Furuta pendulum is an underactuated nonlinear mechanism very broadly used in academy and research to prove and test control algorithms and techniques. The Furuta pendulum consists on a inverted pendulum connected to a horizontal rotating arm, where the rotating arm is actuated by a direct current motor drive, Figure 1 is a representation of the Furuta pendulum. The non-linear model of the Furuta pendulum is [11]:

$$0 = \theta_1 \ddot{q}_1 + \theta_2 \cos(q_q)\ddot{q}_2 - \theta_3 \sin(q_1)\cos(q_1)\dot{q}_2^2 - \theta_4 g \sin(q_1), \qquad (1)$$

$$\tau = \theta_2 \cos(q_1)\ddot{q}_1 + (\theta_5 + \theta_3 \sin^2(q_1))\ddot{q}_2 - \theta_2 \sin(q_1)\dot{q}_1^2 + \qquad (2)$$
$$2\theta_3 \sin(q_1)\cos(q_1)\dot{q}_1\dot{q}_2,$$

where $q_1(t)$, $q_2(t)$ are the pendulum angle from the vertical, and the arm angle, respectively, $\dot{q}_1(t)$, $\dot{q}_2(t)$ are the angular velocities of the pendulum and the arm, and g is gravitational acceleration. The control input τ is the applied torque to the shaft of the arm, and $\theta_1 \ldots, \theta_5$ are parameters of the system defined as $\theta_1 = I_1 + m_1 l_1^2$, $\theta_2 = m_1 l_1 L_2$, $\theta_3 = m_1 l_1^2$, $\theta_4 = m_1 l_1$, and $\theta_5 = I_2 + m_2 l_2^2$. The rest of the systems parameters are given in Table 1.

3   Fuzzy Controller Design

3.1   Control Objective

The control objective is to drive the pendulum, from an arbitrary initial condition around the open-loop unstable equilibrium point, to its unstable equilibrium

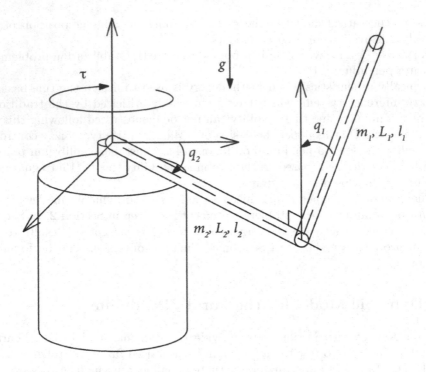

Fig. 1. Schematic of the Furuta pendulum

point (upper vertical position), and hold it even in presence of bounded external disturbances, that is:

$$\lim_{t \to \infty} \|q_{1_d} - q_1(t)\| = 0, \tag{3}$$

where q_{1_d} is the desired position.

Table 1. Parameters for the Furuta pendulum

Symbol	Value	Unit
m_1	67.9×10^{-3}	kg
m_2	0.2869	kg
L_1	0.14	m
L_2	0.235	m
l_1	0.07	m
l_2	0.1175	m
I_1	5.5452×10^{-5}	kg·m^2
I_2	1.9×10^{-3}	kg·m^2

3.2   Synthesis of the Fuzzy Controller

To apply the fuzzy Lyapunov synthesis it is considered that no exist information about the mathematical model of the system. Additionally the following is assumed:

1. The system have indeed only the two degrees of freedom q_1 and $\dot{q}_1$. According with the control objective lets define the error variable as $x_1 = q_1(t) - q_{1_d}$, where $q_{1_d} = \pi$ rad, and $x_2 = \dot{x}_1 = \dot{q}_1(t)$;
2. The angular acceleration $\dot{x}_2$ is proportional to τ, that is, when τ increases (decreases) then $\dot{x}_2$ increases (decreases);
3. The initial condition belongs to a neighborhood around the origin, that is $x(0) \in \mathcal{N} \subset \mathbb{R}^2$ where

$$\mathcal{N} = \left\{ x \in \mathbb{R}^2 : \|x_1\| \le \varepsilon, x_2 = 0 \right\}.$$

Remark 1. Note that position $q_1(t)$ is the only one available information available for the controller synthesis while $\dot{q}_1(t)$ is computed using the Euler's difference formula $\dot{q}_1 = (q_1(t) - q_1(t - \Delta t))/\Delta t$ with $q_1(t) \equiv 0$ for $-\Delta t \le t < 0$ and $\Delta t > 0$ being sufficiently small.

It is proposed the following Lyapunov candidate function

$$V(x_1, x_2) = \frac{1}{2}(x_1^2 + x_2^2). \tag{4}$$

This is a positive defined and radially unbounded function. The time derivative of the Lyapunov candidate function (4) results on

$$\dot{V}(x_1, x_2) = x_1 \dot{x}_1 + x_2 \dot{x}_2 = x_1 x_2 + x_2 \dot{x}_2. \tag{5}$$

Considering the previous knowledge that $\dot{x}_2$ is proportional to $-\tau$, it is possible to make the change of $\dot{x}_2$ by $-\tau$ on (5) giving as result:

$$\dot{V}(x_1, x_2) = x_1 x_2 + x_2(-\tau). \tag{6}$$

Now, to guarantee asymptotical stability of the equilibrium point, $\dot{V} < 0$ must to be satisfied. However, the algorithm increases in complexity in the sense that computationally more conditions must to be evaluated for x_1 and x_2 in (6) to ensure that $\dot{V} < 0$, which imply an automatic increment in the number of rules of the fuzzy rule-base and hence a major number of computations are needed to get inference results, affecting the performance or even making impossible to make implementations to execute real time experiments. Then, the fuzzy controller is designed such that $\dot{V}(x_1, x_2) \le 0$ or:

$$x_1 x_2 + x_2(-\tau) \le 0. \tag{7}$$

Condition (7) is necessary and sufficient to guarantee stability, at least locally, of the equilibrium point (cf. [14]). The Barbalat lemma ([14]) or invariance principle ([14]) can be invoked to guarantee asymptotic stability.

Table 2. Conditions to satisfy $\dot{V}(x_1, x_2) \leq 0$

x_1	x_2	τ
negative	negative	negative such that $\dot{V}(x_1, x_2) \leq 0$
negative	positive	zero
positive	negative	zero
positive	positive	positive such that $\dot{V}((x_1, x_2)) \leq 0$

Table 2 is obtained by inspection, testing the signs for each state variable, schematically can be deduced the qualitative state of the system for each situation, and hence, to find conditions to satisfy (7). Table 2 represents this process in a resumed way.

From Table 2 the rule-base for the fuzzy inference system (fuzzy controller) can be derived as follows:

1. IF x_1 is *negative* AND x_2 is *negative*, THEN τ is *negative big*,
2. IF x_1 is *negative* AND x_2 is *positive*, THEN τ is *zero*,
3. IF x_1 is *positive* AND x_2 is *negative*, THEN τ is *zero*,
4. IF x_1 is *positive* AND x_2 is *positive*, THEN τ is *positive big*.

The type and form of the membership functions have been obtained heuristically, and nonlinear functions are selected over lineal ones to get a soft response. x_1 and x_2 inputs are automatically granulated in the two linguistic labels *negative* and *positive*. For this particular case the sigmoidal membership functions x_{neg} and x_{pos} are selected, defined respectively as

$$x_{\text{neg}} = \frac{1}{1 + \exp\{1.45x\}} \tag{8}$$

and

$$x_{\text{pos}} = \frac{1}{1 + \exp\{-1.45x\}}, \tag{9}$$

that represents the sign that can take a state variable. In both cases, functions are symmetric around zero, see Figure 2.

The domain for input membership functions is $[-2\pi, 2\pi]$, this definition domain is selected in order to contain any possible position in a complete circle.

For output membership functions gaussian functions are selected to represent the linguistic expressions *negative big*:

$$\tau_{\text{negative-big}} = \exp\left\{-(x-5)^2\right\}, \tag{10}$$

zero, defined as

$$\tau_{\text{zero}} = \exp\{-x^2\}, \tag{11}$$

and *positive big*, defined as

$$\tau_{\text{positive-big}} = \exp\left\{-(x+5)^2\right\}. \tag{12}$$

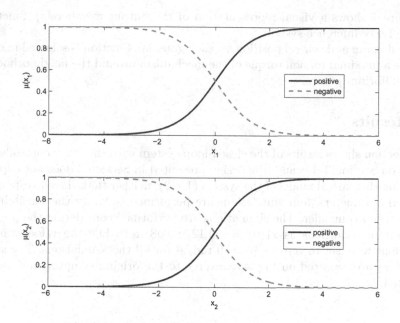

Fig. 2. Input variables membership functions granulation

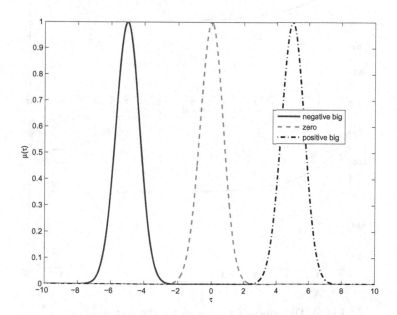

Fig. 3. Output variable membership functions granulation

Figure 3 shows a visual representation of the output membership functions for the fuzzy inference system.

The domain and central position for each gaussian function is selected in order to have a maximal torsion torque of the mechanism around the neighborhood of the equilibrium point.

4   Results

This Section shows results of the closed-loop system with the fuzzy controller designed on Section 3. Because the design presented in Section 3 does not depends on the mathematical model of the system (1)-(2), neither than the corresponding nominal parameters, four simulations are performed to verify the sensibility of the designed controller. The simulations are performed considering the position error initial conditions as $x_1(0) = \pm 0.12, \pm 0.08$ rad while the velocity initial conditions were set to zero ($x_2(0) = 0$ rad/s) for all the simulations. The states x_1 and x_2 are reported on Fig. 4, converge to the origin asymptotically as was expected.

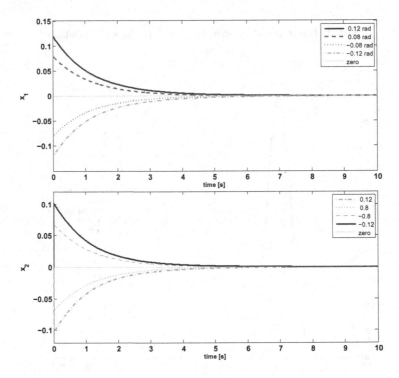

Fig. 4. Dynamics of x_1 and x_2 for the system (1)-(2)

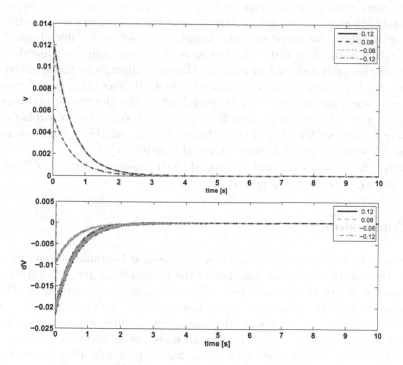

Fig. 5. Dynamics of (4) and (5)

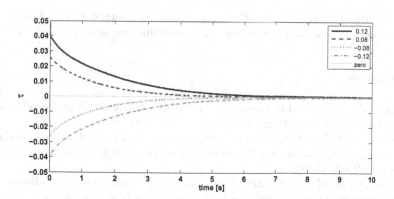

Fig. 6. Control input τ

The time evolution for the Lyapunov function (4) and its time derivative (5) depicted on Fig. 5, are positive and negative, respectively, and both converge to zero when $t \to \infty$, meaning that the closed-loop system is asymptotically stable, which can be demonstrated invoking the invariance principle [14] theorem. It should be noted that the Lyapunov function for initial conditions $(x_1(0), x_2(0)) = (0.12, 0)$ and $(-0.12, 0)$ have the same shape because the same amount of energy is required to stabilize the pendulum from those initial conditions, also $(x_1(0), x_2(0)) = (0.08, 0)$ and $(-0.08, 0)$ show the same Lyapunov function shape, similar cases can be found when the derivative of Lyapunov function is plotted. As can be seen from previous results, the controller solves the control problem for each of the selected initial conditions that means the controller is able to handle a range of initial conditions.

Finally, Fig. 6 shows the control applied to the system (1)-(2), verifying that $\tau \to 0$ while $t \to \infty$ as was expected..

5   Conclusions

The design of a fuzzy controller based on the classical Lyapunov theory has been applied to solve the regulation problem of the Furuta Pendulum, facilitating the analysis of stability that cannot be made with other fuzzy techniques. For the type of membership functions non-linear functions has been preferred over linear functions in order to obtain a smooth control signal while avoiding stress on the actuator that normally is cause of potential damages on motors. In this work it is also shown how the application of the La Salle's principle allows to determine asymptotically stable for the closed-loop system.

Acknowledgments.   This work was partially supported by a DGEST grant "Analisis de problemas de Cauchy en ecuaciones diferenciales difusas" 5424.14-P.

References

1. Andrievsky, B.: Global stabilization of the unstable reaction-wheel pendulum. Automation and Remote Control 72, 1981–1993 (2011)
2. Hernández, V.M.: A combined sliding mode-generalized pi control scheme for swinging up and balancing the inertia wheel pendulum. Asian Journal of Control 5, 620–625 (2003)
3. Qaiser, N., Iqbal, N., Hussain, A., Qaiser, N.: Stabilization of non-linear inertia wheel pendulum system using a new dynamic surface control based technique, pp. 1–6 (2006)
4. Qaiser, N., Iqbal, N., Hussain, A., Qaiser, N.: Exponential stabilization of the inertia wheel pendulum using dynamic surface control. Journal of Circuits, Systems and Computers 16, 81–92 (2007)
5. Ng, W.M., Chang, D.E., Song, S.H.: Four representative applications of the energy shaping method for controlled lagrangian systems. Journal of Electrical Engineering and Technology 8, 1579–1589 (2013)

6. Andary, S., Chemori, A., Krut, S.: Control of the underactuated inertia wheel inverted pendulum for stable limit cycle generation. Advanced Robotics 23, 1999–2014 (2009)
7. Ye, H., Wang, H., Wang, H.: Stabilization of a pvtol aircraft and an inertia wheel pendulum using saturation technique. IEEE Transactions on Control Systems Technology 15, 1143–1150 (2007)
8. Martinez-Soto, R., Rodriguez, A., Castillo, O., Aguilar, L.T.: Gain optimization for inertia wheel pendulum stabilization using particle swarm optimization and genetic algorithms. International Journal of Innovative Computing, Information and Control 8, 4421–4430 (2012)
9. Castillo, O., Aguilar, L., Cazarez, N., Cardenas, S.: Systematic design of a stable type-2 fuzzy logic controller. Applied Soft Computing 8, 1274–1279 (2008)
10. Cazarez-Castro, N.R., Aguilar, L.T., Castillo, O.: Fuzzy logic control with genetic membership function parameters optimization for the output regulation of a servomechanism with nonlinear backlash. Expert Systems with Applications 37, 4368–4378 (2010)
11. Furuta, K., Yamakita, M., Kobayashi, S.: Swing up control of inverted pendulum. In: Proceedings of the 1991 International Conference on Industrial Electronics, Control and Instrumentation, IECON 1991, vol. 3, pp. 2193–2198 (1991)
12. Mamdani, E.H., Assilian, S.: An experiment in linguistic synthesis with a fuzzy logic controller. International Journal of Man-Machine Studies 7, 1–13 (1975)
13. Lyapunov, A.: The General Problem of the Stability of Motion. Phd, Univ. Kharkov (1892) (in Russian)
14. Khalil, H.K.: Nonlinear Systems. 3rd edn. Prentice Hall, EEUU (2002)

A Fast Scheduling Algorithm for Detection and Localization of Hidden Objects Based on Data Gathering in Wireless Sensor Networks

Eugene Levner[1], Boris Kriheli[1], Amir Elalouf[2], and Dmitry Tsadikovich[2]

[1] Ashkelon Academic College, Ashkelon, Israel
elevner@acad.ash-college.ac.il, borisk@hit.ac.il
[2] Bar Ilan University, Ramat Gan, Israel
amir.elalouf@biu.ac.il, dmitrytsadikovich@gmail.com

Abstract. The need for the search and localization of hidden or lost objects arises in many military and civil applications. Suppose a set of underground tunnels is hidden in an area of interest. In order to efficiently detect and neutralize the targets a network of wireless sensors is used which provide acoustic, seismic, electromagnetic, gravimetric and other information about the targets. The information is automatically put together in order to determine position of the targets. The problem considered in this paper is to find optimal routes for mobile agents gathering the information. The problem is formulated as the constrained assignment problem and a fast scheduling algorithm for its solution is developed.

Keywords: Detection-and-localization problem, hidden objects, routing-and-dispatching algorithm, underground tunnels.

1 Introduction

The need for the search and localization of hidden or lost objects arises in many civil and military applications. Suppose, for example, that a set of secret underground tunnels (in what follows, called "targets") are hidden in an area of interest. Until being found, they can cause serious damage and loss to the environment and people, the damage scale being dependent on location of the tunnels and time needed to detect and neutralize them. In order to efficiently detect and neutralize the targets a network of wireless smart sensors is used that provides information about the targets based on fusing various acoustic, seismic, electromagnetic, geological and other data. This information is collected on-line and automatically put together to determine location of the targets. The problem is to find a policy aimed to efficiently collect and process the sensor data in order to effectively detect and neutralize the hidden targets (we refer to [16, 17, 18], [28], [33] for more detailed description of the problem).

A similar situation is often encountered in practice in many areas other than the underground tunnel detection and neutralization. Rescue teams may search for lost people and shipwrecks. Autonomous agents like helicopters or mobile robots are used to find survivors and victims after earthquakes or other natural disasters. In military search

A. Gelbukh et al. (Eds.): MICAI 2014, Part II, LNAI 8857, pp. 436–450, 2014.

operations, patrol aircraft and unmanned aerial vehicles (UAVs) look for hidden targets such as lost submarines, missile launchers, man-made underground channels, or terrorist locations. Similar problems arise in planning risky R&D projects, technical and medical diagnostics, and the search for natural resources (we refer to [20], [31], [39] for more applications). In many applications, the choice of a search strategy has a strong impact on the search costs and losses incurred by the target as well as the chance of finding the target within time and cost limits. Specifically, in this paper we focus on finding a fast scheduling procedure for finding the routes of information-gatherers for detecting hidden human-made underground tunnels.

The automatic information-gathering system sequentially inspect the sensors scattered over a geographical region so that to find the targets in minimum time (or cost) within a priori given level of available resources. We study a discrete search-and-detection process subject to the budget (resource) constraints. We model the problem as a constrained asignment problem for several search teams working in parallel and subject to resource and budget constraints. The general constrained assignment problem is fundamentally hard due to its complex combinatorial structure and proved to be NP-hard [12]. In this work, we restrict ourselves to searching for approximate, "almost-optimal", solutions and develop the approximation algorithm belonging to the family of fully polynomial-time approximation schemes (FPTAS).

The remainder of the paper is organized as follows. In the next section, we provide a review of related works and approaches for using smart sensors for detecting hidden objects, with a focus on detecting hidden man-made underground tunnels. Then in Section 3, we describe the problem and propose its mathematical model. In Section 4 we develop a fast algorithm approximately solving the problem without significant computational load and in Section 6 give brief summary of computational results. A summary of contributions and an outline of future research are provided in Section 6.

2   Related Work

The discrete search-and-detection of hidden objects is one of the oldest problems of Operations Research and Artificial Intelligence. Its initial study was made by Bernard Koopman and his team during the World War II aimed to provide efficient methods for detecting hidden submarines (see a historical survey and the bibliography of the discrete search literature in [4], [31].

In recent years, the problem of underground tunnels detection and localization has become a critical task, particularly for protecting national borders and for monitoring sensitive areas, such as prisons, banks, and power plants. Among numerous examples we can mention the smugglers' tunnels between the U.S. and Mexico, tunnels beneath the Korean demilitarized zone, and a network of tunnels that Palestinian militants have dug from Gaza to Israel. Until being found, they enable unmonitored movement of people, drugs and weapons and pose a very serious threat and damage to homeland security dependent on location of the tunnels and time needed to detect and neutralize them. This has led to the development and testing of a variety of geophysical and surveillance techniques for the detection of these tunnels. In order to efficiently detect and neutralize all the targets a network of wireless smart sensors is used which provide information about the targets based on different acoustic, seismic, electromagnetic, geological and other data.

Tunnel detection is complicated by a large number and variety of factors such, for example, tunnel size and depth, tunnel infrastructure, surrounding soil and water content, and ambient noise from other electrical and seismic sources. The complex nature of these factors and their interactions with various sensors is the heart of the tunnel detection problem. There known four basic methods of detecting tunnels with smart sensors: a) detecting seismic activity (low frequency digging noises and tunnel transit noises), b) detecting acoustic activity (higher frequency noises), c) magnetic and electromagnetic anomalies (electrical power lines in the tunnel, metal digging tools or metal shoring) and finally d) detecting earth density anomalies (the tunnel is a hole and so the amount of earth below the surface changes when one digs a tunnel).

A common type of methods for tracking down tunnels is on acoustic and seismic activities. Geophones are the conventional detectors used by the seismic research community. Passive recording of vibrations or seismic signals is useful for monitoring activities during the construction and use of tunnels, whereas active sensing offers the potential of imaging the structure. In works [26], [35], [37] among many others, used an array of acoustic and seismic sensors placed at various depths to determine the characteristic signatures produced by underground tunneling. Detection of shallow tunnels by using active seismic, gravimetric, passive seismic and passive emit electromagnetic (EM) sensors is investigated in [29]. They concluded that the EM sensors showed the best performances in comparison with others.

Another recently used approach for sensing seismic vibrations is based on a laser vibrometry sensor called ladar vibrometer. The laser vibrometer permits remote sensing of vibrating surfaces over broad ranges of amplitudes and frequencies compares them to a library of target data and can provide a map of what is below the ground [8]. One more promising approach for tunnel detection is the smart sensors of magnetic and electromagnetic fields [8]. Imaging at optical, radar or radio wavelengths is another effective and fast method of obtaining information about underground facilities from the density anomaly viewpoint [13].

An underground detection fence using the Brillouin optical time domain reflectometry (BOTDR) was first implemented in [15]. Their results indicate that the BOTDR system is capable of detecting even small tunnel as deep as at 20 or 30 meter. Recently, [23] developed a system that used a fiber optic cable buried several meters beneath the surface the stress of which is able to detect underground movement. The radio frequency (RF) tomography was implemented in [24] to detect underground tunnels. This method uses a set of low-cost transmitters and receivers deployed on the surface of the ground, or slightly buried.

The success of the tunnel detection cannot rely on a single technology but, rather, on their clever combination. As each of the individual methods has its advantages and disadvantages, in their entirety they should help to detect the tunnels and build a map of underground facilities. While it is impossible to attack this problem by using a collection of all possible sensors, since cost and operational issues make this impractical, the question arises as to how a combination of smart sensors should be deployed within the wireless sensor network (WSN).

Wireless Sensor Network (WSN) is a prospective modern method for detecting hidden objects by collecting diverse data. A comprehensive survey regarding the main factors influencing the WSN design and network topology could be found in [3], [36]. A structure-aware self-adaptive sensor system for the underground monitoring, which provides a feasible framework for underground monitoring in coal mines was presented in [22]. A typical WSN system is distributed within the *Sensor Field* (as shown in Fig. 1) and consists of a number of sensor nodes, such as: a) seismic (white circles), b) acoustic (grey circles) and c) magnetic anomaly (black circles).

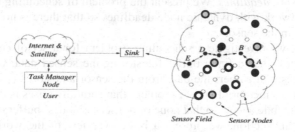

Fig. 1. Sensor nodes scattered in a field (adopted from [3])

The WSN collects thousands of raw data and works as a centralized or decentralized fusion system [38], when in the first case the collected data from the individual sensors is sent through the *sink node* to the central dedicated fusion node (called *Task Manager Node*) in which the information is fused whereas in the second case a set of autonomous devices collect the information.

We consider a situation where the basic functions of the wireless sensor networks are to monitor and control physical and environmental parameters related to the tunnel detection mentioned above and collectively transfer the data obtained through the network either to a central location or to a set of mobile agents called *data-gatherers*. In WSNs, the mobile agents are added into the system to improve its performance and act as automatic carriers of data. We refer the interested reader to [9], for more examples and details of military applications of WSN including the battlefield surveillance, detection of enemy intrusion, detection of hidden hostile targets, rescuing lost people or objects, and so on.

Applied WSN systems serving for tunnel detection (WSN-TD) may run unattended by human operators for long periods of time (sometimes hours, in other cases days or weeks). In these cases, the readings taken by the sensors are relayed to the central base station for processing and decision making using an ad-hoc multi-hop network formed by the sensor nodes. However, this technique for data transfer can create energy problems in the network. Indeed, the sensor nodes located closely to the base station relay the data sent from the nodes located far away. The sensors have limited lifetime due to the battery capacity, and the nodes near the base station are the first to run out of batteries since they are used more intensively. If the batteries of these nodes die, then the entire network becomes practically useless. Periodically replacing the battery of the nodes may be costly, dangerous and impractical in large-scale WSN-TDs. A practical solution to the problem of energy-efficient data gathering is by exploiting autonomous mobile data gatherers, i.e., controlled mobile agents that move on predetermined paths and visit the sensors to collect their data before their buffers are full and batteries are exhausted.

Obviously, the performance of the detection-and-localization system heavily depends on obtaining optimal routing policies allowing the automatic data -gatherers and verification teams to visit each sensor as soon as possible due to the constraint. Since information is available at many different nodes that yield different degrees of quality, the verification team should find a best possible itinerary to visit them. Some nodes need to be visited more frequently than others, which lead to different speed and *dynamic nodes' deadlines*. We present the problem of scheduling multiple mobile agents in the network with dynamic node deadlines so that there is no data loss due to buffer overflow in the sensors.

In this work we investigate a scheduling problem for a set of controlled mobile agents. Each sensor has a finite buffer for storing the sensed data. Once the mobile agent visits a sensor, it gathers the data from the sensor and stores in its own memory making the sensor's memory freed. A problem that naturally arises is the scheduling of the visits of the mobile agents so that none of the sensor nodes' buffer overflows.

Concluding this section, we present a brief overview of the work related to the mobile agent scheduling problem above. The mobile data-gatherers, called also "data mules", physically can be either buses, or robots, or unmanned aerial vehicles. Various types of mobile agents can be roughly classified in two large groups, random or deterministic (controlled). In the work by [30], the mobile agents moves randomly and collect data from the sensor nodes when they come near them. The use of a deterministic mobile agent (mounted on an armored carrier, or a robot, or an unmanned aerial vehicle) was considered in [7], [10], [14], [21]. A sleeping sensor node can "be awakened" when the mobile agent comes near it and starts to transfer its data. The controlled mobile agent moves on a predetermined path and can change its speed depending on the goodness of the wireless channel, density of nodes, or other controlled parameter. The sensors may be sampling at different rates (in particular, the nodes near the populated locations are used more intensively than those far away).

The arising agent scheduling problem is known in literature as the *Traveling Agent Scheduling* (TAS) problem [5], [10] or the *Mobile Agent Scheduling* (MAS) problem [32]. The TAS problem considered here differs from other, earlier known, problems. First of all, the TAS problem is essentially different from the classic traveling salesman problem (TSP) (see, e.g., [19]). In the TSP, the goal is to find a minimum distance/cost closed route in which each node is met exactly once. In contrast, in the TAS problem, any node may be visited several times, and any node must be visited before its pre-specified deadline. In addition, in the TAS the deadlines are dynamically updated, after the agent performs its data gathering operation.

In the related Vehicle Routing Problem - VRP [34], similar to the TSP and TAS problem, a set of nodes needs to be visited, but unlike the TSP and TAS, there many vehicles can be whereas the objective is to find the minimal number of the vehicles and to minimize the sum of the distances travelled by each vehicle. There are many variants to the VRP, for instance the VRP with time windows (VRPW) and the periodic VRP (PVRP). In the VRPW, there are time intervals ("windows") within which each node has to be visited. In spite of some common features, the both latter versions are different from our scheduling problem, as in our case some nodes may need to be visited more than once. In addition, the time windows of the visits are not known in advance but rather are defined dynamically during the data gathering process basing on the current visit time. Our problem can be looked at as a special-type VRP with dynamic time windows and deadlines.

The difference with the model described by [32] is that we consider the case of *multiple* mobile agents rather than as a single agent. Finally, the difference with the work by [10] is that we take into account the WSN specificity, in particular, the resource-saving constraints and node deadlines; besides, we consider a different objective function and corresponding algorithms.

3   Problem Description and Mathematical Formulation

Consider a WSN-TD system in which a set of mobile agents visit the set of sensors until the requested information is gathered. The problem is to find a feasible route for each agent so as to minimize time spent by all the agents to collect the needed information under given budget constraints. The WSN can be represented as a directed graph in which the nodes represent mutually dependent sensors. Each of such nodes is assigned a set of operational attributes like transfer time, deadline, operation costs, etc. whereas each arc linking a pair of sensors has its own transportation attribute, i.e. transportation time.

We are given the following input data:

• A fully connected graph of n nodes: $node[1..n]$.
• A matrix $time[1..n][1..n]$ that denotes the time taken by the data-gatherer to go from one node to another.
• An n-dimensional vector that contains buffer overflow times, $deadline\_time[1..n]$. The i-th element of this vector determines the time at which the buffer in the i-th node will overflow. This value can be computed using the buffer size and sensing rate (see, e.g., [32]). In fact, these values define the deadlines of visiting the nodes by the mobile agents.
• Each sensor requires a given time $transfer[1,n]$ and $budget$ $[1,n]$o carry out the agent's task. It means that, in contrast to the model by [32], the actual data transfer time from the sensor node to the mobile agent is non-negligible.
• A starting node $node_{0k}$, for each agent k.

We make the following assumptions:

• The matrix $time[1..n][1..n]$ and vector $budget[1..n]$ consist of integer entries.
• Each agent is assigned to exactly one destination, so a single path for the agent is to be defined.

In order to further simplify notation, we assume that each sensor node, say, node v, is represented (substituted) by a corresponding arc (v', v'') leading from v' to v''. Such an arc will be called a *sensor arc*. Also, all the arcs depicting agent's pass and leading to any node v (respectively, going out of v) in the initial network are substituted by the arcs leading to v' (respectively, going out of v'') in the transformed graph, for all the sensors. This simple transformation permits us, in what follows, to state that the arcs of two types (namely the link arcs and sensor arcs) are assigned the corresponding attributes and the total path length (budget, time, etc) is defined as the sum of the corresponding individual attributes taken along all the arcs in the path.

The problem of enhancing the efficiency of *multiple* mobile agents then reduces to a non-standard problem of finding budget-constrained extremal paths in a graph for each agent. The main theme of our paper is to show that a combination of the routing and assignment problems may render a realistic model of mobile agent planning in WSNs.

3.1   Mathematical Formulation

The WSN is represented as graph $G = (N, A)$ consisting of a set N of nodes and set A of arcs, where $|N| = n$ and $|A| = m$; a start node s; sets of resources and *times* associated with the arcs; a set of deadlines are associated with the nodes; a set D of destination nodes $D = \{t_1, \ldots, t_{|D|}\}$, and a set Q of agents located at the start node. The arcs in G are denoted by (i, j).

Denote by $r_{ij}(q) = resource_q(i,j)$ and $t_{ij}(q) = time_q[i][j]$ the individual resource (budget) and time, respectively, when agent q traverses arc (i, j), where $1 \leq q \leq |Q|$, and $d_i = deadline\_time[1..n]$ for sensor i. In this multi-agent setting, the graph G is a multi-graph in which any pair of nodes i and j is linked by exactly $|Q|$ parallel arcs, each one with parameters $r_{ij}(q)$ and $t_{ij}(q)$. (For more information about constructing such a network, the reader is referred to [40] [10]).

Let T_q be a given amount of time available for agent q to fulfill its mission. For each agent, define a time $T(p)$ and resource $R(p)$ of path p from a given node s to a given destination t as the sum of the times and resource requirement, respectively, of the arcs in the path (corresponding to that agent). Denote by $p(t_d)$ $(t_d \in D)$ an ordered set of nodes $p(t_d) = (s, v_1, \ldots, t_d)$, which defines a path from s to t_d. Denote by $T(p_d,q)$ and $R(p_d,q)$ the time and resource of traversing path $p(t_d)$ by agent q, respectively:
$$T(p_d, q) = \sum_{(i,j)} t_{ij}(q) \;\&\; R(p_d, q) = \sum_{(i,j)} r_{ij}(q)$$

Path $p(t_d)$ for agent q is called *feasible* if: (1) its resource requirement $R(p_d,q)$ does not exceed a given threshold R_q, and (2) its travel time $T(p_d,i)$ to each sensor node i is less than d_i. The problem is to find a feasible route for each agent so as to minimize time required by all the agents gathering the information.

Without loss of generality, it can be assumed that $|Q| = |D|$. Let X_{qd} be a binary variable equal to 1 if and only if agent q is assigned to destination $t_d \in D$. Then the multi-agent dispatching problem denoted by MDP can be formulated as follows:

$$z = \min_{p_d, X_{qd}} \left(\sum_{d \in D} \sum_{q \in Q} t(p_d, q) \cdot X_{qd} \right) \tag{1}$$

s.t

$$\sum_d X_{qd} = 1, \qquad\qquad 1 \leq q \leq |Q| \tag{2}$$

$$\sum_q X_{qd} = 1, \qquad\qquad 1 \leq d \leq |D| \tag{3}$$

$$R(p_d, q) \cdot X_{qd} \leq R_q, \qquad 1 \leq q \leq |Q|, 1 \leq d \leq |D| \tag{4}$$

$$X_{qd} \in \{0,1\}, \qquad\qquad 1 \leq q \leq |Q|, 1 \leq d \leq |D| \tag{5}$$

The problem (1)-(5) is a version of the assignment problem, which along with the agent-destination assignment constraints (2)-(3) seeks for finding a path satisfying resource constraints (4). Here (4) defines $|Q| \cdot |D|$ constraints for the agent-destination combinations. This problem has two sets of decision variables: (i) $|Q|\cdot|D|$ assignment variables X_{qd} and (ii) unknown paths p_d to be found for all the agents. The constrained assignment problem is known to be NP-hard even for the case of a single agent and a single destination (see [12]).

4   The Solution Algorithms

4.1   The Exact Algorithm for a Single Agent

For any fixed pair (q, d), we can introduce the single-agent routing problem from s to d for agent q, which we denote by ARP(q, d).

$$ARP^*(q,d) = \min_{p_d}\left(t\left(p_d,q\right)\right)$$

$s.t$

$$R\left(p_d,q\right) \le R_q$$
$$R\left(p_d,i\right) \le d_i, \text{ for any node } i \text{ in path } p_d$$

This is an extension of the agent routing problem considered by [10]. The main differences are that (i) the objective is to minimize time rather than to maximize and (ii) path must satisfy the given deadlines in each node. One can observe that in the optimal solution of MDP, if any agent q is assigned to a destination d, it must traverse to d by the constrained min-time path. Then we are able to find the optimal solution to MDP in two stages, as follows:

Stage 1. For all combinations of q and d, find a path that minimizes ARP(q, d). The minimum time for a pair of the agent and destination is denoted by ARP$^*(q, d)$.

Stage 2. In MDP, the individual travel times of separate agents are to be combined together to provide the total min-time of all the agents. The problem is to assign each agent to its proper destination. This is the constrained version of the assignment problem wherein the objective in ARP*(q, d) is the min-time of agent q assigned to mission d. There are many algorithms for its solution in the literature (see, e.g., [25] [1]). We omit their description and in the following section concentrate on solving the sub-problems ARP(q, d) of Stage 1, presenting an exact and an approximation algorithms for their solution.

The exact iterative dynamic programming (DP) algorithm for finding the optimal constrained path for any given agent q and any given destination d for ARP*(q, d) is straightforward, the reader is referred to [10] where a similar algorithm is presented for the maximization routing problem. For each agent, the algorithm returns a correct min-time value (denoted by *ans*) and the corresponding path if and only if the destination is reachable from the start. Step 3 of the algorithm checks this fact and returns "*no answer*" if the destination is unreachable.

Let us associate with each path p a pair (T, R), where $T = T(p)$ is the path time and $R = R(p)$ is the path budget. We deal with sets $S(k)$ of pairs (T, R) arranged in decreasing order of the T values so that every pair in $S(k)$ corresponds to a path from node $s=1$ to node k in the given graph G. In order to restore a path itself corresponding to a pair (T, R), we define a predecessor node to each node and use standard backtracking.

If there are two pairs in $S(k)$, say, $(T1, R1)$ and $(T2, R2)$ such that $T1 \leq T2$ and $R1 \leq R2$, then the pair $(T2, R2)$ is called *dominated* and is discarded. If the partial travel budget $R2$ to a node exceeds the given deadline in (6) for that node then the pair $(T2, R2)$ is also discarded.

The complexity of the DP is $O(mnUB)$, where the upper bound UB is the time of the min-time route from start node s to destination node t_d. The space required for running DP is $O(nUB)$. The proof is similar to that in [10] and is omitted.

Procedure DISPATCHING first runs DP $|Q| \cdot |D|$ times, each time yielding the optimal path and minimum time to a fixed agent and a fixed destination, and then finds the optimal agent-destination assignment. Procedure DISPATCHING is presented in Fig. 2.

Procedure DISPATCHING
1. Input: $G(N, A)$, $|N| = n$, $|A| = m$, $\{(b_{ij}(q), r_{ij}(q)): (i, j) \in A, 1 \leq q \leq Q\}$; R
2. Output: Optimal paths p_q for all the agents $1 \leq q \leq Q$ and all the destinations
3. **Step 1. [Initialization]**
4. OPT_B$(1...Q, 1...D) = 0$
5. for $q = 1$ to Q
6.   for $d = 1$ to D
7.   OPT_B$(q, d) = $ DP1(q, t_d)
8.   end for
9. end for
10. Run the minimization assignment algorithm for data in OPT_B(q, d)..
11. Return the matrix OPT_B(q, d) containing $\max\{Q, D\}$ and Agent, Optimal Destination, Time.
12. Return the min total time, which is the sum of all the items in the column *Times* of OPT_T(q,d).

Fig. 2. Procedure DISPATCHING

Lemma 1. The complexity of DISPATCHING is $O(|Q| \cdot |D| mnT_{min}) + C_{assign}$, where T_{min} is maximin-time among all the min-time single-agent routes from start s to destinations, and C_{assign} is the complexity of solving the assignment problem. The space required is $O(nT_{min} + |Q| \cdot |D|)$.

Proof. Since DISPATCHING runs DP1 $O(|Q| \cdot |D|)$ times and the complexity of DP is $O(mnUB)$, the total complexity of the first part of DISPATCHING is $O(|Q| \cdot |D| mnT_{min})$. The assignment problem can be solved in polynomial time, e.g., in $O(h^3)$, where h denotes max $\{|Q|, |D|\}$ (see, e.g. [2]). The space required by this part of the algorithm is only $O(nT_{min} + |Q| \cdot |D|)$ because at each iteration of DP the results of the previous iterations need not be stored.   □

4.2   The Approximation Algorithm for a Single Agent

We construct a fully polynomial-time approximation scheme (FPTAS). This is an algorithm that, for any given error $\varepsilon > 0$, finds an "almost-optimal" solution (that is, lying within the given ε) in time polynomial with respect to the problem size. An FPTAS was originally proposed by [27] for the knapsack problem, and later was developed by [21] and [10] for solving the routing problem. We further develop two latter algorithms and adjust them to solving the routing problem with deadlines.

Using the DP, we find an approximate solution for each individual agent and a given destination. Then we combine the FPTASs for the individual agents and obtain a complete approximate solution for all the agents. For this aim, we carry out the following three steps, A, B, and C,

Step A. Find a preliminary lower bound LB and an upper bound UB on the optimal solution such that $UB/LB \leq n$.

Step A1. Find the finite shortest (with respect to time) s-i paths and shortest (with respect to time) t-j paths for all those edges (i, j) for which such paths exist. For this aim, we run twice the standard algorithm for finding the shortest path from one source to the entire destinations graph G; during these runs, we treat node s as a source in the first run and node t as a "source" in the second run.

Step A2. For each edge (i, j) in G, add the length of the shortest (in time) s-i path, the length of the shortest (in-time) j-t path, and the length $r(i, j)$ of edge (i, j) itself. Denote the obtained sum by $R(i, j)$

Step A3. Let us call the edge (i, j) *right* if $R(i, j) \leq r$. Scan all the "right" edges and select among them one with the minimum time value. Denote the latter value by b_0. Clearly, $b_0 \leq b^* \leq nb_0$.

The complexity of Step A1 is $O((m+n) \log n)$; the complexity of Steps A2 and A3 is $O(m)$. Therefore, Step A requires $O((m+n) \log n)$ time in total. If we cannot find any right arc in Step A2, the problem has no feasible solution. Then we return "no solution" without performing Steps B and C.

Step B. Find the improved lower and upper bounds such that $UB/LB \leq 2$.

This step uses a test procedure denoted by Test(v, ε). Test(v, ε) is a parametric dynamic-programming type algorithm that has the following property: Given positive parameters v and ε, it either reports that the maximum possible time $t^* \geq v$ or reports that that $t^* \leq v(1+\varepsilon)$.

Associate with each path p a pair (T, R), where $T = T(p)$ is the path time and $R = R(p)$ is the path resource (or budget). We deal with sets $S(k)$ of pairs (B, R) arranged in decreasing order of the T values so that every pair in $S(k)$ corresponds to a path from node s to node k. As in DP, we delete all the dominated pairs in all the $S(k)$ sets. In addition to the dominated pairs, we delete δ-close pairs as follows:

Given inaccuracy δ, if there are two pairs in $S(k)$, say, $(T1, R1)$ and $(T2, R2)$, such that $0 \leq T2 - T1 \leq \delta$, then the pairs are called δ-close. We use the operation called discarding δ-close from set $S(k)$, which means the following:

(a) Let v be a given parameter satisfying $LB \leq v \leq UB$. In each $S(k)$, partition the interval $[0, v]$ into $\lceil (n/\varepsilon) \rceil$ equal sub-intervals of size no greater than $\delta = \varepsilon v/n$; one more interval is $[v, UB]$

(b) If more than one pair from $S(k)$ fall into any one of the above sub-intervals, discard all such δ-close pairs, leaving only one representative pair in each sub-interval, namely the pair with the smallest (in this sub-interval) R-coordinate.

Lemma 2. The complexity of Test(v, ε) is $O(mn^2/\varepsilon)$ and the space required is $O(n^2/\varepsilon)$.

Indeed, since the sub-interval length is $\delta = \varepsilon v/n$, we have $O(n/\varepsilon)$ sub-intervals in the interval $[0, v]$. Therefore there are $O(n/\varepsilon)$ representative pairs in any set W and

$S(k)$. Furthermore, constructing each W requires $O(n/\varepsilon)$ elementary operations.. Merging the sorted sets W and T, as well as discarding all the dominated pairs, is accomplished in linear time (in the number of pairs, which is $O(n/\varepsilon)$). Thus, algorithm Test(v, ε) has a total time complexity of $O(mn^2/\varepsilon)$. The space is $O(n^2/\varepsilon)$ since in each $S(k)$, $k = 1, ..., n$, there are at most $O(n/\varepsilon)$ pairs. □

Now we present a narrowing procedure in this section, which originates from the procedure suggested by [11] for solving the restricted shortest path. Specifically, when running Test(w, ε), we choose ε to be a function of UB/LB changing from iteration to iteration. For the reader's convenience, in order to distinguish between the allowable error (ε) in the FPTAS and an iteratively changing error in the testing procedure, we denote the latter by θ.

The idea is that when UB and LB are far from each other, we choose a large θ; when UB and LB get closer, we choose a smaller θ. More precisely, just as in [11], in each iteration of Test(v, θ), we set $\theta \leftarrow \sqrt{UB/LB}-1$, and a new v-value   is:

$$v=\sqrt{LB \cdot UB/(1+\theta)} \ .$$

Step C. The ε-approximation algorithm. We start Step C with deriving LB and UB, satisfying $UB/LB \leq 2$, and then obtain an ε-approximate path.

The corresponding algorithm is presented in Fig. 3:

The ε-approximation algorithm AA (*LB, UB, ε*)
1.   Input: $G(N, A)$, $|N| = n$, $|A| = m$, $\{(t_{ij}(q), r_{ij}(q)): (i, j) \in A, 1 \leq q \leq Q\}$; R_q
2.   Input ε, v, q, and d
3. $\delta \leftarrow \varepsilon w/n$
4.   **Step 1.** [Initialization]
5.   Set $S(1)=\{(0, 0)\}$
6. $S(k) \leftarrow \varnothing$ for $k=2,...,n$
7.   **Step 2.** [Generate $S(1)$ to $S(t_d)$]
8.   Repeat n-1 times
9.   for each arc (u,k) leading from node u to node k do
10. $W \leftarrow \varnothing$
11.   for each pair $(B, R) \in S(u)$ do
12.   if $R + r_{uk}(q) \leq R_q$, then $W \leftarrow W \cup \{(B+ b_{uk}(q), R + r_{uk}(q))\}$
13.   end for
14. $S(k) \leftarrow$ merge($S(k), W$); during merging eliminate the dominated and δ-close pairs
15.   end for
16.   end Repeat
17.   **Step 3.** [Check cycles]
18.   for each arc (u,k) leading from node u to node k do
19. $W \leftarrow \varnothing$
20.   for each pair $(T, R) \in S(u)$ do
21.   if $R + r_{uk}(q) \leq R_q$, then $W \leftarrow W \cup \{(T+ b_{uk}(q), R + r_{uk}(q))\}$
22.   end for
23. $ST \leftarrow$ merge($S(k), W$); during merging eliminate the dominated pairs
1.   *If $S(k) \neq ST$ return "no answer"*
24.   end for
25.   **Step 4.** [Determine approximate solution]
26.   find min T in $S(t_d)$, denote it by *ans*
27.   Return *ans* as the ε-approximate; use backtracking to find the path.

Fig. 3. The ε-approximation algorithm **AA**

Theorem 1. The complexity of AA(LB, UB, ε) is $O(mn^2/\varepsilon)$. The complexity of the three-step approximation algorithm is $O(mn^2/\varepsilon)$. The space required is $O(n^2/\varepsilon)$.

Proof. Since the sub-interval length is $\delta = \varepsilon LB/n$, we have $O(n(UB/LB)(1/\varepsilon))$ sub-intervals in interval $[0, UB]$ and since $UB/LB \leq 2$, there are $O(n/\varepsilon)$ sub-intervals in interval $[LB, UB]$. Therefore there are $O(n/\varepsilon)$ representative pairs in any set W, and $S(k)$. Constructing each W requires $O(n/\varepsilon)$ elementary operations. Merging the sorted sets W and $S(k)$ as well as discarding all the dominated pairs, is accomplished in linear time (in the number of pairs, which is $O(n/\varepsilon)$). In Step 2 lines 8-16, we have two nested loops: the first begins at line 8 and the second at line 9. Because these loops go over all arcs $n-1$ times, in total we have $O(mn)$ iterations of lines 11-13. Thus, the algorithm has a time complexity of $O(mn^2/\varepsilon)$. Since Step C dominates steps A and B of the algorithm, the complexity of the entire approximation algorithm is $O(mn/\varepsilon)$. The space is $O(n^2/\varepsilon)$ since in each $S(k)$ ($k=1,...,n$) there are at most $O(n/\varepsilon)$ pairs. □

Now we can incorporate the algorithm AA into the integrated algorithm DISPATCHING-Q for solving the multi-agent problem. DISPATCHING-Q runs the AA $|Q|\cdot|D|$ times, each time yielding an approximate path and the time, for a certain agent q and a certain destination d. The return of the total time is the minimum of the individual times of Q mobile agents.

The total time returned by DISPATCHING-Q is at least $(1-\varepsilon)OPT$, where OPT is the total optimal time gathered by all the agents. Since OPT is the minimum of $OPT1(q, d)$ for all agents, we have: $APP = \sum_{q \in Q} APP1(q,d) \geq \sum_{q \in Q} (1-\varepsilon)OPT1(q,d) = (1-\varepsilon)OPT$.

Theorem 2. Complexity of the heuristic DISPATCHING-Q is $O(|Q|\cdot|D|\cdot mn^2/\varepsilon + h^3)$, where $h = \max\{|Q|, |D|\}$.

Proof: Because DISPATCHING-Q runs the FPTAS(q, d) $O(|Q|\cdot|D|)$ times and the FPTAS(q, d) complexity, according to Theorem 1, is $O(m\ n^2/\varepsilon)$, the complexity of DISPATCHING-Q is $O(|Q|\cdot|D|\cdot mn^2/\varepsilon)$. The space required by the algorithm is $O(n^2/\varepsilon + h^2)$ because in each iteration of the FPTAS, the previous iteration data can be discarded. The assignment problem can be solved in polynomial time, e.g., in $O(h^3)$. Therefore the total time of DISPACHING-Q is $O(|Q|\cdot|D|\cdot mn^2/\varepsilon + h^3)$. □

So the heuristic DISPATCHING-Q has a polynomial worst-case complexity.

5   Computational Experiments

We examine the computational properties of the new scheduling algorithm, described in section 3, on an experimental WSN. We varied the number of mobile agents from 4 to 12 and the number of randomly distributed sensors from 50 to 150. We coded the programs from sections 4 and additional program form another paper [6] in Java and ran them on a NEWRON computer with Intel Core i3 CPU, 3.06 GHz, 4 GB memory. The agent attributes were uniformly distributed random numbers in the interval [1; 25]. For each combination of the network size, we randomly generated 30 numerical instances, totally about 600 different network configurations.

Computational results are presented in Table 1 that compares the running time of the algorithm DISPATCHING-Q for $\varepsilon=0.1$ (denoted here by LKET) with those of two other algorithms: the rounding FPTAS developed by [6] for $\varepsilon=0.1$ (denoted by CSA), and the exact dynamic programming algorithm DP.

Table 1. Comparisons of the routing/dispatching algorithms

Network size		Number of agents	Average running time (hours)		
# of nodes	# of edges		LKET	CSA	DP
50	1,000	4	0.01	0.01	0.58
100	2,500	8	0.09	0.24	2.38
150	5,000	12	0.25	1.98	28.50*

* The entry with an asterisk required more than two hours of running time. The value in the table is the extrapolation on the basis of theoretical worst-case estimation.

We can observe that the new algorithm outperforms CSA and DP algorithms.

6   Conclusion

The choice of a search strategy in search-and-detection of hidden targets has a strong impact on the search costs and losses incurred by the target as well as the chance of finding the target within time and cost limits. Specifically, in this paper we focus on finding a fast scheduling/dispatching procedure for detecting hidden human-made underground tunnels by multiple searchers. The makeup of an optimal or near optimal combination of sensors depends on the particular combination of factors for a given scenario. The problem then becomes a problem of determining the optimal combination of sensors, that is, a combination that can perform well for a large number of possible scenarios for different hidden object types.

It is possible that the time complexity of the algorithm presented in this paper can be improved on. The approximation scheme can be combined with the information quality analysis aimed at minimizing the false-negative and false-positive sensor tests. This is a challenging question for our future research.

References

1. Aboudi, R., Jornsten, K.: Resource-constrained assignment problem 26(2-3), 175–191 (1990)
2. Ahuja, R.K., Magnanti, T.L., Orlin, J.B.: Network Flows: Theory, Algorithms, and Applications. Prentice Hall, New Jersey (1993)
3. Akyildiz, I.F., Su, W., Sankarasubramaniam, Y., Cayirci, E.: Wireless sensor networks: a survey. Computer Networks 38(4), 393–422 (2002)
4. Benkoski, S.J., Monticino, M.G., Weisinger, J.R.: A survey of the search theory literature. Naval Research Logistics 38(4), 469–494 (1991)
5. Brewington, B., Gray, R., Moizumi, K.K.: D., Cybenko, G., Rus, D.: Mobile agents in distributed information retrieval. Intelligent Information Agents, 355–395 (1999)

6. Camponogara, E., Shima, R.B.: Mobile agent routing with time constraints: A resource constrained longest-path approach. Journal of Universal Computer Science 16(3), 372–401 (2010)
7. Chakrabarti, A., Sabharwal, A., Aazhang, B.: Using predictable observer mobility for power efficient design of sensor networks. In: Zhao, F., Guibas, L.J. (eds.) IPSN 2003. LNCS, vol. 2634, pp. 129–145. Springer, Heidelberg (2003)
8. Cornwall, J., Despain, A., Eardley, D., Garwin, R., Hammer, D.: Characterization of Underground Facilities. Report No. JSR-97-155. MITRE Corp, New York (1999)
9. Dargie, W., Poellabauer, C.: Fundamentals of Wireless Sensor Networks: Theory and Practice, 330 pages. John Wiley and Sons (2010)
10. Elalouf, A., Levner, E., Cheng, T.C.E.: Routing and dispatching of multiple mobile agents in integrated enterprises. Int. Journal of Prouction Economics 145(1), 96–106 (2013)
11. Ergun, F., Sinha, R., Zhang, L.: An improved FPTAS for restricted shortest path. Information Processing Letters 83, 287–291 (2002)
12. Garey, M.R., Johnson, D.S.: Computers and Intractability, A Guide to the Theory of NP-Completeness. W.H.Freeman and Company (1979)
13. Gonzalez-Valdes, Quivira, F., Martinez-Lorenzo, J.A., Rappaport, C.M.: Tunnel detection using underground-focusing spotlight SAR and rough surface estimation. In: 2012 IEEE Antennas and Propagation Society International Symposium (APSURSI), pp. 1–2 (2012)
14. Kansal, A., Somasundara, A., Jea, D., Srivastava, M., Estrin, D.: Intelligent fluid infrastructure for embedded networks. In: The Second International Conference on Mobile Systems, Applications, and Services (MobiSys), (2004)
15. Klar, Linker, R.: Feasibility study of the automated detection and localization of underground tunnel excavation using Brillouin optical time domain reflectometer. In: SPIE Defense, Security, and Sensing. International Society for Optics and Photonics (2009)
16. Kress, M., Lin, K.Y., Szechtman, R.: Optimal discrete search with imperfect specificity. Mathematical Methods of Operations Research 68(3), 539–549 (2008)
17. Kress, M., Royset, J.O., Rozen, N.: The eye and the fist: Optimizing search and interdiction. European Journal of Operational Research 220(2), 550–558 (2012)
18. Kriheli, B., Levner, E.: Search and detection of failed components in repairable complex systems under imperfect inspections. In: Batyrshin, I., Mendoza, M.G. (eds.) MICAI 2012, Part II. LNCS, vol. 7630, pp. 399–410. Springer, Heidelberg (2013)
19. Lenstra, J.K., Kan, A.R., Shmoys, D.B.: The traveling salesman problem: a guided tour of combinatorial optimization, p. 3. Wiley, New York (1985)
20. Levner, E.: Infinite-horizon scheduling algorithms for optimal search for hidden objects. Int. Trans. Opl. Res. 1(2), 241–250 (1994)
21. Levner, E., Elalouf, A., Cheng, T.C.E.: An improved FPTAS for mobile agent routing with time constraints. Journal of Universal Computer Science 17(13), 1854–1862 (2011)
22. Li, M., Liu, Y.: Underground structure monitoring with wireless sensor networks. In: Proceedings of the 6th International Conference on Information Processing in Sensor Networks, pp. 69–78 (2007)
23. Linker, R., Klar, A.: Detection of tunnel excavation using fiber optic reflectometry: experimental validation. In: SPIE Defense, Security, and Sensing. International Society for Optics and Photonics (2013)
24. Lo Monte, L., Erricolo, D., Soldovieri, F., Wicks, M.C.: Radio frequency tomography for tunnel detection. IEEE Transactions on Geoscience and Remote Sensing 48(3), 1128–1137 (2010)
25. Mazzola, J.B., Neebe, A.W.: Resource-constrained assignment scheduling. Operations Research 34(4), 560–572 (1986)

26. Piwakowski, B., Tricot, J.C., Leonard, C., Ouarradi, N., Delannoy, B.: Underground tunnels detection and location by high resolution seismic reflection. In: 3rd EEGS Meeting (1997)
27. Sahni, S.: Algorithms for scheduling independent tasks. Journal of ACM 23(1), 116–127 (1976)
28. Sato, H., Royset, J.O.: Path optimization for the resource-constrained searcher. Naval Research Logistics 57, 422–440 (2010)
29. Senglaub, M., Yee, M., Elbring, G., Abbott, R., Bonal, N.: Sensor Integration Study for a Shallow Tunnel Detection System. Sandia Report, Sandia National Laboratory, New Mexico, USA (2010)
30. Sugihara, R., Gupta, R.K.: Optimal speed control of mobile node for data collection in sensor networks. IEEE Transactions on Mobile Computing 9(1), 127–139 (2010)
31. Stone, L.D.: Theory of Optimal Search. ORSA, New York (1992)
32. Somasundara, A., Ramamoorthy, A., Srivastava, M.B.: Mobile element scheduling for efficient data collection in wireless sensor networks with dynamic deadlines. In: Proceedings of the 25th IEEE International Real-Time Systems Symposium, RTSS (2004)
33. Song, N.O., Teneketzis, D.: Discrete search with multiple sensors. Math. Methods Oper. Res. 60(1), 1–13 (2004)
34. Toth, P., Vigo, D.: The Vehicle Routing Problem. Society for Industrial & Applied Mathematics (SIAM), New York (2001)
35. Tucker, R.E., McKenna, J.R., McKenna, M.H., Mattice, M.S.: Detecting underground penetration attempts at secure facilities. Army Engineer School, Fort Leonard Wood MO (2007)
36. Verma, R.: A Survey on Wireless Sensor Network Applications, Design Influencing Factors & Types of Sensor Network. International Journal of Innovative Technology and Exploring Engineering 3(5), 2278–3075 (2013)
37. Vesecky, J.F., Nierenberg, W.A., Despain, A.M.: Tunnel detection. Report No. SRI-JSR-79-11. SRI International Arlington VA (1980)
38. Warston, H., Petersson, H.: Ground surveillance and fusion of ground target sensor data in a network based defense. In: Proceedings of the 7th International Conference on Sensors (2004)
39. Washburn, A.R.: Search and Detection. INFORMS, New York (2002)
40. Wu, Q., Rao, N.S.V., Barhen, J., Iyengar, S.S., Veishavi, V.K., Qi, H., Chakrabarty, K.: On computing mobile agent routes for data fusion in distributed sensor networks. IEEE Transactions on Knowledge and Data Engineering 16(6), 1–14 (2004)

A Constraint-Based Planner for Mars Express Orbiter

Martin Kolombo and Roman Barták

Charles University in Prague, Faculty of Mathematics and Physics
Malostranské náměstí 25, 118 00 Praha 1, Czech Republic
kolombomartin@gmail.com, bartak@ktiml.mff.cuni.cz

Abstract. The Mars Express mission is a space exploration mission being conducted by the European Space Agency. The Mars Express Orbiter is extremely successful and is performing scientific experiments since early 2004, generating 2-3Gbit of scientific data per day. It is therefore very important to plan its activities properly to obtain high-quality scientific data outcome. The paper describes a complete constraint-based automated planner of the Mars Express Orbiter activities covering uploading tele-commands, experiments and maintenance activities, and downloading data back to Earth.

Keywords: Planning, scheduling, scientific operations, MEX mission.

1 Introduction

Complete planning and scheduling of all spacecraft operations is a challenging area with the remote agent experiment at Deep Space 1 being a pioneering system [8]. Still the complete approach is rare in practice. For example, in the Mars Express (MEX) mission, planning and scheduling techniques are used to solve some sub-problems namely scheduling command upload and data download. MEXAR 2 [3] and RAXEM [9] are two tools operational at ESA-ESOC. MEXAR 2 was developed to schedule Data Dumping activities while RAXEM schedules Command Uplink activities. However, these tasks (downlink and uplink) are just two types of tasks necessary to operate the spacecraft. The core role of MEX consists of scientific (observation) tasks that are complemented by the command uplink and data downlink activities. There are also maintenance activities necessary to keep the spacecraft in a good condition. Currently the complete planning process is realized through a collaborative problem solving process between the science team and the mission planning team. Two teams of human planners iteratively refine a plan of all activities of the mission. In 2012 this complex planning problem has been proposed as a challenge for the Fourth International Competition on Knowledge Engineering for Planning and Scheduling (ICKEPS 2012) [5]. The goal was to develop a system that takes the description of scientific operations together with operational constraints, ground station visibility, a spacecraft trajectory etc. as its input and generates a complete schedule of all the uplink, science, downlink, maintenance, and auxiliary operations. Notice in particular that the flight dynamics is not part of the solution as the spacecraft trajectory is given as the input. The plan must respect all operational constraints and maximize the scientific outcome.

A. Gelbukh et al. (Eds.): MICAI 2014, Part II, LNAI 8857, pp. 451–463, 2014.
© Springer International Publishing Switzerland 2014

So far only one system was proposed to solve the complete MEX Orbiter planning problem. This was an ad-hoc planner based on incrementally adding observation activities together with their supporting activities (command uplink, data downlink, and change pointing) to a partial plan [7]. Though this approach scales well with the increasing number of observations, its major drawback is extremely hard maintenance at the level of source code. In this paper we propose a planner based on constraint satisfaction techniques. The idea is that the problem is described as a scheduling problem with optional activities and this problem is then modeled as a constraint satisfaction problem. This is possible because the observation activities are known in advance and the unknown activities for changing pointing can be modeled similarly to set-up activities in manufacturing scheduling [2]. The major advantage of the constraint-based approach is its modularity and extendibility as new constraints can be added easily. As we will show experimentally, this approach also generates more compact plans in comparison to the ad-hoc approach.

In the paper we will first introduce the problem solved and describe some simplifications that we took. Then we will briefly introduce the constraint satisfaction technology with the focus on constraints used in the model. After that we will describe the constraint model for the MEX planning problem together with the search strategy. The paper is concluded by experimental evaluation of the model and comparison to the ad-hoc approach.

2   Problem Description

The MEX domain was proposed as a challenge problem for the Fourth International Competition on Knowledge Engineering for Planning and Scheduling (ICKEPS 2012) [5]. We adopted this problem in our work and in this section we will describe the core parts of the problem specification that are necessary to understand the solution.

The Mars Express Orbiter (MEX) is a spacecraft (Figure 1) operating at Mars orbit. The orbiter carries six operating scientific instruments called payloads that collect data about Martians atmosphere, planet's structure and its geology:

- ASPERA - Energetic Neutral Atoms Imager,
- HRSC - High-Resolution Stereo Camera,
- MARSIS - Mars Advanced Radar for Subsurface and Ionosphere Sounding,
- OMEGA - IR Mineralogical Mapping Spectrometer,
- PFS - Planetary Fourier Spectrometer,
- SPICAM - UV and IR Atmospheric Spectrometer.

There is one more instrument VMS (Visual Monitoring Camera) that is not used anymore and hence omitted from planning. The major task is to schedule as many experiments on the payloads as possible. In general, this is an oversubscribed scheduling problem though in the proposed model we will assume that all observations can be scheduled as no information about which experiments are more preferred is given.

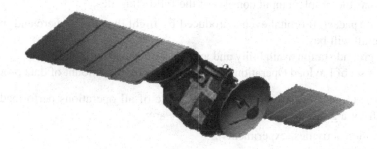

Fig. 1. Mars Express Orbiter

Each payload has an accompanying *data store* with limited capacity, which is used exclusively by a given payload (no sharing). The data produced in the experiments is saved on these data stores and has to be downloaded to Earth before data from another experiment overwrites it. The data size is known for each experiment. The experiments require particular positions of the spacecraft in orbit (see below) and particular *pointings*, which describe the orientation of the spacecraft in orbit. The spacecraft can focus on Mars in the *Inertial* (NAD) and *Fixed* (FIX) pointing – required by certain experiments – or the spacecraft can be directed on Earth in the *Earth* pointing – for uplink, downlink, and maintenance. The spacecraft can maintain NAD and FIX pointings for a limited time only (68 minutes for NAD and 90 minutes for FIX). To transfer from one pointing to another the orbiter needs to perform a *Pointing Transition Action* (PTA) taking 30 minutes.

The main activity of the spacecraft is a scientific experiment that is fully described as a *Payload Operation Request* (POR). A POR activity always has a fixed offset time restricting when it can be scheduled. The offset is tied to the MEX's passage of the orbit's pericenter. A single orbit takes roughly seven hours to complete. It should be noted, that more instruments can perform POR activities in parallel, if the conditions for operating the instruments are met. The only condition considered in our solution is the pointing required by the specific instrument. The required pointing is specified in the Payload Operation Request. It is expected that there will be more PORs than the orbiter can accommodate, but in our current experimental setting, all PORs can be scheduled. In addition to experiments, the spacecraft is expected to perform regular maintenance routines, which need to run every 3 to 5 orbits. A maintenance activity takes 90 minutes; it must be performed in the Earth pointing preferably close to the orbit apocenter. These maintenance activities must be part of the schedule.

The description of every activity taken by the orbiter needs to be uplinked from Earth to the spacecraft as a *TeleCommand* (TC). We expect that there is always enough memory for TCs. Uplink of TCs is one type of communication activities; the other type is downlink of data produced by an experiment and during maintenance. The MEX can downlink and uplink data at the same time. For the communication to be possible the orbiter needs to be in the Earth pointing and a ground station needs to be available at the time of the communication. The description of availability of ground stations as well as their bitrates is one of the problem inputs.

In summary, the problem input consists of the following files:

- EVTM: spacecraft orbital events produced by flight dynamic (where and when the spacecraft will be),
- GSA: ground station availability and antennas transmission bitrates,
- POR: a set of Payload Operation Requests including the amount of data produced.

The goal is to generate a complete plan/schedule of all operations performed by the spacecraft for a given period. In particular there are:

- observation activities (experiments),
- maintenance activities,
- pointing transition activities,
- command uploading activities,
- data downloading activities.

3   Background on Constraint Satisfaction

Constraint satisfaction technology originated in Artificial Intelligence as a technique for declarative modeling and solving of combinatorial optimization problems. Recall that a constraint satisfaction problem (CSP) is a triple (X, D, C), where X is a finite set of decision variables, for each $x_i \in X$, $D_i \in D$ is a finite set of possible values for the variable x_i (the domain), and C is a finite set of constraints [4]. A constraint is a relation over a subset of variables (its scope) that restricts the possible combinations of values to be assigned to the variables in its scope. Constraints can be expressed in extension using a set of compatible value tuples or as a formula. A solution to a CSP is a complete instantiation of variables such that the values are taken from respective domains and all constraints are satisfied.

Constraint satisfaction techniques are frequently based on the combination of inference techniques (called consistency techniques) and search. The most widely used consistency technique is *arc consistency* that maintains consistency of individual constraints by removing values that violate the constraint. As different constraints remove different inconsistencies the choice of right constraints is critical for efficient problem solving. Formulation of a CSP for a given problem is called *constraint modeling*. In the constraint model for the MEX planner we will use arithmetic and table constraints, where the table constraint uses a table of compatible value tuples to define the constraint. We will also use two specific constraints: element and cumulative. In the constraint element(X,List,Y), X and Y are variables and List is a list of variables – element is a (k + 2)-ary constraint, where k is the length of List. The semantics of element(X,List,Y) is as follows: Y equals to the X-th element of List, Y = List_X. For example the constraint element(2, [3, 4, 5], 4) is satisfied, while element(3,[3,4,5],4) is not satisfied. The constraint cumulative(Tasks, Limit) models a cumulative resource with the capacity Limit to which a set of tasks should be allocated. Each task is specified by its start and end times and resource capacity that the task consumes – task(Start, End, Cap). The constraint ensures that the tasks are allocated to times in such a way that the resource capacity limit is never exceeded.

Arc consistency is a local inference technique meaning that in general it does not remove all values that do not belong to the solution. Therefore a search algorithm is necessary to instantiate the variables. The search algorithm is usually integrated with the inference procedure in the following way. After each search decision the problem is made arc consistent. If the problem is still consistent, the inference procedure might remove some inconsistencies (for example, inconsistent values of variables) and hence prune the remaining search space. If the problem is found inconsistent then the search algorithm explores the alternative branch(es) or backtracks (if no alternative branch remains). The *search strategy* defines how the search space is explored, for example by defining in which order the variables will be instantiated (variable selection) and in which order the values will be assigned (value selection). It is also possible to use a disjunction of constraints splitting the search apace, such as the disjunction $X = Y$ or $X \neq Y$ that splits the search space into two disjoint subareas, a so called semantic branching [6]. We will define a specific search strategy for the MEX model.

4   Constraint Model

The MEX problem is a mixed planning and scheduling problem. We know the POR activities (experiments) together with their auxiliary activities (uplink of telecommands and downlink of data) and the task is to allocate them to time while respecting the resource capacities. This is a scheduling problem. However, we do not know in advance the maintenance and PTA (pointing transition) activities as they depend on the allocation of POR and communication activities. Hence we need to plan them. We will use the idea of optional activities where more activities are generated in the input but not all of them will be scheduled.

Recall, that maintenance activities should appear 3 to 5 orbits from each other and each orbit is 7 hours. If D is a total scheduling horizon in hours (frequently it is one week, 168 hours) then the upper bound for the number of maintenance activities is $\lceil D/21 \rceil$. In our model, we use a less conservative estimate $\lceil D/28 \rceil$. The non-used maintenance activities will be allocated after the scheduling horizon. Regarding the PTA activities, we know that pointing may need to be changed before the experiments and before the communication activities. We assume that each POR will require exactly one data downlink activity (all data will be downloaded together). Moreover, command uplink is much shorter than data downlink and as both uplink and downlink operations can run in parallel, we can ignore the uplink operations during scheduling and we add them later during post-processing. Let N be the number of POR activities then we estimate the maximal number of PTA activities as 2N. The idea is that non-used PTA activities will have zero duration (see below).

We showed that we can generate all activities to be scheduled in advance and hence we can see the problem as a scheduling problem. Constraint-based scheduling [1] is a good approach to handle such problems and hence we decided to use it there. In the rest of this section we will specify the constraint model used, that is, the variables, their domains, and constraints.

4.1   Variables

Recall, that we have four types of activities to be scheduled: POR (experiments), data downlink (communication), PTA (pointing transition), and maintenance. TeleCommand uplink activities will be added during post-processing. Each POR activity is allocated to a particular payload. Each payload can process at most one activity at any time, but PORs for different payloads may run in parallel provided that they share the same pointing. Communication, PTA, and maintenance activities occupy the spacecraft completely and cannot run in parallel with any other activity. As resources are pre-allocated to activities we only need to decide the time allocation of all activities. Hence each activity i of type X is modeled using the variables for its start time S_i^X, end time E_i^X, and duration D_i^X that are connected using the constraints:

$$\forall X,i: S_i^X + D_i^X = E_i^X \tag{1}$$

Table 1 shows the names of the variables for all types of activities in the problem. Note that POR, communication, and maintenance activities need to be connected to a particular PTA activity that sets the right pointing for the activity. We use W_i^X variables that specify an index of the PTA activity in the sequence of PTA activities. Note that several activities may share the same pointing so some variables W_i^X may have the same value. On the other hand, there might be pointing activities that are not used by any of these activities. Recall that NAD and FIX pointing can hold for the limited time only so we may need to change pointing to Earth even if there is no particular activity requiring it (see the constraints later).

Table 1. Variables for modeling activities

Activity type	Index i	Start time	End time	Duration	Pointing window
POR (experiment)	$1..N$	S_i^{POR}	E_i^{POR}	D_i^{POR}	W_i^{POR}
Downlink (comm.)	$1..N$	S_i^{COM}	E_i^{COM}	D_i^{COM}	W_i^{COM}
PTA (pointing switch)	$1..2N$	S_i^{PTA}	E_i^{PTA}	D_i^{PTA}	–
Maintenance	$1..\lceil D/28 \rceil$	S_i^{MTN}	E_i^{MTN}	D_i^{MTN}	W_i^{MTN}

Let us now specify the domains of all the variables. Durations of the POR activities are constant and given in the input. Duration of the maintenance activities is 90 minutes. Duration of the PTA activities is 30 minutes, but we set the domain of D_i^{PTA} to be $\{0,30\}$, where 0 means that the pointing activity is not used. Duration of the downlink activities depends on the amount of data and bitrate of used ground station. We know the amount of data for each POR activity i, let us denote it $data_i$. We are given the communication windows and bitrates for each ground station in the input. We do not need to distinguish between the ground stations so we may assume that we have a set of (possibly overlapping) communication windows $[S_j^{GRA}, E_j^{GRA}]$ and corresponding bitrates $bitrate_j^{GRA}$ in the input. Then for each POR activity i we can define a table constraint connecting the possible start time and duration of its communication action (Table 2). For W communication windows, each such table has W lines; each line describes one communication window, that is, the possible start time and duration of the communication activity for the POR activity i.

Table 2. Table constraint for the communication activity i

S_i^{COM}	D_i^{COM}
$[S_1^{GRA}, E_1^{GRA} - \lceil data_i / bitrate_1^{GRA} \rceil]$	$\lceil data_i / bitrate_1^{GRA} \rceil$
...	...
$[S_W^{GRA}, E_W^{GRA} - \lceil data_i / bitrate_W^{GRA} \rceil]$	$\lceil data_i / bitrate_W^{GRA} \rceil$

Note that the above table constraints also define the domains of variables S_i^{COM} while the domain of E_i^{COM} is set via the constraints (1). We set the domains of variables S_i^{PTA} and S_i^{MTN} to be [0,2D] to allow non-used PTA and maintenance activities to appear after the schedule horizon D ([a,b] denotes an interval starting at a and finishing at b). The domain of start-time variables S_i^{POR} of POR activities is defined by a given offset from the pericenter and locations of pericenters given in the input (EVTM). Let p_j be the time when the orbiter reaches j-th pericenter (there are P pericenters) and o_i be the offset of the i-th POR. Then we define the domain of the start times of the POR activity i as follows:

$$\forall i: \text{dom}(S_i^{POR}) = \{ p_j + o_i \mid j \in [1,P] \} \tag{2}$$

Again, the domain of variables E_i^{POR} is set via constraints (1). Finally, the domain for all W_i^X is [1,2N] as these variables denote the indexes of PTA activities.

4.2   Payload Constraints

Recall that each payload can process at most one activity at any time. Let $Payload_j$ be the set of indexes of POR activities assigned of payload j. Then for each payload j we define a resource constraint that forbids overlap of payload activities. Each activity consumes one unit of the resource whose capacity is also one (unary resource):

$$\forall j: \text{cumulative}(\{task(S_i^{POR}, E_i^{POR}, 1) \mid i \in Payload_j \}, 1) \tag{3}$$

Now we need to connect the POR activities with the corresponding communication (data downlink) activities. Obviously, the downlink must start after the experiment finishes:

$$\forall i: E_i^{POR} < S_i^{COM} \tag{4}$$

Moreover, data produced by the experiment must stay in memory until they are downloaded to Earth. We reserve the memory since the start of the experiment (POR) till the end of the communication. Let $PayloadCap_j$ by the capacity of memory assigned to payload j. Then we can model the memory resource as follows:

$$\forall j: \text{cumulative}(\{task(S_i^{POR}, E_i^{COM}, data_i) \mid i \in Payload_j \}, PayloadCap_j) \tag{5}$$

4.3   Maintenance Constraints

The maintenance activities should be scheduled 3 to 5 orbits apart. As all maintenance activities are identical we can order them in time to remove permutation symmetries:

$$\forall i: S_i^{MTN} + 21 < S_{i+1}^{MTN} < S_i^{MTN} + 35 \tag{6}$$

Moreover, we need to schedule the first maintenance activity close to schedule start. We assume that last maintenance finished close to the start of schedule (at most seven hours before the schedule start), but any time in past can be used:

$$S_1^{MTN} < 28 \tag{7}$$

4.4   Pointing Transition Constraints

Finally, we need to define the pointing transition constraints and connect the POR, communication, and maintenance activities with the corresponding PTA activities. For each PTA activity i we introduce two more variables, one defining the object to which the spacecraft points Pt_i (Earth, NAD, FIX) and one defining the duration of the pointing T_i (its domain is $[1,+\infty]$). This duration describes the time when the spacecraft stays in the given pointing after the pointing transition finished. Recall that the spacecraft can stay in NAD and FIX pointings for a limited time only. This restriction is described using a tabular constraint as specified in Table 3.

Table 3. Table constraint for the pointing transition i

Pt_i	T_i
Earth	$[1,+\infty]$
NAD	$[1,68]$
FIX	$[1,90]$

Similarly to maintenance activities we remove the permutation symmetry between the PTA activities by ordering them (this also defines the pointing duration T_i):

$$\forall i: E_i^{PTA} + T_i = S_{i+1}^{PTA} \tag{8}$$

Moreover to keep the "empty" transitions at the end of the sequence we use the following constraint. Briefly speaking if the duration of some PTA is set to zero then all following PTAs will also have zero duration (recall that the domain of PTA duration variables is $\{0,30\}$).

$$\forall i: D_{i+1}^{PTA} \leq D_i^{PTA} \tag{9}$$

Let us call the POR, communication, and maintenance activities the main activities. Now we connect the main activities with the corresponding PTA activities. Briefly speaking, the PTA activity that changes spacecraft pointing to the requested pointing must finish before the main activity and the next pointing activity must start after the end of the main activity. In other words, during the main activity, the pointing will be as requested. This is where the variable W_i^X and element constraints will play a role. Let E^{PTA} be the sequence of variables E_i^{PTA} ordered by i, S^{PTA} be the sequence of variables S_i^{PTA} ordered by i, and SP_i^X and EP_i^X be auxiliary variables denoting the interval when a given pointing holds. Then the following constraints define the requested connection:

$$\forall X,i:\ \text{element}(W_i^X, E^{PTA}, SP_i^X) \wedge SP_i^X \leq S_i^X \tag{10}$$

$$\forall X,i:\ \text{element}(1+W_i^X, S^{PTA}, EP_i^X) \wedge E_i^X \leq EP_i^X$$

We also need to set the requested type of pointing (Earth, NAD, FIX) for the main operation, let us call it RPt_i^X and let Pt be the sequence of variables Pt_i ordered by i. Then the constraint is defined as:

$$\forall X,i:\ \text{element}(W_i^X, Pt, RPt_i^X) \tag{11}$$

4.5 Other Constraints

The constraints (10) and (11) ensure that the PTA activities are not overlapping with the main activities. As maintenance activities require a different pointing (Earth) than POR activities (FIX or NAD) these two types of activities are also not overlapping. Only communication activities may overlap with maintenance activities, which should be forbidden. We will use the following constraint ensuring the activities of different types are not overlapping and at most six POR activities run in parallel (there are six payloads):

$$\begin{aligned}
\text{cumulative}(\{&\text{task}(S_i^{POR}, E_i^{POR}, 1) \mid \forall i\ \} \cup \\
\{&\text{task}(S_i^{COM}, E_i^{COM}, 6) \mid \forall i\ \} \cup \\
\{&\text{task}(S_i^{PTA}, E_i^{PTA}, 6) \mid \forall i\ \} \cup \\
\{&\text{task}(S_i^{MTN}, E_i^{MTN}, 6) \mid \forall i\ \}, 6)
\end{aligned} \tag{12}$$

5 Search Strategy

After specifying the constraint model, we decided to define a search strategy that takes in account specifics of the problem. We used the following core principles for the search strategy. First, the POR activities (experiments) are scheduled as they determine how the schedule will look. We schedule them as early as possible to leave as much as possible space for other experiments. We also assign them the corresponding PTA activities (pointing transition) and after performing the pointing, we suggest to change pointing to Earth. This is motivated by observation of real schedules, where experiments with the same pointing are grouped and then data are downloaded to Earth (hence the Earth pointing). After the POR activities are scheduled, we schedule the PTA activities. Basically we try to omit non-necessary pointing operations by trying the zero duration. For real pointings we try first the Earth pointing (unless the pointing was already decided) because the Earth pointing is safer for the spacecraft (and it has no upper bound for its duration). We try to schedule the Earth pointing as early as possible but the other types of pointings are scheduled as late as possible. This is motivated by having the NAD and FIX pointings with the restricted length as tight around the experiments as possible. Recall that NAD and FIX pointings have restricted duration and are required by experiments so it is better to change to these pointings as late as possible before the experiment. After the PTA activities, we schedule the maintenance activities. These activities fit well between the blocks of POR activities. We find for them the requested pointing and then we allocate them to time. Finally, we schedule the downlink activities again to as early time as possible. As all other activities are already scheduled at that time, we allocate the downlink activities to the earliest possible time in the communication window, as there is no reason to try later times in the same window. We also tried to schedule the communication activities before the maintenance activities, but it worked much worse.

Let us now describe the search procedure formally. We will use the following notation. Up(X) means trying the values for variable X in the increasing order. Down(X) means trying the values for X in the decreasing order. UpInter(X) means trying only the first values in the intervals from the domain of X. For example, if the domain of X is $[1,10] \cup [15,20] \cup [30,40]$ then we try values 1, 15, 30 (in this order) for X. We will also use a general branching of exclusive disjunction constraints denoted using the *or* connector. Each of these assignment procedures defines a choice point of the search procedure so if the assignment fails, the search procedure returns to the previous choice point and tries an alternative branch there. Figure 2 describes the used search procedure.

```
for each i do
    S_i^POR := up(S_i^POR)
    W_i^POR := up(W_i^POR)
    let j = 1+W_i^POR do: (Pt_j := Earth
                              or Pt_j ≠ Earth)
end for
for each i do
    (D_i^PTA := 0
    or (D_i^PTA > 0 ∧ ((Pt_i := Earth ∧ S_i^PTA := up(S_i^PTA))
                       or (Pt_i ≠ Earth ∧ S_i^PTA := down(S_i^PTA)))))
end for
for each i do
    W_i^MTN := up(W_i^MTN)
    S_i^MTN := up(S_i^MTN)
end for
for each i do
    W_i^COM := up(W_i^COM)
    S_i^COM := upInter(S_i^COM)
end for
```

Fig. 2. Search procedure

6   Experimental Evaluation

To evaluate the performance of the proposed model, we compared it experimentally with the ad-hoc planner [7]. We used randomly generated data based on the same distribution as real data. In particular, we generated random schedules so we knew that a schedule exists and then we run the planners to see if they can find the schedules and how these schedules compare to the initial schedule. We tried three different scenarios. First, we focused on scalability with the increased number of POR activities. Second, we evaluated behavior of planners when the communication windows are restricted. Finally, we added the limited memory constraints to see how the planners work when a lot of data are produced. We run the solvers for one minute as if they did not produce any solution within one minute then they did not produce a solution even after running for several hours. Hence we do no compare runtimes, but we focus on quality of schedules. Though no planner was actually doing any optimization and there were no optimization criteria given, we compare compactness of the schedules as it roughly indicates how many experiments can fit in the schedule.

In the first experiment, we used a single ground-station availability window spanning the entire length of the schedule. Downlinks occupied about 75% of time between successive groups of experiments and all data can be downloaded before the next group starts. The amount of data produced was much smaller than available memory. Table 4 shows the results.

Table 4. Scalability experiment

#PORs	horizon	planner	makespan (hours)	unused time (hours)
15	5 days	initial	104	40
		Ad-hoc	103	40
		CSP	59	5
30	5 days	initial	117	40
		Ad-hoc	119	29
		CSP	91	13
50	7 days	initial	117	30
		Ad-hoc	120	24
		CSP	59	5
70	7 days	initial	167	22
		Ad-hoc	166	23
		CSP	-	-
100	7 days	initial	166	29
		Ad-hoc	167	25
		CSP	-	-

The experiment shows that the CSP approach generates much more compact schedules than the ad-hoc approach. However, the CSP approach does not scale well with the increased number of POR activities.

The second experiment added restricted communication windows. In the data sets we used communication windows of size about 4 hours allocated around apocenters. Again, in the initial schedule roughly 75% of time in each window was necessary to download all data produced from experiments in the pericenter preceding the apocenter communication window. Table 5 summarizes the results.

Table 5. Communication capacity experiment

#PORs	horizon	planner	makespan (hours)	unused time (hours)
15	5 days	initial	120	40
		Ad-hoc	102	28
		CSP	114	20
30	5 days	initial	121	31
		Ad-hoc	113	38
		CSP	103	15
50	7 days	initial	169	45
		Ad-hoc	167	38
		CSP	149	16
70	7 days	initial	169	25
		Ad-hoc	168	32
		CSP	132	11
100	7 days	initial	172	27
		Ad-hoc	167	25
		CSP	132	17

Again, the CSP approach generated the most compact schedules. Now the restricted communication windows probably helped the CSP solver to prune the search space and it can solve even the largest problems.

The last experiment used a complete set of constraints. We increased the size of generated data in such a way that each POR required about half of available memory. It means that after two PORs we need to download data before we can continue with experiments for the same payload. Table 6 shows the results.

Table 6. Data capacity experiment

#PORs	horizon	planner	makespan (hours)	unused time (hours)
15	5 days	initial	118	53
		Ad-hoc	117	30
30	5 days	initial	120	54
		Ad-hoc	117	32
50	7 days	initial	171	60
		Ad-hoc	164	40

In this experiment, the CSP model was not able to produce any solution. The reason is that the CSP planner scheduled too many POR operations and discovered only late that downlink operations cannot fit which caused a lot of backtracking.

7   Conclusions

We presented a constraint-based planner to do complete planning and scheduling of MEX Orbiter operations. This planner produces more compact plans than the existing ad-hoc approach so it is a promising direction as it can exploit better available observation time. Moreover, a CSP is modular in the sense that it is easy to add other constraints and for example to modify the planner to cover over-constrained problems where more scientific experiments are requested than the orbiter can actually perform. Unfortunately, the current model does not scale up well and it has a problem when a lot of data are generated. A possible direction to overcome these difficulties is modifying the search strategy for example by using discrepancy search techniques that recover better from the failure of search heuristic. Another alternative is adding redundant constraints that help in pruning infeasible search branches.

Acknowledgments. Research is supported by the Czech Science Foundation under the projects P103/10/1287 and P202/12/G061.

References

1. Baptiste, P., Le Pape, C., Nuijten, W.: Constraint-based Scheduling: Applying Constraints to Scheduling Problems. Kluwer Academic Publishers, Dordrecht (2001)
2. Barták, R.: Visopt ShopFloor: Going beyond traditional scheduling. In: O'Sullivan, B. (ed.) CologNet 2002. LNCS (LNAI), vol. 2627, pp. 185–199. Springer, Heidelberg (2003)
3. Cesta, A., Cortellessa, G., Denis, M., Donati, A., Fratini, S., Oddi, A., Policella, N., Rabenau, E., Schulster, J.: AI solves mission planner problems. IEEE Intelligent Systems 22 (2007)
4. Dechter, R.: Constraint processing. Morgan Kaufmann Publishers Inc. (2003)
5. Fratini, S., Policella, N.: ICKEPS 2012 challenge domain: Planning operations on the Mars Express mission (2012), http://icaps12.poli.usp.br/icaps12/sites/default/files/ickeps/mexdomain/MEXKEPSdomainv12.pdf
6. Giunchiglia, F., Sebastiani, R.: Building decision procedures for modal logics from propositional decision procedures—the case study of modal K(m). In: McRobbie, M.A., Slaney, J.K. (eds.) CADE 1996. LNCS, vol. 1104, pp. 583–597. Springer, Heidelberg (1996)
7. Kolombo, M., Pecka, M., Barták, R.: An Ad-hoc Planner for the Mars Express Mission, In. In: Proceedings of 5th International Workshop on Planning and Scheduling for Space (2013)
8. Muscettola, N.: HSTS: Integrating planning and scheduling. In: Intelligent Scheduling. Morgan Kauffmann (1994)
9. Rabenau, E., Donati, A., Denis, M., Policella, N., Schulster, J., Cesta, A., Cortellessa, G., Fratini, S., Oddi, A.: The RAXEM tool on Mars Express - uplink planning optimisation and scheduling using AI constraint resolution. In: Proceedings of the 10th International Conference on Space Operations, SpaceOps 2008 (2008)

Glucose Oxidase Biosensor Modeling
by Machine Learning Methods

Livier Rentería-Gutiérrez, Félix F. González-Navarro,
Margarita Stilianova-Stoytcheva, Lluís A. Belanche-Muñoz,
Brenda L. Flores-Ríos, and Jorge Eduardo Ibarra-Esquer

Instituto de Ingeniería
Universidad Autonóma de Baja California
Blvd. Benito Juárez y Calle de la Normal s/n
Mexicali, México, C.P. 21280
{livier.renteria,fernando.gonzalez,margarita.stoytcheva
brenda.flores,jorge.ibarra}@uabc.edu.mx
belanche@lsi.upc.edu

Abstract. Biosensors are small analytical devices incorporating a biological element for signal detection. The main function of a biosensor is to generate an electrical signal which is proportional to a specific analyte i.e. to translate a biological signal into an electrical reading. Nowadays its technological attractiveness resides in its fast performance, and its highly sensitivity and continuous measuring capabilities; however, its understanding is still under research. This paper focuses to contribute to the state of the art of this growing field of biotechnology specially on Glucose Oxidase Biosensors (GOB) modeling through statistical learning methods from a regression perspective. It models the amperometric response of a GOB with dependent variables under different conditions such as temperature, benzoquinone, PH and glucose, by means of well known machine learning algorithms. Support Vector Machines(SVM), Artificial Neural Networks (ANN) and Partial least squares (PLS) are the algorithms selected to do the regression task.

Keywords: Machine Learning, SVM, linear regression, Neural Network, PLS, biosensor, glucose oxidase.

1 Introduction

Biosensors are small analytical devices that incorporate a biological element, whose aim is to generate an electrical signal which is proportional to a specific analyte –i.e. the targeted chemical element to be measured. The biosensors acts as a translator mechanism from a biological signal into an electrical reading. The recognition element called electrode usually is an enzyme, tissue, microorganism or an organelle, which is coupled to a physic-chemical transducer which perform this translation –see Figure 1 [8].

Currently, its technological attractiveness resides in its fast performance, and its highly sensitivity, continuous measuring capabilities, range, response time,

A. Gelbukh et al. (Eds.): MICAI 2014, Part II, LNAI 8857, pp. 464–473, 2014.

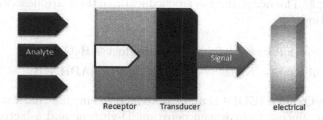

Fig. 1. The analyte is recognized by the bioreceptor followed by the detection of the transducer producing a measurable electric signal

stability, low cost and precision. Table 1 illustrates different types of biosensor construction elements such as receptor types, transducers and physic-chemical signals.

Table 1. Diferent types of biosensor construction elements

Receptor	$Physic - ChemicalSignal$	Transducers
Dye	Protein	Optoelectronic detector
Lectin	Saccharide	Field effect transistors
Enzyme	Glycoprotein	Semiconductor electrode
Apo enzyme	Substrate	Potentiometric electrode
Antibody	Inhibitor	Amperometric electrode
Organelle	Prosthetic group	Thermistors
Microbe	Antigen	
Tissue slice	Hormone	

Biosensors have a wide potential in diverse fields such as biomedicine, food industry, engineering, and environment [7]. Despite growing advances in its design, this technology its still under develompent. One of the emerging scenarios is the biomedical monitoring. In this work we put our attention to the blood sugar sensing trough Glucose-Oxidase biosensors. The accurate determination of blood glucose is highly important for the screening and treatment of the Diabetes Mellitus Disease [4].

2   Electrochemical Biosensors

There exist diverse techniques to measure glucose levels in blood. The most common are the spectrophotometric type using small devices called glucometers. A current alternative is the technology based on electrochemical enzymatic sensors. It works on the basis of oxygen consumption, hydrogen peroxide production or b-nicotinamide adenine obtaining during the process of the catalytic conversion of a substrate [9]. The occurring electrochemical reactions are described by the following equations:

$$\text{Substrate} + O_2 \xrightarrow{\text{Enzyme}} \text{Product} + H_2O_2$$
$$\text{Substrate} + NAD^+ \xrightarrow{\text{Enzyme}} \text{Product} + NADH + H^+$$

The Glucose-Oxidase (GOD) is an oxidoreductase enzyme that catalyzes the oxidation of the glucose to hydrogen peroxide, D-glucone and 5-lactone. Nowadays the GOD is widely used for the assessment of glucose in human body fluids –i.e. blood and urine samples. It is produced by the *penicillium notatum* and other fungi in presence of oxygen and glucose [5].

3 GOB Mathematical Modeling

The biosensors are based on physical process and biological-chemical reactions that can be interpreted by mathematical models. Given some input parameters it is possible to interpret the phenomena taking advantage of modern computational techniques. The goal is to develop a flexible mathematical model which can be used towards a software capable of predicting the behavior of electrochemical biosensor.

Since the first steps in the electrochemical biosensors design and development, mathematical models have been introduced as a powerful tool that provides a better understanding of the main influences of processing biosensor response. Electrode construction features(material), electrical factors (potential, current, charge, impedance), electrolytic factors (pH), and reaction variables (thermodynamic and kinetic parameters) are factors of the electrochemical biosensor design [3]. This information is useful to make decisions and consequently imply a reduction in time and costs.

GOB modeling efforts deal with quantitative descriptions of biosensors kinetic behavior of simple idealized enzymes [2]. Nowadays exist important contributions to GOB modeling by means of machine learning methods, however this field of research it is still under development [6].

4 Experimental Work

4.1 Biosensor Dataset

The GOB incorporates a p-benzoquinone mediated amperometric graphite sensor with covalently linked glucoseoxidase. This mediator is responsible for the electronic transfer between the enzyme and the electrode surface. Additionally, the following reagents were used: glucose oxidase (E.C. 1.1.3.4. from *Aspergillus*, 1000 U/mg), N-cyclohexyl-N'-[2-(methylmorpholino)ethyl] carbodimide-4-toluenesulphonate (Merk) and glucose. Amperometric data acquisition was achieved using a Radelkis OH-105 polarograph. The amperometric or electrical response was analyzed under different conditions of the Glucose

(Glucose), pH (PH), temperature (T) and concentration of the mediator, the p-benzoquinone (Benzoquinone). Values for these input parameters are described in the table 2:

Table 2. GOB Input parameters

Glucose G (mM)	PH	Temperature T (celcius)	p-Benzoquinone (mM)
4	4	20	1
8	5	37	0.8
12	6	47	0.4
20			

The resulting data file consists of 320 rows (observations) and 5 columns, 4 predictive variables and a continuous target variable, which corresponds to the biosensor amperometric response measured in mA. As stated above, the predictive variables are: Glucose, Benzoquinone, T and PH. These predictive variables are standardized to zero mean, unit standard deviation. Finally the data file is shuffled to avoid predefined ordering biases.

4.2 Experimental Settings

The dataset was randomly partitioned into a training set (70 percent) and a test set (30 percent). The training phase was conducted by cross validation in 30x10-Fold fashion. The generalization capacity was assessed by feeding the trained models with the test set. The performance measure used was the Normalized Root Means Square Error (NRMSE) whose definition is as follows:

$$\sqrt{\frac{\sum_{i=1}^{N}\left(\frac{e_i}{1-h_{ii}}^2\right)}{\sum_{i=1}^{N}(\hat{y}-\bar{y})^2}} \tag{1}$$

where e_i are the residuals and h_{ii} are the leverage of the observation x_i.

Three well known regression algorithms were used in the biosensor response prediction, the Partial Least Squares algorithm (PLS), a Support Vector Machine (SVM) with Linear and Radial Basis Function Kernel and a Neural Network (NN) for regression with Levenberg-Marquardt backpropagation learning strategy. Optimal parameters were selected by grid search as follows: the SVM complexity parameter C and the SVM-RBF gamma parameter was varied logarithmically between $10^{-1.5}$ and $10^{1.5}$; for the NN the number of hidden layers was fixed to one with four neurons.

4.3 Results and Discussion

Two experimental modes were analyzed, training and testing learning algorithms with and without applying the natural log to the target variable. Table 3 shows the cvRMSE error for each learner, before LOG and LOG data. The PLS and

Table 3. cvNRMSE error and Regression Coefficient

Regression method	Before LOG NRMSE	R	LOG data NRMSE	R
PLS	0.50	0.509	0.26	0.763
Linear SVM	1.44	0.520	0.28	0.718
RFB SVM	0.03	0.999	0.01	0.999
NN	0.11	0.984	0.05	0.980

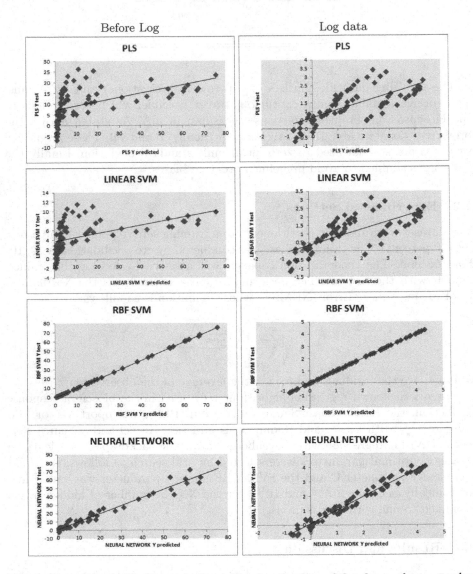

Fig. 2. Plot regression before and after taking log the data of the observed target value vs. predicted target value

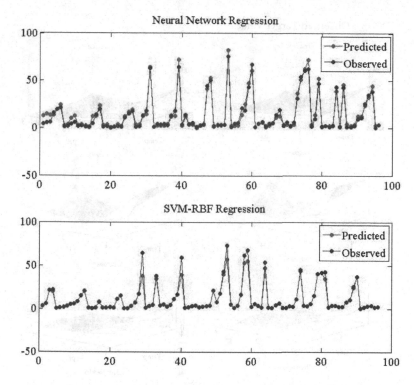

Fig. 3. Observed and predicted values rendered by the NN and RBF SVM models on the data log

the RBF SVM shows the lowest errors, being (in a cautious matter) the RBF SVM the best model according to this performance measure.

It is presented also, in this table, the regression coefficient R rendered by the comparison observed target value vs. predicted target value in the test set. It is clearly seen that the two linear models, PLS and the linear SVM are outperformed by the non-linear models, the NN and the RFB SVM. Figure 2 shows the linear regression plots before LOG and data LOG.

Figure 3 shows the predicted target values vs. observed target values for the RBF SVM and the NN algorithms. Despite that most of the signal is satisfactory predicted, some of the points present divergences w.r.t. the observed target values. A particular phenomenon is seen, models –i.e. NN and RBF SVM– have difficulties to predict high-valued outputs.

Figure 4 and 5 show particular sections of the target value by presenting the observed and predicted values in the test set. The former figure was assembled by fixing the Benzoquinone to 0.2 and different Glucose values. X-Y axis are the T and pH. The later uses Glucose equals to 4 and at different Benzoquinone values. The differences pointed before can be seen in figure 5.

Observed Target Value

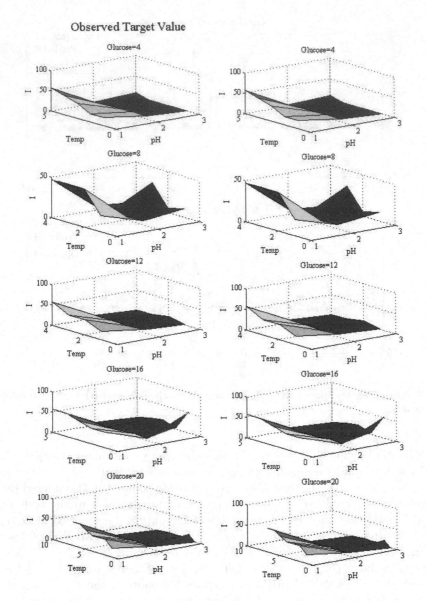

Fig. 4. Observed Target value vs. Predicted Target value with fixed Benzoquinone to 0.2 at different glucose values

Wilcoxon Signed Rank test comparing the NN and the RBF SVM algorithms –in the data LOG– shows no significative differences in testing the null hypothesis that the difference between both cvNRMSE medians is zero –i.e p-value=0.125.

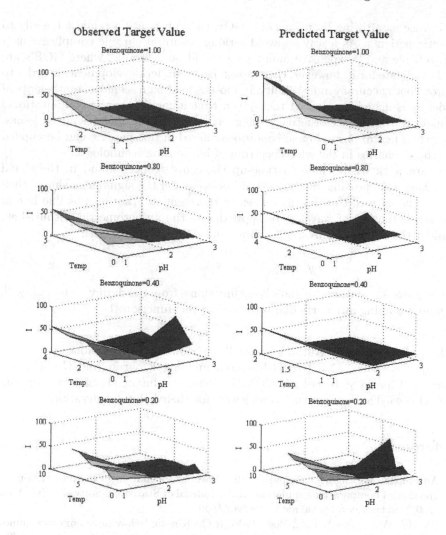

Fig. 5. Observed Target value vs. Predicted Target value with fixed Glucose to 4 at different Benzoquinone values

5   Conclusions and Future Work

Some machine learning methods have been used to model the amperometric response of a GOB. The reported experimental results show a promising very low prediction error of the biosensor output by using Neural Networks and Support Vector Machines. It is shown also that the relationship between predictors –i.e. features or variables– and response –target variable– corresponds to a non-linear behavior. A final RBF-SVM model with parameters C=16, GAMMA=5.6569 and NU=0.95 can be solidly constructed in order to predict the amperometric response.

Glucose monitoring by means of a GOB can constitute a remarkable ally to diabetic patients. As a way to avoid serious collateral chronic complications a fast, reliable and inexpensive monitoring would be desirable, where GOB's are solid candidate for it; however, their design is still under development, in order to improve both accuracy and stability. In biosensors design scenario, mathematical modeling is a highly solicited tool, given that it facilitates the computational simulation avoiding destructive testing, as long as time and resources issues. The experimental proposal and conditions offered in this paper could be applied for other scenarios in the wide spectrum of bio-sensing technology.

Future work will include to tune-up those divergences found in the signal prediction. One possible direction could be to model the signal as a shape, then it could be natural to think in splines to represent it. Another possible line of research is the use of wavelets to approximate the amperometric output. Lets consider the standard univariate nonparametric regression model:

$$y_i = g(t_i) + \sigma \epsilon_i, i = 1, \ldots, n,$$

The goals is to gather the underlying function g from the data $\mathbf{y} = (y_1, \ldots, y_n)'$, without assuming any particular structure of this function [1].

Acknowledgements. Authors gratefully acknowledge Universidad Autónoma de Baja California, 17th UABC Research Funding Program and Consejo Nacional de Ciencia y Tecnología CONACyT for the financial support. Authors also acknowledge the anonymous reviewers for their helpful suggestions.

References

1. Antoniadis, A., Bigot, J., Sapatinas, T.: Wavelet estimators in nonparametric regression: A comparative simulation study. Journal of Statistical Software 6(6), 1–83 (2001), http://www.jstatsoft.org/v06/i06
2. Blaedel, W.J., Kissel, T.R., Boguslaski, R.C.: Kinetic behavior of enzymes immobilized in artificial membranes. Analytical Chemistry 44(12), 2030–2037 (1972), http://pubs.acs.org/doi/abs/10.1021/ac60320a021 pMID: 4657296
3. Borgmann, S., Schulte, A., Neugebauer, S., Schuhmann, W.: Amperometric biosensors. In: Alkire, R., Kolb, D., Lipkowski, J. (eds.) Bioelectrochemistry: Fundamentals, Applications and Recent Developments. Wiley-VCH (2011)
4. Malhotra, B., Turner, A.: Advances in Biosensors: Perspectives in Biosensors. Advances in Biosensors, Elsevier Science (2003), http://books.google.com.mx/books?id=d8i_2uJ4N-oC
5. Prodromidis, M., Karayannis, M.: Enzyme based amperometric biosensors for food analysis. Electroanalysis 14(4), 241–261 (2002), http://dx.doi.org/10.1002/1521-4109(200202)14:4<241: AID-ELAN241>3.0.CO;2-P
6. Rangelova, V., Tsankova, D., Dimcheva, N.: Soft computing techniques in modelling the influence of ph and temperature on dopamine biosensor. In: Somerset, V. (ed.) Intelligent and Biosensors. INTECH (2010)

7. Sadana, A.: Biosensors: Kinetics of Binding and Dissociation Using Fractals: Kinetics of Binding and Dissociation Using Fractals. Elsevier Science (2003), http://books.google.com.mx/books?id=vlnYu7XA_mQC
8. Scheller, F., Schubert, F.: Biosensors. Techniques and Instrumentation in Analytical Chemistry. Elsevier Science (1991), http://books.google.com.mx/books?id=TF7AW4kSY1gC
9. Thévenot, D., Toth, K., Durst, R., Wilson, G.: Electrochemical biosensors: recommended definitions and classification. Biosensors and Bioelectronics 16(1-2), 121–131 (2001)

On the Breast Mass Diagnosis
Using Bayesian Networks

Verónica Rodríguez-López and Raúl Cruz-Barbosa

Universidad Tecnológica de la Mixteca, 69000, Huajuapan de León, Oaxaca, México
{veromix,rcruz}@mixteco.utm.mx

Abstract. Nowadays, breast cancer is considered a significant health problem in Mexico. Mammogram is an effective study for detecting mass lesions, which could indicate this disease. However, due to the density of breast tissue and a wide range of mass characteristic, the mass diagnosis is difficult. In this study, the performance comparison of Bayesian networks models on classification of benign and malignant masses is presented. Here, Naïve Bayes, Tree Augmented Naïve Bayes, K-dependence Bayesian classifier, and Forest Augmented Naïve Bayes models are analyzed. Two data sets extracted from the public BCDR-F01 database, including 112 benign and 119 malignant masses, were used to train the models. The experimental results have shown that TAN, KDB, and FAN models with a subset of only eight features have achieved a performance of 0.79 in accuracy, 0.80 in sensitivity, and 0.77 in specificity. Therefore, these models which allow dependencies among variables (features), are considered as suitable and promising methods for automated mass classification.

1 Introduction

Breast cancer is a disease in which malignant cells are formed in the breast tissues [20]. Nowadays, it is the main cause of death from cancer among women in the world. The highest rates of incidence for this disease are found in Europe, North America, Brazil and Argentina. Although in Mexico it is found at an intermediate level, with incidence rates four times lower than the highest ones, since 2006 breast cancer is the primary cause of death from malignant tumors among women [5].

A mammogram is an X-ray film of the breast that has proven to be an effective tool for early detection of breast cancer. This study usually involves two views of each breast: craniocaudal (CC) that is a head-to-foot view, and mediolateral oblique (MLO) that is an angled side-view [25]. In the visual analysis of radiologists, one of the most important signs of breast cancer that they look for are masses.

The American College of Radiology (ACR) defines a mass as a three-dimensional structure demonstrating convex outward borders, usually evident on two orthogonal views [1]. Some important characteristics of masses are size, shape, margins, and density. Margin refers to the mass border, and density is the amount of fat tissue in the mass compared with the surrounding breast tissue [13].

A. Gelbukh et al. (Eds.): MICAI 2014, Part II, LNAI 8857, pp. 474–485, 2014.

Detection and diagnosis of masses, deduced from a wide range of mass characteristics and density of breast tissue are complex, tedious, and time-consuming tasks. Moreover, the success of these tasks depend on training, experience and judgment of radiologists. For this, Computer Aided Diagnosis Systems (CADx) have been developed in order to help in the mammogram analysis. These systems have demonstrated to improve the performance in mass diagnosis from 75% to 82% [7,25].

In this study, the use of Bayesian networks models for mass diagnosis is presented. Bayesian networks are probabilistic models that can capture expert knowledge and work under conditions of uncertainty. They have a graphical structure that is easy to interpret and validate by experts. Moreover, these models can combine knowledge and data [12].

There are several reports about the use of Bayesian networks for breast diagnosis. Bayesian networks models trained with clinical data and mammogram findings provided by radiologists have been proposed in [3,4,10,14]. However, few works have been discussed about their performance when they are trained from automatically obtained features [22,26,31]. For the above mentioned, and considering the advantages of these kind of probabilistic models, the main aim of this work is the performance evaluation of Bayesian networks models on classification of benign and malignant masses from automatically obtained features.

The paper is organized as follows. In Section 2, we explain the image features used for mass description. A brief review of Bayesian networks classifiers is presented in Section 3. In Section 4, the data sets used in our experiments is described, and the experimental results are presented in Section 5. Finally, conclusions and future work are given in Section 6.

2   Feature Extraction

In this study, the features extracted from mammogram images are used to characterize the shape, margins and density of masses. The considered image descriptors of intensity, shape and texture, are selected from similar works [7,2,9,15,27], and are explained in the following sections.

2.1   Intensity

Intensity features are used to describe the density of masses. From pixels belonging to the mass region, five basic statistics were calculated: mean, median, variance, skewness, and kurtosis [7,9].

2.2   Shape

Shape of masses are investigated by ten features calculated from the pixels located within the mass region area. Nine of them are the basic shape image descriptors: area, compactness, and the seven Hu invariant moments [2,7,26].

The last one, is the linear texture feature proposed in [15] that allows to analyze the degree of mass spiculation.

Perimeter and statistics based on the distribution of the normalized radial length (NRL) are used as margins descriptors. The normalized radial length is defined as the normalized Euclidean distance from a point on the mass boundary to the mass centroid. Six features are calculated from the normalized radial length of the pixels on the mass boundary: mean, standard deviation (STD), entropy, area ratio, zero crossing count, and boundary roughness [9,30].

2.3   Texture

The following statistics of gray-level co-occurrence matrices (GLCM), gray-level difference matrices (GLDM), and gray-level run length matrices (GRLM) are extracted to evaluate the density of masses [7]:

- **GLCM**: An element of the GLCM matrix $P(i, j, d, \theta)$ is defined as the joint probability that the gray levels i and j occur separated by a distance d and along direction θ of the image [21]. From the GLCM matrices, the eleven following statistics are obtained: energy, contrast, correlation, variance, entropy, homogeneity, sum average, sum variance, sum entropy, inverse difference moment, and difference variance.
- **GLDM**: The GLDM vector is the histogram of the absolute difference of pixel pairs which are separated by a given displacement δ [32]. Also, to obtain GLDM features, four forms of the vector δ were considered: $(0, d), (-d, d),$ $(d, 0),$ and $(-d, -d)$. Four measurements are calculated from these vectors: mean, variance, entropy, and contrast.
- **GRLM**: The GRLM method is based on computing the number of gray-level runs of various lengths [29]. A gray-level run is a set of consecutive and collinear pixel points having the same gray-level value. The length of the run is the number of pixels in the run. For an $M \times N$ run length matrix $p(i, j)$, M is the number of gray levels and N is the maximum run length. From these matrices, the following statistics are obtained: Short Run Emphasis (SRE), Long Run Emphasis (LRE), Gray-Level Nonuniformity (GLN), Run Length Nonuniformity (RLN).

All the above mentioned texture statistics are calculated from a sample of 32×32 pixels of the mass center for four directions $\{0°, 45°, 90°, 135°\}$, and $d = 1$. Average and range, in the four directions, of each one of these statistics are used as texture features.

3   Bayesian Networks Classifiers

A Bayesian Network (BN) is a probabilistic graphical model where the nodes represent variables, and the arcs, dependence among variables. BN are recognized as powerful tools for knowledge representation and inference under conditions of uncertainty [8].

A formal definition of BN is as follows: A Bayesian network is a pair (D, P), where D is a directed acyclic graph, and $P = \{p(x_1|\pi_1), p(x_2|\pi_2), ..., p(x_n|\pi_n)\}$ is a set of n conditional probability distributions, one for each variable, and Π_i is the parents set of node X_i in D. The set P defines the associated joint probability distributions as [6],

$$p(x_1, x_2, ..., x_n) = \Pi_{i=1}^{n} p(x_i|\pi_i) \tag{1}$$

Several types of BN models have been proposed as classifiers, some of them are: Naïve Bayes, Tree Augmented Naïve Bayes (TAN), K-dependence Bayesian classifier (KDB), and Forest Augmented Naïve Bayes (FAN).

3.1   Naïve Bayes (NB)

Naïve Bayes model is the simplest form of a Bayesian network, in which the root node of a tree-like structure corresponds to a class variable. Also, the class node is the only parent for each attribute variable. The key assumption of a NB model is that all attributes are independent given the value of the class variable [8].

3.2   Tree Augmented Naïve Bayes (TAN)

A TAN classifier is an extension of the Naïve-Bayes model, and also has a tree-like structure. In this model is allowed that each variable has at most two parents: the class variable, and other attribute. The Friedman method [11] can be applied to learn the structure of a TAN model.

3.3   K-dependence Bayesian Classifier (KDB)

A KDB classifier is a Bayesian Network where each attribute variable has at most k parents. This BN model is also considered as an extension of a Naïve-Bayes, and its structure can be learned with the algorithm proposed by Sahami [24].

3.4   Forest Augmented Naïve Bayes (FAN)

This BN classifier is a variant of TAN where the attribute variables form a forest graph. One of the advantages of this classifier is that eliminates unnecessary relations among attributes. A method to learn the structure of FAN classifiers is proposed by Lucas [17].

4   Datasets

In this study, two datasets extracted from the public BCDR-F01 (Film Mammography dataset number 1) database [18] were used. This database is the first public released dataset of the Breast Cancer Digital Repository (BCDR) which contains craniocaudal and mediolateral oblique mammograms of 190 patients. The mammograms were digitized with a resolution of 720×1167 pixels, using 256 grey levels. For each mammography, the coordinates for the lesion contours, and numerical anonymous identifiers for linking instances and lesions are provided. Besides, a data set including clinical data and image-based descriptors of each lesion, is also available.

The two data sets used in our experiments were named as *BCDR-1* and *BCDR-2*. In order to form the *BCDR-1* dataset, the 231 mammograms images with mass lesion were selected from the BCDR-F01 database. Next, all the image features explained in Section 2 were extracted from each smallest bounding box containing a mass (region of interest-ROI, see Fig. 1). The ROIs were obtained with the help of ImageJ program [23]. In summary, this dataset includes 231 mass cases: 112 benigns and 119 malignants; and each mass is described with sixty features.

The *BCDR-2* dataset consists of mass cases that were extracted from the data included in the BCDR-F01 database. The considered mass cases are the same as *BCDR-1* set. Unlike the *BCDR-1* set, each mass is described with the twenty

Table 1. Features set for the *BCDR-2* set

Type	Feature
Intensity	mean, standard deviation,
	maximum, minimum,
	kurtosis, skewness
Shape	area, perimeter, x-coordinate of center mass,
	y-coordinate of center mass, circularity, elongation,
	form, solidity, extent
GLCM	energy, contrast, correlation, variance
Texture	homogeneity, sum average, sum entropy, sum variance
	entropy, difference variance, difference entropy
	information measure of correlation 1, information measure of correlation 2

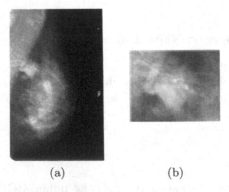

(a)   (b)

Fig. 1. An example of a BCDR image used in this study: (a) original image and (b) the corresponding ROI containing the mass

eight image features provided by the database as shown in Table 1. In summary, this data set includes 231 mass cases: 112 benigns and 119 malignants; and each mass is described with twenty eight features.

5   Experiments and Results

The goal of the experiments is twofold. Firstly, we aim to assess the performance of several Bayesian networks models in terms of three metrics. Secondly, we aim to study the effectiveness of two feature sets in the mass classification task.

In our experiments, four type of Bayesian networks models are analized: Naïve-Bayes, Tree Augmented Naïve Bayes, K-dependence Bayesian classifier (with $K = 2$), and Forest Augmented Naïve Bayes. All models are trained and tested in Matlab®with help of the Bayes Net toolbox [19] and the BNT Structure Learning Package [16]. To train the models, *BCDR-1* and *BCDR-2* sets are used. The values of the extracted features are normalized to have zero mean and unit variance, and then discretized with the Equal width discretization method.

The performance of the Bayesian networks models is evaluated with the Leave-one-out cross validation technique. The metrics used to report the results are accuracy, sensitivity, and specificity. Classification accuracy is the proportion of masses that are correctly classified by the model. The ratio of malignant masses that are correctly identified is the sensitivity; and specificity is the ratio of benign masses that are correctly identified [25].

5.1   Bayesian Networks Models Using the Complete Set of Features

In our first experiment, Bayesian networks models trained with the complete set of features of both data sets (*BCDR-1* and *BCDR-2*) are evaluated. The results are presented in Table 2. From this table, it can be seen that all models obtain a regular performance. The results of the models trained with *BCDR-2* set are slightly better and show similar average performance in accuracy, sensitivity, and specificity. In the case of the models trained with *BCDR-1* set, the results show a slightly higher average performance in specificity than in accuracy and sensitivity. The best model obtained for *BCDR-1* is the simplest NB model, and the KDB model for the case of *BCDR-2*.

Table 2. Performance results of mass classification for the Bayesian networks models using the complete set of features

Model	accuracy		sensitivity		specificity	
	BCDR-1	*BCDR-2*	*BCDR-1*	*BCDR-2*	*BCDR-1*	*BCDR-2*
NB	0.72	0.73	0.70	0.76	0.74	0.70
TAN	0.71	0.74	0.68	0.75	0.73	0.73
KDB	0.70	0.77	0.70	0.72	0.70	0.84
FAN	0.71	0.74	0.68	0.75	0.73	0.73

5.2   Bayesian Networks Models Using Subsets of Features

In our second experiment, Bayesian Networks models trained with different subset of features are evaluated.

Feature selection is applied to each data set before training of the models. In order to find the best subset of features, the following process is applied. First, the total space of features is approximately reduced to a third of it. Here, the most relevant features according to their Fisher score are selected (see Table 3). Then, the best combination of features is found by using the sequential backward selection method. The final subset of features for *BCDR-1* (named *BCDR-1* subset) is presented in Table 4. In the case of the *BCDR-2* set, the most relevant features are selected as the best combination of them by the feature selection method. This feature subset (named *BCDR-2* subset) is shown in Table 5.

The performance results of the Bayesian networks models trained with the best combination of features are summarized in Table 6. From this table, it can be seen that almost all models trained with *BCDR-1* subset outperformed those obtained with *BCDR-2*. NB is the best model obtained for the *BCDR-2* subset, and models with dependences among features (TAN, KDB, and FAN) are the corresponding for the *BCDR-1*.

The topology obtained for all Bayesian networks models using the *BCDR-1* subset are presented in Fig. 2. From this figure, it is shown that the topology

Table 3. First selection of features for *BCDR-1* set which are ordered according to their Fisher score

Feature	Fisher score
compactness	0.76
NRL mean	0.68
skewness	0.46
NRL STD	0.31
median	0.30
perimeter	0.30
variance	0.27
NRL zero crossing count	0.27
GLRM range of GLN	0.17
GLCM average of sum entropy	0.16
GLCM average of entropy	0.16
NRL entropy	0.16
GLCM range of energy	0.15
GLRM average of SER	0.15
GLRM average of RLN	0.13
GLCM average of difference variance	0.12
GLRM range of RLN	0.11
kurtosis	0.11
GLCM average of inverse difference moment	0.10
GLCM average of homogeneity	0.09

Table 4. The best combination of features for *BCDR-1* set which are ordered according to their Fisher score

Feature	Fisher score
compactness	0.76
NRL mean	0.68
skewness	0.46
NRL STD	0.31
median	0.30
NRL entropy	0.16
GLCM range of energy	0.15
kurtosis	0.11

Table 5. The best combination of features for *BCDR-2* set which are ordered according to their Fisher score.

Feature	Fisher score
circularity	1.75
solidity	1.15
extent	0.96
perimeter	0.29
GLCM entropy	0.22
GLCM sum entropy	0.21
GLCM correlation	0.18
GLCM energy	0.15
standard deviation	0.12
GLCM information measure of correlation 2	0.09
GLCM homogeneity	0.07
skewness	0.06
kurtosis	0.05
GLCM difference entropy	0.04
minimum	0.03

of the best models (listed in Table 6) TAN, KDB, and FAN, are almost similar. They only differ in the direction of the arc between NRL mean and compactness, between NRL mean and skewness, and between skewness and kurtosis. These models show a compact structure that is easy to interpret, and validate by experts.

Also from Table 6, it can be seen that for *BCDR-1* subset the results show an acceptable performance on identification of both malignant and benign masses. This feature subset reveals a better ability to capture the inherent characteristics of the malignant masses. In fact, the sensitivity is improved when the dependences among features are captured by the models TAN, KDB and FAN. On the other hand, a regular performance in sensitivity and specificity are observed

Table 6. Performance results of mass classification for the Bayesian networks models using the best combination of features

Model	accuracy		sensitivity		specificity	
	BCDR-1	*BCDR-2*	*BCDR-1*	*BCDR-2*	*BCDR-1*	*BCDR-2*
NB	0.73	0.76	0.65	0.75	0.81	0.77
TAN	0.79	0.69	0.80	0.64	0.77	0.74
KDB	0.79	0.76	0.80	0.65	0.77	0.88
FAN	0.79	0.69	0.80	0.64	0.77	0.74

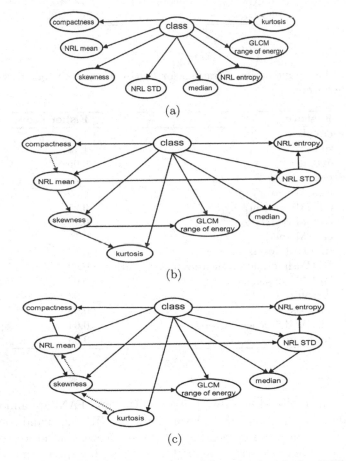

Fig. 2. Topology for the Bayesian network models trained with the *BCDR-1* subset: (a) NB, (b) TAN, (c) KDB and FAN, the former is represented with solid arc lines and the latter is the same structure except where the dotted arcs appear.

in models trained with the *BCDR-2* subset. In summary, the results indicate that *BCDR-2* subset is more appropriate to describe the benign masses than the malignant ones; while *BCDR-1* subset is suitable for identification of both mass type.

The topologies shown in Fig. 2 for TAN, KDB, and FAN using the *BCDR-1* subset suggests that shape, margins, and density are important factors for mass diagnosis: shape is described by the compactness; margins by NRL mean, NRL STD, and NRL entropy; and density by skewness, median, and GLCM energy. Moreover, the dependences among these features captured by the TAN model, reveal that the shape of a mass has influence on margins, and this impact on the density attributes. These findings, factors and their relationships, are consistent with both the analysis followed by experts for mass diagnosis and medical literature [13,28].

6   Conclusions

A performance comparison of Bayesian networks models on classification of benign and malignant masses was presented in this work . The experimental results have shown that TAN, KDB, and FAN models, with performance of 0.79 in accuracy, 0.80 in sensitivity, and 0.77 in specificity, are suitable models for this task. These models have a compact structure and can capture part of the specialized knowledge used by radiologists for mass diagnosis. The accuracy performance obtained by these models is comparable with the average performance (0.82) of experimentals CADx [25]. Also, the experimental results have shown that our proposed feature set (*BCDR-1* subset) when compared with that found in the BCDR-F01 database, is appropriate to identify both types of masses. For these results, it can be concluded that Bayesian networks are promising models for mass classification with automatically obtained features.

As future work, interpretation and validation by experts of the best found models, as well as the construction of models with both clinical data and image descriptors of masses are considered.

References

1. American College of Radiology, ACR: Breast Imaging Reporting and Data System BI-RADS, 4th edn. (2003)
2. Brake, G.T.: Computer Aided Detection of Masses in Digital Mammograms. Ph.D. thesis, University Medical Center Nijmegen (2000)
3. Burnside, E., Rubin, D., Shachter, R.: A Bayesian network for mammography. In: Proceedings of the AMIA Symposium, p. 106. American Medical Informatics Association (2000)
4. Burnside, E.S., Davis, J., Chhatwal, J., Alagoz, O., Lindstrom, M.J., Geller, B.M., Littenberg, B., Shaffer, K.A., Kahn Jr., C.E., Page, C.D.: Probabilistic computer model developed from clinical data in national mammography database format to classify mammographic findings 1. Radiology 251(3), 663–672 (2009)
5. Cárdenas, J.S., Bargalló, E.R., Erazo, A.V., Maafs, E.M., Poitevin, A.C.: Consenso mexicano sobre diagnóstico y tratamiento del cáncer mamario: Quinta Revisión. Elsevier Masson Doyma México (2013)

6. Castillo, E.: Expert systems and probabilistic network models. Springer (1997)
7. Cheng, H., Shi, X., Min, R., Hu, L., Cai, X., Du, H.: Approaches for automated detection and classification of masses in mammograms. Pattern Recognition 39(4), 646–668 (2006)
8. Cheng, J., Greiner, R.: Learning Bayesian belief network classifiers: Algorithms and system. In: Stroulia, E., Matwin, S. (eds.) Canadian AI 2001. LNCS (LNAI), vol. 2056, p. 141. Springer, Heidelberg (2001)
9. Delogu, P., Evelina Fantacci, M., Kasae, P., Retico, A.: Characterization of mammographic masses using a gradient-based segmentation algorithm and a neural classifier. Computers in Biology and Medicine 37(10), 1479–1491 (2007)
10. Fischer, E., Lo, J., Markey, M.: Bayesian networks of BI-RADS descriptors for breast lesion classification. In: 26th Annual International Conference of the IEEE Engineering in Medicine and Biology Society, IEMBS 2004, vol. 2, pp. 3031–3034. IEEE (2004)
11. Friedman, N., Geiger, D., Goldszmidt, M.: Bayesian network classifiers. Machine Learning 29(2-3), 131–163 (1997)
12. Heckerman, D.: A tutorial on learning with Bayesian networks. Springer (1998)
13. Jackson, V., Dines, K., Bassett, L., Gold, R., Reynolds, H.: Diagnostic importance of the radiographic density of noncalcified breast masses: analysis of 91 lesions. American Journal of Roentgenology 157(1), 25–28 (1991)
14. Kahn Jr., C.E., Roberts, L.M., Shaffer, K.A., Haddawy, P.: Construction of a Bayesian network for mammographic diagnosis of breast cancer. Computers in Biology and Medicine 27(1), 19–29 (1997)
15. Karssemeijer, N., Brake, G.T.: Detection of stellate distortions in mammograms. IEEE Transactions on Medical Imaging 15(5), 611–619 (1996)
16. Leray, P., Francois, O.: BNT structure learning package. Tech. Rep. FRE CNRS 2645, Technical Report, Laboratoire PSI-INSA Rouen-FRE CNRS (2004)
17. Lucas, P.J.: Restricted Bayesian network structure learning. In: Gámez, J.A., Moral, S., Salmerón, A. (eds.) Advances in Bayesian Networks. STUDFUZZ, vol. 146, pp. 217–234. Springer, Heidelberg (2004)
18. Moura, D.C., López, M.A.G.: An evaluation of image descriptors combined with clinical data for breast cancer diagnosis. International Journal of Computer Assisted Radiology and Surgery 8(4), 561–574 (2013)
19. Murphy, K.: How to use Bayes net toolbox (2004),
http://www.ai.mit.edu/murphyk/Software/BNT/bnt.html
20. National Cancer Institute, NCI: General Information About Breast Cancer (May 2014),
http://www.cancer.gov/cancertopics/pdq/treatment/breast/Patient/page1 (retrieved)
21. Nixon, M.S., Aguado, A.S.: Feature extraction & image processing for computer vision. Academic Press (2012)
22. Patrocinio, A.C., Schiabel, H., Romero, R.A.: Evaluation of Bayesian network to classify clustered microcalcifications. In: Medical Imaging 2004, pp. 1026–1033. International Society for Optics and Photonics (2004)
23. Rasband, W.: ImageJ: Image processing and analysis in Java. Astrophysics Source Code Library (2012)
24. Sahami, M.: Learning limited dependence Bayesian classifiers. In: KDD, vol. 96, pp. 335–338 (1996)
25. Sampat, M., Markey, M., Bovik, A.: Computer-Aided Detection and Diagnosis in Mammography. In: Handbook of Image and Video Processing, ch. 10.4, pp. 1195–1217. Elsevier Academic Press (2005)

26. Samulski, M.R.M.: Classification of Breast Lesions in Digital Mammograms. Master's thesis, University Medical Center Nijmegen, Netherlands (2006)
27. Samulski, M., Karssemeijer, N., Lucas, P., Groot, P.: Classification of mammographic masses using support vector machines and Bayesian networks. In: Medical Imaging, pp. 65141J–65141J. International Society for Optics and Photonics (2007)
28. Sickles, E.A.: Breast masses: mammographic evaluation. Radiology 173(2), 297–303 (1989)
29. Tang, X.: Texture information in run-length matrices. IEEE Transactions on Image Processing 7(11), 1602–1609 (1998)
30. Tsui, P.H., Liao, Y.Y., Chang, C.C., Kuo, W.H., Chang, K.J., Yeh, C.K.: Classification of benign and malignant breast tumors by 2-d analysis based on contour description and scatterer characterization. IEEE Transactions on Medical Imaging 29(2), 513–522 (2010)
31. Velikova, M., Lucas, P.J., Samulski, M., Karssemeijer, N.: A probabilistic framework for image information fusion with an application to mammographic analysis. Medical Image Analysis 16(4), 865–875 (2012)
32. Weszka, J.S., Rosenfeld, A.: A comparative study of texture measures for terrain classification. NASA STI/Recon Technical Report N 76, 13470 (1975)

Predicting the Occurrence of Sepsis
by *In Silico* Simulation

Flávio Oliveira de Sousa[2], Alcione Oliveira de Paiva[2], Luiz Alberto Santana[1],
Fábio Ribeiro Cerqueira[2], Rodrigo Siqueira-Batista[1], and Andréia Patrícia Gomes[1]

[1] Departamento de Medicina e Enfermagem, Universidade Federal de Viçosa (UFV)
CEP 36570-000 – Viçosa – MG – Brasil
[2] Departamento de Informática, Universidade Federal de Viçosa (UFV)
CEP 36570-000 – Viçosa – MG – Brasil
{flavio7co,alcione,andreiapgomes,frcerqueira}@gmail.com,
luizsantana@ufv.br, rsiqueirabatista@yahoo.com.br

Abstract. From public health and clinical point of view, sepsis is a life-threatening complication and its mechanisms are still not fully understood. This article claims that Multiagent Systems are suitable to help elucidate this phenomenon and that it is possible to carry out simulations that can be used in the observation of emergent behaviors, enabling a better understanding of the disease. Requirements for computational simulation of sepsis in AutoSimmune system are presented as also the simulation results. The results presented when using more aggressive pathogens are compatible with sepsis by simultaneously presenting symptoms such as fever, bacteria in the blood and Leukocytosis as reported in literature.

Keywords: in silico simulation, sepsis prediction, multiagent system.

1   Introduction

From public health and clinical point of view, sepsis is a life-threatening infectious complication and its mechanisms are still not fully understood. Sepsis has great relevance in terms of public health not only because of the high incidence of cases but also due to the high mortality rate pointed in several studies [1]. Three million people in the United States and Europe are estimated to develop severe sepsis and/or septic shock every year and about 35% to 50% come to death [2]. This is therefore a major cause of death in intensive care units (ICU), causing thousands of deaths annually worldwide.

In sepsis, systemic inflammatory response, triggered by suspected or confirmed infection syndrome, occurs the balance rupture between pro and anti-inflammatory mediators [1][3][4]. Then, one can reach a state of intense "immunologic dissonance", called MARS (*mixed antagonistic response syndrome*), where it occurs SIRS (systemic inflammatory response syndrome) and CARS (*compensatory anti-inflammatory response syndrome*) [5]. This context is proposed as the core for explaining the evolution of sepsis [1]. The process of disruption of this complex balance of pro and anti-inflammatory mechanisms disorganizes homeostasis in patients suffering of sepsis[6][7].

A. Gelbukh et al. (Eds.): MICAI 2014, Part II, LNAI 8857, pp. 486–498, 2014.
© Springer International Publishing Switzerland 2014

As a consequence, researches *in vitro*, *in vivo*, and more recently *in silico* (using computational modeling) have been conducted with the aim of contributing to a better understanding of the pathophysiology of sepsis. In the case of sepsis, there are factors, such as bioethical aspects, that hinder research *in vitro* and *in vivo*. For this reason, computational simulations have aided the understanding in pathogenic/man interaction playing an important role in the expansion of knowledge and the construction of scientific hypotheses with a degree of effectiveness consistent with contemporary medical practice [7] [8] [9].

According to Li et al. [10], computational models are not only cheaper than *in vivo* studies, but they are also faster and able to assist in a better understanding of bio-inspired algorithms and the use of these algorithms in improving intelligent and adaptive systems.

The objective of this paper is to present the results obtained in the simulation of Sepsis in a multi-agent system simulator termed AutoSimmune. Next, we introduce the systemic aspects of sepsis that ensure the suitability of the use of multi-agent systems (MAS) in the simulation of this disease. Section 3 describes the general characteristics of the simulator. Section 4 presents the necessary additions to the simulator for simulating the occurrence of *sepsis*. Section 5 presents the simulation results. Finally, Section 6 presents the conclusions of this work.

2   Agent Oriented Computational Modeling of the Human IS

Human immune system (IS) has evolved over millions of years to develop sophisticated mechanisms for maintaining homeostasis in order to protect the organic integrity of the host in relation to microorganisms and their virulence factors [11]. Sometimes, however, imperfections in tolerance mechanisms give rise to so-called autoimmune diseases. Furthermore, inappropriate immune responses can cause tissue damage and development of diseases rather than protection [12]. Knowledge of the structure, function and regulation of IS is key to understanding the pathogenesis of many diseases and the development procedures that allows its regulation [12].

In addition to the specific characteristics of IS, general systems theory, proposed by Bertalanffy[13], lists some of the common characteristics of complex systems that are perfectly matched to IS. These characteristics indicate the scale of the challenge of understanding a systemic event, revealing, through a careful analysis what are the best approaches to be used. Such analyzes converge to the understanding of these systems as bottom-up systems where complex behavior emerges from the iterations of its most basic elements. Given these characteristics, agent oriented systems are perfectly matched to create systems that simulate these problems. In them, the agents that reside on a lower level on the scale start producing behavior that lies on a scale above them: ants create colonies; citizens create communities; simple pattern-recognition software learns how to recommend new books. The movement of low-level rules to higher-level sophistication is what is called *emergent behavior* [14]. However, currently there are some limitations that restrict the use of multi-agent systems. The main one is to maintain a system capable of handling millions of agents that communicate continuously, as is the case of IS. Current research seeks to allow the use of GPU to ensure the scalability of such systems [15].

3   The AutoSimmune Simulator

AutoSimmune is an Immune System simulator with original focus on autoimmunity. In its basic version it simulates the bone marrow, thymus, lymph nodes, blood circulation and parenchymal tissue region. The regions are simulated as a discrete space in a form of a two-dimensional grid in which each agent has a position (i,j). More than one agent can occupy the same position, which somehow simulates a 3D space. The movement of the agent is done by changing its position to a new position in the *Moore neighborhood*[1]. Thus, an agent cannot "jump" positions, i.e., it needs to move one position at a time. In such a structure in the form of two-dimensional grid, the Moore neighborhood (of radius one) comprises the eight neighboring position to a central position. If allowed in their specification, an agent can move from one region to another by means of special elements called *portals*, as proposed in [16]. The simulation of substances such as cytokines are performed by means of layers of data provided by the framework repast, called *ValueLayer*. Substances, as they are released by cells, undergo a process of diffusion, spreading in the surroundings of the site in which they were released, decreasing its concentration, and also undergo a process of decay, decreasing its amount with time [17]. *ValueLayer* is an abstract layer of data that, at the time of its creation, is associated with a region of the grid. Combination of multiple layers of data at the same grid is possible. Thus, an agent can know the concentration of a given substance at that time instant at position (i,j).

Passage of time is modeled using the concept of discrete time unit called *tick* provided by the framework. Each agent defines when to start to be called and the interval of each call. *Ticks* are the time intervals necessary for the transition from a state of the environment to the next. Therefore, all events scheduled to be executed must be completed before the next round occurs. Thus, during a *tick*, all agents scheduled for the given time will change their positions, release substance and analyze its neighborhood, based on information from the previous tick. Only when every agent has made its actions the *tick* ends and the information is updated [17].

In the simulator, the affinity (which is the recognition strength of an antigen by a receptor) is simulated by the number of matching bits between two bit sequences: one belonging to a cell receptor and another belonging to the antigen. The greater the length of the matching, the greater the affinity. For the calculation of the affinity we used the method suggested by [22], called the "length of the longest common subsequence", whose goal is to compute, given two patterns of bit sequences A and B, the size of the largest contiguous subsequence of bits that are contained in A and B simultaneously, in the same order.

AutoSimmune have been successfully used to simulate various biological phenomena related to the human immune system, such as the development of autoimmunity [17]; verifying the role of mast cells in infections [23] and to study the immune response in the post-infectious glomerulonephritis (GnPE) by *Streptococcus pyogenes* [11].

---

[1] http://mathworld.wolfram.com/MooreNeighborhood.html

4   Simulation of Sepsis

Given the granularity of the simulator, we focused our modeling at the cellular level by adding the necessary elements for the simulation of sepsis. For this, it is necessary to identify and model the main cells and mechanisms that play a predominant role in the simulation of sepsis. They are bacteria, neutrophil, macrophage and their interactions, including interactions outside the *Tissue* zone, such as blood circulation. These elements worked as important markers of diagnosis in cases of sepsis. Moreover it was necessary to insert the *Neutrophil* agent and to adapt the *Macrophage* agent to simulate the behaviour related with pro inflammatory substances   (denoting IL1, IL2 and TNF-a),   and anti-inflammatory.   The *Bacterium* agent was also modified to respond to anti and pro-inflammatory mechanisms and provide indicators of sepsis compatible with literature.

4.1   The Computational Model of Neutrophil

Neutrophils are the most numerous cells contained in blood, distinguished morphologically by a nucleus segmented into three to five connected lobules and by abundant granules present in their cytoplasm [19]. Such cells have an increase in bacterial infectious processes, when the production and release by the bone marrow are increased, and are markers of occurrence of such infections, being fundamental to understand their roles and interactions with microorganisms, in order to unravel the complex mosaic of illness by such etiologies [18]. Neutrophils are represented in the simulator by the agent *Neutrophil*. The implementation of the agent seeks to reflect aspects of the immune response in the occurrence of diseases such as sepsis. These agents are inserted in the *BoneMarrow* zone and migrate to *Circulation* zone where they circulate randomly or move according to the gradient of concentration of the substance PK1 when they change to the *tecidual* state, simulating in this way, the chemotaxis of these cells. When *Neutrophil* agent find and identify a *Bacterium* agent, it phagocytes the latter and then die due to the microorganism destruction process. It can phagocyte more than one bacterium before its own cell death. If the life span expires the agent is eliminated. The states of Neutrophil agent are illustrated in Figure 1 and was presented in a previous article [26].

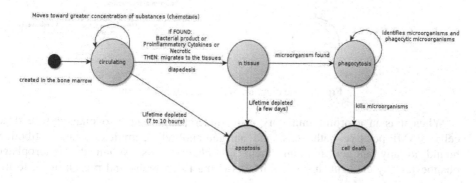

Fig. 1. State diagram of the *Neutrophil* agent [26]

When its lifetime expires, the *Neutrophil* agent changes its State to apoptosis. Upon finding microorganisms or inflammatory substances it goes into proinflammatory state, performing its function of phagocytosis and elimination of bacteria.

4.2   Macrophage

Macrophages are cells originating from blood monocytes migrating from the circulation into the tissues and from proliferation of precursor on site. They are responsible for phagocytosis of tumor cells opsonized by antibodies, bacteria, and other microorganisms. They produce mediators such as prostaglandins, leukotrienes, platelet activating factor, interleukin 1, 6 and 12, attracting other cells and triggering the immune response. They also participate in regulatory events as well as the interaction of the innate immune response with acquired immunity [20]. Figure 2 shows a state machine describing the behavior of the agent representing the macrophage. The implemented behavior sought to simulate the immune response in the occurrence of diseases such as sepsis. It is based on Macrophage agent defined by Folcik [16] and is created by *TissuePortal* class when it detects the presence of MK1 and are inserted in the *Tissue* zone. Thus, is represented the attraction of macrophages to the site of infection. Upon entering the Tissue zone, the agent follows the substance of cellular stress signaling PK1 to find the site of infection and the presence of the NECROSIS substance. When this occurs the agent switches to the proinflammatory state since it found evidence that the cells are actually being damaged. Once in this state, it begins to produce pro-inflammatory cytokine MK1, simulating the function of macrophages in initiating the inflammatory process by recruiting other elements of immunity.

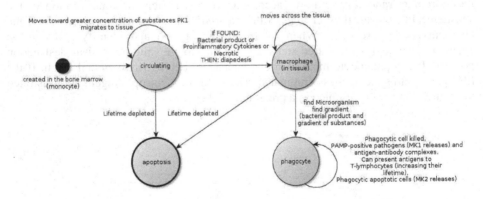

Fig. 2. State diagram of the *macrophage* agent

When it is in a proinflammatory state, macrophage can also phagocytose dead cells, PAMP-positive pathogens, and antigen-antibody complexes, i.e., antibodies bound to any antigen marking them for phagocytosis. When the macrophage phagocytes any element, it renders it, extracting its antigens and presenting it to the main histocompatibility complex class II (MHC II). At that point, it goes to the activated state.

When they encounter T lymphocytes that recognize the antigen that it is presenting, the macrophage receives survival factors (increasing its activated life time) and also provides survival factors for the lymphocyte that recognized it. Macrophage have a limited lifespan in both pro-inflammatory state and in the activated state. If it does not get surviving factors to extend that time, it undergoes a process of programmed cell death, apoptosis, and is eliminated from the simulation.

Macrophage anti-inflammatory states were not modelled, because the model is based only on the hypothesis that the decline in immune response happens due to the absence of antigen stimulation. On the other hand, there are other studies cited in the model described by Folcik [16], pointing to the existence of suppressor T cells or regulatory, which would be responsible for the decline and suppression of the immune response.

4.3   The Computational Model of Bacteria

The *Bacterium* agent simulates a generic bacterium and is inserted in the *Tissue* zone where it randomly moves until be found by an agent that it can connect with. Following recognition and connection, if the agent represents a cell that has the target pattern (cell tissue) and if the cell is no longer infected, then the bacterium attaches to the cell and multiplies. When the multiplication process occurs, the cell is lysed. If the bacterium could not recognize the agent as a target or if the cell is already infected, the bacterium agent starts again to move randomly in the tissue. If the lifetime of the bacterium runs out it is eliminated. Bacteria can also bump into a portal and, in this case, may fall into the bloodstream. In the circulation bacteria do not multiply, however, they can return to tissue through a portal. Figure 3 displays the state machine of the *Bacterium* agent.

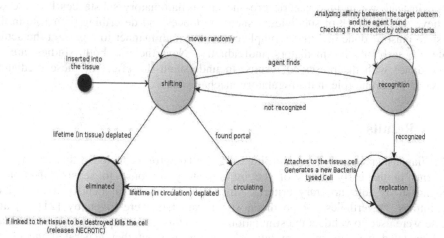

Fig. 3. State diagram of the *bacterium* agent

5   Related Works

Some works can be found on *in silico* studies of sepsis [8]. They bring a general review of the subject and the computational tools available, such analyzes (e.g. proteomics) made by computer and the use of data mining on datasets collected in hospitals. In [24] was proposed an agent-based simulation model combined with systemic dynamic mathematical model to execute a simulation of the initial stage of a typical sepsis episode, often leading to severe sepsis or septic shocks. Based on the computational studies, the simulated behavior of the agent-based model conforms to the mechanisms described by the system dynamics mathematical models established in previous research. They used the NetLogo framework for the model implementation. They used a generic agent such as phagocyte and pathogen as well as mediator substances modeled as agents. Our approach uses more specific agents and does not model substances as agents.

The article [25] made a comparison between two models: a system dynamics mathematical model (SDMM) and a multiagent based model (MABM), which model and simulate the human's innate immune responses of sepsis. When comparing the results of the two models, the paper concludes that the models based on multiagent systems are the most realistic approaches to simulate the progression of sepsis. The results between the MAS and mathematical models differ because of the stochastic nature of the immune response. SMA model sought to maintain the same characteristics of the hypothetical scenarios of acute response at the interface between the blood vessels and cells within tissues. Our work uses the MAS approach and the interactions among cells of immune system and the pathogen, mediated by pro and anti-inflammatory substances, in order to elucidate through computer simulations some of the complex mechanisms of sepsis. Although our simulation involves a larger number of immune cells and use slightly different mechanisms for simulating zones (e.g. tissue and circulation), we do not use the same level of detail of mediator as in [25]. Instead, we include generic pro-and anti-inflammatory substances because we believe that the work of subdividing such substances and describing their role in the system must be done in a more complete and thorough manner to represent the actual role of each of the mediators individually. Nevertheless, both studies are in accordance with the presented results, to understand the effect of these mediators plays an important role in the regulatory mechanisms.

6   Results

The diagnosis is not trivial. According to [21], "The group concluded that few, if any, patients in the early stages of the inflammatory response to sepsis infection is diagnosed by four arbitrary criteria." Instead, one needs to identify a myriad of symptoms. Nevertheless, some diagnostic parameters were given by [21] [1] and these were used to validate the simulation results. Given the capacity of the simulator and modeled mechanisms, simulations were carried out that generated the charts contained in this section. Such charts relate to the presence of macrophages and neutrophils in the circulation (indicating the presence or absence of leukocytosis), bacteria in the circulation and bacteria in the tissue and tissue damage.

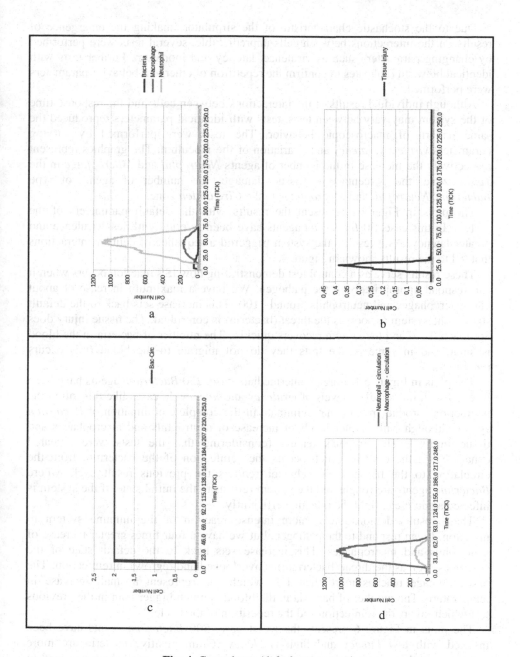

Fig. 4. Control test (default parameters)

Due to the stochastic characteristic of the simulator, making the emergence of results on the interactions between cells unpredictable, several tests were performed by changing parameters such as virulence, latency and inoculum. Further tests with identical between replicates to confirm the repetition of emergent behavior parameters were performed.

Although individual results of the interactions between cells and the response time of the system may vary between tests, tests with identical parameters reproduced the same pattern of macroscopic behavior. The tests were performed by varying parameters *virulency*, *latency* and variation of the inoculum. The graphics represent respectively the increase in the number of agents *Neutrophil* and *Macrophage* in the *Tissue* zone, the percentage of tissue damage, the number of agents of type *Bacterium*, *Neutrophil* and *Macrophage* in the *Circulation* zone.

The plots in Figure 4 represent the results with the default parameters of the system. In this case, 50 *Bacterium* agents have been inserted with less virulence and greater latency. As a result, the system triggered a sequence of cellular interactions that led to the results shown in Figure 4.

These results serve as a control test demonstrating how IS's reaction occurs when it can respond appropriately to the pathogen. We have a maximum increase of about 180 macrophages and neutrophils around 1100. This increase sets back to the default state of the system as soon as the threat (bacteria) is controlled. The tissue injury does not reach 0.4% and the system recovers quickly. The number of bacteria in the blood is small and in some of the tests they do not migrate to the blood (this occurs randomly).

The plots in Figure 5 feature an intermediate case. 250 *Bacterium* agents have been inserted with intermediate levels of *virulency* and *latency*. In cases like this, often the interactions produce results that culminate in the complete elimination of *Bacterium* agents although with greater levels of increase of neutrophils and macrophages and tissue injury. The graphics feature (considering that the tests were repeated exhaustively) the case in which occurs the reinfection of the bacterium from the circulation to the tissue. This behavior renders the previous result cycle where *Bacterium* agents are fought and the system returns to the initial state. If the system is infected again it can fight the infection efficiently.

These results demonstrate a more intense reaction of the immune system to infection. It can respond to the pathogen, but we have a four times greater increase of neutrophils and macrophages. This increase sets back to the default state of the system as soon as the threat (bacterium) is overlooked and regrows in reinfection. The tissue damage reaches more than 1%, which can represent a small increase in temperature. The number of bacteria in the blood is much bigger than in the previous test which favors the reinfection and the repetition of the cycle.

The plots in Figure 6 presents the worst case. 500 *Bacterium* agents have been inserted with low *latency* and high *virulency* (Gram positive bacteria are more aggressive and is expected to generate a larger immune response, which can lead to sepsis). The system triggered a sequence of cellular interactions that led to the results that can be seen in Figure 6.

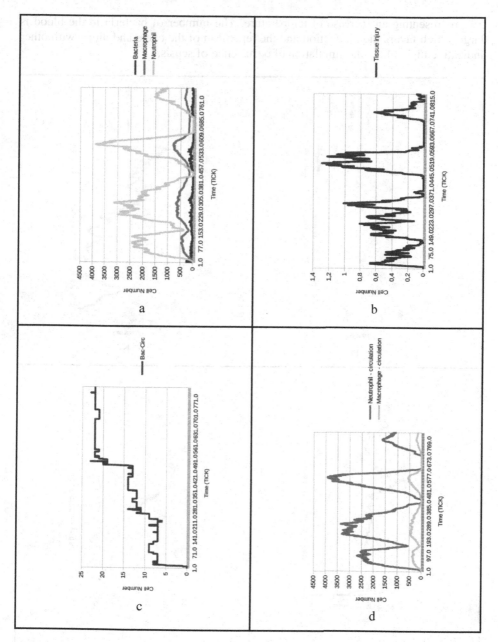

Fig. 5. Intermediate case tests

These results demonstrate a critically serious reaction from the system, which is unable to respond to infection in an appropriate manner. It cannot fight the pathological agent efficiently. The increase of neutrophils and macrophages does not cease or at most stabilizes. This increase does not retreat, generating high levels of phagocytic cells (macrophages and neutrophils). Tissue damage reaches more than

5%, representing an increase of temperature. The number of bacteria in the blood is large which favors the reinfection and the repetition of the cycle and along with other indicative highlights   the simulation of occurrence of sepsis.

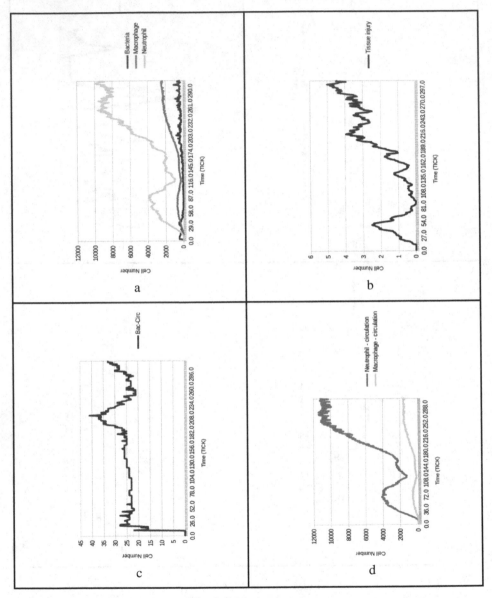

Fig. 6. Critical case tests

The results presented when using more aggressive pathogens are compatible with sepsis by simultaneously presenting symptoms such as fever, bacteria in the blood and Leukocytosis as confirms the literature   [21][1]. Among variations between virulence and latency parameters, the latter was more relevant for triggering a more aggressive immune response probably due to the fact that it triggers mediators faster and with greater frequency, in addition to cause tissue injury in short time, contributing to the symptoms of the disease.

7   Conclusion

Computational investigation of the immune system may lead to new hypotheses as well as conducting preliminary tests before using *in vitro* and *in vivo* experiments, contributing to the development of knowledge about the pathophysiology of human diseases. It also allows the deepening of the studies in the area of immunology and the improvement of the model – AutoSimmune – in computational terms.

Extend the model to simulate situations of sepsis is a complex challenge due to the systemic aspect of the disease. However, as our computational procedure is extended to deal with other diseases, including the expansion of cells involved in infectious processes and the expansion of mechanisms as mediator substances, it will allow the model to approach more and more of what happens in the human immune system. Research on the cell T-reg (T CD4+CD25+), for example, is being held in parallel because there is evidence that such a cell can have a decisive role in sepsis, considering that it has a strong role in regulating the human immune system. Therefore, the agent T-reg can also be included in the template, which adds one more test variable to the elucidation of the mechanisms involved in the disease.

Acknowledgments. This research is supported in part by the funding agencies FAPEMIG, CNPq, CAPES and by the Gapso company.

References

1. Siqueira-Batista, R., Gomes, A.P., Calixto-Lima, L., Vitorino, R.R., Perez, M.C.A., Mendonça, E.G.D., Oliveira, M.G.A., Geller, M.: Sepsis: an update. Revista Brasileira de Terapia Intensiva 23(2), 207–216 (2011)
2. Gogos, C., Kotsaki, A., Pelekanou, A., Giannikopoulos, G., Vaki, I., Maravitsa, P., Skouras, V.: Early alterations of the innate and adaptive immune statuses in sepsis according to the type of underlying infection. Critical Care 14(3), 1–12 (2010)
3. Martin, G.: Epidemiology studies in critical care. Critical Care 10(2), 136 (2006)
4. Hotchkiss, R.S., Karl, I.E.: The pathophysiology and treatment of sepsis. New England Journal of Medicine 348(2), 138–150 (2003)
5. Perez, M.C.A.: Epidemiologia, diagnóstico, marcadores de imunocompetência e prognóstico da sepse. Rio de Janeiro: Faculdade de Ciências Médicas da Universidade do Estado do Rio de Janeiro. Phd thesis (2009)
6. Ceccon, M.E.J., Vaz, F.A., Diniz, E.M., Okay, T.S.: Interleucina interleucina 6 e proteína c reativa no diagnóstico diagnóstico diagnóstico de sepse tardia no recém-nascido. Rev. Assoc. Med. Bras. 52(2), 79–85 (2006)
7. Siqueira-Batista, R., et al.: CD4+ CD25+ T lymphocytes and regulation of the immune system: perspectives for a pathophysiological understanding of sepsis. Rev. Bras. Ter. Intensiva 24(3), 294–301 (2012)
8. Vodovotz, Y., Billiar, T.R.: In silico modeling: methods and applications to trauma and sepsis. Critical Care Medicine 41(8), 2008–2014 (2013)

9. Song, S.O., Hogg, J., Peng, Z.Y., Parker, R., Kellum, J.A., Clermont, G.: Ensemble models of neutrophil trafficking in severe sepsis. PLoS Computational Biology 8(3), e1002422 (2012)
10. Wang, L.X.H., Lu, Z.X., Che, T.Y., Modelling, X.J.: immune system: Principles, models, analysis and perspectives. Journal of Bionic Engineering 6(1), 77–85 (2009)
11. Bastos, C.A., et al.: Simulação do sistema imunológico por meio de sistemas multiagentes: um estudo da resposta imune na glomerulonefrite pós-infecciosa (GnPE) por Streptococcus pyogenes. In: WIM 2013 - XIII Workshop de Informática Médica - XXXIII Congresso da Sociedade Brasileira de Computação, pp. 1093–1102 (2013)
12. Calich, V.L.G., Vaz, C.A.C., Abrahamsohn, I.D.A., Barbuto, J.A.M., Isaac, L., Rizzo, L.V., Jancar, S.: Imunologia. Revinter, Rio de Janeiro (2001)
13. Von Bertalanffy, L.: General system theory. General Systems 1(1), 11–17 (1956)
14. Johnson, S.: Emergence: The connected lives of ants, brains, cities, and software. Simon and Schuster (2002)
15. Paul, R., Daniela, R.: Template driven agent based modelling and simulation with CUDA. In: Hwu, W.-M. (ed.) GPU Computing Gems Emerald Edition, pp. 313–324. Morgan Kaufmann (2011)
16. Folcik, V.A., An, G.C., Orosz, C.G.: The Basic Immune Simulator: an agent based model to study the interactions between innate and adaptive immunity. Theoretical Biology and Medical Modelling 4, 39 (2007)
17. Possi, M.A., Oliveira, A.P., et al.: An in-silico immune system model for investigating human autoimmune diseases. In: XXXVII Conferencia Latinoamericana de Informática, XXXVII CLEI (2012)
18. Siqueira-Batista, R., et al.: The artificial neutrophil and a proposal of an in silico research of the immune response in human bacterial diseases. Abakós 2(2), 79–91 (2014)
19. Abbas, A.K., Lichtman, A.H., Pillai, S.: Imunologia celular e molecular. Elsevier, Brasil (2008)
20. Jantsch, J., Binger, K.J., Müller, D.N., Titze, J.: Macrophages in homeostatic immune function. Frontiers in Physiology 5 (2014)
21. Levy, M.M., Fink, M.P., Marshall, J.C., Abraham, E., Angus, D., Cook, D., Ramsay, G.: 2001 sccm/esicm/accp/ats/sis international sepsis definitions conference. Intensive Care Medicine 29(4), 530–538 (2001)
22. Floreano, D., Mattiussi, C.: Bio-inspired artificial intelligence: theories, methods, and technologies. MIT Press (2008)
23. Da Silva, C.C., Oliveira, A.P., Possi, M.A., Cerqueira, F.R., Gomes, A.P., Santana, L.A., Siqueira-Batista, R.: Immune system simulation: Modeling the mast cell. In: 2012 IEEE International Conference on Bioinformatics and Biomedicine (BIBM), pp. 1–4. IEEE (2012)
24. Wu, J., Ben-Arieh, D., Shi, Z.: An Autonomous Multi-Agent Simulation Model for Acute Inflammatory Response. In: Investigations Into Living Systems, Artificial Life, and Real-world Solutions, p. 218 (2013)
25. Shi, Z., Wu, J., Ben-Arieh, D.: A Modeling Comparative Study on Sepsis. In: Guan, Y., Liao, H. (eds.) Proceedings of the Industrial and Systems Engineering Research Conference (2014)
26. Sousa, F.O., et al.: Imunologia da sepse: investigação por meio de simulação computacional com sistemas multiagentes. In: WIM 2013 - XIII Workshop de Informática Médica. Anais do XXXIII Congresso da Sociedade Brasileira de Computação, pp. 1123–1126 (2013)

Data Mining and Machine Learning on the Basis from Reflexive Eye Movements Can Predict Symptom Development in Individual Parkinson's Patients

Andrzej W. Przybyszewski[1,2], Mark Kon[3], Stanislaw Szlufik[4], Justyna Dutkiewicz[4], Piotr Habela[2], and Dariusz M. Koziorowski[4]

[1]University of Massachusetts Medical School, Dept Neurology, Worcester, MA 01655, USA,
Andrzej.Przybyszewski@umassmed.edu
[2]Polish-Japanese Institute of Information Technology, 02-008 Warszawa, Poland
{przy,piotr.habela@pjwstk.pl
[3]Mathematics and Statistics, Boston University, Boston, MA 02215, USA
mkon@bu.edu
[4]Neurology, Faculty of Health Science, Medical University Warsaw, Poland
stanislaw.szlufik@gmail.com, justyna_dutkiewicz@wp.pl,
dkoziorowski@esculap.pl

Abstract. We are still not in a position to understand most of the brain's deeper computational properties. As a consequence, we also do not know how brain processes are affected by nerve cell deaths in neurodegenerative diseases (ND). We can register symptoms of ND such as motor and/or mental disorders (dementias) and even provide symptomatic relief, though the structural effects of these are in most cases not yet understood. Fortunately, with early diagnosis there are often many years of disease progression with symptoms that, when they are precisely monitored, may result in improved therapies. In the case of Parkinson's disease, measurements of eye movements can be diagnostic. In order to better understand their relationship to the underlying disease process, we have performed measurements of reflexive eye movements in Parkinson's disease (PD) patients. We have compared our measurements and algorithmic diagnoses with experts' diagnoses. The purpose of our work was to find universal rules, using rough set theory, to classify how condition attributes predict the neurologist's diagnosis. Prediction of individual UPDRS values only from reflexive saccade (RS) latencies was not possible. But for n = 10 patients, the patient's age, latency, amplitude, and duration of RS gave a global accuracy in individual patients' UPRDS predictions of about 80%, based on cross-validation. This demonstrates that broadening the spectrum of physical measurements and applying data mining and machine learning (ML) can lead to a powerful biomarker for symptom progression in Parkinson's.

Keywords: Neurodegenerative disease, rough set, decision rules.

1 Introduction

The majority of neurologists use their experience based largely on statistical intuition to analyze symptom development in Parkinson's disease (PD) patients. By applying

A. Gelbukh et al. (Eds.): MICAI 2014, Part II, LNAI 8857, pp. 499–509, 2014.
© Springer International Publishing Switzerland 2014

statistics based on analysis of large databases one can find significant information about the specificity of PD. But, due to a variety of cares, some results obtained even from the most prominent experts might be inconsistent. Applying standard, statistical averaging methods to such inconsistent information may give confusing results even leading to conclusions that a specific care does not effectively work in "averaged" PD patient. We might face similar challenges when studying factors that might lead to longer, better, and more active lives for people with Parkinson's. Various neurologists may also interpret differently the meanings of the UPDRS that result different therapies. These problems are articulated in the popular statement "No two people face Parkinson's in quite the same way." People vary substantially in their combination of symptoms, rate of progression, and reaction to treatment. As mentioned, averaging patients' symptoms to measure effects of different therapies can give very crude approximation of actual outcomes. If we want to improve such analyses, we must take into account the great variety of patients' symptoms and inconsistent effects of care in different PD cases.

For this reason, we propose to extend statistical analysis of PD outcomes using data mining and machine learning (ML) methods that give a more standardized interpretation of individual patient's symptoms and development. As a consequence it is possible that these methods may suggest specific treatments adjusted to different individual patients that may lead to slowing of symptoms and improvements in quality of life. Such analysis is proposed on the basis of learning algorithms that intelligently process data of individual patients in a standardized and specific ways. Our symptom classification method strives to emulate other means of complex object recognition such as those in visual systems. The ability of natural vision to recognize objects arises in the afferent, ascending pathways that classify properties of objects' parts from simple attributes in lower sensory areas, to more complex ones, in higher analytic areas. The resulting classifications are compared and adjust by interaction with whole object ("holistic") properties (representing the visual knowledge) at all levels using interaction with descending pathways [1] that was confirmed in animal experiments [2]. These interactions at multiple levels between measurements and prior knowledge can help to differentiate individual patient's symptoms and response treatments variability in a way similar to a new, complex object inspection [3, 4]. Machine learning algorithms for analyzing subtle signal variations will hopefully lead to better analysis of individual patients' conditions.

Diagnostic findings of neurologists are based on interaction of their measurements and experience. In the most cases, they estimate values of the Hoehn and Yahr scale and the UPDRS (Unified Parkinson's Disease Rating Scale). However, these are not always precise and can be partially subjective. In our data mining approach we use the neurologist's diagnosis as decision attributes and measurements as condition attributes.

2   Methods

Our experiments were performed on ten Parkinson Disease (PD) patients who had undergone the Deep Brain Stimulation (DBS) surgery mainly for treatment of their motor symptoms. They were qualified for the surgery and observed postoperatively in the Dept. of Neurology and got surgical DBS implementation in the Institute of

Neurology and Psychiatry WUM [5]. We conducted horizontal RS (reflexive saccades) measurements in ten PD patients during four sessions designed as S1: MedOffDBSOff, S2: MedOffDBSOn, S3: MedOnDBSOff, S4: MedOnDBSOn. During the first session (S1) the patient was off medications (L-Dopa) and DBS stimulators was OFF; in the second session (S2) the patient was off medication, but the stimulator was ON; in the third session (S3) the patient was after his/her doses of L-Dopa and the stimulator was OFF, and in the fourth session (S4) the patient was on medication with the stimulator ON. Changes in motor performance, behavioral dysfunction, cognitive impairment and functional disability were evaluated in each session according to the UPDRS. The reflexive saccades (RS) were recorded by head-mounted saccadometer (Ober Consulting, Poland). We have used an infrared eye track system coupled with a head tracking system (JAZZ-pursuit – Ober Consulting, Poland) in order to obtain high accuracy and precision in eye tracking and to compensate possible subjects' head movements relative to the monitor. Thus subjects did not need to be positioned in an unnatural chinrest.

A patient was sited at the distance of 60-70 cm from the monitor with head supported by a headrest in order to minimize head motion. We measured fast eye movements in response to a light spot switched on and off, which moved horizontally from the straight eye fixation position (0 deg) to 10 deg to the left or 10 deg to the right after arbitrary time ranging between 0.5–1.5 s. When the patient fixated eyes on the spot in the middle marker (0 deg) the spot then changed color from white to green, indicating a signal for performance of RS (reflexive saccades); or from white to red meaning a signal for performing AS (antisaccades). Then the central spot was switched off and one of the two peripheral targets, selected at random with equal probability, was illuminated instead. Patients had to look at the targets and follow them as they moved in the RS task or made opposite direction saccades in the AS task. After making a saccade to the peripheral target, the target remained on for 0.1 s after which another trial was initiated.

In each test the subject had to perform 20 RS and 20 AS in a row in Med-off (medication off) within two situations: with DBS off (S1) and DBS on (S2). In the next step the patient took medication and had a break for one half to one hour, and then the same experiments were performed, with DBS off (S3) and DBS on (S4). In this work we have analyzed only RS data using the following population parameters averaged for both eyes: delay mean (+/-SD –standard deviation); amplitude mean (+/-SD); max velocity mean (+/-SD); duration mean (+/-SD).

2.1 Theoretical Basis

The structure of data is an important point of our analysis. Here we represent it in the form of information system or a decision table. We define such an information system (after Pawlak [6]) as a pair $S = (U, A)$, where U, A are nonempty finite sets called the *universe of objects* and the *set of attributes*, respectively. If $a \in A$ and $u \in U$, the value $a(u)$ is a unique element of V (where V is a value set).

The *indiscernibility relation* of any subset B of A or $IND(B)$, is defined [6] as follows: $(x, y) \in IND(B)$ or $xI(B)y$ if and only if $a(x) = a(y)$ for every a $\in B$, where $a(x)$ $\in V$. $IND(B)$ is an equivalence relation, and $[u]_B$ is the equivalence class of u, or a B-*elementary granule*. The family of all equivalence classes of $IND(B)$ will be denoted $U/I(B)$ or U/B. The block of the partition U/B containing u will be denoted by $B(u)$.

We define a **lower approximation** of symptoms set $X \subseteq U$ in relation to a symptom attribute B as $\underline{B}X = \{u \in U: [u]_B \subseteq X \}$, and the **upper approximation** of X as

$\overline{B}X = \{u \in U: [u]_B \cap X \neq \phi\}$. In other words, all symptoms are classified into two categories (sets). The lower movement approximation set X has the property that all symptoms with certain attributes are part of X, and the upper movement approximation set has property that only some symptoms with attributes in B are part of X (for more details see [5]). The difference of $\overline{B}X$ *and* $\underline{B}X$ is defined as the boundary region of X i.e., $BN_B(X)$. If $BN_B(X)$ is empty set than X is *exact* (*crisp*) with respect to B; otherwise if $BN_B(X) \neq \phi$ and X is not *exact* (i.e., it is *rough*) with respect to B. We say that the B-lower approximation of a given set X is union of all B-*granules* that are included in X, and the B-upper approximation of X is of the union of all B-*granules* that have nonempty intersection with X.

The system S will be called a decision table $S = (U, C, D)$ where C **is the condition** and D **is the decision attribute** [6]. In the table below (Table 2), as an example, the decision attribute D, based on the expert opinion, is placed in the last column, and condition attributes measured by the neurologist, are placed in other columns. **On the basis of each row in the table, rules describing the condition of each patient can be proposed.** As the number of rules is same as the number of rows, these rules can have many particular conditions. The main concept of our approach is to describe different symptoms in different patients by using such rules. On the basis of such rules, using the **modus ponens principle** we wish to find universal rules to relate symptoms and treatments in different patients.

However, symptoms even for the same treatments are not always the same; therefore **our rules must have certain "flexibility", or granularity, which can be interpreted as the probability of finding certain symptoms in a group of patients under consideration. The granular computation simulates the way in which neurologists interact with patients.** This way of thinking relies on the ability to perceive a patient's symptoms under various levels of granularity (i.e., abstraction) in order to abstract and consider only those symptoms that serve to determine a specific treatment and thus to switch among different granularities. By focusing on different levels of granularity, one can obtain different levels of knowledge, as well as a greater understanding of the inherent knowledge structure. Granular computing is thus essential in human intelligent problem solving behaviors in *problem-specific* tasks.

We define the notion of a reduct $B \subset A$. The set B is a reduct of the information system if $IND(B) = IND(A)$ and no proper subset of B has this property. In case of decision tables decision reduct is a set $B \subset A$ of attributes which cannot be further reduced and $IND(B) \subset IND(d)$. A decision rule is a formula of the form $(a_{i1} = v_1) \wedge ... \wedge (a_{ik} = v_k) \Rightarrow d = v_d$, where $1 \le i_1 < ... < i_k \le m$, $v_i \in Va_i$. Atomic subformulas $(a_{i1} = v_1)$ are called conditions. We say that rule r is applicable to object, or alternatively, the object matches rule, if its attribute values satisfy the rule. With a rule we can connect some numerical characteristics such as matching and support. We can replace the original attribute a_i with new, binary attributes which indicate whether actual attribute value for an object is greater or lower than c (see [7]), we define c as a cut. Thus a cut for an attribute $a_i \in A$, with V_{ai} will be a value $c \in V_{ai}$. A template of A is a propositional formula $v_i \in V_{ai}$. A generalized template is a formula of the form $\wedge(a_i \in T_i)$ where $T_i \subset V_{ai}$. An object satisfies (matches) a template if for every attribute a_i we have $a_i = v_i$ where $a_i \in A$. The template is a natural way to split the original information system into two distinct sub-tables. One of these sub-tables consists of the objects that satisfy the template, while the second contains all others. A *decomposition tree* is defined as a binary tree, whose every internal node is labeled by some template and external node (leaf) is associated with a set of objects matching all templates in a path from the root to a given leaf [8].

In a second test we have divided our data into two or more subsets. By training on all but one of these subsets (the training set) using machine learning (ML), we obtained classifiers that when applied to the remaining (test) set gave new numerical decision attributes, well correlated with neurologist decision attributes (based on a confusion matrix).

3   Results

The patients' mean age was 51.1 ± 10.2(SD) years, mean disease duration was 11.3 ± 3.2 years, mean UPDRS (related to all symptoms): S1: 66.6 ± 13.8 S2: 30.0 ± 16.3; S3: 58.1 ± 13.5; S4: 22.3 ± 13.6; mean UPDRS III (related only to motor symptoms): S1: 42.7 ± 11.3 S2: 17.8 ± 10.6; S3: 34.1 ± 10.8; S4: 10.9 ± 8.3; mean RS latencies: S1:291.2 ± 93.1ms, S2: 199.6 ± 39.5ms, S3: 232.9 ± 82.7ms; S4: 183.2 ± 30ms.

Differences between latencies: S1-S2, and S1-S4 were statistically significant (t-test $p< 0.01$) even when they were variable in individual patients (Fig. 1), while S1-S3 was not statistically significant, this is similar to differences between UPDRS/UPDRS III: S1-S2, and S1-S4 were statistically significant (t< 0.001) and S1-S3 was not statistically significant.

Other parameters of RS did not change significantly with the session number.

3.1   Rough Set and Machine Learning Approach

As described above we have used the RSES 2.2 (Rough System Exploration Program) [8] in order to find regularities in our data. At first our data was placed in the information table as originally proposed by Pawlak [6].

The full table has 15 attributes and 36 objects (measurements). In the Table 1 are values of 11 attributes for two patient: P# - patient number, age – patient's age, sex – patient's sex: 0 - female, 1 – male, t_dur – duration of the disease, S# - Session number, UPDRS – total UPDRS, HYsc – Hoehn and Yahr scale all measured by the neurologist and saccades measurements: SccDur - saccade duration; SccLat - saccade latency; SccAmp – saccade amplitude, and SccVel – saccade velocity.

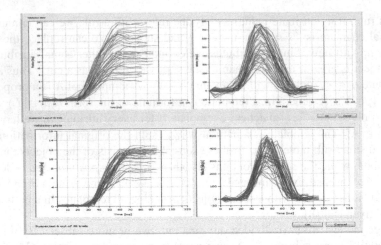

Fig. 1. An example of experimental recordings from Pat #38 in two sessions: upper plots from session S1: MedOFF & StimOFF; lower plots from session S4: MedON & StimON; left plots show latency measurements, right plots – saccades' amplitude and velocity. Notice change in variability of responses between S1 and S4.

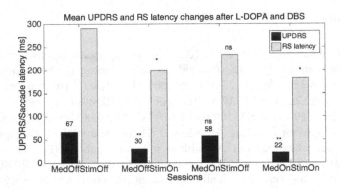

Fig. 2. This graph shows parallel changes in UPDRS and reflexive saccade latencies as effects of medication and stimulation. Changes between control and MedOnStimOn were significantly different for UPDRS p<0.001 (**), RS p<0.01 (*).

Table 1. Extract from the information table

P#	age	sex	t_dur	S#	UPDRS	HYsc	SccDur	SccLat	SccAmp	SccVel
28	54	1	8	1	58	2.0	43	402	12	566,9
28	54	1	8	2	40	1.0	46	297	11	474,5
28	54	1	8	2	40	1.0	49	227	10	431,2
28	54	1	8	4	16	1.0	47	198	9	376,2
38	56	0	11	1	49	2.5	42	285	14	675,2
38	56	0	11	2	22	1.5	48	217	12	509,7
38	56	0	11	3	37	2.5	43	380	14	638,9
38	56	0	11	4	12	1.5	45	187	10	482,6

In the next step, we have performed reduction of attributes (see reduct in the Method section) to a minimum number of attributes describing our results. We have also created a discretization table: here single values of measurements were replaced by their range (as describe in the Method section on cut sets). As the result we have obtained the decision table (Table 2 –see below).

Table 2. Part of the decision discretized-table

Pat#	age	t_dur	S#	HYsc	SccDur	SccLat	SccAmp	UPDRS
28	"(-Inf,55.0)"	*	1	*	"(-Inf,45.5)"	"(260.0,Inf)"	"(10.5,Inf)"	"(55.0,Inf)"
28	"(-Inf,55.0)"	*	2	*	"(45.5,Inf)"	"(260.0,Inf)"	"(10.5,Inf)"	"(22.5,55.0)"
28	"(-Inf,55.0)"	*	2	*	"(45.5,Inf)"	"(-Inf,260.0)"	"(-Inf,10.5)"	"(22.5,55.0)"
28	"(-Inf,55.0)"	*	4	*	"(45.5,Inf)"	"(-Inf,260.0)"	"(-Inf,10.5)"	"(14.0,22.5)"
38	"(55.0,Inf)"	*	1	*	"(-Inf,45.5)"	"(260.0,Inf)"	"(10.5,Inf)"	"(22.5,55.0)"
38	"(55.0,Inf)"	*	2	*	"(45.5,Inf)"	"(-Inf,260.0)"	"(10.5,Inf)"	"(14.0,22.5)"
38	"(55.0,Inf)"	*	3	*	"(-Inf,45.5)"	"(260.0,Inf)"	"(10.5,Inf)"	"(22.5,55.0)"
38	"(55.0,Inf)"	*	4	*	"(-Inf,45.5)"	"(-Inf,260.0)"	"(-Inf,10.5)"	"(-Inf,14.0)"

In the first column is the patient's number, in the second the patient's age divided in our group into patients below (Pat#28) or above (Pat#38) 55 years of age; disease duration and Hoehn and Yahr scale were not considered important (stars), along with session number; and other parameters of saccades were also divided into ranges. It is interesting to note how the UPDRS were divided into different ranges: above 55, 22.5 to 55, 14 to 22.5, and below 14 (the last column). On the basis of this decision table we can write the following rule:

('Pat'=28)&('age'="(-Inf,55.0)")&('Sess'=1)&('SccDur'="(-Inf,45.5)")&('SccLat' ="(260.0,Inf)")& (' SccAmp')="(10.5,Inf)") => ('UPDRS'="(55.0,Inf)")   (1)

We read this formula above (eq. 1), as stating that each row of the table (Table 1) can be written in form of this equation (eq. 1). It states that if we evaluate patient #28 *and* with age below 55 *and* in session #1 *and* with saccade duration below 45.5 *and* saccade latency above 260 *and* ... *and* saccade amplitude above 10.5 *then* patient's UPDRS is above 55.

These equations are parts of a data mining system bases on rough set theory [6]. We have tested our rule using the machine-learning concept. Randomly dividing our data into 6 groups, we took 5 groups as training set and tested the fourth. By changing groups belonging to the training and test sets, we have removed the effect of accidental group divisions. The results of each test were averaged – thus we have performed a 6-fold cross-validation. The results are gives as a confusion matrix (Table 3). As a machine-learning algorithm we have used the decomposition tree (see Methods).

We have performed several tests trying to predict UPDRS values on the basis of measures saccades properties. As changes in UPDRS and saccade latencies were similar when the session number was changed (Fig.2) we tried to predict individual UPDRS values only from RS latencies. Here however, we did not get good results. When to the session number, patient age, RS: latency, amplitude, and duration were added, the global accuracy in UPRDS prediction was about 80% (ML: decomposition tree, cross-validation-method). This is good result for such a small population showing power of the data mining and machine learning methods in this type of neurological analysis. As UPDRS is a standard measurement in PD, the above results give the possibility of at least partly replace or augmenting neurologist estimates with the eye movements (EM) measurement results.

Table 3. Confusion matrix for different session numbers (S1-S4)

Predicted

	55.0, Inf	22.5, 55.0	-Inf, 14.0	14.0, 22.5	ACC
55.0, Inf	0.3	0.3	0	0	**0.2**
22.5, 55.0	0	1.5	0	0	1
-Inf, 14.0	0.0	0.3	0	0.2	0
14.0, 22.5	0	0	0	0	0
TPR	0.2	0.8	0	0	

(Actual — row label for the first four data rows)

TPR: True positive rates for decision classes, ACC: Accuracy for decision classes: the global coverage was 0.44, the **global accuracy was 0.79**, coverage for decision classes: 0.2, 0.5, 0.3, 0.0.

Another question that result is, whether EM can help to estimate possible effects of different treatments in individual patients? In order to demonstrate an answer, we have removed EM measurements and added other typically measured attributes such as: the Schwab and England ADL Scale, and UPDRS III and UPDRS IV to the decision table and tried to predict the effects of different treatments as represented by sessions 1 to 4 (medication and stimulation effects). Table 4 is a part of full decision discretized-table with decision attributes – the session number placed in the last column. On the basis of this table we have formulated rules using a rough set system and tested them with randomly divided data into 6 groups. We took 5 as training set (using ML protocol) and tested with sixth. In order to remove effect of the accidental division we have exchanged training and test groups and averaged results placed in the confusion matrix (Tabel 5).

Table 4. Part of the decision discretized-table **without** eye movement measurements

Pat#	age	t_dur	SEngs	UPDRS III	UPDRS IV	UPDRS	Sess#
"(27.5,41.5)"	"(43.5,Inf)"	*	"(-Inf, 75)"	"(36.0,46.0)"	"(10.5,Inf)"	"(1.75,Inf)"	1
"(27.5,41.5)"	"(43.5,Inf)"	*	"(75, Inf)"	"(13.0,26.0)"	"(10.5,Inf)"	"(-Inf,1.75)"	2
"(27.5,41.5)"	"(43.5,Inf)"	*	"(75, Inf)"	"(-Inf,6.0)"	"(10.5,Inf)"	"(-Inf,1.75)"	4
"(27.5,41.5)"	"(43.5,Inf)"	*	"(-Inf, 75)"	"(26.0,36.0)"	"(10.5,Inf)"	"(1.75,Inf)"	1
"(27.5,41.5)"	"(43.5,Inf)"	*	"(75, Inf)"	"(13.0,26.0)"	"(10.5,Inf)"	"(-Inf,1.75)"	2
"(27.5,41.5)"	"(43.5,Inf)"	*	"(-Inf, 75)"	"(13.0,26.0)"	"(10.5,Inf)"	"(1.75,Inf)"	3
"(27.5,41.5)"	"(43.5,Inf)"	*	"(75, Inf)"	"(-Inf,6.0)"	"(10.5,Inf)"	"(-Inf,1.75)"	4

Table 5. Confusion matrix for different session numbers (S1-S4)

		Predicted			
	1	**2**	**3**	**4**	**ACC**
1	0.5	0	0.5	0	**0.3**
2	0	0.5	0	0.3	**0.4**
Actual **3**	0.8	0	0.2	0	**0.2**
4	0	0.5	0	0.5	**0.4**
TPR	**0.3**	**0.3**	**0.2**	**0.4**	

TPR: True positive rates for decision classes, ACC: Accuracy for decision classes: the global coverage was 0.64, the **global accuracy was 0.53**, coverage for decision classes: 0.5, 0.5, 0.75, 0.7.

We have performed the same procedures once more to test results of patients' eye movement influence on our predictions.

Table 6. Part of the decision discretized-table **with** eye movement measurements

Pat#	age	SccVel	UPDRS III	HYsc	SccDur	SccLat	SccAmp	Ses#
"(27.5,34.5)"	*	"(458.5,578.0)"	"(36, Inf)"	"(1.75,Inf)"	"(38,Inf)"	"(308.5,Inf)"	*	1
"(27.5,34.5)"	*	"(458.5,578)"	"(11.5,36)"	"(-Inf,1.75)"	"(38.0,Inf)"	"(-Inf,308.5)"	*	2
"(27.5,34.5)"	*	"(341.5,403)"	"(-Inf,11.5)"	"(-Inf,1.75)"	"(38,Inf)"	"(-Inf,308.5)"	*	4
"(34.5,Inf)"	*	"(665.5,Inf)"	"(11.5,36.0)"	"(1.75,Inf)"	"(38.0,Inf)"	"(-Inf,308.5)"	*	1
"(34.5,Inf)"	*	"(458.5,578)"	"(11.5,36)"	"(-Inf,1.75)"	"(38.0,Inf)"	"(-Inf,308.5)"	*	2
"(34.5,Inf)"	*	"(578.0,665.5)"	"(11.5,36)"	"(1.75,Inf)"	"(38.0,Inf)"	"(308.5,Inf)"	*	3
"(34.5,Inf)"	*	"(458.5,578)"	"(-Inf,11.1)"	"(-Inf,1.75)"	"(38, Inf)"	"(-Inf,308.5)"	*	4

Table 7. Confusion matrix for different session numbers (S1-S4)

		Predicted			
	1	**2**	**3**	**4**	**ACC**
1	0.8	0	0	0	**0.7**
2	0	0.7	0	0	**0.7**
Actual **3**	0.2	0	0.8	0	**0.6**
4	0	0.2	0	0.3	**0.25**
TPR	**0.7**	**0.7**	**0.6**	**0.25**	

TPR: True positive rates for decision classes, ACC: Accuracy for decision classes, the global coverage was 0.5; the **global accuracy was 0.91**; coverage for decision classes: 0.6, 0.6, 0.6, 0.25.

As above, results of each test were averaged in a 6-fold cross-validation giving as the confusion matrix (Table 3). As a machine-learning algorithm we have used the decomposition tree (see Methods).

In summary, two last results have demonstrated that adding eye movement (EM) results to classical measurements performed by the most neurologists, can result in improved predictions of disease progression measured, as measured by improvement in global accuracy from 0.53 to 0.91. The EM measurements may also partly replaces neurological measurements such as the UPDRS, as global accuracy of the total UPDRS predictions taken from EM data was 0.79 for the above 10 PD patients.

4   Discussion

In current therapeutic protocols, even with the large numbers of approaches and clinical trials, there have still been few conclusive results on therapeutic identification and measurement of PD symptoms. There are multiple reasons for such failures: first, the shortcomings of current disease models in target validation and testing; second, difficulties in choosing clinical endpoints; third difficulties in finding sensitive biomarkers of disease progression. One clear problem is that the disease starts long before motor symptoms are observed, and another is that individual pathological mechanisms form a large spectrum. We have given an example comparing classical neurological diagnostic protocols with a new approach. The main difference between these types of measures is in their precision and objectivity. Our approach is doctor-independent and can be performed automatically. In the near future it may help in transforming some hospital-based to home-based treatments. In this scenario it will be possible to measure patient symptoms at home, and send these for consultation by neurologists. Such methods will be faster, more precise and can help with more frequent measurements. In consequence, they may help not only to determine more objectively a patient's symptoms, but also to follow up disease progression in more frequent intervals, something not possible currently, with the limited time resources of neurologists. If we obtain such information, it may lead to more appropriate therapies and the slowing down of disease progression. It is one of the purposes of this work to try to extract knowledge from symptoms in order further on to develop more appropriate therapies to stem disease progression.

5   Conclusions

We have presented a comparison of classical statistical averaging methods for PD diagnosis with rough set (RS) approaches. We used processed neurological data from PD patients in four different treatments and we have plotted averaged effects of the medication and brain stimulation in individual patients. As these effects are strongly patient dependent they could not give enough information to predict new patient's behavior. The RS and ML approaches are more universal giving general rules for predicting individual patient responses to treatments as demonstrated in UPDRS predictions.

Acknowledgements. This work was partly supported by projects Dec-2011/03/B/ ST6/03816 and NN 518289240 from the Polish National Science Centre.

References

1. Przybyszewski, A.W.: The Neurophysiological Bases of Cognitive Computation Using Rough Set Theory. In: Peters, J.F., Skowron, A., Rybiński, H. (eds.) Transactions on Rough Sets IX. LNCS, vol. 5390, pp. 287–317. Springer, Heidelberg (2008)
2. Przybyszewski, A.W., Gaska, J.G., Foote, W., Pollen, D.A.: Striate cortex increases contrast gain of macaque LGN neurons. Visual Neuroscience 17, 1–10 (2000)
3. Przybyszewski, A.W.: Logic in Visual Brain: Compute to Recognize Similarities: Formalized Anatomical and Neurophysiological Bases of Cognition. Review of Psychology Frontier 1, 20–32 (2010) (open access)
4. Przybyszewski, A.W.: Logical rules of visual brain: From anatomy through neurophysiology to cognition. Cognitive Systems Research 11, 53–66 (2012)
5. Pizzolato, T., Mandat, T.: Deep Brain Stimulation for Movement Disorders. Frontiers in Integrative Neuroscience 6, 2 (2012), doi:10.3389/fnint.2012.00002
6. Pawlak, Z.: Rough sets: Theoretical aspects of reasoning about data. Kluwer, Dordrecht (1991)
7. Bazan, J., Son, N.H., Trung, T., Nguyen, S.A., Stepaniuk, J.: Desion rules synthesis for object classification. In: Orłowska, E. (ed.) Incomplete Information: Rough Set Analysis, pp. 23–57. Physica – Verlag, Heidelberg (1998)
8. Bazan, J., Szczuka, M.: RSES and RSESlib - A Collection of Tools for Rough Set Computations. In: Ziarko, W.P., Yao, Y. (eds.) RSCTC 2000. LNCS (LNAI), vol. 2005, pp. 106–113. Springer, Heidelberg (2001)

Agents That Help to Avoid Hyperthermia in Young Children Left in a Baby Seat Inside an Enclosed Car

Juan Pablo Soto, Julio Waissman, Pedro Flores-Pérez,
and Gilberto Muñoz-Sandoval

Universidad de Sonora, Blvd. Luis Encinas y Rosales S/N, Col Centro
83000 Hermosillo, México
{jpsoto,juliowaissman,pflores}@mat.uson.mx

Abstract. Despite the public education efforts to alert parents about the safety threat hyperthermia poses for young children left unattended inside a car, the number of victims each year is increasing. For this reason, this work focuses on using current technology to help prevent such fatalities. One proposed solution is provide a trustworthy mechanism that permits to alerts parents or caregivers whom accidentally leave their children in a baby seat inside an enclosed car, we propose a multi-agent system to monitor the baby seats inside cars.

Keywords: Hyperthermia, Baby car seats, Software agents.

1 Introduction

In recent years, the number of children that die from hyperthermia after being left unattended in closed cars has increased [1, 2]. In addition to those who die, it is estimated that annually, hundreds of children experience varying degrees of heat illness from being left in cars [3]. One explanation attributes this rise to increasing stress levels in daily life [2, 4].

In the United States, child deaths by hyperthermia have been on the rise since the early '90s, when new safety regulations mandated that children, often injured by front-seat, passenger-side airbags, should always ride in the backseat. The laws did successfully reduce airbag injuries to kids, but they also inadvertently made children less visible in the car, and they're one of the factors often cited to explain the eightfold increase in hyperthermia deaths since the regulations passed [4].

Hyperthermia is a dramatic and devastating medical condition [5, 6]. It strikes healthy people suddenly, and many of them die [1]. Those who survive may sustain permanent neurologic damage and other vital organs if emergency treatment is not provided [5, 7]. Hyperthermia it is characterized by a body temperature above 40°C and is accompanied by mental status changes (disorientation, lethargy, delirium, and coma) [8, 9]. Individuals who are most at risk for hyperthermia are the elderly and young children [9]. A study conducted to investigate the thermoregulation of young children compared to that of adults points out that the sweating and skin temperature responses of the children are not enough to prevent a rise in body temperature [10].

A. Gelbukh et al. (Eds.): MICAI 2014, Part II, LNAI 8857, pp. 510–517, 2014.

According to the National Highway Traffic Safety Administration (NHTSA), heatstroke is the leading cause of non-crash vehicle fatalities in children aged 14 and under [11]. A car parked in the sun can reach 51°C in minutes, even when the windows are partially open [1, 11]. The critical temperature for lethal thermal cellular injury is around 42.2°C [12]. In [1], the authors demonstrated that on sunny days, even when the ambient temperature is mild or relatively cool, there is a rapid and significant heating of the interior of vehicles [1]. On days when the ambient temperature was 22°C, that study showed that the internal vehicle temperature can reach 47°C within 60 minutes, with 80% of the temperature rise occurring in the first 30 minutes [1].

In order to resolve this issue, we propose a multi-agent system that detects when young children left in child safety seats inside cars are at high risk of hyperthermia and sends an alert message to the driver's smartphone.

The remainder of this paper is organized as follows. Section 2 we briefly describe how we are using the INGENIAS methodology [13] to develop the multi-agent system. Section 3 describes the implementation of the proposed system based on Arduino microcontroller and Raspberry pi mini-computer. Finally, in Section 4, we outline the conclusions obtained.

2   Multi-agent System

The system has two main types of agencies: Monitoring Agency and User Agency (Figure 1).

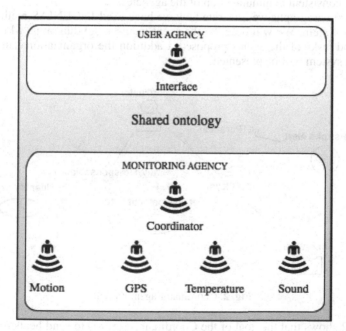

Fig. 1. Multi-agent architecture

The Monitoring Agency is in charge of monitoring the conditions facing young children left by error in a baby seat inside a vehicle. It consists of the Coordinator agent, the Temperature agent, the GPS agent, the Sound agent and the Motion agent.

- The temperature agent is responsible for reading the temperature inside the vehicle using a temperature sensor. It executes a proactive monitoring process to obtain the measure.
- The GPS agent is in charge of advice when there is a change in routine of the driver. This happens when the driver breaks a well-established routine.
- The sound agent is in charge of identifying the sound inside the vehicle. This data is collected to confirm the presence of a baby in a car.
- The motion agent is responsible for identifying whether there is motion inside the baby seat car.
- The coordinator agent is responsible for identifying conditions in which there is a high risk of heatstroke for the child. To do this, the agent receives data from the temperature agent, sound agent, GPS agent and motion agent. Based on this data the coordinator agent must make a decision to alert the driver or not.

The User Agency is formed by the Interface Agent. The interface agent is the mediator between the users and the agents. It is in charge of sending a heatstroke risk alert to the driver's smartphone.

Another component of the multi-agent system is the Shared Ontology, which provides a conceptualization of the hyperthermia risk domain. The Shared Ontology is used for the consistent communication of the agencies.

In the next paragraphs we illustrate how we have used INGENIAS methodology to develop our system. We will describe the agent meta-model diagrams, which describe the roles and tasks of the agents proposed. I addition the organizational model of the multi-agent system will be presented.

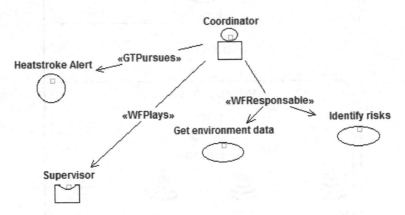

Fig. 2. Coordinator agent model

Figure 2 shows that the goal of the Coordinator agent is to send heatstroke alerts to the Interface agent. For this, the Coordinator agent must to identify and create the type of notification to be sent to the user, in order to alert about a possible risk. For this, the agent uses the model notices CANoE, which to be explained in section 3.

Its role is "Supervisor" since it must receive the information sent by other agents that make up the monitoring agency.

In the following lines, we describe each of the tasks carried out by this agent.

Get environment data: this task consists of obtaining available information provided by the Temperature Agent, GPS Agent, Motion Agent and Sound Agent (Monitoring agents).

Identify risks: the agent must analyze the information obtained from the monitoring agents in order to determine the existence of a heatstroke risk.

Figure 3 shows the Temperature agent diagram, whose goal is called "Get temperature" since the agent must obtain the environmental temperature of the baby car seat. To do this, the agent uses a temperature sensor.

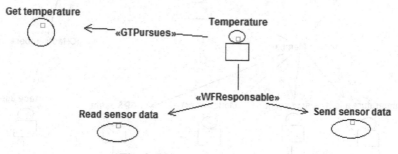

Fig. 3. Temperature agent model

In order to attain this goal it should carry out the following tasks:

Read sensor data: this task consists of getting the data provided by the temperature sensor.

Send sensor data: the agent must send the temperature obtained with the temperature sensor to the Coordinator agent.

Figure 4 shows the Motion agent diagram, whose goal is called "Body movement detect". To do this, the agent must detect movement of the child in the baby car seat using a body movement detect sensor.

Finally, in Figure 5 the organizational model is presented. In this model the basis for the multi-agent system definition and construction is defined.

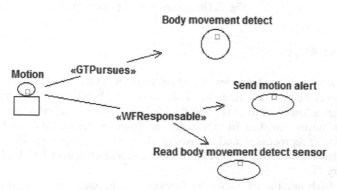

Fig. 4. Motion agent model

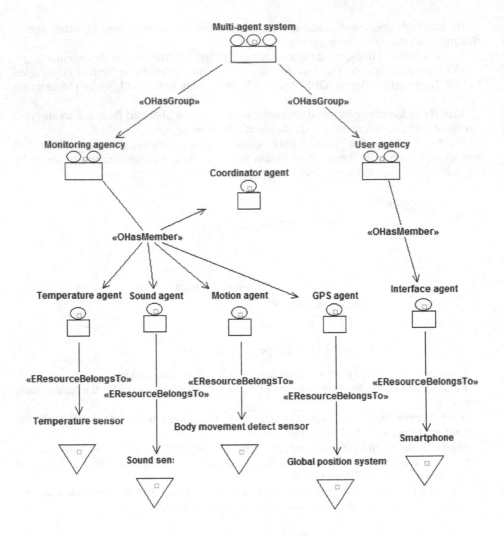

Fig. 5. Organization model diagram

3   Prototype

A prototype system has been developed on an Android based smartphone. We are also using a micro-controller Arduino [14] and Raspberry Pi [15] computer. Both technologies allowed us to create the device that will be attached to the baby car seat. Arduino acquires raw data from the sensors (motion, temperature and sound) and a GPS device, preprocesses and transmits them to a Raspberry Pi computer. The platform that we are using to develop the multi-agent system is JADE [16] running on a Raspberry Pi.

Figure 6 shows the exchange of information between the agents that form the multi-agent system proposed using the JADE framework.

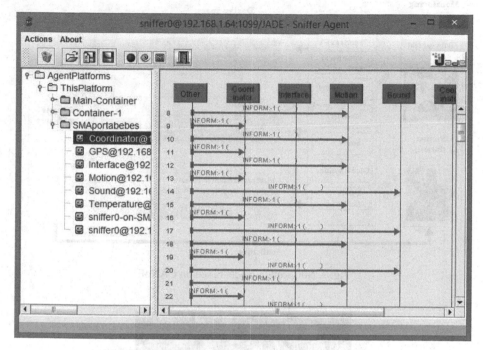

Fig. 6. Exchange of information between agents in JADE

The user interface consists of two parts: a notification area and a message area.

A notification area shows the notification of potential risk of hyperthermia by a small icon on the top of a display, which is realized by the Android notification framework. This notification is based on CANoE, a model for the design of context-aware notifications in critical environments [17]. CANoE has been designed to be used in critical environments by taking into consideration three sources of context for adaptation: the recipient of the notification; the issuer of the notification; and the characteristics of the environment where the notification occurs.

Figure 7 shows a schematic view of the notification model, which considers as inputs the actual situation of baby car seat inside a car, the context of the children involved in the situation of negligence. The model adapts the message content, the delivery and determines the presentation mechanism based on the context through the following three design guidelines: Configure the Content (1), Assign Response Priority to the Parents as the receiver of the notification (2), and Adapt the presentation of the notification to the parents (3). Finally, the outputs of each of these adaption processes (Message, Priority and Mechanism) are integrated to form a notification.

A user can receive a notification while he/she is utilizing other applications. Once a notification is sent, a user can obtain more information by tapping the notification bar downward to show the message area implemented as an "Activity" in the Android programming model (Figure 8).

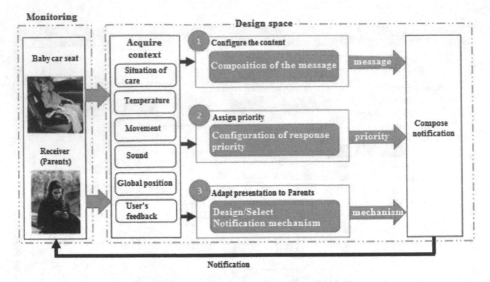

Fig. 7. Notification model based on CANoE

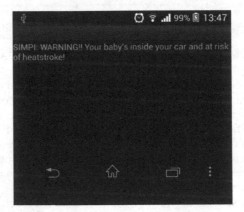

Fig. 8. Alert message in a smartphone

4   Conclusions

The main contribution of this paper is the design of a multi-agent system to avoid hyperthermia in young children left in baby car seats inside cars. In addition, this work describes how the INGENIAS methodology was used to develop our multi-agent system.

One important contribution of this paper is the prototype, as it helps to alert parents and save lives in situations in which they forget that their child is in the baby car seat. At the same time, parents must understand that, while requiring children to ride in the baby car seat has saved many lives, it also requires drivers to take extra precautions to avoid children from being left alone in a car. Prevention of heat illness in children is crucial, and leaving a children accidentally in parked car not only on hot days but also on cool, sunny days, may subject the child to significant risk of mortality due to hyperthermia.

References

1. McLaren, C., Null, J., Quinn, J.: Heat Stress From Enclosed Vehicles: Moderate Ambient Temperatures Cause Significant Temperature Rise in Enclosed Vehicles. Pediatrics 116(1), 109–112 (2005)
2. Ferrara, P., Vena, F., Caporale, O., Del Vogo, V., et al.: Children left unattended in parked vehicles: a focus on recent italian cases and a review of literature. Italian Journal of Pediatrics 39(1) (2013)
3. Null, J.: Hyperthermia deaths of children in vehicles, http://ggweather.com/heat
4. Ford, A.: Locked In: Why Child Car Deaths Are on the Rise (August 11, 2014), http://www.divinecaroline.com/life-etc/culture-causes/locked-why-child-car-deaths-are-rise
5. Clowes, G., O'Donnell, Y.: Heat stroke. New England Journal of Medicine 291, 564–567 (1974)
6. Semenza, J., Rubin, C., Falter, K., et al.: Heat-related deaths during heat wave in Chicago. New England Journal of Medicine 335, 84–90 (1995)
7. Knochel, J.: Heatstroke and related heatstress disorders. Disease-a-Month 35(5), 306–377 (1989)
8. Amore, M., Cerisoli, M.: Heatstroke and hypertermias. The Italian Journal of Neurological Sciences 13(4), 337–341 (1992)
9. Ozcetin, M., Arslan, M., Yilmaz, R., Yildirim, A.: Rare Cause of Cerebral Damage: Child with Heatstroke found inside an enclosed Vehicle. Hong Kong Journal of Emergency Medicine 9(2), 126–129 (2012)
10. Tsuzuki-Hayakawa, K., Tochihara, Y., Ohnaka, T.: Thermoregulation during heat exposure of young children compared to their mothers. Eur. J. Appl. Physiol. 72, 12–17 (1995)
11. National Highway Traffic Safety Administration (NHTSA), http://www.nhtsa.gov
12. Ash, C., Kashmeery, A.: Heatstroke: marathons to mecca. In: Yearbook of Intensive Care and Emergency Medicine, pp. 971–981. Springer (1995)
13. Pavón, J., Gómez-Sanz, J.: Agent Oriented Software Engineering with INGENIAS. In: Mařík, V., Müller, J.P., Pěchouček, M. (eds.) CEEMAS 2003. LNCS (LNAI), vol. 2691, p. 394. Springer, Heidelberg (2003)
14. Arduino, http://arduino.cc
15. Raspberry Pi, http://www.raspberrypi.org
16. Java Agent Development Framework (JADE), http://jade.tilab.com
17. Nava-Muñoz, S., Morán, A.: CANoE: A Context-Aware Notification Model to Support the Care of Older Adults in a Nursing Home. Sensors 12, 11477–11504 (2012)

Author Index

Abud-Figueroa, Ma. Antonieta   II-296
Acosta-Guadarrama, Juan Carlos   I-28
Acuña, Gonzalo   II-160, II-198
Aguilar, Luis T.   II-426
Alarcón, Teresa E.   I-316, I-327
Ali, Imtiaz   II-206
Alor-Hernández, Giner   I-494, II-296
Amin, Adnan   II-206
André, Leanderson   II-61
Anwar, Sajid   II-206
Araya, Beatriz   II-198
Avilés-Cruz, Carlos   I-281

Baltazar, María del Rosario   II-152
Baptista, Jorge   I-37
Barrón Estrada, María Lucía   I-483, I-494
Barták, Roman   II-451
Baruch, Ieroham   II-95
Batyrshin, Ildar   I-9
Bedoya, Carol   II-382
Belanche-Muñoz, Lluís A.   II-464
Belghazi, Ouissam   II-105, II-116
Benitez, Antonio   II-128
Benois-Pineau, Jenny   I-336
Bergler, Sabine   I-139
Bessa Maia, José Everardo   II-25
Biere, Armin   I-431
Bravo, Maricela   I-443
Brychcín, Tomáš   I-70

Calvo, Hiram   I-1
Camarena-Ibarrola, Jose Antonia   II-219
Canul, Juana   I-233
Cappelle, Cindy   I-257, I-304
Carballido, José Luis   I-407
Cardenas-Maciel, Selene L.   II-426
Cardona, Carlos   II-160
Carpio, Juan Martín   II-152
Caseli, Helena de Medeiros   I-99
Castillo, Oscar   II-331, II-345
Castro-Espinoza, Felix A.   II-285
Cazarez-Castro, Nohe Ramon   II-426
Ceballos, Héctor G.   II-272

Cervantes-Ojeda, Jorge   II-85
Chacón, Max   II-160
Chaparro-Altamirano, Daniel   II-392
Cherkaoui, Mohamed   II-105, II-116
Cobos, Carlos   I-80, I-125
Contreras Vega, Gerardo   I-293
Cruz-Barbosa, Raúl   II-474
Cubillos, Francisco   II-198
Curilem, Millaray   II-160, II-198

Dalmau, Oscar S.   I-269, I-316, I-327
Dávila-Pérez, Rogelio   I-28
Dĕdek, Jan   I-51
de la Calleja, Jorge   II-128
De la Vega, Erick   II-50
Del Bosque, Laura P.   I-221
de Luna, Carlos   I-233
Díaz, Juan   I-419
Douiri, Moulay Rachid   II-105, II-116
Dragan, Ioan   I-431
Dutkiewicz, Justyna   II-499

Elalouf, Amir   II-436
Escalante, Hugo Jair   I-151

Fang, Yong   I-257
Ferfra, Mohamed   II-105, II-116
Fernandez-Vazquez, Alfonso   I-349
Fierro-Radilla, Atoany   I-336
Flores-Pérez, Pedro   II-510
Flores-Ríos, Brenda L.   II-464
Flores, Juan J.   II-1, II-50
Fonollosa, José A.R.   I-92
Formiga, Lluís   I-92
Fraire, Héctor Joaquín   II-152
Franco, Luis   II-160
Franco-Arcega, Anilu   II-285
Franco-Sánchez, Kristell D.   II-285
Fuentealba, Gustavo   II-160

Galicia-Haro, Sofía N.   I-175
García, Uriel A.   II-184
García-Islas, Luis H.   II-285
García-Nájera, Abel   II-13

Garrido, Fernanda   II-198
Garrido, Leonardo   II-357
Garza, Sara Elena   I-221
Gelbukh, Alexander   I-1, I-175, II-263
Goddard-Close, John   II-252
Gomes, Andréia Patrícia   II-486
Gomes Nepomuceno Da Silva, Thiago
    II-25
Gómez-Fuentes, María del Carmen
    II-13, II-85
Gonzalez, Ivan   II-357
Gonzalez-Garcia, Gustavo   I-349
González Hernández, Francisco   I-483
Gonzalez Mendoza, Miguel   II-319
González-Navarro, Félix F.   II-464
Gonzalez-Sua, Luis Carlos   II-357
Goribar-Jimenez, Carlos A.   II-426
Graff, Mario   II-1, II-50
Guerrero Casas, José de Jesús   I-316
Gutiérrez, Guadalupe   I-233

Habela, Piotr   II-499
He, Ping   II-310
Heidarzadegan, Ali   II-140
Hernández Manzano, Sergio Miguel
    II-95
Hernández-Zavala, Antonio   II-370
Herrera-Viedma, Enrique   I-80, I-125
Hladká, Barbora   I-51, I-113
Huenupan, Fernando   II-160
Huerta-Ruelas, Jorge Adalberto   II-370
Hussain, Ayyaz   II-231

Ibargüengoytia, Pablo H.   II-184
Ibarra-Esquer, Jorge Eduardo   II-464
Isaza-Narvaez, Claudia Victoria   II-382
Ismail, Saad M.   I-393
Ivanov, Vladimir   I-18

Jaffar, M. Arfan   II-231
Jamnejad, Mohammad Iman   II-140
Jiménez-Salazar, Héctor   I-245

Khan, Changez   II-206
Knap, Tomáš   I-113
Kolombo, Martin   II-451
Kon, Mark   II-499
Kovács, Laura   I-431
Koziorowski, Dariusz M.   II-499
Král, Pavel   I-70
Kriheli, Boris   II-436

Kříž, Vincent   I-51, I-113
Kuri-Morales, Angel Fernando   II-72

Lahlouhi, Ammar   I-472
Larranaga-Cepeda, Ander   I-368
Lazo-Cortés, Manuel S.   II-128
León, Elizabeth   I-125
Levner, Eugene   II-436
Lima Vieira, Thiago   I-99
López, Manuel Guillermo   I-269
Lopez Sanchez, Ivan Adrian   II-319
Lozano, Manuel   I-125
Lyashin, Andrey   I-201

Mabrouki, El Batoul   II-105
Mamede, Nuno   I-37
Manic, Milos   I-80
Manzo-Martínez, Alain   II-219
Margain, Lourdes   I-233
Marin Hernandez, Antonio   I-293
Markov, Ilia   I-37
Martinez-Licona, Alma   II-252
Martinez-Licona, Fabiola   II-252
Masood, Sohail   II-231
Mazzucchi-Augel, Pablo N.   II-272
Mederos, Boris   I-269
Mejri, Salah   I-191
Melin, Patricia   II-331, II-345
Méndez-Gurrola, Iris Iddaly   I-443
Méndez Rosiles, José Roberto   II-38
Mendoza, Martha   I-80, I-125
Mendoza-Martinez, Cyntia   I-356
Meurie, Cyril   I-380
Mihalcea, Rada   I-163
Miranda, Rodrigo   II-198
Molano, Viviana   I-80
Mollineda, Ramón A.   II-128
Montes-y-Gómez, Manuel   I-151
Mora Gutiérrez, Roman Anselmo   II-38
Morales, Eduardo F.   II-184
Mora Vargas, Jaime   II-319
Moshki, Mohsen   II-140
Motta-Avila, Carlos Alberto   I-368
Muñoz-Sandoval, Gilberto   II-510
Murgia, Julian   I-380

Nakano-Miyatakea, Mariko   I-336
Nečaský, Martin   I-51, I-113

Ochoa, Alberto   I-233
Oliva, Francisco E.   I-327

Oliva-Juarez, Gabriela   II-252
Oliveira de Paiva, Alcione   II-486
Oliveira de Sousa, Flávio   II-486
Olvera-López, J. Arturo   II-128
O'Reilly, Philip   I-104
Oramas Bustillos, Raúl   I-483
Oropeza Rodríguez, José Luis   II-242
Osorio, Mauricio   I-28, I-407, I-419

Padierna, Luis Carlos   II-152
Padilla, Alejandro   I-233
Padilla, Ricardo   II-172
Pakray, Partha   II-263
Panagiotopoulos, Alexandra   I-139
Parvin, Sajad   II-140
Pech, David   II-184
Pedraza-Ortega, Jesus Carlos   I-356
Peláez-Camarena, S. Gustavo   II-296
Pellegrin, Luis   I-151
Perez-Daniel, Karina   I-336
Perez-Meana, Hector   I-336
Pérez-Rosas, Verónica   I-163
Petit, Jordi   I-92
Pinto, David   I-191
Ponce, Hiram   II-172
Ponce, Julio   I-233
Ponsich, Antonin   II-38
Posadas-Duran, Juan-Pablo   I-9
Prasath, Rajendra   I-104
Priego Sánchez, Belém   I-191
Pronoza, Ekaterina   I-201
Przybyszewski, Andrzej W.   II-499
Puga, Héctor José   II-152

Qiao, Yongliang   I-304

Rakib, Abdur   I-453
Ramírez-de-la-Rosa, Gabriela   I-245
Ramírez-Mendoza, Ricardo A.   II-392
Ramirez-Torres, Jose Gabriel   I-368
Ramos-Arreguin, Juan Manuel   I-356
Rentería-Gutiérrez, Livier   II-464
Reyes, Alberto   II-184
Reyes-García, Carlos Alberto   I-494
Ribeiro Cerqueira, Fábio   II-486
Rincón García, Eric Alfredo   II-38
Rios Figueroa, Homero Vladimir   I-293
Rodríguez, Francisco   I-125
Rodríguez-López, Verónica   II-474
Rodriguez-Maya, Noel E.   II-1

Rodríguez-Mazahua, Lisbeth   II-296
Rodríguez-Salas, Dalia   II-128
Rodríguez-Zalapa, Omar   II-370
Romero-Herrera, Rodolfo   I-349
Romero-Leon, Inés   II-184
Ruichek, Yassine   I-257, I-304, I-380
Ruiz Costa-jussà, Marta   I-92

Sampaio Rocha, Leonardo   II-25
Sánchez, Daniela   II-345
Sanchez Garcia, Angel Juan   I-293
Sánchez-Sánchez, Christian   I-245
San Martin, Cesar   II-160
Santana, Luiz Alberto   II-486
Santos, Cipriano A.   II-319
Santoyo, Alejandro   I-419
Sarkar, Sudeshna   I-104
Sheikh Abdullah, Siti Norul Huda   I-393
Sidorov, Grigori   I-9
Silva-López, Mónica   I-443
Silva-López, Rafaela Blanca   I-443
Siqueira-Batista, Rodrigo   II-486
Soto, Ismael   II-231
Soto, Juan Pablo   II-510
Soto, Rogelio   II-357
Stilianova-Stoytcheva, Margarita   II-464
Stubs Parpinelli, Rafael   II-61
Suárez Guerra, Sergio   II-242
Sucar, Luis Enrique   II-184
Surynek, Pavel   II-410
Szlufik, Stanislaw   II-499

Tsadikovich, Dmitry   II-436

Ul Haque, Hafiz Mahfooz   I-453
Uribe, Diego   I-62

Valdez, Fevrier   II-331
Velasco Vazquez, Maria de Lourdes   I-293
Villanueva-Escudero, Carla   I-281
Villatoro-Tello, Esaú   I-245
Villegas-Cortez, Juan   I-281
Volskaya, Svetlana   I-201
Voronkov, Andrei   I-431

Waissman, Julio   II-510
Waissman-Villanova, Julio   II-382

Xu, Xiaohua   II-310

Yagunova, Elena   I-201

Zaldivar, Victor Hugo   I-28
Zamudio, Adalberto   I-316
Zataraín Cabada, Ramón   I-483, I-494

Zavala-Yoé, Ricardo   II-392
Zepeda, Claudia   I-407
Zúñiga-López, Arturo   I-281